Psychologists' Psychotropic Drug Reference

Pharmacology Texts and Reference Books by the Pagliaros

Clinical Psychopharmacotherapeutics for Psychologists. Philadelphia, PA: Brunner/Mazel, (in preparation).

Drug Reference Guide to Brand Names and Active Ingredients. St. Louis, MO: C. V. Mosby, (1986).

Pharmacologic Aspects of Aging. St. Louis, MO: C. V. Mosby, (1983).

Pharmacologic Aspects of Nursing. St. Louis, MO: C. V. Mosby, (1986).

The Pharmacologic Basis of Psychotherapeutics: An Introduction for Psychologists. Washington, DC: Brunner/Mazel, (1998).

Problems in Pediatric Drug Therapy. Hamilton, IL: Drug Intelligence Publications, Washington, DC: American Pharmaceutical Association Books, (1979, 1987, 1995).

Psychologists' Neuropsychotropic Drug Reference. Philadelphia, PA: Brunner/Mazel, (in press).

Psychologists' Psychotropic Drug Reference. Philadelphia, PA: Brunner/Mazel, (1999).

Substance Use Among Children and Adolescents: Its Nature, Extent, and Effects from Conception to Adulthood. New York, NY: John Wiley & Sons, (1996).

Psychologists' Psychotropic Drug Reference

by

Louis A. Pagliaro, MS, PharmD, PhD, FPPR
Professor, Department of Educational Psychology
University of Alberta
President, College of Alberta Psychologists
Edmonton, Alberta, Canada

and

Ann Marie Pagliaro, BSN, MSN, PhD Candidate, FPPR
Professor, Faculty of Nursing
Director, Substance Abusology Research Unit
University of Alberta
Edmonton, Alberta, Canada

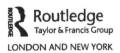
Routledge
Taylor & Francis Group
LONDON AND NEW YORK

PSYCHOLOGISTS' PSYCHOTROPIC DRUG REFERENCE

First published 1999 by
BRUNNER/MAZEL

Published 2014 by Routledge
2 Park Square, Milton Park, Abingdon, Oxfordshire OX14 4RN
711 Third Avenue, New York, NY 10017

First issued in paperback 2014

Routledge is an imprint of the Taylor & Francis Group, an informa business

Library of Congress Cataloging-in-Publication Data available from the publisher.

ISBN 978-0-87630-964-3 (hbk)
ISBN 978-1-13800-969-1 (pbk)

Dedication

This book, the second in a series of pharmacopsychology texts specifically written for psychologists and graduate psychology students, is dedicated to the advancement of the profession of psychology with the hope and trust that this advancement will be accompanied by commensurate improvements in the psychological health of those who seek, require, and receive psychotropic pharmacotherapy as an integral adjunct to their psychotherapy.

Contents

Contents

Editorial Advisory Committee

Rosalie J. Ackerman, PhD
Co-Chair of the Task Force on Prescription Privileges
Division 35 (Psychology of Women)
American Psychological Association
Research and Development Division
ABackans Diversified Computer Processing, Inc.
Uniontown, Ohio

Robert K. Ax, PhD
Midlothian, Virginia

Martha E. Banks, PhD
Co-Chair of the Task Force on Prescription Privileges
Division 35 (Psychology of Women)
American Psychological Association
Research and Development Division
ABackans Diversified Computer Processing, Inc.
Uniontown, Ohio

John Bolter, PhD
The Neuromedical Center
Baton Rouge, Louisiana

Ron L. Cohorn, PhD
Co-Chair, Task Force on Prescription Privileges
Texas Psychological Association
Clinical Associate Professor
Texas Tech Health Science Center
Department of Pediatrics
Malone & Hogan Clinic
Big Spring, Texas

Joseph E. Comaty, PhD
Director of Special Programs
East Louisiana State Hospital
Jackson, Louisiana
Adjunct Assistant Professor
Department of Psychology
Louisiana State University
Baton Rouge, Louisiana

Charles A. Faltz, PhD
Director of Professional Affairs
California Psychological Association
Sacramento, California

Samuel A. Feldman, PhD, FAPM, FPPR
Board-Certified Diplomate and Fellow and President
Prescribing Psychologists' Register, Inc.
North Miami Beach, Florida

Eldridge E. Fleming, PhD, FPPR
Past President, Mississippi Psychological Association
Chair, Task Force on Psychopharmacology
Mississippi Psychological Association
Tupelo, Mississippi

Raymond A. Folen, PhD, ABPP
Chief, Behavioral Medicine and Health Psychology Service
Department of Psychology
Tripler Army Medical Center
Honolulu, Hawaii

Ronald E. Fox, PhD
Former President, American Psychological Association
Executive Director
Division of Organizational and Management Consulting
Human Resource Consultants
Chapel Hill, North Carolina

Alan R. Gruber, DSW, PhD
Co-Chair, Psychopharmacology Committee
Massachusetts Psychological Association
Neurobehavioral Associates
Hingham, Massachusetts

C. Alan Hopewell, PhD, ABPP
Medical Support Psychology
Dallas Neuropsychological Institute, PC
Dallas, Texas

Lawrence E. Klusman, PhD
Director, Psychopharmacology Demonstration Project
Chief, Department of Psychology
Walter Reed Army Medical Center
Washington, DC

Joan C. Martin, PhD
Member, Task Force on Psychopharmacology Training
Levels I and II, American Psychological Association

Maxine L. Stitzer, PhD
Professor of Psychiatry and Behavioral Science
Johns Hopkins University School of Medicine
Baltimore, Maryland

Michael F. Wesner, PhD
Associate Professor of Psychology
Lakehead University
Thunder Bay, Ontario

Jack G. Wiggins, PhD
Former President, American Psychological Association
Fountain Hills, Arizona

James P. Zacny, PhD
Assistant Professor
Department of Anesthesia and Critical Care
The University of Chicago
Chicago, Illinois

Preface

The purpose of the *Psychologists' Psychotropic Drug Reference* (or the *PPDR*) is to provide prescribing psychologists and psychology graduate students with an accurate and authoritative reference for the psychotropic drugs that are commonly available for prescription in North America. The authors believe strongly that *all* clinical, health, and school psychologists should have a knowledge of the therapeutic action of the psychotropics and their associated ADRs and toxicities, which can be confused with, or be exacerbated by, virtually every psychological disorder. This reference text is particularly directed for use by psychologists and psychology graduate students who already have, or who are currently developing their, professional expertise and responsibilities in the prescription and management of psychotropic pharmacotherapy as an *adjunct* to psychotherapy.

The *PPDR* presents, in alphabetical order, detailed drug monographs for over 100 different prescription psychotropic drugs available in North America.[1] Thus, this reference is the most comprehensive, currently available, psychotropic drug reference designed for psychologists. The psychotropic drugs presented include the antidepressants, antimanics, antipsychotics, CNS stimulants, opiate analgesics, and sedative-hypnotics.[2] Monographs also are provided for the benzodiazepine and opiate analgesic antagonists. Emphasis is on current guidelines for the prescription of these psychotropics as adjuncts to psychotherapy for the symptomatic management of psychological disorders. Anticonvulsants, antiparkinsonians, and nootropics (i.e., drugs that enhance learning and memory among patients who have neurological disorders) are not included in this reference volume because their prescription is not generally considered to be primarily within the general expertise of practicing psychologists. However, they will be included as the primary topic of another reference in this series, *Psychologists' Neuropsychotropic Drug Reference*.

Each psychotropic monograph is clearly and concisely written to reflect only essential and important data that are commonly required by prescribing psychologists. Monographs are organized by generic name in alphabetical order.[3] Whenever available and appropriate, each monograph includes the following information: phonetic pronunciation guide; up to five common trade or brand names; pharmacologic or therapeutic classification and subclassification; United States Drug Enforcement Agency schedule designation for abuse potential (C-I, "high abuse potential," through C-V, "limited abuse potential;" see Appendix B); specific indications for prescription by psychologists;[4] recommended dosages for adults, women

---

[1] *Only* single active ingredient products have been included. The use of fixed-dosage combination psychotropics is not generally recommended because of the lack of flexibility in appropriately adjusting the dosage of the component drugs to meet individual patient requirements. However, relevant information regarding the fixed-dosage combination products can be obtained using this text by separately accessing required information for each drug.

[2] See Appendix A for a pharmacologic classification of the psychotropics and a complete listing of the drugs for which monographs are included in the *PPDR*.

[3] The generic names used in this text are those that have been officially designated by the United States Adopted Names Council. International drug names, such as those used by the British Pharmacopeia (British Adopted Names), are cross-referenced for convenience as secondary headings.

[4] The FDA allows physicians to prescribe approved drugs for any indication, whether or not the indication is part of the approved labeling. Thus, a physician could prescribe the antibiotic tetracycline for the treatment of depression if he or she so wished. In the absence of any scientific data to substantiate the efficacy of tetracycline for the treatment

who are pregnant, including Food and Drug Administration (FDA) pregnancy codes (see Appendix C), women who are breast-feeding, the elderly, and children and adolescents; guidelines for the initiation, maintenance, and discontinuation of psychotropic pharmacotherapy; available dosage forms and storage instructions; helpful and important notes regarding methods of administration; proposed mechanism(s) of drug action; pharmacokinetic/pharmacodynamic parameters, including therapeutic drug monitoring (TDM) parameters for specific drugs for which TDM is recommended; relative contraindications to use; cautions and comments to be considered when prescribing and managing adjunctive psychotropic pharmacotherapy; clinically significant drug interactions currently reported in the literature; the most commonly occurring ADRs and their general management; and signs and symptoms of overdosage.[5,6]

The *PPDR* integrates for each monograph important and essential information under these major headings in a specially designed taxonomy. For example, information that is helpful to prescribing psychologists for making decisions regarding the administration of a particular psychotropic is included under "Usual Dosage and Administration." Dosage forms and storage considerations are identified in a specific "Available Dosage Forms, Storage, and Compatibility" section in each monograph. This integrated organization of these clinical psychotropic drug data should greatly facilitate the rapid retrieval of needed information. The use of the *PPDR* should enable prescribing psychologists to develop and enhance their abilities to prescribe, manage, and discontinue optimal, safe, and effective psychotropic pharmacotherapy as an important adjunct to psychotherapy.

Each of the monographs has been reviewed for form, style, and content by the members of the Editorial Advisory Committee for this series of texts. The members of this international group of distinguished psychologists from across North America have given freely of their time and expertise to improve and advance the clinical practice of psychology. We are extremely grateful for their valuable contributions and support. All psychologists, as well as their patients, who will benefit directly from the clinical application of the information and knowledge gained from this and the other texts in this series, owe the Editorial Advisory Committee a profound

---

of depression, we would consider this use to be irrational and professionally negligent. Therefore, indications for use, as adjunctive pharmacotherapy for psychological disorders, are limited to those indications that have received FDA and/or Health Protection Branch (HPB) approval *and* for which efficacy has been established in the published clinical literature. For example, although some sedative-hypnotics have received FDA and/or HPB approval for the symptomatic management of anxiety associated with depression, they all may cause depression as an adverse drug reaction. In fact, both the published literature and clinical experience indicate that sedative-hypnotics usually exacerbate the existing depression and that this action is much more pronounced and clinically significant than is the relief of any associated anxiety. In this clinical context, the appropriate selection of an antidepressant that is indicated for the symptomatic management of depression, the underlying disorder, and its associated anxiety would be considered to be a more rational therapeutic decision. Thus, for these sedative-hypnotics, the indication "anxiety associated with depression," although officially approved, is *not* included in this reference text.

[5]Signs and symptoms of psychotropic overdosages are presented to assist prescribing psychologists to recognize possible overdosage among their patients so that pharmacotherapy can be appropriately discontinued and patients referred for emergency symptomatic medical management. The clinical management of overdosages is considered to be within the practice realm of medicine. Therefore, a discussion of the actual emergency symptomatic medical management of overdosage (e.g., selection and dosage of specific drugs used to facilitate elimination; use of adjunctive measures, such as hemodialysis; support of body systems [e.g., mechanical ventilation, provision of fluids and electrolytes]; and laboratory monitoring parameters) has not been included in this text. Whenever overdosage is *suspected*, clinical psychologists should directly refer their patients for emergency medical evaluation and management.

[6]The data included in these monographs have been derived from several sources, including references listed in the first volume in this series, *The Pharmacologic Basis of Psychotherapeutics: An Introduction for Psychologists* (Pagliaro & Pagliaro, 1998); current (1998) official FDA- and HPB-approved drug monographs for each of the psychotropics listed; previous textbooks by the authors (see listing in the front material of this text); the authors' current graduate lectures for the "Series of Hierarchical Graduate and Post-Graduate Courses in Pharmacopsychology;" and the authors' clinical experiences. These available data were content analyzed and synthesized into the monographs presented.

debt of gratitude. In all cases, responsibility for the completeness and accuracy of the data in this and in the other texts in the series remains with the authors.[7]

As previously noted, the psychotropics discussed in this reference are referred to by their generic (nonproprietary) USAN names. However, psychologists who use brand or trade names may access needed information by consulting the general index located at the end of this reference. All dosages included in this reference are average dosages derived, using population-based statistical models, from data obtained from sample patient groups and groups of research subjects. Therefore, these dosages are approximate dosages. In all cases, variability in *individual* patient response may necessitate alterations in drug dosages or frequency of dosing. Accepted guidelines for the use of each psychotropic drug, including drug information centers, current manufacturer patient and product package inserts, or other authoritative references, should be consulted whenever there is further question about a particular use or dose of a drug. For example, psychologists who require additional information or review concerning the basic principles of clinical pharmacology are referred to the companion volume and first text in this series, *The Pharmacologic Basis of Psychotherapeutics: An Introduction for Psychologists* (Pagliaro & Pagliaro, 1998).[8] In addition, psychologists who require additional information or review regarding the indications and use of the psychotropics as adjuncts to psychotherapy and other therapeutic modalities (e.g., biofeedback or electroconvulsive therapy) that are most appropriate for the symptomatic management of specific psychological disorders are referred to the companion volume and fourth text in this series, *Clinical Psychopharmacotherapeutics for Psychologists* (Pagliaro & Pagliaro, in preparation).[9]

When additional age-specific information regarding pharmacotherapy is required for children and adolescents or the elderly, psychologists are referred to Pagliaro and Pagliaro (1995), *Problems in Pediatric Drug Therapy*, 3rd edition, or to Pagliaro and Pagliaro (in preparation), *Problems in Geriatric Drug Therapy*, respectively. For a more detailed discussion of abusable psychotropic exposure and use among infants, children, and adolescents, psychologists are referred to Pagliaro and Pagliaro (1996), *Substance Use Among Children and Adolescents: Its Nature, Extent, and Effects from Conception to Adulthood*. Several appendices, including a list of abbreviations used in the *PPDR* can be found at the end of this text for further assistance.

It is hoped that, by using the information presented in the *Psychologists' Psychotropic Drug Reference*, prescribing psychologists and graduate psychology students, as they strive to significantly improve psychological health, will be better able to provide their patients with the maximum benefits of adjunctive pharmacotherapy with a minimum of adverse and toxic effects.

LAP/AMP
1998

---

[7] However, readers of this text have a professional responsibility to actively seek and obtain clarification whenever information seems to them to be unclear or incomplete.

[8] *The Pharmacologic Basis of Psychotherapeutics: An Introduction for Psychologists* is the first text in this series from both a temporal publication perspective and a pedagogical hierarchical perspective. For this reason, it is expected that readers of the *PPDR* are already familiar with the terms (e.g., akathisia, anorexiant), concepts (e.g., methods of drug administration, therapeutic drug monitoring), and basic principles of pharmacology (e.g., basic mechanisms of drug action, similarities and differences between and among the various classes of antidepressants). If not, they should first review *The Pharmacologic Basis of Psychotherapeutics: An Introduction for Psychologists*. See the Preface to *The Pharmacologic Basis of Psychotherapeutics*, which has been reproduced in the front material of this text, for further details and information about that text and the series.

[9] *Clinical Psychopharmacotherapeutics for Psychologists* discusses, in the context of specific psychological disorders that are amenable to adjunctive pharmacotherapy, the currently available treatment modalities (e.g., alternative, such as acupuncture; medical, such as surgery; and psychological, such as biofeedback, hypnotherapy, pharmacotherapy, and psychotherapy). The treatment modalities are evaluated in terms of their demonstrated efficacy. The criteria and parameters for selecting the best single or combination therapy for specific individual patients are presented with an emphasis upon empirically validated psychotherapeutic modalities.

Preface to *The Pharmacologic Basis of Psychotherapeutics: An Introduction for Psychologists*

We are in a time of significant economic, political, and social change. This time of change is affecting the professional practice of psychology in a variety of ways, as traditional disciplinary lines are dissolving and new boundaries are being drawn. Major practice issues, such as prescription and hospital admitting privileges for psychologists, need to be expediently and adequately addressed. Naturally, it is to be expected that some psychologists, perhaps because they are content with the status quo or because they are fearful of change, may wish that things be left as they are. Unfortunately, things cannot be left as they are. As noted by Chesterton almost 90 years ago, "If you leave a thing alone you leave it to a torrent of change" (*Orthodoxy*, 1908). Thus, our only logical and rational alternative is to become involved with the changes and to view the process of change not as a threat but as an opportunity to broaden the professional practice of psychology and, in so doing, improve the health and well-being of people who require psychological services.

As many psychologists have come to realize, appropriate pharmacotherapy can be a useful adjunct to appropriate psychotherapy and, as such, is a welcome tool for psychologists. Certainly, the optimal professional practice of psychology requires, if not prescription privileges for psychologists, at least a minimum significant degree of specialized knowledge about the propensity for psychotropics to affect behavior, cognition, learning, memory, and psychological health. Even those psychologists who choose not to prescribe psychotropics as part of their professional practice require an understanding of the use and effects of these drugs.

Such understanding is essential for all psychologists to meet more competently and comprehensively the needs of their patients, many of whom will be prescribed a psychotropic by a family physician or another prescriber (e.g., advanced practice nurse, cardiologist, clinical pharmacist, dentist, or psychiatrist). For example, even psychologists considered to be the best *psychotherapists* in the world would more than likely be unsuccessful in the treatment of a depression if they were unaware that the clinical depression was a direct adverse result of the use of a benzodiazepine (e.g., Ativan®, Halcion®, Valium®) with the adverse drug reaction of depression. In another example, school psychologists, considered to be the best learning specialists in the world, would be unable to plan optimal programs for learning disabled children if they were unaware that the children's learning problems were a direct result of anticonvulsant drug therapy, which some children require for the treatment of seizure disorders, or too high a dosage of methylphenidate (Ritalin®), which is commonly prescribed to children for the treatment of attention-deficit/hyperactivity disorder (A-D/HD). This argument becomes even more relevant when it is recognized that virtually *every* psychological disorder, whether characterized by the *Diagnostic and Statistical Manual of Mental Disorders*, 4th edition (American Psychiatric Association, 1994), or other relevant criteria (e.g., ICD), can have its signs and symptoms mimicked by the adverse drug reactions of the various psychotropics.

The preface of the first text in the series of pharmacopsychology texts for psychologists is reproduced here in order to place the current text, which is a continuation of that series, in both historical and pedagogical perspective.

Prescription privileges and related issues are being actively addressed by the profession of psychology in several countries, including Canada, South Africa, New Zealand, and the United Kingdom. In these countries, professional practice acts are increasingly being rewritten to incorporate a *nonexclusive* scope of practice for all health professions. By providing nonexclusive scopes of practice, these acts appropriately and correctly recognize that no one individual or group "owns" exclusively knowledge of a particular area of mental health practice (e.g., prescription authority). However, nowhere has this issue received more scrutiny and active debate within the profession of psychology than in the United States, where it has received the official endorsement of the American Psychological Association, the largest psychological association in the world. The Foreword to this text, written by Patrick DeLeon and Morgan Sammons, provides a historical overview of the debate and progress surrounding this crucial issue for psychologists.

The Ad Hoc Task Force on Psychopharmacology of the American Psychological Association has recommended the following three levels of psychopharmacology education: Level 1, "basic psychopharmacology education," would provide a minimal level of psychopharmacology education for all psychologists in clinical practice. Level 2, "collaborative practice," would provide additional education to enable psychologists to participate actively as partners with physicians and other prescribers in determining the need for and the monitoring of psychotropic therapy for patients they "share." Level 3, "prescription privileges," would provide the education necessary for psychologists to have independent psychotropic prescription privileges.

In accordance with these developments in psychology and the need for related formal advanced education, the authors of this text developed, at the University of Alberta, the "Hierarchical Integrated Series of Graduate/Postgraduate Courses in Pharmacopsychology," which they have taught since 1990 to both graduate psychology students and postgraduate psychologists in private practice.[1,2] The development of the "hierarchical series" was based on three basic assumptions: (1) that no single profession or group "owns" exclusively any given knowledge; (2) that psychologists, who as a group are the highest academically prepared health care professionals, are able to comprehend and to apply appropriately in clinical contexts the information and concepts of clinical pharmacology relevant to the promotion of mental health; and (3) that appropriate pharmacotherapy, when prescribed by psychologists, should be used only as an adjunct to appropriate psychotherapy.[2,3]

The current series of textbooks, of which this text is the first, is based on the authors' experience in teaching the hierarchical series of pharmacopsychology courses to a variety of graduate students in psychology and to postgraduate psychologists in independent practice in many different settings. The development of this series of textbooks also reflects the authors' concern that psychologists be provided with reference texts that are pharmacologically correct and that specifically reflect the expanded professional practice of psychology. Although each of the three initial textbooks in the series can be used alone, they have been developed as a complementary set to delineate the pharmacopsychologic knowledge required for the optimal professional prac-

---

[1]Interested readers can contact the authors for a copy of the syllabus "A Hierarchical Integrated Series of Graduate/Postgraduate Courses in Pharmacopsychology."

[2]For example, when treating a depressed patient, a psychologist would use appropriate pharmacotherapy to complement or augment established psychotherapy (e.g., cognitive therapy). In this example, if the psychologist believed that psychotherapy was unnecessary and that only pharmacotherapy was required, then the patient should be referred to another prescriber (e.g., advanced practice nurse, family physician, or psychiatrist).

[3]The third assumption is predicated upon the following rationale: First, psychotherapy is the core foundational aspect of clinical psychology treatment services (i.e., whereas psychologists may provide additional forms of treatment, such as biofeedback and hypnotherapy, psychotherapy remains the *raison d'etre* for the existence of clinical psychology as a distinct treatment-providing health care profession). Second, although research studies examining the relative therapeutic benefits of pharmacotherapy and psychotherapy have provided mixed results, a growing consensus is that combined pharmacotherapy and psychotherapy result in greater success (i.e., better therapeutic outcome) than the use of either modality alone.

tice of psychology (i.e., basic principles of pharmacotherapy, synopses of psychotropic drugs, and clinical psychopharmacotherapeutics).

The first volume in the series, *The Pharmacologic Basis of Psychotherapeutics: An Introduction for Psychologists*, introduces psychology students and psychologists to the basic principles and concepts of pharmacotherapy. As such, it assumes no prior knowledge of the principles and concepts of pharmacotherapy and should be readily amenable for use by the graduate psychology student or postgraduate psychologist in clinical practice. The second volume in the series, *Psychologists' Psychotropic Desk Reference*, provides psychologists with a valuable synopsis of all of the clinically relevant data currently available for each of the psychotropics marketed in North America. These data have been subsumed and arranged within individual drug monographs to facilitate the conceptualization and rapid retrieval of desired information when needed. The optimal use of this text requires a knowledge of the basic principles and concepts of psychotherapeutics, discussed in the first volume in the series. The third volume in the series, *Clinical Psychopharmacotherapeutics for Psychologists*, now in press, will critically discuss each of the major psychological disorders that is amenable to pharmacotherapy as an adjunct to psychotherapy. Thus, emphasis is on the validated effectiveness of these combined therapeutic approaches and related issues, including their empirical validation.[4] The optimal use of this text requires mastery of the information presented in the first and second volumes in the series, which have been designed to facilitate retrieval and review of required material.

Thus, the present volume is the foundational text that provides the pharmacologic basis of psychotherapeutics that is required for optimal use of the second and third volumes in this series. Together, these three volumes reflect all three levels of pharmacopsychology education.

The Pharmacologic Basis of Psychotherapeutics: An Introduction for Psychologists is divided into six chapters. The Foreword, "Prescription Privileges for Psychologists: A Historical Overview," coauthored by Patrick DeLeon, a champion of prescription drug privileges for psychologists, and Morgan Sammons, one of the first graduates of the Department of Defense Psychopharmacology Fellowship Program, provides a brief history of the major events leading to prescription privileges for psychologists. It also provides a precis of the arguments that have been made both for and against this expanded role for psychologists.[5] Chapter 1, "Introduction to the Basic Principles of Pharmacotherapy," describes and discusses the various purported mechanisms by which psychotropic drugs elicit their effects in the human body. Chapter 2, "The Psychotropics," introduces readers to the psychotropic drugs, including their differentiation according to abuse liability and pharmacologic classification. In addition, an overview of the remaining chapters in the textbook, in terms of their relevance to the central theme of the text and their application to clinical practice, is presented. Chapter 3, "Pharmacokinetics and Pharmacodynamics," deals with the processes of absorption, distribution, and elimination (i.e., metabolism and excretion) of psychotropic drugs from the human body. In addition, the concept of therapeutic drug monitoring and the influences of age and disease states on pharmacokinetic and pharmacodynamic processes are presented and discussed. Related mathematical modeling, including graphical representations and formulas, is included. Chapter 4, "Administration of Psychotropics," provides an overview of the various formulations of psychotropic drugs (e.g., injectables, tablets, transdermal delivery systems) and their methods of administration (e.g., intramuscular injection, oral ingestion). Attention is given to optimizing drug delivery and therapeutic response.

---

[4]The three-volume series of texts focuses exclusively on the therapeutic uses of the psychotropics. Psychologists who require additional specific information regarding the problematic patterns of abusable psychotropic use (i.e., those patterns associated with addiction and habituation) are referred to *Substance Use Among Children and Adolescents: Its Nature, Extent, and Consequences From Conception to Adulthood* (Pagliaro & Pagliaro, 1996) and *Substance Use Among Women* (Pagliaro & Pagliaro, in preparation).

[5]We are extremely grateful to Patrick DeLeon and Morgan Sammons, who took time from extremely busy schedules to write the Foreword for this first text in the series.

Chapter 5, "Adverse Drug Reactions," discusses the nature and extent of adverse drug reactions involving the psychotropic drugs. Adverse drug reactions that mimic the various psychological disorders, including those related to the use of non-psychotropic drugs (e.g., antibiotics, antiulcer drugs), are also discussed. Several comprehensive tables have been included to facilitate retrieval of relevant information. Chapter 6, "Drug Interactions," discusses the general mechanisms and sites of drug interactions that are known to occur in the human body. Individual monographs for each clinically significant drug interaction known to involve the psychotropics are provided, with attention to the specific nature, mechanisms, and clinical consequences of the drug interactions. Methods used to prevent or manage each of these interactions also are discussed.

As a means for ensuring that each chapter is as comprehensive, well-written, and up-to-date as humanly possible, the chapters have been subjected to a rigorous process of writing and revision. This has been done by the authors' taking into consideration their extensive academic and clinical backgrounds, in terms of both clinical pharmacology and psychology, and the related, relevant published literature. In addition, an Editorial Advisory Committee, composed of distinguished academics, researchers, and clinical psychologists from across North America, was established to help to ensure that the focus and leveling of the series of textbooks was appropriately directed to the needs and abilities of graduate psychology students and psychologists.[6] Each chapter has been independently reviewed by several members of the Editorial Advisory Committee, who have given freely of their time and expertise to help produce a series of textbooks that should become a proud standard for psychologists. The authors, and all psychology students and psychologists who use these texts, owe a profound debt of gratitude to the Advisory Committee members.[7]

It is hoped that, by using the information presented in this specially developed three-volume series of pharmacopsychologic texts, psychologists will be better able to provide their patients who have various psychological disorders with optimal psychotropic pharmacotherapy as an appropriate adjunct to psychotherapy and, thus, optimize the benefit derived by all patients who seek professional treatment from psychologists. In our earnest attempt to provide the best possible series of pharmacopsychology texts for psychologists, we are humbly reminded of the following words and sentiment paraphrased from Adlai Stevenson:

> *We have not done as well as we would have liked to have done, but*
> *we have done our best, honestly and forthrightly.*
> *No one can do more and you (our colleague psychologists) are*
> *entitled to no less.*

LAP/AMP
1998

---

[6]For example, to assist with this goal, the Editorial Advisory Committee identified terms with which psychologists might not be readily familiar. The most common terms were then defined and arranged in a glossary that can be found in Appendix 2 at the end of this text. In relation to leveling, it should be noted that the three-volume series, although in many regards introductory to the subject matter, was written for psychologists at a graduate level of education. Therefore, the "series" is significantly more comprehensive and at a higher scholarly level than will be found in related undergraduate texts, including those generally written for medical students.

[7]The responsibility for the completeness and accuracy of all information provided within this text remains with the authors.

Acknowledgment

The authors gratefully acknowledge the assistance of a number of people whose concerted efforts made this text and this series of texts possible. First, Herb Reich, for bringing us together with the publisher, Brunner/Mazel (a member of the Taylor & Francis group). What began as a working relationship several books ago has developed into a wonderful friendship. Next, we would again like to thank the members of the Editorial Advisory Committee for their help and encouragement throughout this entire process. A deep expression of gratitude is extended both to the Dean of Nursing, Marilynn J. Wood, for her continuing support of our textbook writing, particularly in an era of diminishing academic resources, and to Leona B. Laird for her typing of seemingly countless revisions. Last, but certainly not least, we would like to formally acknowledge the assistance and extend our sincerest thanks to all at Brunner/Mazel, including Bernadette Capelle and Alison Labbate, for their faith in us and this series of new textbooks for psychologists, for their commitment to excellence in publishing, and for their continuing assistance and support at every phase of this project.

Psychotropic
Drug
Monographs

ALPRAZOLAM

(al pray'zoe lam)

TRADE NAMES

Apo-Alpraz®
Novo-Alprazol®
Xanax®

CLASSIFICATION

Sedative-hypnotic (benzodiazepine) (C-IV)

See also Benzodiazepines General Monograph

APPROVED INDICATIONS FOR PSYCHOLOGICAL DISORDERS

Adjunctive pharmacotherapy for the short-term symptomatic management of:

- Anxiety Disorders: Acute anxiety. *Note*: Alprazolam pharmacotherapy is *not* indicated for the management of everyday anxiety or tension or for that anxiety that can be managed with psychotherapy alone. Alprazolam also is *not* recommended for the management of anxiety associated with depression because it has the potential to exacerbate the depression while alleviating the anxiety. The anxiety associated with depression generally resolves with appropriate adjunctive pharmacotherapy (i.e., the use of antidepressants) and psychotherapy.
- Anxiety Disorders: Panic disorder with or without agoraphobia.

USUAL DOSAGE AND ADMINISTRATION

Acute Anxiety

Adults: Initially, 0.75 to 1.5 mg daily orally in three divided doses. Increase the dosage at three- or four-day intervals to achieve maximal therapeutic benefit.

MAXIMUM: 4 mg daily orally

Women who are, or who may become, pregnant: FDA Pregnancy Category D. Safety and efficacy of alprazolam pharmacotherapy for women who are pregnant have not been established. Benzodiazepine pharmacotherapy during pregnancy has been associated with teratogenic effects (i.e., birth defects). Although alprazolam has not been directly implicated with fetal harm, it is assumed that alprazolam also may cross the placenta and cause teratogenic effects if prescribed during the first three months of pregnancy because of its similarity to other benzodiazepines. In addition, long-term benzodiazepine pharmacotherapy during pregnancy, or regular personal use, may result in the neonatal benzodiazepine withdrawal syndrome. This syndrome has been associated with flaccidity and respiratory problems among neonates. Avoid prescribing alprazolam pharmacotherapy to women who are pregnant. If alprazolam pharmacotherapy is required during pregnancy, advise patients of the potential benefits and possible risks to themselves and the embryo, fetus, or neonate. Collaboration with the patient's obstetrician is indicated.

Women who are breast-feeding: Safety and efficacy of alprazolam pharmacotherapy for women who are breast-feeding and their infants have not been established. Benzodiazepines are known to be excreted in breast milk. It is assumed that alprazolam also may be excreted in breast milk because of its similarity to other benzodiazepines. Benzodiazepine pharmacotherapy (i.e., diazepam) among women who are breast-feeding has resulted in lethargy and weight loss among their infants. It also may result in addiction among these infants. If alprazolam pharmacotherapy is required, breast-feeding should be discontinued. If desired, lactation may be maintained and breast-feeding resumed following the discontinuation of short-term alprazolam pharmacotherapy. Collaboration with the patient's pediatrician may be indicated.

Elderly, frail, or debilitated patients and those who have liver dysfunction: Initially, 0.25 to 0.375 mg daily orally in two or three divided doses. Increase the dosage gradually, if needed, according to individual patient response. Generally prescribe lower dosages for elderly, frail, or debilitated patients. These patients may be more sensitive to the pharmacologic actions of alprazolam than are younger or healthier adult patients. Also prescribe lower dosages for patients who have severe liver dysfunction.

Children: Safety and efficacy of alprazolam pharmacotherapy for children have not been established. Alprazolam pharmacotherapy is *not* recommended for this age group.

Notes, Acute Anxiety

Initiating and maintaining alprazolam pharmacotherapy: Prescribe the lowest possible effective dosage to avoid incoordination (ataxia) or over-sedation, which may be particularly troublesome for elderly, frail, or debilitated patients. Adjust the dosage according to individual patient response. Safety and efficacy of alprazolam pharmacotherapy for longer than four months have not been established. Reevaluate patients who appear to require alprazolam pharmacotherapy for the symptomatic management of anxiety for longer than four months.

Discontinuing alprazolam pharmacotherapy: Signs and symptoms of the alprazolam withdrawal syndrome may occur when alprazolam pharmacotherapy is abruptly discontinued or when the dosage is decreased for any reason (e.g., prescribed reduction of dosage, patient misses a dose because of forgetfulness, hospitalization of patient). Thus, discontinue alprazolam pharmacotherapy gradually. Reduce the daily dosage by no more than 0.5 mg every three days. Some patients may require a more gradual reduction of dosage (e.g., 0.25 mg weekly).

Panic Disorder

Adults: Initially, 1.5 mg daily orally in three divided doses. Increase the dosage gradually at three- or four-day intervals by increments of no more than 1 mg daily. A gradual increase in dosage allows better achievement of full pharmacologic benefit. Divide the daily dosage evenly throughout the waking hours. Dosing three or four times daily minimizes the possible occurrence of the signs and symptoms of interdose withdrawal.

MAXIMUM: 10 mg daily orally

Women who are, or who may become, pregnant: FDA Pregnancy Category D. Safety and efficacy of alprazolam pharmacotherapy for women who are pregnant have not been established. Benzodiazepine pharmacotherapy during pregnancy has been associated with teratogenic effects (i.e., birth defects). Although alprazolam has not been directly implicated in fetal harm, it is assumed that alprazolam also may cross the placenta and cause teratogenic effects if prescribed during the first three months of pregnancy because of its similarity to other benzodiazepines. Long-term benzodiazepine pharmacotherapy during pregnancy, or regular personal use, also may result in the neonatal benzodiazepine withdrawal syndrome. This syndrome has been associated with flaccidity and respiratory problems among neonates. Avoid prescribing alprazolam pharmacotherapy to women who are pregnant. If alprazolam pharmacotherapy is required during pregnancy, advise patients of the potential benefits and possible risks to themselves and the embryo, fetus, or neonate. Collaboration with the patient's obstetrician is indicated.

Women who are breast-feeding: Safety and efficacy of alprazolam pharmacotherapy for women who are breast-feeding and their neonates and infants have not been established. Benzodiazepines are known to be excreted in breast milk. It is assumed that alprazolam also may be excreted in breast milk because of its similarity to other benzodiazepines. Benzodiazepine pharmacotherapy (i.e., diazepam) among women who are breast-feeding has resulted in lethargy and weight loss among their infants. It also may result in addiction among these infants. If alprazolam pharmacotherapy is required, breast-feeding should be discontinued. If desired, lactation may be maintained and breast-feeding resumed following the discontinuation of alprazolam pharmacotherapy. Collaboration with the patient's pediatrician may be indicated.

Elderly, frail, or debilitated patients and those who have liver dysfunction: Initially, 0.5 to 0.75 mg daily orally in two or three divided doses. Increase the dosage gradually, if needed, according to individual patient response. Generally prescribe lower dosages for elderly, frail, or debilitated patients. These patients may be more sensitive to the pharmacologic actions of alprazolam than are younger or healthier adult patients. Also prescribe lower dosages for patients who have severe liver dysfunction.

Children and adolescents younger than 18 years of age: Safety and efficacy of alprazolam pharmacotherapy for children and adolescents younger than 18 years of age have not been established. Alprazolam pharmacotherapy is *not* recommended for this age group.

Notes, Panic Disorder

Initiating alprazolam pharmacotherapy: The goal of alprazolam pharmacotherapy for the symptomatic management of panic disorder is a substantial reduction in panic attacks or their total elimination. Alprazolam pharmacotherapy for the management of panic disorder may require dosages ranging from 4 mg daily to a maximum of 10 mg daily. Generally initiate alprazolam pharmacotherapy at a lower dosage to minimize the occurrence of common ADRs. Increase the dosage to the maximal recommended dosage according to individual patient response. Alprazolam's half-life of elimination can be used as a guide. The dosage may be increased at intervals equal to at least five times the elimination half-life (approximately 11 hours for young adults and 16 hours for elderly adults). Longer intervals are recommended because maximal therapeutic benefit may not be achieved until the alprazolam blood levels achieve steady state.

Maintaining alprazolam pharmacotherapy: Monitor patients for a reduction in panic attacks or their total elimination. Also monitor for anxiety and other ADRs. Early morning anxiety and the emergence of signs and symptoms of anxiety between doses have been reported among patients receiving alprazolam pharmacotherapy at recommended maintenance dosages. These signs and symptoms may indicate that the daily dosing interval is longer than the duration of action or that tolerance to alprazolam has developed. The prescribed dosing interval may not be short enough to maintain adequate blood levels to prevent the recurrence of signs and symptoms of panic attacks (i.e., rebound or relapse), or the alprazolam withdrawal syndrome during the inter-dosing interval. In these situations, the same total daily dosage probably should be divided more frequently throughout the day.

Discontinuing alprazolam pharmacotherapy: Once the control of panic attacks has been achieved, discontinue alprazolam pharmacotherapy gradually. Reduce the dosage by no more than 0.5 mg every three days. Some patients may require a more gradual reduction of dosage. Monitor patients carefully for the recurrence of the signs and symptoms of panic attacks (i.e., rebound or relapse) or the alprazolam withdrawal syndrome. If signs and symptoms of panic or withdrawal are observed, reinitiate alprazolam pharmacotherapy at the previous dosage. After patients have once again stabilized, attempt a more gradual reduction of dosage. Some patients, reportedly, may be resistant to all attempts at discontinuation of alprazolam pharmacotherapy. These patients will generally require psychotherapy alone or in combination with adjunctive pharmacotherapy for the symptomatic management of alprazolam addiction and habituation.

Rebound (i.e., the return of the signs and symptoms of the panic disorder but in a more severe form and occurring more frequently than those seen before pharmacotherapy was initiated) is differentiated from relapse (i.e., the return of the signs and symptoms of the panic disorder equal in severity or frequency to those seen before pharmacotherapy was initiated). These signs and symptoms may resemble those of the alprazolam withdrawal syndrome, which include anorexia, blurred vision, confusion, diarrhea, distortion of normal smell perception (i.e., dysosmia), impaired concentration, muscle cramps, numbness or tingling of the extremities (i.e., paresthesias), twitching, and weight loss. Anxiety and insomnia also may be observed in relation to rebound, relapse, or withdrawal.

The recurrence of the signs and symptoms of the panic disorder and the signs and symptoms of the benzodiazepine withdrawal syndrome may be difficult to differentiate. However, the time course and the nature of the signs and symptoms of the alprazolam withdrawal syndrome usually include new signs and symptoms. These signs and symptoms appear generally toward the end of the gradual discontinuation of alprazolam pharmacotherapy or shortly after pharmacotherapy has been completely discontinued. These signs and symptoms generally decrease over time. The signs and symptoms of rebound or relapse are similar to those observed before the initiation of alprazolam pharmacotherapy. These signs and symptoms may recur early or late and will persist.

Seizures also have been associated with the discontinuation of alprazolam pharmacotherapy or upon abrupt reduction of dosage. The risk for seizures appears to be greatest among patients who were receiving dosages of 2 to 10 mg daily over eight or more weeks and during the first 24 to 72 hours after alprazolam pharmacotherapy has been discontinued. Consultation with an appropriate specialist (e.g., neurologist) may be required when long-term alprazolam pharmacotherapy is discontinued because of the increased risk for seizures.

AVAILABLE DOSAGE FORMS, STORAGE, AND COMPATIBILITY

Tablets, oral: 0.25, 0.5, 1, 2 mg

Notes

The 2 mg tablets are multi-scored and can be divided into two 1 mg segments or four 0.5 mg segments.

General Instructions for Patients Instruct patients who are receiving alprazolam pharmacotherapy to

- ingest each dose of the alprazolam oral tablets with food to avoid or minimize associated GI irritation.
- safely store alprazolam tablets out of the reach of children in tightly closed, light- and child-resistant containers at controlled room temperature (15° to 30°C; 59° to 86°F).
- obtain an available patient information sheet regarding alprazolam pharmacotherapy from their pharmacist at the time that their prescription is dispensed. Encourage patients to clarify any questions that they may have concerning alprazolam pharmacotherapy with their pharmacist or, if needed, to consult their prescribing psychologist.

PROPOSED MECHANISM OF ACTION

Alprazolam and other benzodiazepines cause a dose-related CNS depression varying from mild depression of cognitive and psychomotor performance to hypnosis. The exact mechanism of action for the anxiolytic and antipanic actions of alprazolam has not yet been fully determined. However, it appears to involve an interaction with benzodiazepine receptors (i.e., BZD-1 and BZD-2) at several sites within the CNS, particularly in the cerebral cortex and the limbic system. It also may be mediated by, or work in concert with, gamma-aminobutyric acid, an inhibitory neurotransmitter. See also Benzodiazepines General Monograph.

PHARMACOKINETICS/PHARMACODYNAMICS

Alprazolam is rapidly and well absorbed following oral ingestion (F = 0.9). Blood levels are proportional to the dose ingested. Peak blood levels are obtained within 1 to 2 hours. Alprazolam is approximately 80% bound to plasma proteins and has an apparent volume of distribution of approximately 1 L/kg. Alprazolam is extensively metabolized in the liver to an active metabolite, alphahydroxyalprazolam, and is excreted primarily in the urine (~20% in unchanged form). It has a mean half-life of elimination of approximately 12 hours (range 7 to 16 hours). The mean total body clearance is 50 ml/minute.

RELATIVE CONTRAINDICATIONS

Depression
Glaucoma, acute narrow-angle. Alprazolam pharmacotherapy may be prescribed for patients who have open-angle glaucoma and who are receiving appropriate pharmacotherapy. Collaboration with the patient's ophthalmologist is indicated.
Hypersensitivity to alprazolam or other benzodiazepines
Itraconazole (Sporanex®) pharmacotherapy, concurrent
Ketoconazole (Nizoral®) pharmacotherapy, concurrent
Pain, severe uncontrolled
Pregnancy
Respiratory depression, severe

CAUTIONS AND COMMENTS

Alprazolam is addicting and habituating. A rapid decrease in dosage or abrupt discontinuation of long-term pharmacotherapy, or regular personal use, may result in the benzodiazepine withdrawal syndrome. Signs and symptoms of the benzodiazepine withdrawal syndrome range from mild dysphoria and insomnia to abdominal and muscle cramps, sweating, tremors, convulsions, and vomiting. The severity and duration of the withdrawal syndrome appear to be related to dosage and duration of pharmacotherapy or personal use. However, signs and symptoms of the withdrawal syndrome, including life-threatening seizures, have been reported among patients who were receiving short-term alprazolam pharmacotherapy at dosages within the recommended range for the management of anxiety (i.e., 0.75 to 4 mg daily). The risk for withdrawal seizures may be increased at dosages higher than 4 mg daily. Monitor all patients closely, particularly those who have histories of epilepsy or other seizure disorders, who require dosage reduction and discontinuation of pharmacotherapy. Discontinue alprazolam pharmacotherapy gradually.

Immediate management of the signs and symptoms of withdrawal may require reinstitution of alprazolam pharmacotherapy at a dosage sufficient to relieve the signs and symptoms of withdrawal (other benzodiazepines may not be effective because of incomplete cross-tolerance or difficulty establishing equivalent dosage).

Habituation has been associated with all benzodiazepine pharmacotherapy, including alprazolam pharmacotherapy. Habituation is generally associated with long-term, high-dosage pharmacotherapy and may be more commonly observed among patients who have a history of problematic patterns of alcohol or other abusable psychotropic use. These patients may have considerable difficulty reducing their dosages and discontinuing their alprazolam pharmacotherapy, particularly long-term, high-dosage pharmacotherapy.

Prescribe alprazolam pharmacotherapy cautiously to patients who

- have histories of chronic alcoholism. A decreased alprazolam elimination rate (increased plasma half-life) has been observed among these patients. This decreased elimination rate has been related to the liver dysfunction commonly associated with chronic alcoholism. (See also previous discussion regarding addiction and habituation.)
- have histories of problematic patterns of benzodiazepine or other abusable psychotropic use. These patients require careful monitoring for the development of problematic patterns of alprazolam use. Repeat prescriptions should be provided only for patients who also are receiving psychotherapy and for whom missed appointments are not a problem.
- have histories of severe respiratory dysfunction. Death has been rarely associated with the initiation of alprazolam pharmacotherapy among these patients.

- have kidney or liver dysfunction. The elimination of alprazolam may be slowed among these patients and result in toxicity.

Caution patients who are receiving alprazolam pharmacotherapy against

- increasing their dosage or using alprazolam more often, or for a longer period, than prescribed. Long-term regular use of alprazolam may result in addiction and habituation. The risk for addiction and habituation may be higher for patients who are receiving alprazolam pharmacotherapy as an adjunct to their psychotherapy for the symptomatic management of panic disorder. These patients often require average daily dosages exceeding 4 mg.
- performing activities that require alertness, judgment, and physical coordination (e.g., driving an automobile, operating dangerous equipment, supervising children). Alprazolam has CNS depressant actions that may affect these mental and physical functions. For the same reason, caution patients against concurrent ingestion of alcohol or other drugs that have CNS depressant actions. The use of alcohol or other CNS depressants can result in excessive CNS depression.

In addition to these general precautions for patients, caution women to inform their prescribing psychologist if they become or intend to become pregnant while receiving alprazolam pharmacotherapy so that their pharmacotherapy can be safely discontinued.

CLINICALLY SIGNIFICANT DRUG INTERACTIONS

Concurrent alprazolam pharmacotherapy and the following may result in clinically significant drug interactions:

Alcohol Use

Concurrent alcohol use may increase the CNS depressant action of alprazolam. Advise patients to avoid, or limit, their use of alcohol while receiving alprazolam pharmacotherapy.

Pharmacotherapy With Central Nervous System Depressants or Other Drugs That Produce Central Nervous System Depression

Concurrent alprazolam pharmacotherapy with opiate analgesics, other sedative-hypnotics, or other drugs that produce CNS depression (e.g., antihistamines, phenothiazines, TCAs) may result in additive CNS depression.

Pharmacotherapy With Drugs That Inhibit Hepatic Microsomal Enzyme Metabolism

Hepatic microsomal enzyme inhibitors (e.g., cimetidine [Tagamet®], fluoxamine [Luvox®], itraconazole [Sporanex®], Ketoconazole [Nizoral®], and nefazodone [Serzone®]) may decrease alprazolam metabolism and, consequently, increase its blood concentration (sometimes several-fold). This interaction may result in excessive CNS depression and toxicity.
See Benzodiazepines General Monograph

ADVERSE DRUG REACTIONS

The ADRs associated with alprazolam pharmacotherapy, when they occur, generally occur upon the initiation of pharmacotherapy. They generally remit upon the discontinuation of pharmacotherapy. The most common ADRs associated with alprazolam pharmacotherapy are generally extensions of its CNS depressant actions and include drowsiness or lightheadedness. Alprazolam pharmacotherapy also has been associated with the following ADRs, listed according to body system:

CNS: confusion, depression, dizziness, headache, incoordination (ataxia), oversedation, unsteadiness, and, rarely, paradoxical reactions (e.g., agitation, hallucinations, increased muscle spasticity, sleep disturbances). The occurrence of these paradoxical ADRs requires the discontinuation of alprazolam pharmacotherapy.
GI: constipation, diarrhea, nausea, and vomiting
Ocular: blurred vision

See also Benzodiazepines General Monograph

OVERDOSAGE

Signs and symptoms of alprazolam overdosage include coma, confusion, diminished reflexes, incoordination, and somnolence. Death has been associated with alprazolam overdosage alone or in combination with alcohol. Alprazolam overdosage requires emergency symptomatic medical support of body systems with attention to increasing alprazolam elimination. The benzodiazepine receptor antagonist flumazenil (Anexate®, Romazicon®) may be required.

AMITRIPTYLINE

(a mee trip′ti leen)

TRADE NAMES

Elavil®
Endep®
Levate®
Novo-Tryptin®

CLASSIFICATION

Antidepressant (tricyclic)

See also Tricyclic Antidepressants General Monograph

APPROVED INDICATIONS FOR PSYCHOLOGICAL DISORDERS

Adjunctive pharmacotherapy for the symptomatic management of:

Mood Disorders: Depressive Disorders: Major Depressive Disorder. Endogenous depression is likely to be more responsive to amitriptyline pharmacotherapy than are other depressive disorders (i.e., melancholic; neurotic-psychotic). In addition, amitriptyline may be of benefit for the symptomatic management of anxiety associated with depression because of its sedative action. It also may be of benefit during the depressed phase of bipolar disorder.

Note: Amitriptyline pharmacotherapy is *not* indicated for the symptomatic management of mild depression. Patients who have transient mood disturbances or normal grief reactions are not expected to benefit from amitriptyline pharmacotherapy.

USUAL DOSAGE AND ADMINISTRATION

Major Depressive Disorder

Adults (hospitalized, severely depressed):   Initially, 100 mg daily orally or intramuscularly in three divided doses. Increase the dosage gradually to 200 mg daily, if needed, according to individual patient response. Replace injectable pharmacotherapy with oral pharmacotherapy as soon as possible.

MAINTENANCE: Severely depressed or hospitalized patients may require up to 200 mg daily.

MAXIMUM: Some hospitalized patients may require up to 300 mg daily.

Adults (non-hospitalized):   Initially, 75 mg daily orally or intramuscularly in three divided doses. Increase the dosage gradually to 150 mg daily, as needed, according to individual patient response. Replace injectable pharmacotherapy with oral pharmacotherapy as soon as possible. When satisfactory improvement is noted, reduce the dosage to the lowest effective dosage that will manage the patient's signs and symptoms of depression. If a single daily dose is preferred, 50 to 100 mg orally 30 minutes before retiring for bed in the evening. The single daily dosage may be increased by 25 to 50 mg, as needed, to a total of 150 mg per dose.

MAINTENANCE: 50 to 100 mg daily in divided doses or as a single daily dose 30 minutes before retiring for bed in the evening. Some patients may be maintained on a lower dosage of 40 mg daily.

MAXIMUM: 150 mg daily

Women who are, or who may become, pregnant: FDA Pregnancy Category D. Safety and efficacy of amitriptyline pharmacotherapy have not been established. Amitriptyline appears to cross the placenta. CNS effects, limb deformities, and developmental delay have been reported among infants whose mothers received amitriptyline pharmacotherapy during pregnancy. Avoid prescribing amitriptyline pharmacotherapy to women who are pregnant. If amitriptyline pharmacotherapy is required, advise patients of potential benefits and possible risks to themselves and the embryo, fetus, neonate, or infant. Collaboration with the patient's obstetrician is indicated.

Women who are breast-feeding: Safety and efficacy of amitriptyline pharmacotherapy for women who are breast-feeding and their neonates and infants have not been established. Amitriptyline is excreted in breast milk. Avoid prescribing amitriptyline pharmacotherapy to women who are breast-feeding. If amitriptyline pharmacotherapy is required, breast-feeding should be discontinued because of the potential for the occurrence of serious ADRs among breast-fed infants. For women who desire to continue breast-feeding, an alternative drug should be selected.

Elderly, frail, or debilitated patients: Initially, 30 mg daily orally in three divided doses and an additional dose of 20 mg orally 30 minutes before retiring for bed in the evening. Generally prescribe lower dosages for elderly, frail, or debilitated patients. Increase the dosage gradually, if needed, according to individual patient response. These patients may be more sensitive to the pharmacologic actions of amitriptyline than are younger or healthier adult patients.

Children younger than 12 years of age: The safety and efficacy of amitriptyline pharmacotherapy for the symptomatic management of depressive disorders among children younger than 12 years of age have not been established. Amitriptyline pharmacotherapy for this indication is *not* recommended for this age group.

Adolescents: Initially, 30 mg daily orally in three divided doses and an additional dose of 20 mg orally 30 minutes before retiring for bed in the evening. Increase the dosage gradually, if needed, according to individual patient response. Generally prescribe lower dosages for adolescent patients. Adolescent patients may be more sensitive to the pharmacologic actions of amitriptyline than are adult patients.

Notes, Major Depressive Disorder

Initiating Amitriptyline Pharmacotherapy   Prescribe a lower daily dosage initially. Increase the dosage gradually according to individual patient response. When increasing the daily dosage, prescribe increases for the late afternoon and evening doses because of amitriptyline's sedative action. Full therapeutic benefit for the symptomatic management of depression may not be achieved for two to three weeks following the initiation of pharmacotherapy. Some patients may require up to four weeks. The sedative action may be observed before the antidepressant action. The possibility of suicide among depressed patients remains high until significant clinical improvement of the depressive episode occurs. Prescribe for dispensing a limited supply of amitriptyline (i.e., prescriptions should not exceed a 14-day supply). Other suicide precautions may be indicated.

INTRAMUSCULAR PHARMACOTHERAPY   The pharmacologic action of amitriptyline is generally more rapid following intramuscular injection than with oral ingestion. When intramuscular pharmacotherapy is prescribed for patients who are unable to ingest oral dosage forms, replace with an oral dosage form as soon as possible.

Maintaining Amitriptyline Pharmacotherapy   Maintenance pharmacotherapy is required throughout the active phase of depression and for the expected duration of the depressive episode. Generally continue maintenance pharmacotherapy for three months or longer to decrease the possibility of relapse.

Discontinuing Amitriptyline Pharmacotherapy   Avoid abruptly discontinuing long-term, high-dosage amitriptyline pharmacotherapy.

AVAILABLE DOSAGE FORMS, STORAGE, AND COMPATIBILITY

Injectable, intramuscular: 10 mg/ml
Suspension, oral: 10 mg/5 ml
Tablets, oral: 10, 25, 50, 75, 100, 150 mg

Notes

Injectable Formulations   Injectable is for intramuscular use only. Store safely below 30°C (86°F). Protect from freezing.

General Instructions for Patients   Instruct patients who are receiving amitriptyline pharmacotherapy to do the following:

- safely store their amitriptyline oral dosage forms out of the reach of children in a tightly closed child-resistant container below 30°C (86°F). Elavil® 10 mg tablets must be protected from light.
- obtain an available patient information sheet regarding amitriptyline pharmacotherapy from their pharmacist at the time that their prescription is dispensed. Encourage patients to clarify any questions that they may have concerning amitriptyline pharmacotherapy with their pharmacist or, if needed, to consult their prescribing psychologist.

PROPOSED MECHANISM OF ACTION

Amitriptyline produces antidepressant and sedative actions. Although the exact mechanism of its antidepressant action is not yet fully understood, it appears to be related to its ability to potentiate the actions of CNS biogenic amines, specifically norepinephrine and serotonin. Amitriptyline appears to block their re-uptake at the presynaptic nerve terminals. This inhibition of re-uptake increases the amount of norepinephrine and serotonin at the synapses and, consequently, results in increased activity at the postsynaptic neuron receptor sites. Although the TCAs generally affect both serotonin and norepinephrine re-uptake, amitriptyline has a greater affinity for blocking the re-uptake of serotonin. It is thought that amitriptyline inhibits the membrane pump mechanism responsible for the uptake of norepinephrine and serotonin in adrenergic and serotonergic neurons. This pharmacologic action may potentiate or prolong neuronal activity because re-uptake of these biogenic amines is important in terminating transmission activity. See also Tricyclic Antidepressants General Monograph.

PHARMACOKINETICS/PHARMACODYNAMICS

Amitriptyline is well-absorbed following oral ingestion. However, its bioavailability is only between 30% and 60% because of its extensive first-pass hepatic metabolism. Amitriptyline is highly plasma protein bound (~96%) and it has a mean apparent volume of distribution of 15 L/kg. Peak blood concentrations are achieved between 2 and 12 hours after ingestion.

Amitriptyline is extensively metabolized in the liver, primarily to an active metabolite, nortriptyline (see Nortriptyline Monograph). Small amounts are excreted in bile. Less than 2% is excreted in unchanged form in the urine. The mean half-life of elimination of amitriptyline is approximately 20 hours (range 9 to 46 hours), and the mean total body clearance is 770 ml/minute.

Therapeutic Drug Monitoring

The dosage must be determined by individual patient response and not by amitriptyline blood levels because it is difficult to correlate blood levels with therapeutic response and ADRs for this drug. Absorption and distribution in body fluids are variable. However, blood levels may be useful for monitoring the patient's correct use of amitriptyline or possible overdosage.

It is generally recommended that blood samples be obtained approximately 12 hours following the last dose (i.e., trough concentrations). However, in cases of suspected overdosage, blood samples can be obtained at anytime. The usual therapeutic blood concentration range is from 430 to 900 nmol/L. Note that these values include the sum total of both amitriptyline and its active metabolite, nortriptyline.

RELATIVE CONTRAINDICATIONS

Glaucoma, narrow-angle
Hypersensitivity to amitriptyline or other TCAs
MAOI pharmacotherapy, concurrent or within 14 days. Concurrent TCA and MAOI pharmacotherapy may result in hyperpyretic crises, severe convulsions, and deaths. However, patients who have refractory depression have been maintained on concurrent TCA and MAOI pharmacotherapy without significant ADRs. If concurrent pharmacotherapy is required, prescribe oral formulations, avoid high dosages, and carefully monitor individual patient response. When replacing MAOI pharmacotherapy with amitriptyline pharmacotherapy, allow a minimum of 14 days to elapse after discontinuing the MAOI pharmacotherapy. Initiate amitriptyline pharmacotherapy cautiously. Increase the dosage gradually until optimal therapeutic benefit is achieved.
Myocardial infarction, acute recovery phase

CAUTIONS AND COMMENTS

Prescribe amitriptyline pharmacotherapy cautiously to patients who

- have bipolar disorders. These patients may experience a shift to mania or hypomania. Prescribe lower dosages for these patients.
- have cardiovascular disease (e.g., congestive heart failure, myocardial infarction). Amitriptyline is contraindicated during the acute recovery phase of post-myocardial infarction or when myocardial infarction is complicated by congestive heart failure. Dysrhythmias (e.g., sinus tachycardia, prolongation of conduction time) have been reported with high dosages. Unexpected death may occur rarely among patients who have cardiovascular disorders. Myocardial infarction and stroke have been reported among patients who were receiving TCA pharmacotherapy. Collaboration with the patient's family physician or a specialist (e.g., cardiologist) may be required.
- have histories of seizure disorders, organic brain syndrome, or are predisposed to seizures. Amitriptyline may lower the seizure threshold among these patients. Collaboration with the patient's family physician or a specialist (e.g., neurologist) may be required.

- have hyperthyroidism or are receiving levothyroxine or other thyroid pharmacotherapy. Concurrent TCA and thyroid pharmacotherapy has been associated with cardiac dysrhythmias. Levothyroxine may increase the therapeutic action and the ADRs of both drugs. If concurrent pharmacotherapy is required, closely monitor patients. Collaboration with the patient's family physician may be required.
- have liver dysfunction. Amitriptyline is extensively metabolized in the liver. Patients who have liver dysfunction may require lower dosages. Monitor these patients closely for amitriptyline toxicity. Collaboration with the patient's family physician may be required.
- require elective surgery. When possible, discontinue amitriptyline pharmacotherapy several days prior to elective surgery. Collaboration with the patient's surgeon or anesthesiologist may be required.
- require ECT. Concurrent amitriptyline pharmacotherapy and ECT may increase the hazards associated with the latter. Prescribe only concurrent amitriptyline pharmacotherapy and ECT for patients for whom it is essential.
- have respiratory dysfunction. The sedative action of amitriptyline may cause respiratory failure among these patients. Collaboration with the patient's family physician or a respiratory specialist may be required.
- have schizophrenia. These patients may display increased signs and symptoms of psychosis, including the exaggeration of paranoid symptomatology.
- have urinary retention, benign prostatic hypertrophy, narrow-angle glaucoma, or increased intraocular pressure. Amitriptyline's anticholinergic action may exacerbate these conditions. Even usual dosages of amitriptyline for patients who have angle closure glaucoma may precipitate an attack. Collaboration with the patient's family physician or a specialist (e.g., ophthalmologist, urologist) may be required.

CLINICALLY SIGNIFICANT DRUG INTERACTIONS

Concurrent amitriptyline pharmacotherapy and the following may result in clinically significant drug interactions:

Alcohol Use

Concurrent alcohol use may increase the CNS depressant action of amitriptyline and result in additive CNS depression. The CNS depression may increase the risk for suicide among depressed patients who have histories of problematic patterns of alcohol use. Advise patients to avoid or limit their use of alcohol while receiving amitriptyline pharmacotherapy.

Anticoagulant (Oral) Pharmacotherapy, Warfarin

Amitriptyline may increase the prothrombin time among patients stabilized with warfarin (Coumadin®) pharmacotherapy. Bleeding may result.

Cimetidine Pharmacotherapy

The initiation of cimetidine (Tagamet®) pharmacotherapy may affect amitriptyline and other TCA pharmacotherapy. Cimetidine may reduce the hepatic metabolism of amitriptyline and other TCAs. Thus, this interaction may result in the delay of their elimination and increase their steady-state blood concentrations. Clinically significant effects include an increased frequency and severity of ADRs, particularly those associated with the anticholinergic action of amitriptyline and other TCAs (e.g., blurred vision, constipation, confusion, drowsiness, dry mouth, urinary retention). The discontinuation of cimetidine pharmacotherapy among patients who are receiving amitriptyline and other TCA pharmacotherapy may decrease the blood levels of the antidepressant and its therapeutic benefit. Collaboration with the prescriber of the cimetidine is required so that cimetidine pharmacotherapy can be replaced with ranitidine (Zantac®) or another appropriate histamine-2 receptor antagonist (antiulcer drug) that does not interact with amitriptyline or other TCAs.

Clonidine (Catapres®), Guanethidine, and Methyldopa (Aldomet®) Pharmacotherapy

Amitriptyline may block the antihypertensive action of guanethidine (Ismelin®) or similar antihypertensives. If amitriptyline pharmacotherapy is required, collaboration with the prescriber of the antihypertensive is necessary so that alternative antihypertensive pharmacotherapy can be prescribed.

Pharmacotherapy With Anticholinergics and Other Drugs That Produce Anticholinergic Actions

Concurrent amitriptyline pharmacotherapy with anticholinergics (e.g., atropine) or other drugs that produce anticholinergic actions (e.g., antihistamines, antiparkinsonians, glutethimide, or phenothiazines) may result in additive anticholinergic actions. These actions, particularly during hot weather, also may cause hyperpyrexia.

Pharmacotherapy With Central Nervous System Depressants or Other Drugs That Produce Central Nervous System Depression

Concurrent amitriptyline pharmacotherapy with opiate analgesics, sedative-hypnotics, or other drugs that produce CNS depression (e.g., antihistamines, phenothiazines) may result in additive CNS depression.

Disulfiram Pharmacotherapy

Delirium has been associated with concurrent amitriptyline and disulfiram (Antabuse®) pharmacotherapy. Patients must be monitored closely.

Fluconazole Pharmacotherapy

Concurrent amitriptyline and fluconazole (Diflucan®; an antifungal) pharmacotherapy may increase amitriptyline blood concentrations 2-fold to 5-fold with resultant amitriptyline toxicity.

The mechanism of this drug interaction is believed to involve the inhibition by fluconazole of the hepatic microsomal enzyme CYP2C9. Collaboration with the prescriber of the fluconazole is required so that it can be replaced with a "non-azole" antifungal in order to avoid this interaction. If concurrent pharmacotherapy cannot be avoided, a reduction of the amitriptyline dosage by as much as 75% may be necessary. In this case, the patient must be more frequently monitored for both loss of therapeutic effect and ADRs, and the dosage of the amitriptyline accordingly adjusted.

Fluoxetine Pharmacotherapy

Concurrent amitriptyline and fluoxetine (Prozac®) pharmacotherapy may result in amitriptyline toxicity. A reduction of the amitriptyline dosage by as much as 75% may be necessary. This interaction also may occur when amitriptyline pharmacotherapy is initiated up to several weeks after the discontinuation of fluoxetine. Paralytic ileus may occur among patients, particularly elderly or bedridden patients, as a result of the additive actions of these drugs. Plan to prevent constipation and monitor for its early signs and symptoms among these patients.

Monoamine Oxidase Inhibitor Pharmacotherapy, Phenelzine (Nardil®) and Tranylcypromine (Parnate®) Pharmacotherapy

Concurrent amitriptyline and MAOI pharmacotherapy is contraindicated. Hyperpyretic crises, severe convulsions, and deaths have occurred among patients who were concurrently receiving TCA and MAOI pharmacotherapy. When replacing MAOI pharmacotherapy with amitriptyline pharmacotherapy, allow a minimum of 14 days following the discontinuation of the MAOI pharmacotherapy before initiating the amitriptyline pharmacotherapy. Initiate amitriptyline pharmacotherapy cautiously, and increase the dosage gradually according to individual patient response.

See also Tricyclic Antidepressants General Monograph

ADVERSE DRUG REACTIONS

The most common ADRs associated with amitriptyline pharmacotherapy are associated with its anticholinergic actions (e.g., blurred vision, confusion, constipation, drowsiness, dry mouth, disturbances of visual accommodation, and urinary retention). When compared to other TCAs, amitriptyline has stronger central and peripheral anticholinergic actions. Amitriptyline pharmacotherapy also has been associated with the following ADRs, listed according to body system:

Cardiovascular: tachycardia and other ADRs involving the cardiovascular system. Although ADRs involving the cardiovascular system may be more serious than other ADRs, they generally occur less frequently.
CNS: cognitive impairment, disturbed concentration, insomnia, lightheadedness, and sedation
Cutaneous: sweating (excessive)
Musculoskeletal: mild tremors
Miscellaneous: weight gain

See also Tricyclic Antidepressants General Monograph

OVERDOSAGE

See Tricyclic Antidepressants General Monograph

AMOXAPINE

(a mox'a peen)

TRADE NAME

Asendin®

CLASSIFICATION

Antidepressant (tricyclic)

See also Tricyclic Antidepressants General Monograph

APPROVED INDICATIONS FOR PSYCHOLOGICAL DISORDERS

Adjunctive pharmacotherapy for the symptomatic management of:

Mood Disorders: Depressive Disorders: Major Depressive Disorder. Patients who have failed to benefit from other adjunctive antidepressant pharmacotherapy may benefit from amoxapine pharmacotherapy.

USUAL DOSAGE AND ADMINISTRATION

Major Depressive Disorder

Adults (hospitalized, severely depressed):   Initially, 150 mg daily orally in three divided doses. Increase the dosage, according to individual patient response, to 200 to 300 mg daily orally in two or three divided doses. The optimal daily dosage is usually 150 to 300 mg. Some patients may require up to 600 mg daily. These higher dosages should *not* be prescribed to patients who have histories of seizure disorders (see Cautions and Comments).

MAXIMUM: 300 mg/dose; 600 mg daily

Adults (non-hospitalized):   Initially, 100 mg daily orally in two divided doses. Increase the dosage to 150 mg daily, according to individual patient response, as early as the third day of pharmacotherapy. If a single daily dose is preferred, 100 to 300 mg daily orally 30 minutes before retiring for bed in the evening.

MAINTENANCE: Prescribe the lowest effective dosage that will manage the signs and symptoms of depression. If the signs and symptoms of depression reappear, increase the dosage to the previous effective dosage until the signs and symptoms of depression are once again managed.

MAXIMUM: 400 mg daily

Women who are, or who may become, pregnant: FDA Pregnancy Category C. Safety and efficacy of amoxapine pharmacotherapy for women who are pregnant have not been established. Amoxapine crosses the placental barrier. Avoid prescribing amoxapine pharmacotherapy to women who are pregnant. If amoxapine pharmacotherapy is required, advise patients of potential benefits and possible risks to themselves and the embryo, fetus, or neonate. Collaboration with the patient's obstetrician is indicated.

Women who are breast-feeding: Safety and efficacy of amoxapine pharmacotherapy for women who are breast-feeding and their neonates and infants have not been established. Amoxapine and its active metabolite 8-hydroxyamoxapine are excreted in breast milk. Avoid prescribing amoxapine pharmacotherapy to women who are breast-feeding. If amoxapine pharmacotherapy is required, breast-feeding probably should be discontinued. Collaboration with the patient's pediatrician is indicated.

Elderly, frail, and debilitated patients: Initially, 37.5 mg daily orally in three divided doses. Initiate pharmacotherapy slowly, and increase the dosage gradually to 100 to 150 mg daily orally in two or three divided doses. Adjust the dosage carefully according to individual patient response. If a single daily dose is preferred, 50 to 75 mg daily orally 30 minutes before retiring for bed in the evening.

MAXIMUM: 150 mg daily

Children younger than 16 years of age: Safety and efficacy of amoxapine pharmacotherapy for children younger than 16 years of age have not been established. Amoxapine pharmacotherapy is *not* recommended for this age group.

Notes, Major Depressive Disorder

Initiating and Maintaining Amoxapine Pharmacotherapy   Dosage must be individualized. Initially prescribe the lowest recommended daily dosage in two divided doses (three doses for severely depressed hospitalized patients and elderly, frail, or debilitated patients). Increase the dosage gradually while monitoring individual patient response. Full therapeutic benefit may not be achieved for one to two weeks following the initiation of amoxapine pharmacotherapy. After therapeutic benefit is achieved, which establishes the optimal dosage for a patient, prescribe the total daily dosage as a single daily dose 30 minutes before retiring for bed in the evening.

Single daily dosing should *not* exceed 300 mg daily. Dosages exceeding 300 mg daily should be prescribed in two or three divided doses. Avoid increasing the dosage if extrapyramidal signs and symptoms are observed or reported. Tardive dyskinesia has been associated with amoxapine pharmacotherapy.

Discontinuing Amoxapine Pharmacotherapy   Withdrawal emergent neurological signs (WENS) have been associated with the discontinuation of amoxapine maintenance pharmacotherapy. Signs and symptoms of WENS are similar to those of tardive dyskinesia. However, they are less persistent. Whether the gradual discontinuation of amoxapine maintenance pharmacotherapy will decrease the incidence of WENS has not been established. However, it appears to be advisable. Discontinue amoxapine maintenance pharmacotherapy gradually.

AVAILABLE DOSAGE FORMS, STORAGE, AND COMPATIBILITY

Tablets, oral: 25, 50, 100, 150 mg

Notes

General Instructions for Patients   Instruct patients who are receiving amoxapine pharmacotherapy to

- safely store amoxapine tablets out of the reach of children in tightly closed, child-resistant containers at controlled room temperature (15° to 30°C; 59° to 86°F).
- obtain an available patient information sheet regarding amoxapine pharmacotherapy from their pharmacist at the time that their prescription is dispensed. Encourage patients to clarify any questions that they may have concerning amoxapine pharmacotherapy with their pharmacist or, if needed, to consult their prescribing psychologist.

PROPOSED MECHANISM OF ACTION

The exact mechanism by which amoxapine produces its antidepressant action is not yet fully understood. It appears to be primarily related to the potentiation of the biogenic amines in the CNS, specifically norepinephrine and serotonin, and the inhibition of their re-uptake at the presynaptic nerve terminals. The latter increases the concentrations of norepinephrine and serotonin in the synapses and, consequently, results in their increased activity at the post-synaptic neuron receptor sites.

PHARMACOKINETICS/PHARMACODYNAMICS

Amoxapine is rapidly and well absorbed following oral ingestion. Peak blood levels are achieved within 90 minutes. Amoxapine is approximately 90% plasma protein bound. It has an apparent volume of distribution of 0.9 to 1.2 L/kg. Amoxapine is almost completely metabolized in the liver, primarily to its major active metabolite, 8-hydroxyamoxapine. The mean half-life of elimination of amoxapine is approximately 8 hours (approximately 30 hours for 8-hydroxyamoxapine). Most of the drug is excreted in the urine as metabolites (~2% is excreted in unchanged form).

RELATIVE CONTRAINDICATIONS

Congestive heart failure, acute

Glaucoma, narrow-angle

Hypersensitivity to amoxapine or other TCAs

MAOI pharmacotherapy, concurrent or within 14 days. When MAOI pharmacotherapy is being replaced with amoxapine pharmacotherapy, allow a minimum of 14 days between the discontinuation of MAOI pharmacotherapy and the initiation of amoxapine pharmacotherapy. Initiate amoxapine pharmacotherapy cautiously. Increase the dosage gradually according to individual patient response.

Myocardial infarction, acute recovery phase

CAUTIONS AND COMMENTS

Prescribe amoxapine pharmacotherapy cautiously to patients who

- are receiving ECT. The combination of amoxapine pharmacotherapy and ECT may be hazardous. Prescribe only concurrent amoxapine pharmacotherapy and ECT to patients for whom potential benefit outweighs possible risks.
- have cardiovascular disease.
- have histories of increased intraocular pressure or urinary retention. Amoxapine may increase intraocular pressure or urinary retention among these patients as a result of its anticholinergic actions. Extreme caution is advised when amoxapine pharmacotherapy is prescribed to these patients. Collaboration with the patient's family physician or a specialist (e.g., ophthalmologist, urologist) may be required.
- have hyperthyroidism.
- have schizophrenia. Amoxapine may exacerbate the signs and symptoms of psychosis, including paranoid symptomatology.
- have seizure disorders. Amoxapine can lower the seizure threshold among these patients. Grand mal seizures have occurred among patients who were receiving therapeutic dosages. Avoid prescribing higher dosages to these patients.

CLINICALLY SIGNIFICANT DRUG INTERACTIONS

Concurrent amoxapine pharmacotherapy and the following may result in clinically significant drug interactions:

Pharmacotherapy With Drugs That Inhibit the Hepatic Microsomal Enzyme (CYP2D6)

Hepatic microsomal enzyme (CYP2D6) inhibitors (e.g., cimetidine [Tagamet®], SSRIs) decrease the metabolism of amoxapine and other TCAs. This interaction may result in clinically significant increases in the blood levels of amoxapine and resultant toxicity.

See also Tricyclic Antidepressants General Monograph

ADVERSE DRUG REACTIONS

Amoxapine pharmacotherapy has been associated with ADRs related to its anticholinergic action (e.g., blurred vision, constipation, drowsiness, dry mouth, or urinary retention). It also has been associated with the following ADRs, listed according to body system. Chemical and pharmacological similarities among the TCAs also require that each of the ADRs generally associated with the TCAs be considered when amoxapine pharmacotherapy is prescribed.

See Tricyclic Antidepressants General Monograph

Cardiovascular: cardiac arrest, heart block, postural hypotension, stroke, or tachycardia

CNS: cognitive impairment, sedation, and seizures. Amoxapine pharmacotherapy also has been associated with EPRs, including akathisia, akinesia, chorea, cogwheel rigidity, dyskinesia (including tardive dyskinesia), dysarthria, mask-like facies, oculogyric crisis, and torticollis. Dyskinesia, including tardive dyskinesia, may occur during long-term pharmacotherapy or with its discontinuation (i.e., withdrawal tardive dyskinesia). In some instances, tardive dyskinesia may develop after relatively short periods of low-dosage pharmacotherapy.

Tardive dyskinesia is characterized by rhythmical involuntary movements of the face, jaw, mouth, and tongue (e.g., puffing of the cheeks, chewing movements, puckering of the mouth, or protrusion of the tongue), but it also may involve abnormal involuntary movements of the extremities and other EPRs (e.g., akathisia). Fine vermicular movements of the tongue may be an early sign of the syndrome, and if pharmacotherapy is discontinued at this time, the full syndrome may not develop. Although the dyskinetic syndrome may remit partially or completely upon the discontinuation of amoxapine pharmacotherapy, it may be irreversible among some patients. Prescribe long-term amoxapine pharmacotherapy only for patients for whom there is no available alternative pharmacotherapy.

Irreversible tardive dyskinesia appears to be associated with the total dosage and duration of pharmacotherapy. Thus, the risk for developing tardive dyskinesia may be reduced by prescribing lower dosages for shorter periods of time, as consistent with the therapeutic management of the signs and symptoms of depression. For patients who are receiving long-term amoxapine pharmacotherapy, periodically reevaluate the need for continued amoxapine pharmacotherapy.

Monitor patients, especially women, elderly patients, and patients who are receiving high-dosage amoxapine pharmacotherapy for EPRs, including tardive dyskinesia.

Musculoskeletal: see CNS

OVERDOSAGE

Signs and symptoms of amoxapine overdosage differ significantly from those associated with overdosages involving the other TCAs. The signs and symptoms of amoxapine overdosage include delirium, drowsiness, grand mal seizures, and lethargy with diminished deep tendon reflexes. Kidney failure may develop within a few days of amoxapine overdosage among patients who may otherwise appear recovered. Coma and acidosis also are associated with overdosages involving large amounts of amoxapine.

Amoxapine overdosage requires emergency symptomatic medical support of body systems with attention to increasing amoxapine elimination and the prevention and control of seizures. Status epilepticus may develop, constituting a serious medical emergency. Amoxapine overdosage has been associated with permanent neurological damage, cardiovascular and renal toxicity, and death. Age, concomitant ingestion of other drugs, and especially, the interval between amoxapine overdosage and the initiation of emergency medical treatment are important determinants for patient recovery. There is no known antidote.

AMPHETAMINES

(am fet′a meens)

GENERIC NAMES

(for trade names, see individual drug monographs)

Amphetamines, mixed *
Benzphetamine *
Dextroamphetamine
Methamphetamine

CLASSIFICATION

CNS stimulant (amphetamine) (C-II)

See also individual amphetamine monographs

APPROVED INDICATIONS FOR PSYCHOLOGICAL DISORDERS

Adjunctive pharmacotherapy for the symptomatic management of:

• Attention-Deficit/Hyperactivity Disorder
• Eating Disorders: Exogenous Obesity
• Sleep Disorders: Narcolepsy

USUAL DOSAGE AND ADMINISTRATION

Attention-Deficit/Hyperactivity Disorder

Adults: See individual amphetamine monographs

Women who are, or who may become, pregnant: FDA Pregnancy Category C. Safety and efficacy of amphetamine pharmacotherapy for women who are pregnant have not been established. Avoid prescribing amphetamine pharmacotherapy to women who are pregnant. If amphetamine pharmacotherapy is required, advise patients of potential benefits and possible risks to themselves and the embryo, fetus, or neonate. Collaboration with the patient's obstetrician is indicated.

Women who are breast-feeding: Safety and efficacy of amphetamine pharmacotherapy for women who are breast-feeding and their neonates and infants have not been established. Amphetamines are excreted in breast milk. Neonates and infants may display expected pharmacologic effects (e.g., irritability, weight loss). Avoid prescribing amphetamine pharmacotherapy to women who are breast-feeding. If amphetamine pharmacotherapy is required, breast-feeding should be discontinued. If desired, lactation may be maintained and breast-feeding resumed following the discontinuation of short-term amphetamine pharmacotherapy. Collaboration with the patient's pediatrician is indicated.

Elderly, frail, or debilitated patients: Generally prescribe lower dosages for elderly, frail, or debilitated patients. Increase the dosage gradually, if needed, according to individual patient response. These patients may be more sensitive to the pharmacologic actions of the amphetamines than are younger or healthier adult patients.

Children and adolescents: Dosages for children and adolescents generally should *not* exceed adult dosages, except where specifically indicated. See individual amphetamine monographs.

Notes, Attention-Deficit/Hyperactivity Disorder

Initiating Amphetamine Pharmacotherapy Pharmacotherapy is not indicated for all children diagnosed with A-D/HD. Prescribe adjunctive pharmacotherapy only after the child has had a complete psychological assessment with attention to the severity and appropriateness of his or her signs and symptoms. Collaboration with the parents, pediatrician, teachers, and other professionals involved in the child's care (e.g., social worker) is indicated. A comprehensive multidisciplinary (e.g., psychological, educational, and family) therapeutic program is generally required. This program should be guided by the goal of achieving optimal symptomatic management of A-D/HD among children 3 years of age and older with a minimum of ADRs.

Decrements in predicted growth (i.e., height or weight) have been associated with long-term mixed amphetamines pharmacotherapy among children. Monitor children who require long-term pharmacotherapy closely. Whenever possible, interrupt mixed amphetamines pharmacotherapy occasionally to reevaluate the need for continued pharmacotherapy.

Before prescribing amphetamine pharmacotherapy for the symptomatic management of A-D/HD:

- assure an accurate diagnosis of the psychological disorder.
- refer patients for medical evaluation of general physical health and body system function and to rule out any medical disorders that may mimic the signs and symptoms of A-D/HD.
- identify any problematic patterns of abusable psychotropic use, including any heavy alcohol, cocaine, LSD, marijuana, or nicotine use.
- note any previous amphetamine or other related pharmacotherapy (e.g., methylphenidate or pemoline pharmacotherapy) and the patient's response.
- identify possible hypersensitivity to amphetamines or other sympathomimetics.
- note any contraindications, cautions, and potential drug interactions.
- assess the patient's (or parent or legal guardian's in regard to the patient) abilities to manage his or her amphetamine pharmacotherapy. Children will generally require parental guidance and supervision. Assure adequate and appropriate assistance is available for children when doses are required during the day while at school.
- assure children and their parents (or legal guardians), as appropriate, have an understanding of the planned course of amphetamine pharmacotherapy when prescribed for the symptomatic management of A-D/HD. In this regard, provide realistic information regarding the benefits and risks of amphetamine pharmacotherapy for the symptomatic

management of A-D/HD. Children, their parents (or legal guardians), and their teachers, as appropriate, should have a realistic view of what to expect in relation to amphetamine pharmacotherapy. They should understand that amphetamine pharmacotherapy will not cure the mental disorder, but will help the child to better manage associated problems. They should understand that amphetamine pharmacotherapy will not improve judgment, poor socialization, or interpersonal skills or change personality. However, they can expect that adjunctive amphetamine pharmacotherapy will help the child to focus better on learning tasks in school and decrease disruptive behavior at home (see individual amphetamine monographs).

Provide realistic information regarding amphetamine pharmacotherapy, including its associated benefits and risks, when prescribed for the symptomatic management of A-D/HD. Children, as appropriate, and their parents (or legal guardians) should be made aware that

- dosage selection depends on several factors, such as the child's age, sex, weight, body metabolism, and previous response to amphetamine or related pharmacotherapy (e.g., methylphenidate pharmacotherapy or pemoline pharmacotherapy).
- long-term amphetamine pharmacotherapy may be associated with addiction or habituation.
- the prescribed pharmacotherapy can be enhanced by concurrent participation in individual and family psychotherapy and other appropriate therapy (e.g., behavioral interventions) and an individualized classroom program.

Children and their parents (or legal guardians) should be encouraged to ask questions about the prescribed amphetamine pharmacotherapy as active consumers of comprehensive psychologic services. In this regard, they also should know

- the exact name of the amphetamine prescribed, its general action, purpose, dosage, storage, administration, and associated contraindications and cautions. They should be able to monitor therapeutic response and be able to identify possible ADRs. They also need to know how to manage common ADRs and know what signs and symptoms may indicate an overdosage or that they should consult their psychologist or family physician for emergency medical services. They also should be appropriately directed to available support groups for additional help. Family members, teachers, and others, as appropriate, should be involved whenever possible in developing a comprehensive therapeutic plan aimed at assisting the child to manage A-D/HD.

Maintaining Amphetamine Pharmacotherapy Monitor children who are prescribed amphetamine pharmacotherapy for the symptomatic management of A-D/HD for initial and continued therapeutic response:

- improved ability to attend to and perform learning tasks in the classroom
- decreased disruptive behavior at school and at home
- decreased frequency or severity of other signs and symptoms

Monitor also for ADRs, particularly overstimulation (e.g., insomnia or irritability). Assist children and their parents (or legal guardians in regard to the child) to manage common or troublesome ADRs, such as insomnia and weight loss. Collaboration with the child's advanced practice nurse, pediatrician, or nutritional consultant may be required in order to help children, as appropriate, follow a balanced diet (e.g., maintain a daily diet sufficient in calories, fats, proteins, carbohydrates, and vitamins and minerals).

Interrupt amphetamine pharmacotherapy periodically (at least once annually) to determine if behavioral signs and symptoms sufficiently persist to justify the continuation of amphetamine pharmacotherapy.

Discontinuing Amphetamine Pharmacotherapy　Abrupt discontinuation following long-term high-dosage pharmacotherapy, or regular personal use, may result in extreme fatigue, mental depression, and sleep pattern changes on EEG. Discontinue long-term amphetamine pharmacotherapy or regular personal use gradually.

Eating Disorders: Exogenous Obesity

Adults:　For the short-term symptomatic management of exogenous obesity, generally prescribe divided doses 30 to 60 minutes before meals. To avoid or minimize associated insomnia, instruct patients to ingest the last dose of the day at least 6 hours before retiring for bed in the evening. Do not prescribe anorexiant pharmacotherapy for longer than recommended (see individual amphetamine monographs).

Women who are, or who may become, pregnant:　See Attention-Deficit/Hyperactivity Disorder. See also individual amphetamine monographs.

Women who are breast-feeding:　See Attention-Deficit/Hyperactivity Disorder. See also individual amphetamine monographs.

Elderly, frail, or debilitated patients:　See Attention-Deficit/Hyperactivity Disorder. See also individual amphetamine monographs.

Children and adolescents:　See Attention-Deficit/Hyperactivity Disorder. See also individual amphetamine monographs.

Notes, Eating Disorders: Exogenous Obesity

Initiating Amphetamine Pharmacotherapy　Before prescribing amphetamine pharmacotherapy for the symptomatic management of exogenous obesity:

- assure an accurate diagnosis of the eating disorder.
- refer patients for medical evaluation of general physical health and body system function to rule out any medical disorders that may mimic the signs and symptoms of exogenous obesity (e.g., endogenous obesity).
- identify any problematic patterns of abusable psychotropic use, including any heavy alcohol, cocaine, LSD, nicotine, or marijuana use.
- note any previous amphetamine or other related pharmacotherapy (e.g., fenfluramine pharmacotherapy) and the patient's response.
- identify possible hypersensitivity to amphetamines or other sympathomimetics and any contraindications, cautions, and potential drug interactions.
- assess the patient's understanding of and ability to manage his or her amphetamine pharmacotherapy. Patients, as appropriate, should understand that amphetamine pharmacotherapy is only indicated for short-term pharmacotherapy. When prescribed for the symptomatic management of exogenous obesity, it is prescribed as adjunctive therapy to a weight reduction program that includes caloric restriction and exercise.

Provide realistic information regarding amphetamine pharmacotherapy, including its associated benefits and risks, when prescribed for the symptomatic management of exogenous obesity. Patients should be aware

- that amphetamines may cause addiction or habituation.
- that dosage selection depends on several factors, such as age, sex, weight, metabolism, and response to previous amphetamine or related pharmacotherapy (e.g., fenfluramine pharmacotherapy).
- that the prescribed pharmacotherapy can be enhanced by concurrent participation in psychotherapy and other appropriate therapy, as indicated for the specific disorder. Patients, as appropriate, should be encouraged to ask questions about the therapeutic plan as active consumers of comprehensive psychologic services.
- of the exact name of the amphetamine prescribed, its general action, purpose, dosage, storage, administration, associated contraindications, cautions, adverse drug reactions, and signs and symptoms of overdosage. They should know how to monitor therapeutic response, identify signs that indicate that the prescribing psychologist should be contacted or that emergency medical care be obtained.
- direct patients, as appropriate, to available support groups for additional help for the management of the mental disorder. Involve family members, as appropriate, in treatment planning whenever possible and provide them with adequate evaluation of the patient's progress.

Maintaining Short-Term Amphetamine Pharmacotherapy

- Monitor patients for initial and continued therapeutic response to amphetamine pharmacotherapy and common ADRs, particularly overstimulation (e.g., insomnia or irritability).
- Assist patients to manage common or troublesome ADRs, such as insomnia. Advise patients, as appropriate, to follow a balanced diet and exercise program to maintain their normal weight, to monitor their daily caloric intake, and to eat nutritious low-calorie snack foods. Collaboration with the patient's advanced practice nurse or a nutritional consultant may be required.

Discontinuing Amphetamine Pharmacotherapy   Abrupt discontinuation following long-term high-dosage pharmacotherapy, or regular personal use, may result in extreme fatigue, mental depression, and sleep pattern changes on EEG. Discontinue long-term amphetamine pharmacotherapy or regular personal use gradually.

Sleep Disorders: Narcolepsy

Adults: See individual amphetamine monographs.

Women who are, or who may become, pregnant: See Attention-Deficit/Hyperactivity Disorder. See also individual amphetamine monographs.

Women who are breast-feeding: See Attention-Deficit/Hyperactivity Disorder. See also individual amphetamine monographs.

Elderly, frail, or debilitated patients: See Attention-Deficit/Hyperactivity Disorder. See also individual amphetamine monographs.

Children and Adolescents: See Attention-Deficit/Hyperactivity Disorder. See also individual amphetamine monographs.

Notes, Sleep Disorders: Narcolepsy

Initiating Amphetamine Pharmacotherapy   Before prescribing amphetamine pharmacotherapy for the symptomatic management of narcolepsy:

- assure an accurate diagnosis of the psychological disorder.
- refer patients for medical evaluation of general physical health and body system function in order to rule out any medical disorders that may mimic the signs and symptoms of narcolepsy.
- identify any problematic patterns of abusable psychotropic use, including any heavy alcohol, cocaine, LSD, marijuana, or nicotine use.
- note any previous amphetamine or other related pharmacotherapy and the patient's response.
- identify possible hypersensitivity to amphetamines or other sympathomimetics, and note any contraindications, cautions, and potential drug interactions.
- assess the patient's knowledge of and ability to manage his or her amphetamine pharmacotherapy.
- assure that patients, as appropriate, have an understanding of the planned course of amphetamine pharmacotherapy when prescribed for the symptomatic management of narcolepsy, and provide realistic information regarding the benefits and risks of amphetamine pharmacotherapy for this indication.

Patients should be aware

- that amphetamines may cause addiction or habituation
- that dosage selection depends on several factors, such as age, sex, weight, metabolism, and response to previous amphetamine or related pharmacotherapy
- that the prescribed pharmacotherapy can be enhanced by concurrent participation in psychotherapy and other appropriate therapy

Patients, as appropriate, should be encouraged to ask questions about the therapeutic plan as active consumers of comprehensive psychologic services. In addition, they should be aware of

- the exact name of the amphetamine prescribed, its general action, purpose, dosage, storage, administration, associated contraindications, cautions, ADRs, and signs and symptoms of overdosage. They should know how to monitor therapeutic response and be able to identify signs that indicate that the prescribing psychologist should be contacted or that emergency medical care be obtained.
- available support groups for additional help for the management of the psychological disorder. Involve family members, as appropriate, in treatment planning whenever possible, and provide them with adequate evaluation of the patient's progress.

Maintaining Amphetamine Pharmacotherapy   Monitor patients for the following:

- initial and continued therapeutic response to amphetamine pharmacotherapy
- ADRs, particularly overstimulation (e.g., insomnia or irritability)

- common or troublesome ADRs, such as weight loss. Collaboration with the patient's advanced practice nurse, family physician, or a sleep consultant may be required in helping the patient to manage these ADRs.
- interrupt amphetamine pharmacotherapy periodically (at least once annually) to determine if signs and symptoms sufficiently persist to justify the continuation of pharmacotherapy.

Discontinuing Amphetamine Pharmacotherapy   Abrupt discontinuation of long-term high-dosage pharmacotherapy, or regular personal use, may result in extreme fatigue, mental depression, and sleep pattern changes on EEG. Discontinue long-term amphetamine pharmacotherapy or regular personal use gradually.

AVAILABLE DOSAGE FORMS, STORAGE, AND COMPATIBILITY

The amphetamines are administered orally.
    See individual amphetamine monographs

Notes

General Instructions for Patients   Instruct patients who are receiving amphetamine pharmacotherapy (or parents/legal guardians when patients are children) to

- safely store amphetamine capsules and tablets in child-resistant containers out of the reach of children.
- obtain an available patient information sheet regarding their amphetamine pharmacotherapy from their pharmacist at the time that their prescription is dispensed. Encourage patients to clarify any questions that they may have concerning amphetamine pharmacotherapy with their pharmacist or, if needed, to consult their prescribing psychologist.

PROPOSED MECHANISM OF ACTION

The amphetamines are chemical members of the phenylisopropylamine family. They are non-catechol, sympathomimetic amines and, when compared to epinephrine and the other catecholamines, produce greater CNS stimulation. As such, the amphetamines are indirect-acting CNS stimulants. They stimulate the release of biogenic amines (e.g., dopamine, norepinephrine, and serotonin) from presynaptic nerve terminal storage vesicles and/or inhibit their re-uptake. These actions result in expected pharmacologic effects, including abnormal dilation of the pupils (mydriasis), bronchodilation, CNS stimulation, contraction of the urinary bladder sphincter, increased blood pressure, and loss of appetite (anorexia). The amphetamines also inhibit, to varying degrees, monoamine oxidase. However, the clinical significance of this action has not yet been clearly established.

    The exact mechanism of action of the amphetamines, when prescribed as adjunctive pharmacotherapy for the symptomatic management of A-D/HD, is unknown. The amphetamines are commonly referred to as anorexiants, anorectics, or anorexigenics when prescribed as adjunctive pharmacotherapy for the symptomatic management of exogenous obesity. Their exact action in regard to this indication has not been clearly established. It is thought that the amphetamines suppress the appetite by such mechanisms of action as CNS stimulation (see previous discussion) and increasing general metabolism. Their exact mechanism of action in regard to the symptomatic management of narcolepsy is related to their CNS stimulant actions.

PHARMACOKINETICS/PHARMACODYNAMICS

The amphetamines are readily absorbed following oral ingestion. They are widely distributed in body tissues, with the highest concentrations in the CNS. Urinary excretion is pH dependent. Amphetamine elimination is increased in acidic urine and decreased in alkaline urine.

See individual amphetamine monographs

RELATIVE CONTRAINDICATIONS

Addiction or habituation to the amphetamines or any other abusable psychotropics, history of
Agitation
Arteriosclerosis, advanced
Breast-feeding
Hypersensitivity to amphetamines or other sympathomimetic amines
Hypertension, moderate to severe
Hyperthyroidism
MAOI pharmacotherapy, concurrent or within 14 days. Concurrent pharmacotherapy has been associated with the development of the serotonin syndrome which is potentially fatal.
Pregnancy, particularly the first trimester

CAUTIONS AND COMMENTS

The amphetamines are addicting and habituating. Tachyphylaxis and tolerance have been demonstrated for all drugs in this class. Patients have reportedly increased their dosage to many times the recommended dosage. Thus, the amphetamines require cautious prescription. Prescribe the lowest effective dosage and the smallest amount for dispensing at one time to minimize the possible development of problematic patterns of use. Although an amphetamine withdrawal syndrome has not been specifically identified, abrupt discontinuation following long-term high-dosage pharmacotherapy, or regular personal use, may result in extreme fatigue, mental depression, and sleep pattern changes on EEG. Signs and symptoms of long-term high-dosage pharmacotherapy, or regular personal use, include cardiomyopathy, dermatoses (severe), hyperactivity, insomnia (marked), irritability, and personality changes. One of the most severe personality changes is psychosis. Amphetamine psychosis is often clinically indistinguishable from schizophrenia. Amphetamine psychosis also may occur with excessive short-term personal use (i.e., "amphetamine run").

Prescribe amphetamine pharmacotherapy cautiously to patients who

- have hypertension, including mild hypertension. Amphetamine pharmacotherapy may increase the blood pressure excessively among these patients.
- have insulin-dependent diabetes mellitus and also are receiving concurrent dietary restrictions. Psychological disturbances have been reported among these patients. Insulin requirements also may be altered.

Caution patients who are receiving amphetamine pharmacotherapy against

- performing activities that require alertness, judgment, and physical coordination (e.g., driving an automobile, operating dangerous equipment, or supervising children) until their response to amphetamine pharmacotherapy is known
- giving, selling, or trading this drug to any relatives, friends, or others

In addition to these general precautions, caution patients to

- carry a card in case of an emergency indicating that they are receiving amphetamine pharmacotherapy. The card also should include other relevant information such as the name of a family member to contact in case of an emergency and the name of the prescribing psychologist.
- inform their advanced practice nurse, dentist, physician, or other health care providers that they are receiving amphetamine pharmacotherapy.

In addition to these general precautions for patients, caution women to inform their prescribing psychologist if they become or intend to become pregnant while receiving amphetamine pharmacotherapy so that their pharmacotherapy can be safely discontinued.

CLINICALLY SIGNIFICANT DRUG INTERACTIONS

Concurrent amphetamine pharmacotherapy and the following may result in clinically significant drug interactions:

Antihypertensive Pharmacotherapy

Amphetamines may decrease the hypotensive action of antihypertensive drugs.

Monoamine Oxidase Inhibitor Pharmacotherapy

See Relative Contraindications

Pharmacotherapy With Drugs That Acidify the Urine

Urinary acidifiers (e.g., ammonium chloride) decrease amphetamine blood concentrations by increasing the renal excretion of the amphetamines.

Pharmacotherapy With Drugs That Alkalinize the Urine

Urinary alkalinizers (e.g., acetazolamide [Diamox®] or sodium bicarbonate) increase amphetamine blood concentrations by decreasing their renal excretion.

Tricyclic Antidepressant Pharmacotherapy

Amphetamines may potentiate the actions of the TCAs.

ADVERSE DRUG REACTIONS

Amphetamine pharmacotherapy has been associated with the following ADRs, listed according to body system:

Cardiovascular: increased blood pressure, palpitation, and tachycardia
CNS: dizziness, euphoria, headache, hyperexcitability, insomnia, irritability, nervousness, psychosis, restlessness, talkativeness, tics, and tremor
Cutaneous: flushing
Genitourinary: increased sex drive
GI: abdominal cramps, constipation, diarrhea, dry mouth, loss of appetite (anorexia), nausea, vomiting, and weight loss
Metabolic/Endocrine: see Genitourinary
Ocular: abnormal dilation of the pupils (mydriasis) and blurred vision
Miscellaneous: chills

OVERDOSAGE

Signs and symptoms of acute amphetamine overdosage include the following: constipation, panic, overstimulation, restlessness, rapid respirations (tachypnea), and tremor. Depression and fatigue usually follow the CNS stimulation. Other signs and symptoms include abdominal cramps, circulatory collapse, diarrhea, dysrhythmias, hypertension or hypotension, nausea, and vomiting. Hyperpyrexia and rhabdomyolysis (i.e., an acute, sometimes fatal, reaction caused by the destruction of skeletal muscle) can result in other complications. Fatal amphetamine overdosage is usually preceded by convulsions and coma. Acute amphetamine overdosage requires emergency symptomatic medical support of body systems with attention to increasing amphetamine elimination. Sedation with a barbiturate may be required. There is no known antidote.

AMPHETAMINES, MIXED *

(am fet′a meens)

TRADE NAME

Adderall®

CLASSIFICATION

CNS stimulant (amphetamine) (C-II)

See also Amphetamines General Monograph

APPROVED INDICATIONS FOR PSYCHOLOGICAL DISORDERS

Adjunctive pharmacotherapy for the symptomatic management of:

- Attention-Deficit/Hyperactivity Disorder
- Sleep Disorders: Narcolepsy

USUAL DOSAGE AND ADMINISTRATION

Attention-Deficit/Hyperactivity Disorder

Adults: Safety and efficacy of mixed amphetamines pharmacotherapy for the symptomatic management of A-D/HD among adults have not been established. Mixed amphetamines pharmacotherapy is *not* recommended for this age group.

Children younger than 3 years of age: Safety and efficacy of mixed amphetamines pharmacotherapy for children younger than 3 years of age have not been established. Mixed amphetamines pharmacotherapy is *not* recommended for this age group.

Children 3 to 5 years of age: Initially, 2.5 mg daily orally in a single morning dose. Increase the daily dosage at weekly intervals by 2.5 mg until optimal therapeutic response is achieved. Avoid prescribing late afternoon or evening doses because of associated insomnia.

Children 6 years of age and older: Initially, 5 mg daily orally upon awakening. Increase the daily dosage at weekly intervals by 5 mg until optimal therapeutic response is achieved. Depending upon patient response, the daily dosage may be divided into two or three doses administered at four to six hour intervals. Avoid prescribing late afternoon or evening doses because of associated insomnia.

MAXIMUM: 40 mg daily orally

Notes, Attention-Deficit/Hyperactivity Disorder

Pharmacotherapy is *not* indicated for all children diagnosed with A-D/HD. Prescribe adjunctive pharmacotherapy only after the child has had a complete psychological assessment with attention to the severity and appropriateness of his or her signs and symptoms. Collaboration with the parents, pediatrician, teachers, and other professionals involved in the child's care (e.g., social worker) is indicated. A comprehensive multidisciplinary (e.g., psychological, educational, and family) therapeutic program is generally required. This program should be guided by the goal of achieving optimal symptomatic management of A-D/HD among children 3 years of age and older with a minimum of ADRs.

Decrements in predicted growth (i.e., height or weight) have been associated with long-term mixed amphetamines pharmacotherapy among children. Monitor children who require long-term pharmacotherapy closely. Whenever possible, interrupt mixed amphetamines pharmacotherapy occasionally to reevaluate the need for continued pharmacotherapy.

Sleep Disorders: Narcolepsy

Adults: 15 to 60 mg daily orally in a single or divided dose

Women who are, or who may become, pregnant: FDA Pregnancy Category C. Safety and efficacy of mixed amphetamines pharmacotherapy for women who are pregnant have not been established. Neonates born to mothers who are addicted to amphetamines have an increased risk for premature delivery and low birth weight. During the neonatal period, these neonates also may display signs and symptoms of the amphetamine withdrawal syndrome, including agitation or lassitude. Avoid prescribing mixed amphetamines pharmacotherapy to women who are pregnant. If mixed amphetamines pharmacotherapy is required, advise patients of potential benefits and possible risks to themselves and the embryo, fetus, or neonate. Collaboration with the patient's obstetrician is indicated.

Women who are breast-feeding: Safety and efficacy of mixed amphetamines pharmacotherapy for women who are breast-feeding and their neonates and infants have not been established. Amphetamines are excreted into breast milk. Avoid prescribing mixed amphetamines pharmacotherapy to women who are breast-feeding. If mixed amphetamines pharmacotherapy is required, breast-feeding probably should be discontinued. Collaboration with the patient's pediatrician may be indicated.

Children 6 to 12 years of age: Initially, 5 mg daily orally in a single dose upon awakening in the morning. Increase the daily dosage at weekly intervals by 5 mg until optimal therapeutic response is achieved. Narcolepsy seldom occurs among children who are younger than 12 years of age.

Children 12 years of age and older: Initially, 10 mg daily orally in a single dose upon awakening in the morning. Increase the daily dosage at weekly intervals by 10 mg until optimal therapeutic response is achieved.

Notes, Sleep Disorders: Narcolepsy

Prescribe the lowest effective dosage. Adjust the dosage according to individual patient response. Late evening doses should be avoided because of associated insomnia.

AVAILABLE DOSAGE FORMS, STORAGE, AND COMPATIBILITY

Tablets, oral: 10, 20 mg

Notes

Each mixed amphetamines tablet contains	10 mg Tablet	20 mg Tablet
amphetamine aspartate	2.5 mg	5 mg
amphetamine sulfate	2.5 mg	5 mg
dextroamphetamine saccharate	2.5 mg	5 mg
dextroamphetamine sulfate	2.5 mg	5 mg
Total amphetamine base equivalent	6.3 mg	12.6 mg

General Instructions for Patients Instruct patients who are receiving mixed amphetamines pharmacotherapy to

- safely store mixed amphetamines tablets out of the reach of children in tightly closed child- and light-resistant containers at controlled room temperature (15° to 30°C; 59° to 86°F).
- obtain an available patient information sheet regarding mixed amphetamines pharmacotherapy from their pharmacist at the time that their prescription is dispensed. Encourage patients to clarify any questions that they may have concerning mixed amphetamines pharmacotherapy with their pharmacist or, if needed, to consult their prescribing psychologist.

PROPOSED MECHANISM OF ACTION

The mixed amphetamines are members of the amphetamine group of sympathomimetic amines that have CNS stimulant action. Peripheral actions include elevation of systolic and diastolic blood pressures and weak bronchodilator and respiratory stimulant action. The mixed amphetamines appear to primarily elicit their stimulant actions by increasing the release of norepinephrine from presynaptic storage vesicles in central adrenergic neurons. A direct effect on α- and β-adrenergic receptors, inhibition of the enzyme amine oxidase, and the release of dopamine also may be involved. However, the exact mechanism of action has not yet been fully determined.

PHARMACOKINETICS/PHARMACODYNAMICS

Data are unavailable.

RELATIVE CONTRAINDICATIONS

Addiction and habituation to amphetamines or other abusable psychotropics, history of
Agitation
Arteriosclerosis, advanced
Glaucoma
Heart disease, symptomatic
Hypersensitivity to amphetamines or other sympathomimetic amines (e.g., ephedrine)
Hypertension, moderate to severe
Hyperthyroidism
MAOI pharmacotherapy, concurrent or within 14 days. Mixed amphetamines and MAOI
    pharmacotherapy, concurrent or within 14 days, may result in hypertensive crisis.

CAUTIONS AND COMMENTS

Amphetamines have a high abuse potential. Prescribe mixed amphetamines cautiously as adjunctive pharmacotherapy for the symptomatic management of A-D/HD and narcolepsy. Long-term amphetamine pharmacotherapy, or regular personal use, may lead to addiction and habituation. Thus, attention must be given to the possibility that some patients may become addicted or habituated to mixed amphetamines as a result of their pharmacotherapy. Attention also must be given to the possibility that some patients may seek mixed amphetamines prescriptions to support their addiction or habituation to amphetamines or other CNS stimulants.

The amphetamines have been associated with problematic patterns of use since their synthesis, including patterns of abuse and compulsive use. Reportedly, patients have increased their dosage to many times the usual recommended dosage. The signs and symptoms of amphetamine toxicity or intoxication include hyperactivity, irritability, marked insomnia, personality changes, psychosis, and severe dermatoses. Psychosis is probably one of the most severe signs and symptoms of amphetamine intoxication and is often clinically indistinguishable from paranoid schizophrenia.

Abrupt discontinuation of high-dosage long-term amphetamine pharmacotherapy, or regular personal use, may result in the amphetamine withdrawal syndrome. Signs and symptoms of this syndrome include the following: EEG changes during sleep, fatigue, and mental depression. Prescribe amphetamine pharmacotherapy cautiously and monitor patients closely. Limit prescriptions to the smallest amount that is feasible for dispensing at one time to minimize the possible development of problematic patterns of use.

Prescribe mixed amphetamines pharmacotherapy cautiously to patients who

- have histories of cardiovascular disorders, including mild hypertension. Amphetamine pharmacotherapy has been associated with cardiac dysrhythmias and increased hypertension among these patients.
- have histories of schizophrenia or other psychotic disorders, particularly in children. Amphetamine pharmacotherapy for children who have psychotic disorders may exacerbate the signs and symptoms of behavior disturbance and thought disorder. Amphetamines reportedly exacerbate motor and phonic tics and Tourette's disorder (Gilles de la Tourette's syndrome). Clinical assessment of children for tics and Gilles de la Tourette's syndrome should precede the prescription of mixed amphetamines pharmacotherapy.

CLINICALLY SIGNIFICANT DRUG INTERACTIONS

Concurrent mixed amphetamines pharmacotherapy and the following may result in clinically significant drug interactions:

Guanethidine Pharmacotherapy

Mixed amphetamines pharmacotherapy may decrease the neuronal uptake of guanethidine (Ismelin®) and, thus, decrease its antihypertensive action.

Insulin Pharmacotherapy

Mixed amphetamines pharmacotherapy may alter the insulin requirements of patients who have insulin-dependent diabetes mellitus, particularly those patients who also have a restricted caloric diet.

Monoamine Oxidase Inhibitor Pharmacotherapy

Mixed amphetamines may interact with MAOIs (e.g., phenelzine [Nardil®]) and cause the release of large amounts of catecholamines. This interaction may result in hypertensive crises characterized by severe headache and hypertension. Thus, mixed amphetamines pharmacotherapy, concurrent or within 14 days of MAOI pharmacotherapy, is contraindicated.

Pharmacotherapy With Drugs That Acidify the Urine

Concurrent mixed amphetamines pharmacotherapy with drugs that acidify the urine (e.g., ammonium chloride) may increase the urinary excretion of mixed amphetamines.

Pharmacotherapy With Drugs That Alkalinize the Urine

Concurrent mixed amphetamines pharmacotherapy with drugs that alkalinize the urine (e.g., acetazolamide [Diamox®] or sodium bicarbonate) may decrease the urinary excretion of mixed amphetamines.

Phenothiazine Pharmacotherapy

Concurrent mixed amphetamines and phenothiazine pharmacotherapy can result in the diminished action of the mixed amphetamines. Phenothiazines antagonize the CNS stimulatory actions of the amphetamines.

Tricyclic Antidepressant Pharmacotherapy

Concurrent mixed amphetamines and TCA pharmacotherapy may result in the potentiation of CNS stimulant actions. As with other amphetamine or sympathomimetic pharmacotherapy, monitor patients closely and adjust the dosage of both drugs carefully when concurrent pharmacotherapy is required.

See also Amphetamines General Monograph

ADVERSE DRUG REACTIONS

Mixed amphetamines pharmacotherapy has been associated with the following ADRs, listed according to body system:

Cardiovascular: increased blood pressure, palpitations, and tachycardia

CNS: dizziness, dysphoria, euphoria, headache, insomnia, and overstimulation. Psychotic episodes have been rarely reported at recommended dosages.

Cutaneous: hives (urticaria)

Genitourinary: changes in sex drive and impotence

GI: constipation, diarrhea, dry mouth, gastrointestinal complaints, loss of appetite (anorexia), and unpleasant taste

Metabolic/Endocrine: weight loss

Musculoskeletal: restlessness and tremor. Suppression of growth also has been reported among children who have received long-term amphetamine pharmacotherapy.

See also Amphetamines General Monograph

OVERDOSAGE

Signs and symptoms of mixed amphetamines overdosage, because it is a combination amphetamine product, resemble those associated with any acute amphetamine overdosage. These signs and symptoms include assaultiveness, cardiovascular reactions (e.g., dysrhythmias, hypertension or hypotension, and circulatory collapse), confusion, gastrointestinal complaints (e.g., abdominal cramps, diarrhea, nausea, and vomiting), hallucinations, hyperpyrexia, hyperreflexia, panic, rapid respirations, restlessness, rhabdomyolysis, and tremor. Depression and fatigue usually follow the central stimulation. Fatal amphetamine overdosage is usually preceded by convulsions and coma.

Mixed amphetamines overdosage requires emergency symptomatic medical support of body systems with attention to increasing mixed amphetamines elimination. There is no known antidote. Chlorpromazine pharmacotherapy may be of benefit because it blocks dopamine and norepinephrine re-uptake, which inhibits the central stimulant actions of the amphetamines.

ANILERIDINE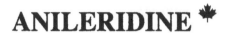

(an i leer'i deen)

TRADE NAME

Leritine®

CLASSIFICATION

Opiate analgesic (C – "not established")

See also Opiate Analgesics General Monograph

APPROVED INDICATIONS FOR PSYCHOLOGICAL DISORDERS

Adjunctive pharmacotherapy for the symptomatic management of:

Pain Disorders: Acute Pain, Moderate to Severe

USUAL DOSAGE AND ADMINISTRATION

Acute Pain, Moderate to Severe

Adults: 25 to 50 mg orally every six hours, as needed; or 25 to 75 mg intramuscularly or subcutaneously every four to six hours, as needed. More frequent dosing may be required for the symptomatic management of severe pain. However, hospitalization is required unless adequate monitoring and assistance are available in the home setting.

MAXIMUM: 200 mg daily

Women who are, or who may become, pregnant: FDA Pregnancy Category "not established." Safety and efficacy of anileridine pharmacotherapy for women who are pregnant have not been established. Avoid prescribing anileridine pharmacotherapy to women who are pregnant. If anileridine pharmacotherapy is required, advise patients of potential benefits and possible risks to themselves and the embryo, fetus, or neonate. Collaboration with the patient's obstetrician is indicated.

Women who are breast-feeding: Safety and efficacy of anileridine pharmacotherapy for women who are breast-feeding and their neonates and infants have not been established. Avoid prescribing anileridine to women who are breast-feeding. If anileridine pharmacotherapy is required, breast-feeding probably should be discontinued. Collaboration with the patient's pediatrician may be required.

Elderly, frail, or debilitated patients and those who have respiratory dysfunction: Prescribe anileridine pharmacotherapy cautiously to elderly, frail, or debilitated patients. Respiratory depression occurs most frequently among these patients and those who have respiratory dysfunction accompanied with hypoxia or hypercapnia. These medical disorders can be further compromised by even moderate therapeutic dosages of anileridine. Collaboration with the patient's family physician or a respiratory specialist is indicated.

Children younger than 12 years of age: Safety and efficacy of anileridine pharmacotherapy for children who are younger than 12 years of age have not been established. Anileridine pharmacotherapy is *not* recommended for this age group.

Notes, Acute Pain, Moderate to Severe

The injectable formulation of anileridine is for intramuscular or subcutaneous injection. Intravenous injection is generally not recommended. Rapid intravenous injection of a dose exceeding 10 mg has been associated with apnea, hypotension, and cardiac arrest.

AVAILABLE DOSAGE FORMS, STORAGE, AND COMPATIBILITY

Injectable, intramuscular or subcutaneous: 25 mg/ml ampules
Tablets, oral: 25 mg

Notes

The injectable formulation contains sodium bisulfite. Sulfites have been associated with hypersensitivity reactions, including anaphylactic reactions, among susceptible patients. Although relatively uncommon, these reactions appear to occur with a higher incidence among patients who have asthma.

General Instructions for Patients   Instruct patients who are receiving anileridine pharmacotherapy to

- safely store anileridine tablets out of the reach of children in tightly closed child- and light-resistant containers.

- obtain an available patient information sheet regarding anileridine pharmacotherapy from their pharmacist at the time that their prescription is dispensed. Encourage patients to clarify any questions that they may have concerning anileridine pharmacotherapy with their pharmacist or, if needed, to consult their prescribing psychologist.

PROPOSED MECHANISM OF ACTION

Anileridine is a relatively strong, centrally acting, synthetic opiate analgesic. Although the exact mechanism of action is not yet fully understood, anileridine appears to elicit its analgesic action primarily by binding to the endorphin receptors in the CNS.

See also Opiate Analgesics General Monograph

PHARMACOKINETICS/PHARMACODYNAMICS

Anileridine is well absorbed after oral ingestion and intramuscular and subcutaneous injection. Its onset of analgesic action is generally within 15 minutes. Its duration of action is approximately two to three hours. Anileridine is virtually completely metabolized in the liver. Only a small amount is excreted in unchanged form in the urine. Additional data are unavailable.

RELATIVE CONTRAINDICATIONS

Hypersensitivity to anileridine
Respiratory depression, including that associated with head injury or brain tumor

CAUTIONS AND COMMENTS

Anileridine is addicting and habituating. Anileridine can counteract the morphine withdrawal syndrome. Long-term anileridine pharmacotherapy over two to three weeks has been associated with addiction and habituation equal to that observed with morphine. Prescribe anileridine pharmacotherapy only when required for the symptomatic management of acute moderate to severe pain, and do not unnecessarily prolong pharmacotherapy.

Prescribe anileridine pharmacotherapy cautiously to patients who

- have acute alcoholism, delirium tremens, or seizures
- have Addison's disease (i.e., medical disorder associated with a deficiency in the secretion of adrenocortical hormones)
- are receiving MAOI pharmacotherapy
- have CNS depression, coma, or are in shock. Anileridine's respiratory depressant action may further reduce the circulating blood volume, cardiac output, and blood pressure among these patients. If severe respiratory depression and circulatory collapse are eminent, the opiate antagonist naloxone (Narcan®) may assist in counteracting these effects.
- have head injuries or other conditions associated with increased intracranial pressure. Anileridine pharmacotherapy can further increase intracranial pressure among these patients.
- have liver dysfunction (severe). The metabolism of anileridine may be decreased among these patients and result in toxicity. Extreme caution is recommended.
- have myxedema (i.e., medical disorder associated with dysfunction of the thyroid gland)

CLINICALLY SIGNIFICANT DRUG INTERACTIONS

Concurrent anileridine pharmacotherapy and the following may result in clinically significant drug interactions:

Alcohol Use

Concurrent alcohol use may increase the CNS depressant action of anileridine. Advise patients to avoid, or limit, their use of alcohol while receiving anileridine pharmacotherapy.

Pharmacotherapy With Central Nervous System Depressants and Other Drugs That Produce Central Nervous System Depression

Concurrent anileridine pharmacotherapy with other opiate analgesics, sedative-hypnotics, or other drugs that produce CNS depression (e.g., antihistamines, phenothiazines, or TCAs) may cause additive CNS, respiratory, or circulatory depression.

See also Opiate Analgesics General Monograph

ADVERSE DRUG REACTIONS

Respiratory depression and, to a lesser extent, circulatory depression are the most serious ADRs associated with anileridine pharmacotherapy. Anileridine pharmacotherapy also has been associated with the following ADRs, listed according to body system:

Cardiovascular: bradycardia and hypotension (transient, slight)
CNS: dizziness, euphoria, excitement, nervousness, and restlessness
Cutaneous: sweating (excessive)
GI: dry mouth, nausea, and vomiting
Ocular: visual difficulty
Miscellaneous: sensations of warmth

See also Opiate Analgesics General Monograph

OVERDOSAGE

The signs and symptoms of anileridine overdosage include severe respiratory depression with circulatory depression and related sequelae. Anileridine overdosage requires emergency symptomatic medical support of body systems with attention to increasing anileridine elimination and maintaining respiratory function. Respiratory depression can be treated with the opiate antagonist naloxone (Narcan®). The use of an opiate antagonist may precipitate an acute opiate withdrawal syndrome among patients addicted to opiate analgesics. The severity of this syndrome depends on the amount of opiate analgesic used, the duration of long-term use, and the amount of antagonist injected.

BARBITURATES

(bar bit'oo rates)

GENERIC NAMES

(for trade names, see individual drug monographs)

Butabarbital
Mephobarbital
Pentobarbital
Phenobarbital
Secobarbital

CLASSIFICATION

Sedative-hypnotic (barbiturate) (C-II, C-III)

See also individual barbiturate monographs

APPROVED INDICATIONS FOR PSYCHOLOGICAL DISORDERS

Adjunctive pharmacotherapy for the short-term symptomatic management of:

- Anxiety Disorders, including Panic Disorder, With or Without Agoraphobia
- Sleep Disorders: Insomnia

USUAL DOSAGE AND ADMINISTRATION

Anxiety Disorders

Adults: See individual barbiturate monographs.

Women who are, or who may become, pregnant: FDA Pregnancy Category D. Barbiturate pharmacotherapy during pregnancy has been associated with teratogenic effects (i.e., birth defects). Following oral ingestion, barbiturates cross the placental barrier readily and are distributed throughout the placenta and embryonic and fetal tissues. The highest concentration is in the brain and liver.

Barbiturate pharmacotherapy, or regular personal use, during pregnancy has been associated with a significantly increased incidence of hemorrhagic disease of the newborn. This disorder is generally readily correctable with appropriate vitamin K (phytonadione) pharmacotherapy for the neonate. Neonates born to mothers who received barbiturate pharmacotherapy, or personally used barbiturates, throughout the last trimester of pregnancy may also display signs and symptoms of the barbiturate withdrawal syndrome. These signs and symptoms include irritability and seizures.

A delayed onset of the signs and symptoms of the barbiturate withdrawal syndrome may occur for up to 14 days after delivery.

Do *not* prescribe barbiturate pharmacotherapy to women who are pregnant. If barbiturate pharmacotherapy is required, advise patients of the potential benefits and possible risks to themselves and the embryo, fetus, or neonate. Collaboration with the patient's obstetrician and pediatrician is required.

Women who are breast-feeding: Safety and efficacy of barbiturate pharmacotherapy for women who are breast-feeding and their neonates or infants have not been established. Small amounts of barbiturates are excreted in breast milk. Breast milk concentrations may be sufficient to cause expected pharmacologic actions among breast-fed neonates and infants, including drowsiness and lethargy. Concentrations also may be sufficient to cause addiction among breast-fed neonates and infants or to stimulate the hepatic microsomal enzymes. Avoid prescribing barbiturate pharmacotherapy to women who are breast-feeding. If barbiturate pharmacotherapy is required, breast-feeding should be discontinued because of the potential for these ADRs among breast-fed neonates and infants. If desired, lactation may be maintained and breast-feeding resumed following the discontinuation of short-term barbiturate pharmacotherapy. Collaboration with the patient's pediatrician is indicated.

Elderly, frail, or debilitated patients and those who have kidney or liver dysfunction: Prescribe generally lower dosages for elderly, frail, and debilitated patients. Increase the dosage gradually, if needed, according to individual patient response. These patients may be more sensitive to the CNS depressant action of the barbiturates than are younger or healthier adult patients. Elderly, frail, or debilitated patients may react to barbiturate pharmacotherapy with marked confusion, depression, or excitement. Lower dosages also should be prescribed for patients who have kidney or liver dysfunction.

Children: Safety and efficacy of barbiturate pharmacotherapy for the symptomatic management of anxiety disorders (or sleep disorders) for children have not been established. Barbiturate pharmacotherapy for these indications is *not* recommended for this age group.

Notes, Anxiety Disorders

Barbiturate pharmacotherapy for the short-term symptomatic management of anxiety has been generally replaced with benzodiazepine pharmacotherapy. However, barbiturate pharmacotherapy for this indication may be of benefit for patients who are hypersensitive to the benzodiazepines or who for any other reason are unable to receive benzodiazepine pharmacotherapy.

Initiating Barbiturate Pharmacotherapy *Before* prescribing barbiturate pharmacotherapy:

- assure an accurate diagnosis of the disorder.
- assess the patient's perception of his or her condition and need for adjunctive pharmacotherapy.
- identify any previous problematic patterns of abusable psychotropic use, including any heavy alcohol, barbiturate, or benzodiazepine use.
- note any previous barbiturate or other sedative-hypnotic pharmacotherapy for the symptomatic management of anxiety (or insomnia) and the patient's response.

- identify possible hypersensitivity to the barbiturates and potential contraindications, cautions, and drug interactions.
- assess the patient's abilities to manage his or her barbiturate pharmacotherapy.

Encourage patients to ask questions about their pharmacotherapeutic plan as active consumers of comprehensive psychological services. They should know the exact name of their prescribed barbiturate, its general action, purpose, dosage, storage, and administration. They also should be advised in relation to associated potential ADRs. They should know how to monitor therapeutic response, identify and manage common ADRs, and know the signs and symptoms that indicate that the prescribing psychologist should be contacted or emergency medical evaluation sought. Also direct patients and their families, as appropriate, to support groups for additional help.

Maintaining Barbiturate Pharmacotherapy   Prescribing psychologists should do the following in regard to appropriately managing barbiturate pharmacotherapy:

- Monitor patients for the desired therapeutic response to the prescribed barbiturate pharmacotherapy (i.e., relief of anxiety [or insomnia]).
- Avoid concurrent use of interacting drugs.
- Monitor patients for ADRs, particularly over-sedation, which can result in falls or trauma. Assure safety precautions (e.g., supervised ambulation) are implemented, as needed. Elderly, frail, or debilitated patients and those who have histories of chronic alcoholism may be particularly sensitive to the barbiturates.

Discontinuing Barbiturate Pharmacotherapy   Abrupt discontinuation of long-term barbiturate pharmacotherapy, or regular personal use, may result in the barbiturate withdrawal syndrome. Signs and symptoms of the barbiturate withdrawal syndrome, which may be fatal, include convulsions and delirium. Discontinue barbiturate pharmacotherapy gradually for patients who have received long-term barbiturate pharmacotherapy or have personally used excessive dosages over long periods of time.

Sleep Disorders: Insomnia

Adults: See Anxiety Disorders. See also individual barbiturate monographs.

Women who are, or who may become, pregnant: See Anxiety Disorders. See also individual barbiturate monographs.

Women who are breast-feeding: See Anxiety Disorders. See also individual barbiturate monographs.

Elderly, frail, or debilitated patients and those who have kidney or liver dysfunction: See Anxiety Disorders. See also individual barbiturate monographs.

Children: See Anxiety Disorders. See also individual barbiturate monographs.

Notes, Sleep Disorders: Insomnia

When prescribed for the short-term symptomatic management of insomnia, barbiturate pharmacotherapy produces various changes in normal sleep patterns. Barbiturate sleep differs from normal sleep in that the amount of time spent in the REM stage, or dreaming stage of the normal sleep cycle, is reduced. Stages III and IV also are reduced. Patients may experience markedly increased dreaming, insomnia, and nightmares when long-term or high-dosage barbiturate pharmacotherapy is abruptly discontinued. Reduce the dosage gradually over a period of five to six days to lessen REM rebound and other associated disturbances in sleep.

The barbiturates are of limited value for the long-term symptomatic management of sleep disorders. Pentobarbital and secobarbital appear to lose their effectiveness for inducing and maintaining sleep by the end of the second week of pharmacotherapy. Other barbiturates also may lose their effectiveness for inducing and maintaining sleep after approximately two weeks. Do not prescribe barbiturate pharmacotherapy for the management of sleep disorders for longer than two weeks.

See also Notes, Anxiety Disorders

AVAILABLE DOSAGE FORMS, STORAGE, AND COMPATIBILITY

See individual barbiturate monographs.

Notes

General Instructions for Patients Instruct patients who are receiving barbiturate pharmacotherapy to

- safely store barbiturate capsules and tablets out of the reach of children in child-resistant containers.
- obtain an available patient information sheet regarding barbiturate pharmacotherapy from their pharmacist at the time that their prescription is dispensed. Encourage patients to clarify any questions that they may have concerning barbiturate pharmacotherapy with their pharmacist or, if needed, to consult their prescribing psychologist.

PROPOSED MECHANISM OF ACTION

The barbiturates are chemical members of the family of substituted pyrimidines. They are structurally derived from barbituric acid, which has no intrinsic CNS activity of its own. The barbiturates depress the sensory cortex, decrease motor activity, and alter cerebellar function. In addition, they can produce, through their dose-related CNS action, all levels of CNS depression, ranging from mild sedation and hypnosis to anesthesia, deep coma, and death.

Anxiety

The exact mechanism of action of the barbiturates in producing sedative or anxiolytic actions has not yet been fully determined. However, it appears to involve binding to barbiturate receptors within the GABA receptor complex. This binding results in the retention of GABA at its receptor and an increased influx of chloride ions through the associated chloride channels, which produces neuronal inhibition.

Insomnia

The exact mechanism of action by which the barbiturates produce hypnosis has not yet been fully determined. However, it appears to be a dose-dependent extension of their sedative action.

PHARMACOKINETICS/PHARMACODYNAMICS

Barbiturates display wide variability in regard to absorption following oral ingestion. The onset of action generally occurs within 10 to 60 minutes. They are rapidly distributed to all body fluids and tissues, and because they are weak acids, they attain high concentrations in the brain, kidney, and liver. Their lipid solubility is the main factor in their wide distribution. Barbiturates are bound to plasma and tissue proteins. The degree of binding associated with the various barbiturates is also a direct function of their lipid solubility. Thiopental, which is used as a general anesthetic, is the most lipid soluble barbiturate and is ~65% plasma protein bound. Their duration of action, which is related to the rate by which they are distributed throughout the body, varies among patients and in the same patient from time to time. Barbiturates have been classified as short-acting (6 to 8 hours; e.g., thiopental), intermediate-acting (8 to 12 hours; e.g., secobarbital), and long-acting (12 to 48 hours; e.g., phenobarbital). They are metabolized primarily by the hepatic microsomal enzyme system. Their metabolites are excreted in the urine and, to a lesser extent, in the feces. The inactive metabolites are excreted as conjugates of glucuronic acid.

See also individual barbiturate monographs.

RELATIVE CONTRAINDICATIONS

Hepatic coma
Hypersensitivity to barbiturates
Porphyria, history of latent or manifest

CAUTIONS AND COMMENTS

Barbiturates are addicting and habituating, particularly long-term, high-dosage pharmacotherapy or regular personal use. For example, a dosage of 400 mg or more daily of pentobarbital or secobarbital over three months is likely to produce addiction. A dosage of 600 to 800 mg daily of pentobarbital or secobarbital over one month may produce seizures upon discontinuation of use. People who have developed addiction to the barbiturates may require up to 1500 mg daily of barbiturates to prevent the barbiturate withdrawal syndrome. As increased tolerance to the barbiturates develops, the amount of barbiturate needed to maintain desired actions increases. However, tolerance to dosages fatal to people who are not addicted to barbiturates does not increase more than 2-fold. As this ceiling effect is approached, the margin between desired actions and fatal overdosage becomes narrower.

The signs and symptoms of acute barbiturate intoxication include unsteady gate, slurred speech, and sustained nystagmus. Signs and symptoms of chronic barbiturate intoxication include confusion, poor judgment, irritability, insomnia, and somatic complaints. These signs and symptoms are similar to those associated with chronic alcoholism. In this regard, if a patient appears intoxicated with alcohol to a degree that is radically disproportionate to his or her blood alcohol concentration, barbiturate intoxication should be suspected. The lethal dose of barbiturates is reduced significantly when alcohol is concurrently ingested.

The abrupt discontinuation of barbiturates may be fatal to patients who are addicted to barbiturates. Signs and symptoms of withdrawal may appear 8 to 12 hours after the last use of a barbiturate. These signs and symptoms generally occur in the following order: anxiety, muscle twitching, tremor of the hands and fingers, progressive weakness, dizziness, distortion in visual perception, nausea and vomiting, insomnia, and postural hypotension. More severe signs and symptoms of barbiturate withdrawal include convulsions and delirium. These signs and symptoms may occur within 16 hours of the last use of a barbiturate and may last up to 5 days. The intensity of these signs and symptoms declines gradually over approximately 15 days. Patients who are susceptible to barbiturate addiction and habituation usually have histories of problematic patterns of alcohol, amphetamine, opiate analgesic, or other abusable psychotropic use.

Barbiturate addiction and habituation are associated with the regular long-term use of a barbiturate in amounts generally exceeding recommended therapeutic dosages. People who have problematic patterns of barbiturate use may have a strong desire or need to continue using the barbiturate, a tendency to increase the dose, habituation characterized by a craving to use the barbiturate, and a desire for or an appreciation of its actions. They also have a need for increasingly higher dosages to prevent the barbiturate withdrawal syndrome, the signs and symptoms of which are immediately relieved by the use of the barbiturate.

Barbiturate addiction and habituation generally require cautious and gradual discontinuation of the barbiturate. Patients who are addicted to short-acting barbiturates often require 30 mg of phenobarbital for each 100 mg of short-acting barbiturate. Patients who are addicted to pentobarbital usually require the total daily dosage of pentobarbital divided into four doses. However, this dosage should not exceed 600 mg daily. If signs and symptoms of barbiturate withdrawal occur during the first day of treatment, a loading dose of phenobarbital 200 mg intramuscularly may be required with an increase in the daily oral dosage. After patients have been stabilized with phenobarbital, the total daily dosage of phenobarbital may be decreased by 30 mg daily according to individual patient response. An alternative approach for managing barbiturate withdrawal is to decrease by 10% per day the daily dosage of the barbiturate to which the patient is addicted.

Neonates born to mothers addicted to barbiturates may require phenobarbital pharmacotherapy for the management of the neonatal withdrawal syndrome (e.g., hyperactivity, disturbed sleep, tremors, or hyperreflexia). Phenobarbital pharmacotherapy for the management of the signs and symptoms of withdrawal may be required for a two-week period. During this time, the dosage should be gradually reduced until the phenobarbital pharmacotherapy is completely discontinued.

Prescribe barbiturate pharmacotherapy cautiously to patients who

- have acute or chronic pain. Paradoxical excitement may occur among these patients. Barbiturate pharmacotherapy also may mask the signs and symptoms important for the monitoring of their pain management.
- have depression or histories of attempted suicide.
- have histories of problematic patterns of abusable psychotropic use. Patients who become addicted or habituated to barbiturates may increase the dosage or decrease the dosage interval without consulting with their prescribing psychologist. To minimize the possible development of addiction and habituation, prescribe the smallest quantity of barbiturates feasible for dispensing (i.e., limit the prescribed quantity to the amount required between appointments).

- have histories of severe respiratory dysfunction. Therapeutic dosages of barbiturates have been associated with changes in respiratory function among normal subjects. However, high therapeutic dosages among patients who have chronic obstructive lung disease (e.g., asthma, bronchitis, or emphysema) may result in respiratory distress. Barbiturate overdosage also may result in respiratory distress. The barbiturates depress alveolar ventilation and decrease hypoxic drive. These actions may result in respiratory acidosis. Apnea generally does not occur unless another CNS depressant (e.g., alcohol or an opiate analgesic) has been concurrently used.
- have sleep apnea. Avoid prescribing barbiturates to these patients. If barbiturate pharmacotherapy is required, prescribe the lowest effective dosage. Monitor patients for potential exacerbation of sleep apnea.

Caution patients who are receiving barbiturate pharmacotherapy against

- drinking alcohol or using other drugs that produce CNS depression. Barbiturates may produce drowsiness and other effects that can be potentiated by these drugs. Advise patients to report the use of any other drugs (prescription or nonprescription) while receiving barbiturate pharmacotherapy.
- exceeding the prescribed dosage or using the barbiturate for a longer period of time than prescribed. Advise patients regarding the addiction and habituation potential of the barbiturates.
- giving, selling, or trading their barbiturates to any relatives, friends, or others.
- performing activities that require alertness, judgment, and physical coordination (e.g., driving an automobile, operating dangerous equipment, or supervising children). The CNS depressant action of barbiturates may adversely affect these mental and physical functions.

In addition to these general precautions for patients, caution women to inform their prescribing psychologist if they become or intend to become pregnant while receiving barbiturate pharmacotherapy so that their pharmacotherapy can be safely discontinued.

CLINICALLY SIGNIFICANT DRUG INTERACTIONS

Most of the clinically significant drug interactions involving the barbiturates have occurred with phenobarbital. However, these data appear to be applicable to the other barbiturates because of the general pharmacologic similarities shared by the barbiturates.

Concurrent barbiturate pharmacotherapy and the following may result in clinically significant drug interactions:

Alcohol Use

Concurrent alcohol use may increase the CNS depressant action of the barbiturates. Advise patients to avoid, or limit, their use of alcohol while receiving barbiturate pharmacotherapy.

Anticoagulant (Oral) Pharmacotherapy

Barbiturates can induce the hepatic microsomal enzymes and, thus, increase the metabolism of oral anticoagulants (e.g., warfarin [Coumadin®]). This interaction results in a decreased anticoagulant response. Patients who are stabilized on oral anticoagulant pharmacotherapy may require dosage adjustments if concurrent barbiturate pharmacotherapy is initiated or discontinued. Collaboration with the prescriber of the oral anticoagulant is indicated.

Corticosteroid Pharmacotherapy

Barbiturates appear to increase the metabolism of exogenous corticosteroids, probably through the induction of hepatic microsomal enzymes. Patients who have been stabilized on corticosteroid pharmacotherapy may require dosage adjustments if concurrent barbiturate pharmacotherapy is initiated or discontinued. Collaboration with the prescriber of the corticosteroid is indicated.

Disulfiram Pharmacotherapy

Disulfiram (Antabuse®) pharmacotherapy may decrease the metabolism of the barbiturates. This interaction may increase the incidence and severity of the ADRs associated with the barbiturates.

Estrogen Pharmacotherapy

Concurrent barbiturate pharmacotherapy may decrease the action of the estrogen present in oral contraceptives by increasing the metabolism of the estrogen. This interaction may result in contraception failure. Alternative contraception may be required. Collaboration with the prescriber of the oral contraceptive is indicated.

Pharmacotherapy With Central Nervous System Depressants and Other Drugs That Produce Central Nervous System Depression

Concurrent barbiturate pharmacotherapy with opiate analgesics, other sedative-hypnotics, or other drugs that produce CNS depression (e.g., antihistamines, opiate analgesics, phenothiazines, or TCAs) may produce additive CNS depression.

Pharmacotherapy With Drugs That Are Metabolized Primarily by the Liver

Barbiturates do not impair normal liver function. However, they may induce liver microsomal enzymes and, thus, alter the metabolism of drugs that are primarily metabolized by the liver (e.g., anticoagulants [oral], corticosteroids, or estrogens). Thus, concurrent barbiturate pharmacotherapy may affect pharmacotherapy with drugs that are susceptible to hepatic microsomal enzyme metabolism. This potential interaction may require therapeutic drug monitoring of drug blood levels to determine the need to adjust the dosages of these drugs. Collaboration with other prescribers may be required.

Phenytoin Pharmacotherapy

Barbiturates appear to have varying effects on phenytoin (Dilantin®). When concurrent barbiturate and phenytoin pharmacotherapy is required, monitor the blood levels of both drugs and adjust dosages, as needed. Collaboration with the prescriber of the phenytoin is required.

Valproic Acid Pharmacotherapy

Valproic acid (Depakene®) and its derivatives (i.e., divalproex sodium or sodium valproate) appear to decrease barbiturate metabolism. When concurrent pharmacotherapy is required, monitor barbiturate blood levels, and adjust the dosage as needed.

See also individual barbiturate monographs

ADVERSE DRUG REACTIONS

Barbiturate pharmacotherapy for the symptomatic management of sleep disorders has been associated with dose-dependent respiratory depression. This respiratory depression is similar to the respiratory depression that occurs during normal sleep. Hypnotic dosages also have been associated with a slight decrease in blood pressure and heart rate. Regardless of the indication, barbiturate pharmacotherapy is commonly associated with severe drowsiness (somnolence). Among some patients, barbiturates reportedly produce excitement rather than depression. In addition, barbiturate pharmacotherapy has been associated with the following ADRs, listed according to body system:

Cardiovascular: bradycardia, fainting (syncope), and hypotension

CNS: anxiety, abnormal thinking, agitation, CNS depression, confusion, dizziness, hangover effects, headache, hallucinations, incoordination (ataxia), insomnia, lethargy, mental depression, nightmares, and paradoxic excitement (particularly among children, the elderly, and patients who have severe pain)

Cutaneous: angioedema (hives and edema involving areas of the skin, mucous membranes, or body organs), exfoliative dermatitis (Stevens–Johnson syndrome), and rash (particularly with mephobarbital and phenobarbital)

GI: constipation, diarrhea, nausea, and vomiting

Hematologic: megaloblastic anemia (following long-term phenobarbital pharmacotherapy or regular personal use)

Musculoskeletal: abnormally increased muscular movement and physical activity (hyperkinesia), joint pain, and muscle pain (myalgia)

Respiratory: apnea, bronchospasm, coughing, hypoventilation, and laryngospasm. *Note:* The ADRs affecting the respiratory system are generally associated with either overdosage or too rapid intravenous injection.

Miscellaneous: fever

See also individual barbiturate monographs

OVERDOSAGE

The ingestion of 1 gram of most barbiturates produces generally serious overdosage among adults. The signs and symptoms of barbiturate overdosage may be confused with alcohol intoxication or various neurological disorders. The ingestion of 2 to 10 grams of barbiturates is generally fatal. The signs and symptoms of acute barbiturate overdosage include CNS and respiratory depression, which may progress to Cheyne–Stokes respiration, areflexia, slightly constricted pupils (in severe overdosage, pupils may show paralytic dilation), decreased urine production (oliguria), tachycardia, hypotension, lowered body temperature, and coma. A typical shock syndrome (i.e., apnea, circulatory collapse, respiratory arrest, and death) may occur. In addition to other complications (e.g., pneumonia), extreme barbiturate overdosage may result in the cessation of all electrical activity in the brain. This effect is reportedly fully reversible unless hypoxic damage has occurred. Barbiturate overdosage requires emergency symptomatic medical support of body systems with attention to increasing barbiturate elimination. There is no known antidote.

BENZODIAZEPINES

(ben zoe dye az'e peens)

GENERIC NAMES

(for trade names, see individual benzodiazepine monographs)

Alprazolam
Bromazepam *
Chlordiazepoxide
Clorazepate
Diazepam
Estazolam *
Flurazepam
Lorazepam
Nitrazepam *
Oxazepam
Quazepam *
Temazepam
Triazolam

CLASSIFICATION

Sedative-hypnotic (benzodiazepine) (C-IV)

See also individual benzodiazepine monographs

APPROVED INDICATIONS FOR PSYCHOLOGICAL DISORDERS

Adjunctive pharmacotherapy for the short-term symptomatic management of:

- Anxiety Disorders
- Sleep Disorders: Insomnia
- Substance-Related Disorders: Alcohol Withdrawal. Benzodiazepine pharmacotherapy is prescribed to ease the signs and symptoms of alcohol withdrawal and to avoid the risk for seizures during the acute withdrawal phase. Long-acting benzodiazepines, such as chlordiazepoxide (Librium®) and diazepam (Valium®), are preferred.

See individual benzodiazepine monographs

USUAL DOSAGE AND ADMINISTRATION

Anxiety, Insomnia, and Alcohol Withdrawal

Adults: See individual benzodiazepine monographs

Women who are, or who may become, pregnant: FDA Pregnancy Category D. Safety and efficacy of benzodiazepine pharmacotherapy for women who are pregnant have not been established. The benzodiazepines readily cross the placental barrier and often achieve fetal blood concentrations that are equal to or higher than those of the maternal blood. Avoid prescribing benzodiazepine pharmacotherapy to women who are pregnant. If benzodiazepine pharmacotherapy is required, advise patients of potential benefits and possible risks to themselves and the embryo, fetus, and neonate. Collaboration with the patient's obstetrician is indicated.
See also individual benzodiazepine monographs

Women who are breast-feeding: Safety and efficacy of benzodiazepine pharmacotherapy for women who are breast-feeding and their neonates and infants have not been established. Benzodiazepines are excreted in breast milk, generally in concentrations sufficient to cause sedation and potential addiction among breast-fed neonates and infants. Avoid prescribing benzodiazepine pharmacotherapy to women who are breast-feeding. If benzodiazepine pharmacotherapy is required, breast-feeding probably should be discontinued. If desired, lactation may be maintained and breast-feeding resumed following the discontinuation of short-term benzodiazepine pharmacotherapy.
See also individual benzodiazepine monographs

Elderly, frail, or debilitated patients: Generally prescribe lower dosages for elderly, frail, or debilitated patients. Increase the dosage gradually, if needed, according to individual patient response. These patients may be more sensitive to the pharmacologic actions of the benzodiazepines than are younger or healthier adult patients. Generally the benzodiazepines, other than lorazepam, oxazepam, and temazepam, which are conjugated and excreted in the urine, have prolonged half-lives of elimination among these patients.
See also individual benzodiazepine monographs

Children and adolescents: Safety and efficacy of benzodiazepine pharmacotherapy for the symptomatic management of anxiety disorders, sleep disorders, or alcohol withdrawal for children and adolescents have not been established. Benzodiazepine pharmacotherapy for these indications is generally *not* recommended for this age group. When prescribed for children and adolescents, dosages generally should *not* exceed adult dosages, except where specifically indicated.
See also individual benzodiazepine monographs

Notes, Anxiety, Insomnia, and Alcohol Withdrawal

Initiating Benzodiazepine Pharmacotherapy   Generally prescribe the lowest effective dosage to avoid over-sedation and other associated ADRs, which may be particularly troublesome for elderly, frail, or debilitated patients. Adjust the dosage according to individual patient response. Safety and efficacy of benzodiazepine pharmacotherapy for longer than four months have not been established. Reevaluate patients who appear to require pharmacotherapy for longer than this period of time.

See individual benzodiazepine monographs
Before prescribing benzodiazepine pharmacotherapy:

- assure an accurate diagnosis of the psychological disorder.
- assess the patient's perception of his or her condition and the need for adjunctive pharmacotherapy.
- identify any previous problematic patterns of abusable psychotropic use, including any heavy alcohol, barbiturate, benzodiazepine, or other sedative-hypnotic use.
- note any previous benzodiazepine or other sedative-hypnotic pharmacotherapy and the patient's response.
- identify possible hypersensitivity to the benzodiazepines and potential contraindications, cautions, and drug interactions.
- assess the patient's ability to manage his or her benzodiazepine pharmacotherapy.
- assure patients have an understanding regarding the course of their pharmacotherapy. Patients should be made aware that benzodiazepines may cause addiction and habituation. In addition, they should know the exact name of the benzodiazepine required, its general action, purpose, dosage, storage, administration, and associated cautions. They also should know how to monitor therapeutic response, identify and manage common ADRs, and identify signs that indicate that the clinical psychologist should be contacted or emergency medical services sought. Direct patients and their families, as appropriate, to support groups for additional help for the management of the psychological disorder being treated.

Maintaining Benzodiazepine Pharmacotherapy

- Monitor patients for therapeutic response to benzodiazepine pharmacotherapy (e.g., relief of anxiety or insomnia).
- Monitor patients for ADRs. Observe for over-sedation and other associated ADRs. Elderly, frail, or debilitated patients, or those who have histories of chronic alcoholism, may be particularly sensitive to sedation and postural (orthostatic) hypotension, which can result in falls or trauma. Assure that safety precautions (e.g., supervised ambulation) are implemented, as needed.
- Avoid concurrent use of interacting drugs.

Discontinuing Benzodiazepine Pharmacotherapy   A benzodiazepine withdrawal syndrome has been associated with the abrupt discontinuation of long-term benzodiazepine pharmacotherapy, or regular personal use. Signs and symptoms of the withdrawal syndrome range from mild dysphoria and insomnia to more severe signs and symptoms, including abdominal and muscle cramps, convulsions, sweating, tremors, and vomiting. Signs and symptoms of the withdrawal syndrome also may include life-threatening seizures at dosages within the recommended range for some benzodiazepines (e.g., alprazolam). The severity of the withdrawal syndrome and its duration appear to be related to dosage and duration of pharmacotherapy, or regular personal use.

Signs and symptoms of the benzodiazepine withdrawal syndrome have been associated with rapid reductions in dosage and abrupt discontinuation of pharmacotherapy. Avoid rapid reductions in dosage and abrupt discontinuation of benzodiazepine pharmacotherapy. Monitor all patients closely who require a dosage reduction or discontinuation of benzodiazepine pharmacotherapy. Cautious reductions in dosage and discontinuation of benzodiazepine pharmacotherapy is particularly recommended for patients who have histories of epilepsy or other seizure disorders. The signs and symptoms of benzodiazepine withdrawal may be managed by the reinstitution of benzodiazepine pharmacotherapy. The dosages should be sufficient to relieve the signs and symptoms of withdrawal.

AVAILABLE DOSAGE FORMS, STORAGE, AND COMPATIBILITY

See individual benzodiazepine monographs

Notes

Injectable Benzodiazepine Pharmacotherapy　Injectable benzodiazepine pharmacotherapy is associated with apnea, bradycardia, cardiac arrest, and hypotension, particularly among elderly, frail, or debilitated patients or those who have cardiovascular or respiratory disorders. An increased incidence of these ADRs is associated with high dosages and rapid intravenous injection.

General Instructions for Patients　Instruct patients who are receiving benzodiazepine pharmacotherapy to do the following:

- safely store benzodiazepines out of the reach of children in child-resistant containers.
- obtain an available patient information sheet regarding benzodiazepine pharmacotherapy from their pharmacist at the time that their prescription is dispensed. Encourage patients to clarify any questions that they may have concerning benzodiazepine pharmacotherapy with their pharmacist or, if needed, to consult their prescribing psychologist.

PROPOSED MECHANISM OF ACTION

The benzodiazepines cause a dose-related CNS depression ranging from mild impairment of cognitive and psychomotor functions to hypnosis. The exact mechanism of action for their anxiolytic, antipanic, and other related actions has not yet been fully determined. However, benzodiazepines appear to act at the benzodiazepine receptors (i.e., BZD-1 and BZD-2). These receptors are found at several sites within the CNS, particularly in the cerebral cortex and the limbic system. The benzodiazepine receptors are found primarily in conjunction with the GABA receptor complex and predominantly in association with the $GABA_{(A)}$ receptor. Thus, it appears that the benzodiazepines elicit their pharmacologic actions by potentiating the actions of GABA, a major inhibitory neurotransmitter, within the CNS.

See also individual benzodiazepines monographs

PHARMACOKINETICS/PHARMACODYNAMICS

The benzodiazepines are generally well absorbed following oral ingestion. Food can sometimes delay the rate, but generally not the extent, of oral absorption. Some benzodiazepines (e.g., flurazepam) undergo extensive first-pass hepatic metabolism. The benzodiazepines are highly bound to plasma proteins and widely distributed throughout body tissues. The benzodiazepines and their metabolites readily cross the blood-brain and placental barriers and are excreted in breast milk.

Most benzodiazepines are mainly metabolized by the hepatic microsomal enzyme system. Therefore, liver dysfunction can significantly affect metabolism and predispose patients to toxicity. Exceptions include lorazepam, oxazepam, and temazepam. These benzodiazepines are primarily metabolized by urinary conjugation to more water-soluble (i.e., polar) glucuronide derivatives that are subsequently excreted in the urine.

On the basis of their duration of action, the benzodiazepines are commonly classified as short-acting (triazolam), intermediate-acting (alprazolam, bromazepam, lorazepam, oxazepam, and temazepam), and long-acting (chlordiazepoxide, clorazepate, diazepam, and flurazepam). The duration of action is generally well correlated with the volume of distribution of the various benzodiazepines, which in turn, is correlated with their degree of lipid solubility.

See individual benzodiazepine monographs

RELATIVE CONTRAINDICATIONS

Alcohol intoxication, acute with depressed cardiovascular and respiratory function
Depression
Glaucoma, acute narrow-angle. This contraindication is noted by most drug manufacturers. However, the benzodiazepines do *not* increase intraocular pressure nor do they possess anticholinergic activity. In addition, glaucoma has *not* been directly associated with benzodiazepine pharmacotherapy.
Hypersensitivity to any of the benzodiazepines
Pain, severe uncontrolled
Pregnancy
Respiratory depression, severe

See also individual benzodiazepine monographs

CAUTIONS AND COMMENTS

The benzodiazepines are addicting and habituating. Addiction and habituation are generally associated with long-term, high-dosage pharmacotherapy, or regular personal use. Addiction and habituation may be more commonly observed among patients who have histories of problematic patterns of alcohol or other abusable psychotropic use. These patients may have considerable difficulty decreasing their dosages and discontinuing their benzodiazepine pharmacotherapy.

Prescribe benzodiazepine pharmacotherapy cautiously to patients who

- have histories of chronic alcoholism. A decreased benzodiazepine elimination rate (increased plasma half-life) has been observed among these patients. This decreased elimination rate has been associated with the liver dysfunction commonly associated with chronic alcoholism (i.e., alcoholic cirrhosis).
- have histories of problematic patterns of alcohol or other abusable psychotropic use. These patients require careful monitoring for the development of problematic patterns of benzodiazepine use. When needed, repeat prescriptions should be provided only for patients who also are receiving psychotherapy and for whom missed appointments are not a problem.
- have histories of severe respiratory dysfunction. Therapeutic dosages of the benzodiazepines have been associated with changes in respiratory function among normal subjects. High therapeutic dosages among patients who have chronic obstructive lung disease (e.g., asthma, bronchitis, emphysema) may result in respiratory distress. Benzodiazepine overdosage also may result in respiratory distress. The benzodiazepines depress alveolar ventilation and decrease hypoxic drive, resulting in respiratory acidosis. Apnea does not generally occur unless other CNS depressants (e.g., alcohol, opiate analgesics) have been concurrently used.
- have kidney or liver dysfunction. The elimination of benzodiazepines may be slowed among these patients and result in toxicity.

- have sleep apnea. Avoid prescribing benzodiazepine pharmacotherapy for these patients. If benzodiazepine pharmacotherapy is required, prescribe the lowest effective dosage. Monitor patients for potential exacerbation of sleep apnea.

Caution patients who are receiving benzodiazepine pharmacotherapy against

- abruptly discontinuing benzodiazepine pharmacotherapy or regular personal use. Abrupt discontinuation of benzodiazepine pharmacotherapy, particularly long-term high-dosage pharmacotherapy, or regular personal use, may result in the benzodiazepine withdrawal syndrome.
- drinking alcohol or using other drugs that have CNS depressant actions. The concurrent use of alcohol or other drugs that depress the CNS can result in severe CNS depression.
- giving, selling, or trading this drug to any relatives, friends, or others.
- increasing their dosage or using benzodiazepines more often or for a longer period of time than prescribed. Long-term regular personal use of the benzodiazepines may result in addiction and habituation. The risk for addiction and habituation may be greater for patients who are receiving benzodiazepine pharmacotherapy as an adjunct to their psychotherapy for the management of panic disorder (e.g., alprazolam pharmacotherapy). These patients often require higher daily dosages.
- performing activities that require alertness, judgment, and physical coordination (e.g., driving an automobile, operating dangerous equipment, supervising children). The benzodiazepines have CNS depressant actions that may affect these mental and physical functions.

In addition to these general precautions, caution patients to inform their advanced practice nurse, dentist, physician, and other health care providers that they are receiving benzodiazepine pharmacotherapy.

CLINICALLY SIGNIFICANT DRUG INTERACTIONS

Concurrent benzodiazepine pharmacotherapy and the following may result in clinically significant drug interactions:

Alcohol Use

Concurrent alcohol use may increase the CNS depressant action of the benzodiazepines. Advise patients to avoid, or limit, their use of alcohol while receiving benzodiazepine pharmacotherapy.

Disulfiram Pharmacotherapy

Concurrent disulfiram (Antabuse®) pharmacotherapy may inhibit the metabolism of the benzodiazepines. This interaction may result in an increase in the incidence and severity of the ADRs associated with benzodiazepine pharmacotherapy.

Pharmacotherapy With Central Nervous System Depressants and Other Drugs That Produce Central Nervous System Depression

Concurrent benzodiazepine pharmacotherapy with opiate analgesics, other sedative-hypnotics, and other drugs that produce CNS depression (e.g., antihistamines, phenothiazines, TCAs) may result in severe additive CNS depression.

Pharmacotherapy With Drugs That Inhibit Hepatic Microsomal Enzyme Metabolism, Particularly Isoenzyme CYP3A4

Hepatic microsomal enzyme inhibitors (e.g., cimetidine [Tagamet®], diltiazem [Cardizem®], erythromycin [E-Mycin®], fluvoxamine [Luvox®], fluoxetine [Prozac®], grapefruit juice, itraconazole [Sporanex®], ketoconazole [Nizoral®], miconazole [Micatin®], nefazodone [Serzone®], omeprazole [Prilosec®], and quinidine [Biquin®]) may decrease benzodiazepine metabolism. This interaction may result in an increase in benzodiazepine blood concentrations (sometimes severalfold) and associated CNS depression (e.g., confusion, dizziness, drowsiness, somnolence).

Ritonavir Pharmacotherapy

Ritonavir (Norvir®), an antiretroviral drug indicated for the pharmacologic management of HIV infection, can significantly inhibit the hepatic microsomal enzyme metabolism of the benzodiazepines that are highly metabolized by the liver (i.e., alprazolam [Xanax®], clorazepate [Tranxene®], diazepam [Valium®], flurazepam [Dalmane®], midazolam [Versed®], and triazolam [Halcion®]). This interaction can result in severe sedation and respiratory depression. Concurrent benzodiazepine and ritonavir pharmacotherapy with the highly metabolized benzodiazepines is contraindicated. Concurrent pharmacotherapy with the other benzodiazepines (i.e., oxazepam [Serax®]) also should probably be avoided among patients who are receiving ritonavir pharmacotherapy. If concurrent pharmacotherapy with these other benzodiazepines cannot be avoided, carefully monitor patients for excessive CNS and respiratory depression. Adjust the benzodiazepine dosage according to individual patient response.

Tobacco Smoking

Concurrent tobacco smoking may increase the metabolism of the benzodiazepines. Patients who smoke tobacco may require higher dosages of the benzodiazepines.

See also individual benzodiazepine monographs

ADVERSE DRUG REACTIONS

Benzodiazepine pharmacotherapy has been commonly associated with amnesia, confusion, depression, psychoses, and rebound insomnia. Each of these ADRs is discussed briefly.

Amnesia

Anterograde amnesia, transient global amnesia, and "traveler's" amnesia have been associated with benzodiazepine pharmacotherapy. Anterograde amnesia, which may vary in severity, appears to be dose-related. However, it also has occurred among patients who were using thera-peutic dosages of the benzodiazepines. Elderly, frail, or debilitated patients may be at particular risk. The occurrence of transient global amnesia and "traveler's" amnesia (i.e., amnesia reported among patients who have ingested a sedative-hypnotic, often in the middle of the night, to in-duce sleep while traveling) is unpredictable and does not appear to be dose-dependent. Caution patients against ingesting a benzodiazepine (e.g., temazepam) when a full night's sleep and clear-ance of the drug from the body are not possible before resuming full daily activities.

Confusion

Benzodiazepine pharmacotherapy has been associated with confusion. The risk for confu-sion is greater among elderly patients who have cerebral dysfunction.

Depression

The benzodiazepines are CNS depressants. Depressive disorders may be exacerbated by benzodiazepine pharmacotherapy. The potential for suicide (i.e., intentional overdosage) is high among patients who are depressed. Prescribe limited quantities of the benzodiazepines for these patients (i.e., do not exceed a two-week supply). Other suicide precautions may be needed.

Psychoses

Although rarely associated with some benzodiazepines (e.g., temazepam), abnormal think-ing and psychoses, often characterized by decreased inhibition (e.g., aggressiveness or extro-version similar to that associated with alcohol or other CNS depressants), have been associated with benzodiazepine pharmacotherapy. The psychoses may be characterized by bizarre behavior, depersonalization, and hallucinations. Although it has been more generally associated with high-dosage long-term pharmacotherapy, or regular personal use, it may occur during the initiation, maintenance, or discontinuation of benzodiazepine pharmacotherapy. Patients who have histo-ries of violent behavior and unusual reactions to the sedative-hypnotics, including alcohol and the benzodiazepines, appear at particular risk. The emergence of any new signs and symptoms among patients receiving benzodiazepine pharmacotherapy requires careful and immediate eval-uation. It is unknown whether this ADR is drug-induced, spontaneous in origin, or a result of an underlying mental disorder. Psychosis also can occur during acute benzodiazepine withdrawal.

Rebound Insomnia

Rebound insomnia is a transient syndrome characterized by the signs and symptoms that led to the prescription of adjunctive benzodiazepine pharmacotherapy for the symptomatic manage-ment of insomnia. These signs and symptoms recur in an exacerbated form upon the discontinu-ation of benzodiazepine pharmacotherapy.

See also individual benzodiazepine monographs

OVERDOSAGE

Signs and symptoms of benzodiazepine overdosage include coma, confusion, diminished re-flexes, incoordination, and somnolence. Generally benzodiazepine overdosage is not fatal because benzodiazepines possess a high LD_{50}. However, death commonly occurs when benzodiazepines are used in combination with alcohol. Benzodiazepine overdosage requires emergency symptomatic medical support of body systems with attention to increasing benzodiazepine elimination. The benzodiazepine receptor antagonist flumazenil (Anexate®, Romazicon®) may be required.

See Flumazenil monograph

BENZPHETAMINE *

(benz'fet a meen)

TRADE NAME

Didrex®

CLASSIFICATION

CNS stimulant (amphetamine) (C-III)

See also Amphetamines General Monograph

APPROVED INDICATIONS FOR PSYCHOLOGICAL DISORDERS

Adjunctive pharmacotherapy for the short-term (i.e., three months or less) symptomatic management of:

Eating Disorders: Exogenous Obesity

USUAL DOSAGE AND ADMINISTRATION

Exogenous Obesity

Adults: 25 to 50 mg daily orally in a single dose mid-morning or, if preferred, in two or three divided doses. For optimal therapeutic benefit, and to minimize associated insomnia, mid-morning or mid-afternoon dosing is recommended, depending on the patient's eating habits.

MAXIMUM: 150 mg daily orally

Women who are, or who may become, pregnant: FDA Pregnancy Category C. Safety and efficacy of benzphetamine pharmacotherapy for women who are pregnant have not been established. Benzphetamine has been implicated in fetal harm when used by pregnant women.

Thus, benzphetamine pharmacotherapy is contraindicated for women who are, or who may become, pregnant. If benzphetamine pharmacotherapy is required, advise patients of potential benefits and possible risks to themselves and the embryo, fetus, or neonate. Collaboration with the patient's obstetrician is indicated.

Women who are breast-feeding: Safety and efficacy of benzphetamine pharmacotherapy for women who are breast-feeding and their neonates and infants have not been established. Avoid prescribing benzphetamine pharmacotherapy to women who are breast-feeding. If benzphetamine pharmacotherapy is required, breast-feeding probably should be discontinued. If desired, lactation may be maintained and breast-feeding resumed following the discontinuation of short-term benzphetamine pharmacotherapy.

Children younger than 12 years of age: Safety and efficacy of benzphetamine pharmacotherapy for the symptomatic management of eating disorders among children younger than 12 years of age have not been established. Benzphetamine pharmacotherapy for this indication is *not* recommended for this age group.

Notes, Exogenous Obesity

Generally benzphetamine pharmacotherapy is prescribed as one component of a comprehensive weight reduction program based on caloric restriction. Discontinue benzphetamine pharmacotherapy when tolerance to its anorexiant action occurs. Do *not* increase the recommended dosage in an attempt to prolong the anorexiant action.

AVAILABLE DOSAGE FORMS, STORAGE, AND COMPATIBILITY

Tablets, oral: 25, 50 mg

Notes

The 25 mg tablets contain tartrazine. Tartrazine has been associated with allergic-type reactions among susceptible patients. Patients who have aspirin hypersensitivity appear to be at particular risk.

General Instructions for Patients Instruct patients who are receiving benzphetamine pharmacotherapy to

- safely store benzphetamine tablets in tightly closed child-resistant containers at controlled room temperature (15° to 30°C; 59° to 86°F).
- obtain an available patient information sheet regarding benzphetamine pharmacotherapy from their pharmacist at the time that their prescription is dispensed. Encourage patients to clarify any questions that they may have concerning benzphetamine pharmacotherapy with their pharmacist or, if needed, to consult their prescribing psychologist.

PROPOSED MECHANISM OF ACTION

Benzphetamine is a sympathomimetic amine that possesses pharmacologic activities similar to those of the amphetamines. The amphetamines are the prototype drugs prescribed for the short-term symptomatic management of exogenous obesity. Similar to the amphetamines, the actions of benzphetamine include CNS stimulation and increased blood pressure. Tachyphylaxis and tolerance have been associated with the amphetamines and also may occur with benzphetamine. The exact mechanism of CNS, respiratory, and sympathomimetic action of benzphetamine has not been fully determined. It is thought to be primarily related to the stimulation of the release of norepinephrine from central adrenergic neurons.

See also Amphetamines General Monograph

PHARMACOKINETICS/PHARMACODYNAMICS

Benzphetamine is readily absorbed following oral ingestion. Pharmacologic activity lasts for approximately four hours. Other pharmacokinetic/pharmacodynamic data are unavailable.

RELATIVE CONTRAINDICATIONS

Addiction and habituation to amphetamines or other abusable psychotropics, history of
Agitation
Cardiovascular disorders, symptomatic, including angina pectoris, arteriosclerosis (advanced), and hypertension (moderate to severe)
Glaucoma
Hypertension, moderate to severe
Hyperthyroidism
Hypersensitivity to benzphetamine, amphetamines, or sympathomimetic amines
MAOI pharmacotherapy, concurrent or within 14 days. Hypertensive crises may result.
Pregnancy

CAUTIONS AND COMMENTS

Benzphetamine is related to the amphetamine class of CNS stimulants and is, thus, addicting and habituating. Benzphetamine should be prescribed cautiously as adjunctive pharmacotherapy for the symptomatic management of exogenous obesity. Attention must be given to the possibility that some patients may become addicted or habituated to benzphetamine as a result of their pharmacotherapy. Attention also must be given to the possibility that some patients may seek benzphetamine prescriptions to support their addiction or habituation (i.e., regular personal use). Other patients may increase their dosage to many times the usual recommended dosage. Prescribe small quantities of benzphetamine and monitor pharmacotherapy closely. Limit prescriptions to the smallest amount that is feasible for dispensing at one time in order to minimize the possible development of problematic patterns of use. Patients who have histories of problematic patterns of amphetamine or other abusable psychotropic use probably should not be prescribed benzphetamine pharmacotherapy because of its addiction and habituation potential.

Prescribe benzphetamine pharmacotherapy cautiously to patients who have histories of cardiovascular disorders, including mild hypertension. Although not directly associated with benzphetamine pharmacotherapy, amphetamine pharmacotherapy has been associated with cardiac dysrhythmias and hypertension among these patients. Caution is indicated because of the similarity between benzphetamine and the other amphetamines.

Caution patients who are receiving benzphetamine pharmacotherapy against performing activities that require alertness, judgment, and physical coordination (e.g., driving an automobile, operating dangerous equipment, supervising children) until their response to benzphetamine pharmacotherapy is known.

CLINICALLY SIGNIFICANT DRUG INTERACTIONS

Concurrent benzphetamine pharmacotherapy and the following may result in clinically significant drug interactions:

Guanethidine Pharmacotherapy

Benzphetamine may decrease the neuronal uptake of guanethidine (Ismelin®) and, thus, decrease its antihypertensive action.

Insulin Pharmacotherapy

Benzphetamine pharmacotherapy may alter insulin requirements among patients who have insulin-dependent diabetes mellitus, particularly those who also have a restricted caloric diet.

Monoamine Oxidase Inhibitor Pharmacotherapy

Benzphetamine may interact with MAOIs (e.g., phenelzine [Nardil®]), resulting in the release of large amounts of catecholamines and associated pharmacologic effects (e.g., headache, hypertension) that can culminate in hypertensive crises. Thus, benzphetamine pharmacotherapy, concurrent or within 14 days of MAOI pharmacotherapy, is contraindicated.

See Relative Contraindications

Pharmacotherapy With Drugs That Acidify the Urine

Concurrent benzphetamine pharmacotherapy with drugs that acidify the urine (e.g., ammonium chloride) may increase the urinary excretion of benzphetamine.

Pharmacotherapy With Drugs That Alkalinize the Urine

Concurrent benzphetamine pharmacotherapy with drugs that alkalinize the urine (e.g., sodium bicarbonate [baking soda]) may decrease the urinary excretion of benzphetamine. Decreased urinary excretion of benzphetamine may result in an increase in benzphetamine blood concentrations and possible toxicity.

Pharmacotherapy With Central Nervous System Stimulants and Other Drugs That Produce Central Nervous System Stimulation

Benzphetamine should not be prescribed concurrently with other CNS stimulants (e.g., amphetamines) or other drugs that produce CNS stimulation (e.g., methylphenidate [Ritalin®], nicotine) because of the potential for additive CNS stimulant actions and related effects.

Phenothiazine Pharmacotherapy

Phenothiazines antagonize the stimulatory actions of the amphetamines. Avoid concurrent benzphetamine and phenothiazine pharmacotherapy.

Tricyclic Antidepressant Pharmacotherapy

Concurrent benzphetamine and TCA pharmacotherapy (as with other amphetamine or sympathomimetic pharmacotherapy) may result in additive or synergistic CNS stimulant actions and associated effects. When concurrent pharmacotherapy is required, monitor patients closely and adjust the dosage carefully according to individual patient response.

See also Amphetamines General Monograph

ADVERSE DRUG REACTIONS

Benzphetamine pharmacotherapy has been associated with the following ADRs, listed according to body system:

Cardiovascular: increased blood pressure, palpitations, and tachycardia
CNS: depression following the discontinuation of pharmacotherapy, dizziness, headache, insomnia, overstimulation, restlessness, sweating (excessive), tremor, and, rarely, psychosis at recommended dosages
Cutaneous: hives (urticaria) and other hypersensitivity reactions involving the skin
Genitourinary: changes in sex drive, initially, usually increased
GI: diarrhea, dry mouth, gastrointestinal complaints, nausea, and unpleasant taste

See also Amphetamines General Monograph

OVERDOSAGE

Information regarding the signs and symptoms of benzphetamine overdosage and its related sequelae is extremely limited. Suspected or actual benzphetamine overdosage requires emergency symptomatic medical support of body systems with attention to increasing benzphetamine elimination. There is no known antidote.

See also Amphetamines General Monograph

BROMAZEPAM ✷

(broe ma'ze pam)

TRADE NAME

Lectopam®

CLASSIFICATION

Sedative-hypnotic (benzodiazepine)

See also Benzodiazepines General Monograph

APPROVED INDICATIONS FOR PSYCHOLOGICAL DISORDERS

Adjunctive pharmacotherapy for the short-term (one week) symptomatic management of:

Anxiety disorders: Excessive anxiety among patients who have anxiety neurosis

Note: Bromazepam pharmacotherapy is *not* indicated for the management of everyday anxiety or tension, or the anxiety that can be managed with psychotherapy alone. Bromazepam also is *not* recommended for the management of anxiety associated with depression because it has the potential to exacerbate the depression while alleviating the anxiety. The depression associated with anxiety generally resolves with appropriate adjunctive pharmacotherapy (i.e., antidepressant pharmacotherapy and psychotherapy). Bromazepam is *not* recommended for patients who have depressive or psychotic disorders.

USUAL DOSAGE AND ADMINISTRATION

Anxiety Disorders: Excessive Anxiety Among Patients who have Anxiety Neurosis

Adults: Initially, 6 to 18 mg daily orally in two or three divided doses. Initiate pharmacotherapy at lower dosages. Adjust the dosage, as needed, according to the severity of signs and symptoms and individual patient response. Optimal dosage may range from 6 to 30 mg daily orally in two or three divided doses.

MAXIMUM: 60 mg daily orally

Women who are, or who may become, pregnant: FDA Pregnancy Category "not established." Safety and efficacy of bromazepam pharmacotherapy for women who are pregnant have not been established. An increased risk for congenital malformations (birth defects)

has been associated with benzodiazepine (e.g., chlordiazepoxide; diazepam) pharmacotherapy. Avoid prescribing bromazepam pharmacotherapy to women who are pregnant. If bromazepam pharmacotherapy is required, advise patients of potential benefits and possible risks to themselves and the embryo, fetus, or neonate. Collaboration with the patient's obstetrician is indicated.

Women who are breast-feeding: Safety and efficacy of bromazepam pharmacotherapy for women who are breast-feeding and their neonates and infants have not been established. Bromazepam and its metabolites are probably excreted in breast milk because of their similarities to other benzodiazepines. Avoid prescribing bromazepam to women who are breast-feeding. If bromazepam pharmacotherapy is required, breast-feeding probably should be discontinued. If desired, lactation may be maintained and breast-feeding resumed following the discontinuation of short-term bromazepam pharmacotherapy.

Elderly, frail, or debilitated patients and those who have organic brain syndrome: Initially, 3 mg daily orally in two divided doses. Adjust dosage according to individual patient response. Elderly, frail, and debilitated patients, or those who have organic brain syndrome, may be more sensitive to the CNS depressant actions of bromazepam than are younger or healthier adult patients, even when lower dosages are prescribed.

Children and adolescents younger than 18 years of age: Safety and efficacy of bromazepam pharmacotherapy for children and adolescents have not been established. Bromazepam pharmacotherapy is *not* recommended for this age group.

Notes, Anxiety Disorders

Bromazepam is indicated for the short-term symptomatic management of excessive anxiety among patients who have anxiety neurosis. Adjust the dosage carefully according to individual patient response in order to avoid excessive sedation and associated cognitive and motor impairment.

Initiating Bromazepam Pharmacotherapy Initiate pharmacotherapy with attention to the general recommendation that bromazepam pharmacotherapy *not* be prescribed for longer than one week. If necessary, the dosage can be adjusted for specific patients after one week of pharmacotherapy. Limited continuation of pharmacotherapy for longer than one week requires reevaluation of patients. Prescribe no more than one week's supply of bromazepam, and do not provide automatic renewals for prescriptions. Limit subsequent prescriptions, when required, for short-term pharmacotherapy. Do not prescribe bromazepam pharmacotherapy for patients who have histories of problematic patterns of alcohol, benzodiazepine, or other abusable psychotropic use. These patients may be at increased risk for problematic patterns of bromazepam use.

Discontinuing Bromazepam Pharmacotherapy A bromazepam withdrawal syndrome that is similar to the withdrawal syndrome associated with alcohol and other benzodiazepines has been associated with the abrupt discontinuation of long-term bromazepam pharmacotherapy, or regular personal use. This syndrome is characterized by abdominal cramps, irritability, memory impairment, nervousness, and vomiting. Patients may appear to be suffering a relapse in regard to their presenting anxiety disorder because of the similarity of signs and symptoms. Thus, discontinue bromazepam pharmacotherapy gradually, particularly if high dosages have been used over an extended period of time and addiction and habituation are suspected.

AVAILABLE DOSAGE FORMS, STORAGE, AND COMPATIBILITY

Tablets, oral: 1.5, 3, 6 mg

Notes

General Instructions for Patients   Instruct patients who are receiving bromazepam pharmacotherapy to

- safely store bromazepam tablets in tightly closed child-resistant containers at controlled room temperature (15° to 30°C; 59° to 86°F).
- obtain an available patient information sheet regarding bromazepam pharmacotherapy from their pharmacist at the time that their prescription is dispensed. Encourage patients to clarify any questions that they may have concerning bromazepam pharmacotherapy with their pharmacist or, if needed, to consult their prescribing psychologist.

PROPOSED MECHANISM OF ACTION

Bromazepam is a benzodiazepine with anxiolytic and sedative actions. The exact proposed mechanism of action of bromazepam has not yet been fully determined. However, it appears to work in concert with the inhibitory neurotransmitter GABA.

See also Benzodiazepines General Monograph

PHARMACOKINETICS/PHARMACODYNAMICS

Bromazepam is completely and rapidly absorbed from the gastrointestinal tract following oral ingestion. Peak blood levels are achieved within 1 to 4 hours. Its mean half-life of elimination is approximately 12 hours (range 8 to 19 hours). Bromazepam is metabolized in the liver and is excreted in the urine in the form of conjugated metabolites. It has no active metabolites. Additional data are unavailable.

RELATIVE CONTRAINDICATIONS

Glaucoma, acute narrow-angle. (*Note:* bromazepam pharmacotherapy may be prescribed for patients who have open-angle glaucoma and who are receiving appropriate medical treatment.) Collaboration with the patient's family physician or ophthalmologist may be indicated.

Hypersensitivity to bromazepam or other benzodiazepines

Myasthenia gravis

CAUTIONS AND COMMENTS

Bromazepam is addicting and habituating. (See Benzodiazepines General Monograph)
 Prescribe bromazepam pharmacotherapy cautiously to patients who

- are elderly or have kidney or liver dysfunction
- have histories of psychotic disorders or tendencies. Bromazepam pharmacotherapy has been associated with excitement and other paradoxical reactions among these patients. If bromazepam pharmacotherapy is required, these patients require hospitalization or close monitoring in the home setting.

Caution patients who are receiving bromazepam pharmacotherapy against

- drinking alcohol or using other drugs (e.g., barbiturates, opiate analgesics) that have CNS depressant actions. Concurrent use of bromazepam and these drugs may result in severe CNS depression.
- performing activities that require alertness, judgment, and coordination (e.g., driving an automobile, operating dangerous equipment, supervising children) until their response to bromazepam pharmacotherapy is known. Bromazepam may adversely affect these mental and physical functions.

In addition to these general precautions for patients, caution women to inform their prescribing psychologist if they become or intend to become pregnant while receiving bromazepam pharmacotherapy so that their pharmacotherapy can be safely discontinued.

CLINICALLY SIGNIFICANT DRUG INTERACTIONS

Concurrent bromazepam pharmacotherapy and the following may result in clinically significant drug interactions:

Alcohol Use

Concurrent alcohol use may increase the CNS depressant action of bromazepam. Advise patients to avoid, or limit, their use of alcohol while receiving bromazepam pharmacotherapy.

Pharmacotherapy With Central Nervous System Depressants and Other Drugs That Produce Central Nervous System Depression

Concurrent bromazepam pharmacotherapy with opiate analgesics, other sedative-hypnotics, or other drugs that produce CNS depression (e.g., antihistamines, phenothiazines, TCAs) may result in additive CNS depression, including memory impairment.
 See also Benzodiazepines General Monograph

ADVERSE DRUG REACTIONS

Bromazepam pharmacotherapy has been frequently associated with dizziness, drowsiness, and incoordination (ataxia). Other ADRs associated with bromazepam pharmacotherapy, listed according to body system, include:

Cardiovascular: hypotension, palpitations, and tachycardia

CNS: agitation, mental confusion, depression, euphoria, headache, irritability, lethargy, nervousness, seizures, sleep disorders, slurred speech, and stupor. Depression of social inhibitions may result in aggressive behavior or hostility. Long-term pharmacotherapy, or regular personal use, may result in addiction and habituation.

Cutaneous: severe itching rash (pruritus)

Genitourinary: urinary incontinence and changes in sex drive

GI: dry mouth, nausea, nonspecific GI complaints, and vomiting

Hematologic: decreased hemoglobin and hematocrit and increased or decreased white blood cell count

Hepatic: elevations in alkaline phosphatase, bilirubin, and liver function tests

Musculoskeletal: muscle spasms or weakness

Ocular: blurred vision and difficulty in depth perception

See also Benzodiazepines General Monograph

OVERDOSAGE

Signs and symptoms of bromazepam overdosage include drowsiness (excessive), incoordination (ataxia), impaired vision, depressed reflexes, and coma. Hypotension and respiratory depression may occur with overdosages involving large amounts of bromazepam. Bromazepam overdosage requires emergency symptomatic medical support of body systems with attention to increasing bromazepam elimination. The benzodiazepine antagonist flumazenil (Anexate®, Romazicon®) may be required.

BUPRENORPHINE *

(byoo pre nor′feen)

TRADE NAME

Buprenex®

CLASSIFICATION

Opiate analgesic (mixed agonist/antagonist) (C-V)

See also Opiate Analgesics General Monograph

APPROVED INDICATIONS FOR PSYCHOLOGICAL DISORDERS

Adjunctive pharmacotherapy for the symptomatic management of:

Pain Disorders: Pain, Moderate to Severe

USUAL DOSAGE AND ADMINISTRATION

Moderate to Severe Pain

Adults: 0.3 mg intramuscularly or intravenously every six hours, as needed. Repeat 0.3 mg dose, if needed, 30 to 60 minutes after the initial dose. Inject intramuscularly into a large healthy muscle site (e.g., dorsogluteal). Inject intravenously slowly over at least two minutes. Extreme caution is required with intravenous injection, particularly with the initial dose until patient response to intravenous buprenorphine pharmacotherapy is known.

Some patients may require single doses of up to 0.6 mg, depending on the severity of the pain and their individual response. *Inject this dose intramuscularly only.* Do *not* inject intravenously. Single doses of up to 0.6 mg are *not* recommended for patients who are at increased risk for respiratory depression (e.g., elderly, frail, or debilitated patients, or those who have respiratory dysfunction).

MAXIMUM: 0.6 mg/dose

Women who are, or who may become, pregnant: FDA Pregnancy Category C. Safety and efficacy of buprenorphine pharmacotherapy for women who are pregnant have not been established. Avoid prescribing buprenorphine pharmacotherapy to women who are pregnant. If buprenorphine pharmacotherapy is required, advise patients of potential benefits and possible risks to themselves and the embryo, fetus, or neonate (see Opiate Analgesics General Monograph). Prescribe buprenorphine during pregnancy only if the potential benefit justifies the potential risk to the embryo, fetus, or neonate. Collaboration with the patient's obstetrician is indicated.

Women who are breast-feeding: Safety and efficacy of buprenorphine pharmacotherapy for women who are breast-feeding and their neonates and infants have not been established. The amount of buprenorphine that is excreted in breast milk is unknown. Avoid prescribing buprenorphine pharmacotherapy to women who are breast-feeding. If buprenorphine pharmacotherapy is required, breast-feeding probably should be discontinued. If desired, lactation may be maintained and breast-feeding resumed following the discontinuation of short-term buprenorphine pharmacotherapy. Collaboration with the patient's pediatrician is indicated.

Elderly, frail, or debilitated patients: Initially, 0.15 mg intramuscularly or intravenously every six hours, as needed. Inject intramuscularly into a large healthy muscle site (e.g., dorsogluteal). Inject intravenously slowly over at least two minutes. Repeat 0.15 mg dose, if needed, 30 to 60 minutes after the initial dose. Note that this recommended dosage is one-half of the usual adult dosage. Generally prescribe lower dosages for elderly, frail, or debilitated patients. These patients may be more sensitive to the pharmacologic actions of buprenorphine pharmacotherapy than are younger or healthier adult patients.

Children 2 to 12 years of age: 2 to 6 μg/kg (0.002 to 0.006 mg/kg) intramuscularly or intravenously every four to eight hours, as needed. Inject intramuscularly into a large healthy muscle site (e.g., dorsogluteal site, vastus lateralis site). Inject intravenously slowly over at least two minutes. Extreme caution is required with intravenous injection, particularly with the initial dose, until the child's response to intravenous buprenorphine pharmacotherapy is known.

Adolescents 13 years of age and older: 0.3 mg intramuscularly or intravenously every six hours, as needed. Repeat 0.3 mg dose, if needed, 30 to 60 minutes after the initial dose. Note that this recommended dosage is the same as the usual adult dosage. Inject intramuscularly into a large healthy muscle site (e.g., dorsogluteal site). Slowly inject intravenously over at least two minutes. Extreme caution is required with intravenous injection, particularly with the initial dose until the adolescent's response to intravenous buprenorphine pharmacotherapy is known.

Notes, Moderate to Severe Pain

The analgesic and respiratory depressant actions of 0.3 mg of buprenorphine (Buprenex®) are approximately equivalent to those produced by 10 mg of morphine.

Inject intramuscularly deeply into healthy muscle sites. Rotate intramuscular injection sites if more than one injection is required to avoid, or minimize, muscle damage.

Extreme caution is required with intravenous injection.

AVAILABLE DOSAGE FORMS, STORAGE, AND COMPATIBILITY

Injectable, intramuscular or intravenous: 0.3 mg/ml (glass ampule)

Notes

Protect injectables from prolonged exposure to light or to temperatures exceeding 40°C (104°F). Injectable formulations that are discolored or contain particulate matter should be returned to the dispensing pharmacy or manufacturer for safe and appropriate disposal. Buprenorphine injectable is *not* compatible with injectable formulations of diazepam or lorazepam. Do not mix these injectables in the same syringe.

General Instructions for Patients　Instruct patients who are receiving buprenorphine pharmacotherapy, as appropriate, to

- obtain an available patient information sheet regarding buprenorphine pharmacotherapy from their pharmacist at the time that their prescription is dispensed. Encourage patients to clarify any questions that they may have concerning buprenorphine pharmacotherapy with their pharmacist or, if needed, to consult their prescribing psychologist.

PROPOSED MECHANISM OF ACTION

Buprenorphine's exact mechanism of action has not been fully determined. However, it probably exerts its analgesic action by binding to mu opiate receptors for which it has high affinity. Although it may be classified as a partial agonist, under conditions of recommended use, it acts much like a classical mu agonist, such as morphine. However, unlike other opiate agonists or agonist/antagonists, buprenorphine appears to dissociate from its receptor sites. This unusual dissociation from receptor sites may account for its longer duration of action when compared to morphine, its unpredictable reversal by opiate antagonists, and its apparently lower addiction potential.

See also Opiate Analgesics General Monograph

PHARMACOKINETICS/PHARMACODYNAMICS

Buprenorphine is rapidly, but variably (i.e., 40% to 90%), absorbed following intramuscular injection. Pharmacologic actions after intramuscular injection occur within approximately 15 minutes. Peak effects are achieved within 1 hour, with analgesic action persisting for 6 hours or longer. Onset and peak actions are shortened with intravenous injection. It is highly (96%) plasma protein bound primarily to α and β globulins with little binding to plasma albumin. Its apparent volume of distribution is ~100 L. Buprenorphine is virtually completely metabolized in the liver. It has a mean half-life of elimination of approximately 2 hours (range 1 to 7 hours) and a total body clearance of 1.3 L/minute. Additional data are unavailable.

RELATIVE CONTRAINDICATIONS

Hypersensitivity to buprenorphine

CAUTIONS AND COMMENTS

Buprenorphine may cause addiction and habituation similar to that associated with morphine, probably because of its opiate-like euphoric action. However, a buprenorphine withdrawal syndrome has not been demonstrated.

Prescribe buprenorphine pharmacotherapy cautiously for patients who

- have acute alcoholism or delirium tremens
- have adrenal cortical insufficiency (Addison's disease)
- are elderly, frail, or debilitated. These patients may be more sensitive to buprenorphine's respiratory and CNS depressant actions.
- have biliary tract dysfunction. Buprenorphine may increase intracholeductal pressure much like other opiate analgesics.
- have CNS depression or coma. These clinical conditions can be exacerbated by buprenorphine's CNS depressant actions.
- have head injuries, intracranial lesions, and other conditions associated with increased cerebrospinal fluid pressure. Buprenorphine may elevate cerebrospinal fluid pressure. Among these patients, the dosage should be reduced by one-half. Note that buprenorphine can produce abnormal contraction of the pupils (i.e., miosis) and changes in the patient's level of consciousness. These actions may interfere with the monitoring of the patient's clinical condition.
- have histories of problematic patterns of abusable psychotropic use. Addiction and habituation may occur with buprenorphine pharmacotherapy. Buprenorphine also may induce the opiate withdrawal syndrome among patients who are currently addicted to opiate analgesics because of its partial action as an opiate antagonist.
- have hypothyroidism (myxedema)
- have lateral curvature and convex prominence of the spine (kyphoscoliosis). This condition may compromise respiratory function.
- have prostatic hypertrophy or urethral stricture
- have respiratory dysfunction. Buprenorphine pharmacotherapy may increase respiratory depression among patients who have medical disorders that compromise respiratory function (e.g., chronic obstructive lung disease). As with other potent opiate analgesics, clinically significant respiratory depression may occur among patients who are receiving usual recommended dosages of buprenorphine. Particular caution is advised when patients are also receiving concurrent pharmacotherapy with other drugs that have CNS and

respiratory depressant actions. The dosage of buprenorphine should be reduced by approximately one-half for these patients. It is important to note that naloxone (Narcan®) may *not* adequately reverse the respiratory depression produced by buprenorphine.
• have severe liver or kidney dysfunction
• have toxic psychoses

Caution patients who are receiving buprenorphine pharmacotherapy against

• drinking alcohol or using other drugs that produce CNS depression. Buprenorphine may produce drowsiness and other effects that can be potentiated by these drugs. Advise patients to avoid or limit their use of alcohol while receiving buprenorphine pharmacotherapy. They also should be advised not to use other drugs (prescription or nonprescription) that produce CNS depression without first checking with their prescribing psychologist and to notify their other prescribers that they are receiving buprenorphine pharmacotherapy.
• performing activities that require alertness, judgment, and physical coordination (e.g., driving an automobile, operating dangerous equipment, supervising children). Buprenorphine may impair these mental and physical abilities by its direct depressant action on the CNS.

In addition to these general precautions, caution patients that buprenorphine is addicting and habituating. Advise patients not to exceed the prescribed dosage or to use buprenorphine more frequently than prescribed without first checking with their prescribing psychologist.

CLINICALLY SIGNIFICANT DRUG INTERACTIONS

Concurrent buprenorphine pharmacotherapy and the following may result in clinically significant drug interactions:

Alcohol Use

Concurrent alcohol use may increase the CNS depressant action of buprenorphine. Advise patients to avoid, or limit, their use of alcohol while receiving buprenorphine pharmacotherapy.

Pharmacotherapy With Drugs That Affect Hepatic Metabolism

Concurrent buprenorphine pharmacotherapy with drugs known to affect hepatic metabolism (e.g., barbiturates, SSRIs) may result in increased or prolonged buprenorphine action. Buprenorphine is metabolized in the liver.

Pharmacotherapy With Central Nervous System Depressants and Other Drugs That Produce Central Nervous System Depression

Concurrent buprenorphine pharmacotherapy with other opiate analgesics, sedative-hypnotics, or other drugs that produce CNS depression (e.g., antihistamines, phenothiazines, TCAs) may result in additive CNS depressant actions. When concurrent pharmacotherapy is required, dosage reductions are indicated.
See also Opiate Analgesics General Monograph

ADVERSE DRUG REACTIONS

Buprenorphine pharmacotherapy has been associated with the following ADRs, listed according to body system:

Cardiovascular: decreased pulse rate and blood pressure (rarely, may be increased)
Cutaneous: sweating (excessive)
CNS: dizziness, drowsiness, headache, and sedation
GI: nausea and vomiting
Ocular: abnormal contraction of the pupils (miosis)
Respiratory: hypoventilation. Buprenorphine produces dose-related respiratory depression similar to morphine. At therapeutic doses (i.e., 0.3 mg), buprenorphine can decrease the respiratory rate to an extent similar to that produced by an analgesic-equivalent dose of morphine (i.e., 10 mg).

See also Opiate Analgesics General Monograph

OVERDOSAGE

Clinical experience with buprenorphine overdosage is limited. Buprenorphine's antagonist action may be observed at dosages somewhat above the usual recommended dosage. Dosages within the therapeutic range may produce clinically significant respiratory depression among certain patients (e.g., patients who are elderly, frail, or debilitated). Buprenorphine overdosage requires emergency symptomatic medical support of body systems with attention to maintaining respiratory and cardiovascular function. Mechanical ventilation may be required because the respiratory depression produced by buprenorphine, a partial opiate agonist/antagonist, may not be effectively reversed by the opiate antagonist naloxone (Narcan®).

BUPROPION *

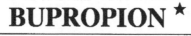

(byoo proe'pee on)

TRADE NAMES

Wellbutrin®
Zyban®

CLASSIFICATION

Antidepressant (monocyclic aminoketone) (CNS stimulant)

APPROVED INDICATIONS FOR PSYCHOLOGICAL DISORDERS

Adjunctive pharmacotherapy for the symptomatic management of:

- Mood Disorders, Depressive Disorders: Major Depressive Disorder
- Substance-Related Disorders: Nicotine Withdrawal Syndrome Associated With the Cessation of Tobacco Smoking

USUAL DOSAGE AND ADMINISTRATION

Major Depressive Disorder

Adults: Initially, 200 mg daily orally in two divided doses, morning and evening. After three days, increase the dosage, if needed, to 300 mg daily orally in three divided doses, morning, noon, and evening. Adjust the dosage according to individual patient response. If therapeutic benefit is not achieved after four weeks of pharmacotherapy, increase the dosage, as needed, to 450 mg daily orally in three divided doses. Adjust the dosage according to individual patient response.

MAXIMUM: 450 mg daily orally

Women who are, or who may become, pregnant: FDA Pregnancy Category B. Safety and efficacy of bupropion pharmacotherapy for women who are pregnant have not been established. Avoid prescribing bupropion pharmacotherapy to women who are pregnant. If bupropion pharmacotherapy is required, advise patients of potential benefits and possible risks to themselves and the embryo, fetus, or neonate. Collaboration with the patient's obstetrician is indicated.

Women who are breast-feeding: Safety and efficacy of bupropion pharmacotherapy for women who are breast-feeding and their neonates and infants have not been established. Avoid prescribing bupropion pharmacotherapy to women who are breast-feeding. If bupropion pharmacotherapy is required, breast-feeding probably should be discontinued. Collaboration with the patient's pediatrician is indicated.

Elderly, frail, or debilitated patients and those who have liver dysfunction: Generally prescribe lower dosages for elderly, frail, or debilitated patients and those who have liver dysfunction. Increase the dosage gradually, if needed, according to individual patient response. These patients may be more sensitive to the pharmacologic actions of bupropion than are younger or healthier adult patients.

Children and adolescents younger than 18 years of age: Safety and efficacy of bupropion pharmacotherapy for children and adolescents have not been established. Bupropion pharmacotherapy is *not* recommended for this age group.

Notes, Major Depressive Disorder

Therapeutic benefit may not be evident for four or more weeks following the initiation of bupropion pharmacotherapy. While awaiting therapeutic benefit, do *not* exceed the recommended dosages. High single doses of bupropion, or daily dosages exceeding the maximum recommended dosage, have been associated with increased risk for seizures. For example, increasing the daily dosage from 450 to 600 mg has been associated with a 10-fold increase in the incidence of bupropion-related seizures (i.e., from 0.4% to 4%). Thus, to avoid or minimize the risk for inducing bupropion-related seizures, do *not* prescribe single adult doses exceeding 150 mg or daily dosages exceeding 450 mg.

The safety and efficacy of long-term bupropion pharmacotherapy (i.e., longer than six weeks) have not been established.

Tobacco Smoking Cessation

Adults: 300 mg daily orally in two divided doses, morning and evening. Prescribe the 150 mg oral extended-release tablet. Continue bupropion pharmacotherapy for seven to twelve weeks while monitoring individual patient response. See also Notes, Tobacco Smoking Cessation for alternative initial dosage schedule.

Women who are, or who may become, pregnant: FDA Pregnancy Category B. Safety and efficacy of bupropion pharmacotherapy for women who are pregnant have not been established. Avoid prescribing bupropion pharmacotherapy to women who are pregnant. If bupropion pharmacotherapy is required, advise patients of potential benefits and possible risks to themselves and the embryo, fetus, or neonate. Collaboration with the patient's obstetrician is indicated.

Women who are breast-feeding: Safety and efficacy of bupropion pharmacotherapy for women who are breast-feeding and their neonates and infants have not been established. Avoid prescribing bupropion pharmacotherapy to women who are breast-feeding. If bupropion pharmacotherapy is required, breast-feeding probably should be discontinued. Collaboration with the patient's pediatrician is indicated.

Elderly, frail, or debilitated patients and those who have liver dysfunction: Generally prescribe lower dosages for elderly, frail, or debilitated patients and those who have liver dysfunction. Increase the dosage gradually, if needed, according to individual patient response. These patients may be more sensitive to the pharmacologic actions of bupropion than are younger or healthier adult patients. See also Notes, Tobacco Smoking Cessation for alternative initial dosage schedule.

Children and adolescents younger than 18 years of age: Safety and efficacy of bupropion pharmacotherapy for children and adolescents have not been established. Bupropion pharmacotherapy is *not* recommended for this age group.

Notes, Tobacco Smoking Cessation

Bupropion is the first non-nicotine drug approved for the symptomatic management of nicotine withdrawal associated with tobacco smoking cessation. Efficacy appears to be greater among smokers who are also depressed. Bupropion can be prescribed alone or in combination with nicotine replacement pharmacotherapy (see Nicotine Monograph). Some dosage regimens begin with 150 mg in the morning for the first three days, increasing to the standard dosage of 150 mg in the morning and another 150 mg in the early evening. The morning and evening doses of bupropion should be taken at least eight hours apart from each other.

AVAILABLE DOSAGE FORMS, STORAGE, AND COMPATIBILITY

Tablets, oral: 75, 100 mg
Tablets, oral extended-release: 100, 150 mg

Notes

General Instructions for Patients   Instruct patients who are receiving bupropion pharmacotherapy to

- safely store bupropion tablets out of the reach of children in tightly closed light- and child-resistant containers at controlled room temperature (15° to 30°C; 59° to 86°F).
- obtain an available patient information sheet regarding bupropion pharmacotherapy from their pharmacist at the time that their prescription is dispensed. Encourage patients to clarify any questions that they may have concerning their bupropion pharmacotherapy with their pharmacist or, if needed, to consult their prescribing psychologist.

PROPOSED MECHANISM OF ACTION

The exact mechanism of the antidepressant action of bupropion has not yet been fully determined. Bupropion does not inhibit monoamine oxidase and is only a relatively weak inhibitor of the neuronal re-uptake of norepinephrine and serotonin. It is structurally related to diethylpropion (see Diethylpropion Monograph) and the phenylethylamines. As such, bupropion is capable of producing dose-related CNS stimulant actions.

Bupropion appears to decrease craving and other signs and symptoms of nicotine withdrawal by increasing dopamine and norepinephrine levels, two of the neurotransmitters that are stimulated by nicotine.

PHARMACOKINETICS/PHARMACODYNAMICS

Bupropion is well absorbed following oral ingestion. Peak blood levels are generally achieved within two hours. However, the absolute bioavailability is low (F = 0.2) because of significant first-pass hepatic metabolism. Bupropion is moderately bound to plasma proteins (~80%) and has a mean apparent volume of distribution of ~7 L/kg. It is extensively metabolized in the liver to several active and inactive metabolites. Less than 1% of bupropion is excreted in unchanged form in the urine. The mean half-life of elimination is 14 hours (range 8 to 24 hours). Total body clearance is approximately 2.25 L/minute.

RELATIVE CONTRAINDICATIONS

Anorexia nervosa. A higher incidence of seizures has been associated with this eating disorder.
Bulimia. A higher incidence of seizures has been associated with this eating disorder.
Hypersensitivity to bupropion
MAOI pharmacotherapy, concurrent or within 14 days
Ritonavir pharmacotherapy
Seizure disorders, history of

CAUTIONS AND COMMENTS

Bupropion pharmacotherapy is not generally associated with the development of addiction and habituation. However, controlled studies among patients who have histories of problematic patterns of abusable psychotropic use, particularly problematic patterns of CNS stimulant use (e.g., amphetamines, cocaine), have associated bupropion use with general feelings of euphoria and craving.

Prescribe bupropion pharmacotherapy cautiously to patients who

- have anorexia, cachexia, or are significantly underweight. Bupropion pharmacotherapy has been associated with significant weight loss among ~30% of patients.
- have bipolar disorder. Bupropion may activate the manic phase of bipolar disorder.

Caution patients who are receiving bupropion pharmacotherapy against

- drinking alcohol. Concurrent use of alcohol can alter the seizure threshold and increase the risk for seizures. The seizure threshold also may be altered among patients who discontinue long-term regular alcohol use. Thus, their risk for seizures may be increased.
- performing activities that require alertness, judgment, and physical coordination (e.g., driving an automobile, operating dangerous equipment, supervising children) until their response to bupropion pharmacotherapy is known.

CLINICALLY SIGNIFICANT DRUG INTERACTIONS

Concurrent bupropion pharmacotherapy and the following may result in clinically significant drug interactions:

Monoamine Oxidase Inhibitor Pharmacotherapy

Concurrent bupropion (Wellbutrin®) and MAOI pharmacology (e.g., phenelzine [Nardil®], tranylcypromine [Parnate®]) may result in acute bupropion toxicity. Concurrent bupropion and MAOI pharmacotherapy is *contraindicated*. At least 14 days should elapse between the discontinuation of MAOI pharmacotherapy and the initiation of bupropion pharmacotherapy (see Relative Contraindications).

Pharmacotherapy With Drugs That Decrease the Seizure Threshold

Bupropion pharmacotherapy may decrease the seizure threshold. Avoid concurrent pharmacotherapy with other drugs that lower the seizure threshold, including other antidepressants and CNS stimulants. The additive actions of these drugs may place patients at increased risk for seizures. If concurrent pharmacotherapy is required, prescribe lower than usual initial dosages and increase the dosage of both drugs gradually according to individual patient response.

Ritonavir Pharmacotherapy

Ritonavir (Norvir®), an antiretroviral drug indicated for the pharmacologic management of HIV infection, may significantly inhibit the hepatic microsomal enzyme metabolism of bupropion. This interaction may result in toxicity and seizures. Concurrent bupropion and ritonavir pharmacotherapy is *contraindicated* (see Relative Contraindications).

ADVERSE DRUG REACTIONS

Bupropion pharmacotherapy has been commonly associated with agitation, anorexia, constipation, dizziness, dry mouth, headache, insomnia, migraine, nausea, tremor, weight loss, and vomiting. Other ADRs associated with bupropion pharmacotherapy are listed according to body system:

> **Cardiovascular:** chest pain, edema, fainting (syncope), hypertension, postural hypotension, palpitations, and tachycardia
>
> **CNS:** anxiety, change in sex drive, confusion, dyskinesia, dystonia, euphoria, hallucinations, hostility, incoordination (ataxia), mania, memory impairment, paranoia, psychosis, sedation, and seizures
>
> **Cutaneous:** dry skin, hair loss (alopecia), itching (severe), and rash
>
> **Genitourinary:** impotence, menstrual complaints, excessive urination during the night (nocturia), painful erection, urinary frequency, and vaginal irritation
>
> **GI:** difficulty swallowing (dysphagia), dyspepsia, esophagitis, gum irritation, and stomatitis
>
> **Metabolic/Endocrine:** abnormal breast enlargement (gynecomastia)
>
> **Musculoskeletal:** arthritis
>
> **Ocular:** blurred vision
>
> **Otic:** hearing impairment
>
> **Respiratory:** bronchitis, difficult or labored breathing (dyspnea), and shortness of breath

OVERDOSAGE

Signs and symptoms of bupropion overdosage include fever, hallucinations, loss of consciousness, seizures, and tachycardia. Although most patients recover from acute overdosages, bupropion overdosage may be fatal. Fatal overdosage is generally preceded by multiple uncontrolled seizures and cardiac arrest. Bupropion overdosage requires emergency symptomatic medical support of body systems with attention to increasing bupropion elimination. There is no known antidote.

BUSPIRONE

(byoo spye'rone)

TRADE NAME

BuSpar®

CLASSIFICATION

Sedative-hypnotic (atypical, azaspirodecanedione)

APPROVED INDICATIONS FOR PSYCHOLOGICAL DISORDERS

Adjunctive pharmacotherapy for the short-term symptomatic management of:

Anxiety Disorders. Buspirone pharmacotherapy is *not* indicated for the management of everyday anxiety or tension, or for anxiety that can be managed with psychotherapy alone. Buspirone also is *not* recommended for the management of anxiety associated with depression because it has the potential to exacerbate the depression while alleviating the anxiety. The depression associated with anxiety generally resolves with appropriate adjunctive pharmacotherapy (i.e., antidepressant pharmacotherapy) and psychotherapy.

USUAL DOSAGE AND ADMINISTRATION

Anxiety Disorders

Adults: Initially, 10 to 15 mg daily orally in two or three divided doses. Increase the dosage gradually by 5 mg every two to three days according to the severity of signs and symptoms and individual patient response.

MAXIMUM: 60 mg daily orally

Women who are, or who may become, pregnant: FDA Pregnancy Category B. Safety and efficacy of buspirone pharmacotherapy for women who are pregnant have not been established. Avoid prescribing buspirone pharmacotherapy to women who are pregnant. If buspirone pharmacotherapy is required, advise patients of potential benefits and possible risks to themselves and the embryo, fetus, or neonate. Collaboration with the patient's obstetrician is indicated.

Women who are breast-feeding: Safety and efficacy of buspirone pharmacotherapy for women who are breast-feeding and their neonates and infants have not been established. Avoid prescribing buspirone pharmacotherapy to women who are breast-feeding. If buspirone pharmacotherapy is required, breast-feeding probably should be discontinued. If desired, lactation may be maintained and breast-feeding resumed following the discontinuation of short-term buspirone pharmacotherapy. Collaboration with the patient's pediatrician is indicated.

Elderly, frail, or debilitated patients: Initially, 5 to 10 mg daily orally in one single or two divided doses. Increase the dosage gradually, if needed, according to individual patient response. These patients may be more sensitive to the pharmacologic actions of buspirone than are younger or healthier adult patients.

MAXIMUM: 30 mg daily orally

Children and adolescents younger than 18 years of age: Safety and efficacy of buspirone pharmacotherapy for children and adolescents younger than 18 years of age have not been established. Buspirone pharmacotherapy is *not* recommended for this age group.

Notes, Anxiety Disorders

The safety and efficacy of buspirone pharmacotherapy for longer than 30 days for the symptomatic management of anxiety disorders have not been established. Reevaluate patients who appear to require buspirone pharmacotherapy for longer than 30 days.

AVAILABLE DOSAGE FORMS, STORAGE, AND COMPATIBILITY

Tablets, oral: 5, 10, 15 mg

Notes

General Instructions for Patients　Instruct patients who are receiving buspirone pharmacotherapy to

- safely store buspirone tablets out of the reach of children in child-resistant containers.
- obtain an available patient information sheet regarding buspirone pharmacotherapy from their pharmacist at the time that their prescription is dispensed. Encourage patients to clarify any questions that they may have concerning buspirone pharmacotherapy with their pharmacist or, if needed, to consult their prescribing psychologist.

PROPOSED MECHANISM OF ACTION

The exact mechanism of action of buspirone has not been fully determined. It is more anxioselective than most other sedative-hypnotics (e.g., buspirone possesses no anticonvulsant or muscle relaxant activity and causes relatively little psychomotor impairment or sedation). Buspirone has high affinity for serotonin (5-HT$_1$) receptors and for dopamine (D$_2$) receptors. This affinity appears to be related to its mechanism of action.

PHARMACOKINETICS/PHARMACODYNAMICS

Buspirone is rapidly absorbed following oral ingestion and undergoes extensive first-pass hepatic metabolism. Food increases the bioavailability of buspirone, presumably by decreasing its first-pass metabolism. Buspirone generally achieves peak blood concentrations within 90 minutes. It is highly plasma protein bound (~95%). Buspirone is extensively metabolized in the liver to several metabolites including pharmacologically active 1-pyrimidinylpiperazine. The mean half-life of elimination is ~3 hours. Additional data are unavailable.

RELATIVE CONTRAINDICATIONS

Hypersensitivity to buspirone
Kidney dysfunction, severe
Liver dysfunction, severe

CAUTIONS AND COMMENTS

Prescribe buspirone pharmacotherapy cautiously to patients who are receiving, or have received within 14 days, MAOI pharmacotherapy (see Clinically Significant Drug Interactions).

Caution patients who are receiving buspirone pharmacotherapy against

- drinking alcohol or using other drugs that depress the CNS because of possible additive CNS depression.
- performing activities that require alertness, judgment, or physical coordination (e.g., driving an automobile, operating dangerous equipment, supervising children). Buspirone's CNS depressant action, while reportedly less than that associated with other sedative-hypnotics, may adversely affect these mental and physical functions.

CLINICALLY SIGNIFICANT DRUG INTERACTIONS

Concurrent buspirone pharmacotherapy and the following may result in clinically significant drug interactions:

Alcohol Use

Concurrent alcohol use may increase the CNS depressant action of buspirone. Advise patients to avoid, or limit, their use of alcohol while receiving buspirone pharmacotherapy.

Erythromycin Pharmacotherapy

Concurrent buspirone and erythromycin (e.g., Ery-Tab®, Erythrocin®) pharmacotherapy may increase buspirone blood concentrations 5-fold with resultant impaired psychomotor performance and increased ADRs. The mechanism of this interaction appears to involve the inhibition by erythromycin of the hepatic microsomal enzyme (i.e., CYP3A4) responsible for the metabolism of buspirone. Avoid prescribing concurrent buspirone and erythromycin pharmacotherapy. If concurrent pharmacotherapy is required, initially prescribe a lower than usual dosage of buspirone and, if necessary, increase the dosage gradually according to individual patient response.

Itraconazole Pharmacotherapy

Concurrent buspirone and itraconazole (e.g., Sporanex®) pharmacotherapy may increase buspirone blood concentrations 13-fold with resultant severely impaired psychomotor performance and increased ADRs. The mechanism of this interaction appears to involve the inhibition by itraconazole of the hepatic microsomal enzyme (i.e., CYP3A4) responsible for the metabolism of buspirone. Avoid prescribing concurrent itraconazole and erythromycin pharmacotherapy. If concurrent pharmacotherapy is required, initially prescribe a lower than usual dosage of itraconazole and, if necessary, increase the dosage gradually according to individual patient response.

Monoamine Oxidase Inhibitor Pharmacotherapy

Concurrent buspirone and MAOI pharmacotherapy have reportedly resulted in several cases of increased blood pressure. Avoid prescribing concurrently, or within 14 days, buspirone and

MAOI pharmacotherapy. Hypertensive crises have been associated with concurrent MAOI and other pharmacotherapy with drugs that are similar to buspirone (see Tranylcypromine Monograph).

ADVERSE DRUG REACTIONS

Buspirone pharmacotherapy has been commonly associated with dizziness, drowsiness, headache, lightheadedness, nausea, and nervousness. Other ADRs, listed according to body system, include:

Cardiovascular: chest pain, palpitations, and tachycardia

CNS: akathisia (feelings of restlessness and an inability to sit down because of associated severe anxiety; may also be associated with feelings of muscle quivering), confusion, and excitement

Cutaneous: blisters, dry skin, easy bruising, hair loss, skin rash, and sweating (excessive)

Genitourinary: changes in sex drive, excessive urination during the night (nocturia), impotence (rare), and involuntary loss of urine (enuresis)

GI: constipation, diarrhea, dyspepsia, nausea, and vomiting

Hematologic: rarely, eosinophilia, leukopenia, and thrombocytopenia

Musculoskeletal: cogwheel rigidity, incoordination (ataxia), joint pain (arthralgia), muscle aches, muscle cramps, numbness, paresthesias, tremor, and weakness (see also CNS)

Ocular: blurred vision and itching of the eyes

Otic: ringing in the ears (tinnitus)

Respiratory: nasal congestion

Miscellaneous: sore throat

OVERDOSAGE

Signs and symptoms of buspirone overdosage include abnormal contraction of the pupils (miosis), a clammy feeling, difficulty thinking, dizziness, drowsiness, hallucinations, headache, hypotension, incoordination (ataxia), insomnia, itching, nausea, and vomiting. Buspirone overdosage requires emergency symptomatic medical support of body systems with attention to increasing buspirone elimination. There is no known antidote.

BUTABARBITAL (Secbutabarbital)

(byoo ta bar′bi tal)

TRADE NAMES

Butalan®
Butisol®

CLASSIFICATION

Sedative-hypnotic (barbiturate) (C-III)

See also Barbiturates General Monograph

APPROVED INDICATIONS FOR PSYCHOLOGICAL DISORDERS

Adjunctive pharmacotherapy for the short-term symptomatic management of:

Sleep Disorders: Insomnia

USUAL DOSAGE AND ADMINISTRATION

Insomnia

Adults: 50 to 100 mg orally 30 minutes before retiring for bed in the evening. Butabarbital pharmacotherapy for the symptomatic management of insomnia for longer than 14 days is *not* recommended. Barbiturates appear to lose their effectiveness for inducing and maintaining sleep after 14 days.

Women who are, or who may become, pregnant: FDA Pregnancy Category D. Safety and efficacy of butabarbital pharmacotherapy for women who are pregnant have not been established. However, other barbiturates have been associated with congenital defects (birth defects) when prescribed during pregnancy. Avoid prescribing butabarbital pharmacotherapy to women who are pregnant. If butabarbital pharmacotherapy is required, advise patients of potential benefits and possible risks to themselves and the embryo, fetus, or neonate (see also Barbiturates General Monograph). Collaboration with the patient's obstetrician is indicated.

Women who are breast-feeding: Safety and efficacy of butabarbital pharmacotherapy for women who are breast-feeding and their neonates and infants have not been clearly established. The amount of butabarbital excreted in breast milk is small and would be unlikely to cause ADRs among breast-fed neonates and infants. However, avoid prescribing butabarbital pharmacotherapy to women who are breast-feeding in order to eliminate the potential for any associated ADRs (e.g., excessive drowsiness, lethargy) among their neonates and infants. If desired, lactation may be maintained and breast-feeding resumed following the discontinuation of short-term butabarbital pharmacotherapy. Collaboration with the patient's pediatrician is indicated.

Elderly, frail, or debilitated patients and those who have kidney or liver dysfunction: Generally prescribe lower dosages for elderly, frail, or debilitated patients. Increase the dosage gradually, if needed, according to individual patient response. These patients may be more sensitive to the pharmacologic actions of the barbiturates than are younger or healthier adult patients. Also reduce the dosage for patients who have kidney or liver dysfunction.

Children: Safety and efficacy of butabarbital pharmacotherapy for the symptomatic management of insomnia among children have not been established. Butabarbital pharmacotherapy for this indication is *not* recommended for this age group.

Notes, Insomnia

Long-term butabarbital pharmacotherapy, or regular personal use, may result in addiction and habituation. Abrupt discontinuation of long-term pharmacotherapy, or regular personal use, may result in the barbiturate withdrawal syndrome. The barbiturate withdrawal syndrome is considered a medical emergency that can be fatal if not appropriately treated.

AVAILABLE DOSAGE FORMS, STORAGE, AND COMPATIBILITY

Capsules, oral: 15, 30 mg
Elixir, oral: 30, 33.3 mg/5 ml (contains 7% alcohol)
Tablets, oral: 15, 30, 50, 100 mg

Notes

Some oral dosage forms (i.e., 30 and 50 mg tablets and the elixir) may contain tartrazine (FD&C Yellow No. 5). Tartrazine has been associated with hypersensitivity reactions (e.g., bronchial asthma) among susceptible patients, particularly those who have a hypersensitivity to aspirin.

General Instructions for Patients   Instruct patients who are receiving butabarbital to

- safely store butabarbital capsules and tablets in tightly closed child-resistant containers at controlled room temperature (15° to 30°C; 59° to 86°F).
- protect butabarbital capsules from moisture.
- obtain an available patient information sheet regarding butabarbital pharmacotherapy from their pharmacist at the time that their prescription is dispensed. Encourage patients to clarify any questions that they may have concerning butabarbital pharmacotherapy with their pharmacist or, if needed, to consult their prescribing psychologist.

PROPOSED MECHANISM OF ACTION

See Barbiturates General Monograph

PHARMACOKINETICS/PHARMACODYNAMICS

Butabarbital is readily absorbed following oral ingestion and has an onset of action of approximately 1 hour. Peak blood levels are obtained within 3 to 4 hours. Its duration of action is approximately 6 to 8 hours. Butabarbital is extensively metabolized in the liver. Less than 2% is excreted in unchanged form in the urine. Butabarbital's mean half-life of elimination is approximately 100 hours. Additional data are unavailable.

Therapeutic Drug Monitoring

Butabarbital blood concentrations of 2 to 3 μg/ml generally produce sedation, concentrations of 7 to 25 μg/ml generally produce sleep, concentrations above 30 μg/ml generally produce coma, and concentrations exceeding 50 μg/ml are potentially fatal.

RELATIVE CONTRAINDICATIONS

Hypersensitivity to butabarbital or other barbiturates
Liver dysfunction, severe

Porphyria, active or latent
Respiratory dysfunction, severe

CAUTIONS AND COMMENTS

Butabarbital is addicting and habituating. See Barbiturates General Monograph.
Prescribe butabarbital pharmacotherapy cautiously to patients who

- are receiving oral anticoagulant pharmacotherapy. Avoid prescribing butabarbital pharmacotherapy to these patients because of the difficulty associated with stabilizing prothrombin times.
- have CNS depression.
- have liver dysfunction.
- have respiratory depression.

Caution patients who are receiving butabarbital pharmacotherapy against

- drinking alcohol or using other drugs that produce CNS depression. Concurrent use of these drugs with butabarbital may result in excessive CNS depression.
- performing activities that require alertness, judgment, and physical coordination (e.g., driving an automobile, operating dangerous equipment, supervising children). Butabarbital pharmacotherapy may adversely affect these mental and physical functions.

CLINICALLY SIGNIFICANT DRUG INTERACTIONS

Concurrent butabarbital pharmacotherapy and the following may result in clinically significant drug interactions:

Alcohol Use

Concurrent alcohol use may increase the CNS depressant action of butabarbital. Advise patients to avoid, or limit, their use of alcohol while receiving butabarbital pharmacotherapy.

Pharmacotherapy With Drugs That Are Primarily Metabolized by the Liver

Butabarbital may stimulate the production of hepatic microsomal enzymes, which are responsible for the metabolism of many different classes of drugs. Whenever butabarbital is added to or removed from a patient's pharmacotherapy, the effect on concurrent pharmacotherapy with drugs that are metabolized by the liver (e.g., corticosteroids, oral anticoagulants, oral contraceptives; quinidine [Biquin®]) must be monitored and their dosages appropriately adjusted, if necessary. Collaboration with other prescribers may be required.

Other Possible Drug Interactions

Although no other clinically significant drug interactions have been documented involving butabarbital pharmacotherapy, they have been reported with other barbiturate pharmacotherapy.

Attention to these clinically significant drug interactions is required because of butabarbital's similarity to the other barbiturates.

See Barbiturates General Monograph

ADVERSE DRUG REACTIONS

Butabarbital pharmacotherapy has been associated with bradycardia, confusion, gastrointestinal complaints, lethargy, and respiratory depression. Other ADRs have been associated with other barbiturate pharmacotherapy. Attention to these ADRs is required because of the chemical and pharmacological similarities among the barbiturates.

See Barbiturates General Monograph

OVERDOSAGE

See Barbiturates General Monograph

BUTORPHANOL

(byoo tore'fan ol)

TRADE NAMES

Stadol®
Stadol NS®

CLASSIFICATION

Opiate analgesic agonist/antagonist

See also Opiate Analgesics General Monograph

APPROVED INDICATIONS FOR PSYCHOLOGICAL DISORDERS

Adjunctive pharmacotherapy for the symptomatic management of:

Pain Disorders: Acute Pain

USUAL DOSAGE AND ADMINISTRATION

Acute Pain

Adults: 1 mg intravenously every three to four hours, as needed; *or* 2 mg intramuscularly every three to four hours, as needed; *or* 1 mg nasal spray (one spray in *one* nostril). If adequate pain relief is not achieved within 60 to 90 minutes following the initial nasal spray, an additional 1 mg nasal spray (one spray in *one* nostril) may be administered. This initial two-dose nasal spray sequence may be repeated in three to four hours, as needed. Adherence to this nasal spray dosage reduces the incidence of associated dizziness and drowsiness. However, for severe pain, an initial nasal spray of 2 mg (one spray in *each* nostril) may be prescribed for patients who are able to remain lying down in the event of associated dizziness or drowsiness. For these patients, do *not* prescribe additional 2 mg nasal sprays for three to four hours.

MAXIMUM: The safety and efficacy of intramuscular doses exceeding 4 mg have not been established.

Women who are, or who may become, pregnant: FDA Pregnancy Category C. Safety and efficacy of butorphanol pharmacotherapy for women who are pregnant have not been established. There are no adequate and well-controlled studies of butorphanol use among pregnant women before 37 weeks of gestation. Avoid prescribing butorphanol pharmacotherapy to women who are pregnant. If butorphanol pharmacotherapy is required, advise patients of potential benefits and possible risks to themselves and the embryo, fetus, or neonate. Collaboration with the patient's obstetrician is indicated.
See also Opiate Analgesics General Monograph

Women who are breast-feeding: Safety and efficacy of butorphanol pharmacotherapy for women who are breast-feeding and their neonates and infants have not been established. Butorphanol has been detected in breast milk. However, the amount that a neonate or an infant would receive from breast-feeding is probably clinically insignificant (estimated as 4 μg/L of breast milk for a mother receiving 2 mg intramuscularly four times a day). Although there are no data regarding the use of the nasal spray among mothers who are breast-feeding, butorphanol is probably excreted in breast milk in similar amounts following nasal use. Avoid prescribing butorphanol pharmacotherapy to women who are breast-feeding. If butorphanol pharmacotherapy is required, breast-feeding probably should be discontinued. If desired, lactation may be maintained and breast-feeding resumed following the discontinuation of short-term butorphanol pharmacotherapy. Collaboration with the patient's pediatrician may be required.

Elderly, frail, or debilitated patients and those who have kidney or liver dysfunction: Generally prescribe lower dosages of butorphanol and increase the dosing interval for elderly, frail, or debilitated patients according to the method of administration.

INJECTABLE PHARMACOTHERAPY: Initially, 0.5 to 1 mg intravenously or 1 mg intramuscularly every six to eight hours, as needed. Note that the initial injectable dose recommended for these patients is half the usual adult dose at twice the usual dosing interval. Prescribe subsequent doses and dosing intervals according to individual patient response.

NASAL PHARMACOTHERAPY: Initially, 1 mg nasal spray (one spray in *one* nostril). Allow 90 to 120 minutes to elapse before deciding whether an additional 1 mg nasal spray (one spray in *one* nostril) is needed. The mean half-life of butorphanol is increased by 25% (to over 6 hours) among patients older than 65 years of age because of age-related changes in the elimination of butorphanol. Elderly patients may be more sensitive to the ADRs associated with the nasal spray formulation (Stadol NS®), particularly dizziness, than are younger or healthier adult patients. Patients who have kidney or liver dysfunction also require lower dosages and increased dosing intervals (see Cautions and Comments).

Children and adolescents younger than 18 years of age: Safety and efficacy of butor-phanol pharmacotherapy for children and adolescents have not been established. Butorphanol pharmacotherapy is *not* recommended for this age group.

Notes, Acute Pain

The injectable and nasal spray are indicated for the symptomatic management of pain when the use of an opiate analgesic is appropriate. Approximate equivalent analgesic action has been reported to be 2 mg butorphanol, 10 mg morphine, 40 mg pentazocine, and 80 mg meperidine. Factors for consideration when determining dosage include age, body weight, general health, presenting clinical condition, and other concurrent pharmacotherapy. Patients receiving intra-muscular or intravenous injections should remain lying down in the event of associated dizziness or drowsiness. Butorphanol is not widely prescribed.

Butorphanol pharmacotherapy is *not* recommended for patients who are addicted or habitu-ated to opiate analgesics. Butorphanol has precipitated the opiate withdrawal syndrome among patients who were receiving long-term opiate analgesic agonist pharmacotherapy. Signs and symptoms of the opiate withdrawal syndrome, include agitation, anxiety, diarrhea, dysphoria, hallucinations, mood changes, and weakness. Prescribe only butorphanol pharmacotherapy for these patients when they have had an adequate period of detoxification from opiates prior to initiating butorphanol pharmacotherapy.

AVAILABLE DOSAGE FORMS, STORAGE, AND COMPATIBILITY

Injectable, intramuscular or intravenous: 1, 2 mg/ml multi-dose vials
Nasal spray, metered: 10 mg/ml (14 to 15 doses, 1 mg/spray); 2.5 ml bottle

Notes

Injectable Formulation Stadol® injectable is supplied in sealed delivery systems that have a low risk for accidental exposure to health care workers. However, care should be taken to avoid aerosol inhalation when preparing a syringe for injection. In the event of inadvertent skin contact, rinse well with cool water. Stadol® injectable has been associated with contact dermatitis.

Store injectables safely at room temperature below 30°C (86°F). Discard cloudy solutions appropriately.

Nasal Spray Formulation Stadol NS® is supplied in a child-resistant prescription vial containing a metered-dose spray pump with protective tip and dust cover, a bottle of nasal spray solution, and patient instructions for use. On average, one 2.5 ml bottle will deliver 14 to 15 doses if no re-priming is required. The patient's pharmacist will assemble the Stadol NS® prior to dispensing to the patient. The nasal spray is administered as a metered spray to the nasal mucosa. The pump reservoir must be fully primed prior to initial use.

After initial priming, each metered spray delivers an average of 1 mg of butorphanol. The unit must be *re-primed* if not used for 48 hours or longer. With intermittent use requiring re-priming before each dose, the 2.5 ml bottle will deliver an average of 8 to 10 doses, depending on the number of times re-priming is required.

Stadol NS® is an open delivery system that may pose increased risk of exposure to health care workers and other people (or pets) who are in the immediate environment (e.g., hospital or home) when the metered-spray pump is initially primed or re-primed. A certain amount of butorphanol may be aerosolized during the priming process. Therefore, the pump sprayer should be aimed away from the face and away from the patient, other people, or pets. The unit should be appropriately disposed of by unscrewing the cap, rinsing the bottle, and placing the parts in a waste container.

General Instructions for Patients   Instruct patients who are receiving butorphanol pharmacotherapy to

- safely store butorphanol nasal spray out of the reach of children at controlled room temperature (15° to 30°C; 59° to 86°F).
- obtain an available patient information sheet regarding butorphanol pharmacotherapy from their pharmacist at the time that their prescription is dispensed. Encourage patients to clarify any questions that they may have concerning their butorphanol pharmacotherapy with their pharmacist or, if needed, to consult their prescribing psychologist.

PROPOSED MECHANISM OF ACTION

Butorphanol is a synthetically derived opiate agonist/antagonist analgesic. Its major metabolites are agonists at kappa-opiate receptors and mixed agonists/antagonists at mu-opiate receptors. The interaction of butorphanol with these receptors in the CNS apparently mediates most of its pharmacologic actions, including abnormal contraction of the pupils (miosis), analgesia, depression of spontaneous respirations and cough, stimulation of the emetic (vomiting) center, and sedation. Other actions possibly mediated by non-CNS mechanisms include alteration in cardiovascular resistance and capacitance, bronchomotor tone, GI secretion and motility, and bladder sphincter activity.

Although butorphanol appears to elicit its analgesic and CNS and respiratory depressant actions primarily by binding to the endorphin receptors in the CNS, the exact mechanism of action has not yet been fully determined. The partial antagonist activity is probably due to competitive inhibition at the receptor sites.

See Opiate Analgesics General Monograph

PHARMACOKINETICS/PHARMACODYNAMICS

Butorphanol is rapidly absorbed following intramuscular injection and obtains peak blood levels within 20 to 40 minutes. After a 1 mg nasal dose, mean peak blood levels occur within 30 to 60 minutes. The absolute bioavailability of the nasal formulation is 60% to 70%. Bioavailability is unchanged among patients who have allergic rhinitis. Among patients using a nasal vasoconstrictor (e.g., oxymetazoline [Dristan Long Lasting Nasal®, Drixoral Nasal®]), the fraction of the dose absorbed reportedly is unchanged, but the rate of absorption is slowed. The peak blood concentrations are approximately half those achieved in the absence of the vasoconstrictor. Following its initial absorption/distribution phase, the single-dose pharmacokinetics of butorphanol by intravenous, intramuscular, or nasal administration have been found to be similar.

Plasma protein binding (~80%) is independent of blood concentration over the range achieved in clinical practice. Its apparent volume of distribution ranges from 4 to 13 L/kg. Butorphanol is transported across the blood-brain barrier and placental barrier. It also is excreted in breast milk. Butorphanol is extensively metabolized in the liver, with less than 5% excreted in unchanged form in the urine. A small amount is excreted in feces. The mean half-life of elimination is approximately 5 hours (range 2 to 9 hours).

The analgesic action of butorphanol is influenced by its method of administration. Onset of analgesia is within a few minutes of intravenous injection (i.e., when used as a preanesthetic). Peak analgesic activity occurs within 30 to 60 minutes following intramuscular injection and within 1 to 2 hours following nasal spray. The duration of analgesia varies, depending on the severity of pain and method of administration, but is generally 3 to 4 hours with intramuscular or intravenous injection. When compared to the injectable formulation and other opiate agonist or agonist/antagonist analgesics, butorphanol nasal spray has a longer duration of action (4 to 5 hours).

RELATIVE CONTRAINDICATIONS

Hypersensitivity to butorphanol or the preservative benzethonian chloride found in some formulations (i.e., Stadol® injectable multi-dose vial and Stadol NS®)

CAUTIONS AND COMMENTS

Butorphanol appears to have a low abuse potential. However, it may precipitate the opiate withdrawal syndrome among patients who are addicted to opiate agonist analgesics. Although the mixed agonist/antagonist opiate analgesics, as a class, have lower abuse potential than morphine, problematic patterns of use, including addiction and habituation, have been associated with these drugs. The discontinuation of long-term injectable butorphanol use has been associated with a mild withdrawal syndrome.

The regular use of Stadol NS® for 2 months or longer has been associated with problematic patterns of use. Upon abrupt discontinuation of use of 16 mg or more daily for longer than 3 months, signs and symptoms of anxiety, agitation, and diarrhea have been observed. These signs and symptoms suggest the opiate analgesic withdrawal syndrome.

Prescribe butorphanol pharmacotherapy cautiously to patients who

- have kidney and liver dysfunction. These patients may have a diminished ability to metabolize and eliminate butorphanol. For these patients, increase the initial dosage interval for the injectable and nasal spray to 6 to 8 hours until their response to butorphanol pharmacotherapy is known. Subsequent doses should be determined by individual patient response rather than fixed dosing intervals.
- have cardiovascular dysfunction. Butorphanol may increase the work load of the heart, especially the pulmonary circuit. The use of butorphanol among patients who have acute myocardial infarction, ventricular dysfunction, or coronary insufficiency should be limited to those situations where the benefits clearly outweigh the risks. Collaboration with the patient's cardiologist is indicated.
- have head injuries or other conditions associated with increased intracranial pressure. Butorphanol pharmacotherapy (and other opiate pharmacotherapy) may be associated with carbon dioxide retention and a secondary increase in cerebrospinal fluid pressure, drug-induced miosis, and alterations in mental function that may obscure the interpretation of the patient's clinical course. Among these patients, butorphanol should only be prescribed if the benefits clearly outweigh the potential risks. Collaboration with the patient's family physician or a specialist (e.g., neurologist) is indicated.

- have histories of addiction and habituation to opiate analgesics or other abusable psychotropics. Evaluate the need for butorphanol pharmacotherapy carefully and assure that these patients have undergone adequate detoxification.
- have recently received repeated doses of opiate agonist analgesics. It is difficult to assess opiate tolerance among these patients.
- have respiratory dysfunction. Butorphanol can produce respiratory depression, especially among patients who are concurrently receiving pharmacotherapy with other drugs that produce CNS depression or who have medical disorders (e.g., sleep apnea) that affect CNS or respiratory function.

CLINICALLY SIGNIFICANT DRUG INTERACTIONS

Concurrent butorphanol pharmacotherapy and the following may result in clinically significant drug interactions:

Pharmacotherapy With Drugs That Affect Hepatic Metabolism

It is unknown whether butorphanol pharmacotherapy is altered by concurrent pharmacotherapy with drugs known to affect hepatic metabolism (e.g., barbiturates, cimetidine [Tagamet®], erythromycin [E-Mycin®], theophylline [Theo-Dur®]). However, clinical psychologists should be alert to the possibility that a lower initial dosage and longer dosing intervals may be needed for patients who are receiving concurrent pharmacotherapy with drugs that affect hepatic metabolism.

Pharmacotherapy With Central Nervous System Depressants and Other Drugs That Produce Central Nervous System Depression

Concurrent butorphanol pharmacotherapy with sedative-hypnotics or other drugs that produce CNS depression (e.g., antihistamines, phenothiazines, TCAs) may result in additive CNS depression. When prescribed concurrently, the dose of butorphanol should be the lowest effective dose, and the frequency of dosing should be extended as much as possible.

Pharmacotherapy With Nasal Vasoconstrictors

The fraction of Stadol NS® absorbed is unaffected by the concomitant use of a nasal vasoconstrictor (e.g., oxymetazoline [Dristan Long Lasting Nasal®, Drixoral Nasal®]), but the rate of absorption is decreased. Therefore, a slower onset of action can be anticipated if Stadol NS® is administered with, or immediately following, a nasal vasoconstrictor.

See also Opiate Analgesics General Monograph

ADVERSE DRUG REACTIONS

The ADRs associated with butorphanol pharmacotherapy, either injectable or nasal spray, are similar to those commonly associated with other mixed opiate agonist/antagonist analgesics. These ADRs include dizziness, drowsiness, nausea, sedation, somnolence, and vomiting. Butorphanol, like pentazocine (Talwin®) and other mixed agonist/antagonists that have a high affinity for the kappa-opiate receptor, may produce unpleasant psychotomimetic reactions among susceptible patients. Nasal administration has been associated with dizziness, drowsiness, insomnia, and nasal congestion.

Severe hypertension has been rarely associated with butorphanol pharmacotherapy. In such cases, discontinue butorphanol pharmacotherapy immediately. Collaboration with the patient's family physician or a specialist (e.g., cardiologist) is indicated for the appropriate medical management of the associated hypertension, which may require antihypertensive pharmacotherapy.

See also Opiate Analgesics General Monograph

OVERDOSAGE

Signs and symptoms of butorphanol overdosage are similar to those associated with other opiate analgesic overdosage. The most serious signs and symptoms are hypoventilation, cardiovascular insufficiency, and coma. Overdosage has occurred with accidental ingestion involving young children who gained access to the drug in the home, and intentional overdosage by suicidal patients. Although butorphanol is more potent than morphine, it appears to have a ceiling effect in terms of respiratory depression. This ceiling effect is a theoretical advantage because an overdosage involving a large amount of butorphanol should not produce a correspondingly excessive respiratory depression.

Suspected or actual butorphanol overdosage requires emergency symptomatic medical support of body systems with attention to increasing butorphanol elimination. The use of the opiate antagonist naloxone (Narcan®) may be required. Repeated dosing with naloxone is usually required because the duration of butorphanol action exceeds that of naloxone.

CARBAMAZEPINE

(kar ba maz'e peen)

TRADE NAMES

Atretol®
Mazepine®
Novo-Carbamaz®
Tegretol®

CLASSIFICATION

Antimanic (anticonvulsant)

APPROVED INDICATIONS FOR PSYCHOLOGICAL DISORDERS

Adjunctive pharmacotherapy for the prophylactic and symptomatic management of:

Mood Disorders, Bipolar (manic-depressive) Disorder: Acute Mania. Carbamazepine pharmacotherapy may be prescribed alone or with lithium pharmacotherapy for the prophylactic and symptomatic management of acute mania.

Note that this indication for use is HPB, but *not* FDA, approved.

USUAL DOSAGE AND ADMINISTRATION

Acute Mania

Adults: Initially, 200 to 400 mg daily orally in two to four divided doses. Increase the dosage gradually, according to individual patient response, until the desired therapeutic effect is achieved.

MAXIMUM: 1600 mg daily

Women who are, or who may become, pregnant: FDA Pregnancy Category C. Safety and efficacy of carbamazepine pharmacotherapy for women who are pregnant have not been established. However, the preponderance of available data suggest that carbamazepine is likely a human teratogen that causes a variety of congenital malformations, including cleft lip, depressed nasal bridge, hypoplastic nails, and mental retardation. Avoid prescribing carbamazepine pharmacotherapy to women who are pregnant. If carbamazepine pharmacotherapy is required, advise patients of potential benefits and possible risks to themselves and the embryo, fetus, or neonate. Concurrent carbamazepine and anticonvulsant pharmacotherapy (e.g., phenytoin) has been associated with significant teratogenic risk. Collaboration with the patient's obstetrician is indicated.

Women who are breast-feeding: Safety and efficacy of carbamazepine pharmacotherapy for women who are breast-feeding and their neonates and infants have not been established. Carbamazepine and its active metabolite, carbamazepine-epoxide, are excreted in breast milk in concentrations equal to approximately 50% of the maternal blood concentration. Lethargy, poor sucking, or sedation may occur among breast-fed neonates and infants. A severe hypersensitivity skin reaction involving a breast-fed infant also has been reported. Avoid prescribing carbamazepine pharmacotherapy to women who are breast-feeding. If carbamazepine pharmacotherapy is required, breast-feeding should be discontinued. Collaboration with the patient's pediatrician is indicated.

Elderly, frail, or debilitated patients: Generally prescribe lower dosages for elderly, frail, or debilitated patients. Increase the dosage gradually, if needed, according to individual patient response. These patients may be more sensitive to the pharmacologic actions of carbamazepine than are younger or healthier adult patients.

Children: Safety and efficacy of carbamazepine pharmacotherapy for the symptomatic management of bipolar disorders for children have not been established. Carbamazepine pharmacotherapy for this indication is *not* recommended for this age group.

Notes, Acute Mania

Initiating Carbamazepine Pharmacotherapy Before initiating carbamazepine pharmacotherapy, obtain baseline blood counts, including platelets, and evaluate kidney and liver function. Carbamazepine pharmacotherapy has been associated with bone marrow depression and serious blood disorders, including aplastic anemia and, rarely, agranulocytosis. It also has been associated with kidney and liver dysfunction.

Maintaining Carbamazepine Pharmacotherapy Prescribe the lowest effective dosage. Therapeutic drug monitoring of carbamazepine blood levels is probably not of assistance for guiding pharmacotherapy for the symptomatic management of bipolar disorder. Collaboration with the patient's family physician or a specialist (e.g., hematologist, internist, nephrologist) is indicated. Monitor patients regularly for signs and symptoms of blood disorders, kidney dysfunction, and liver dysfunction. Discontinue carbamazepine pharmacotherapy immediately if any signs and symptoms suggesting these conditions are noted. Carbamazepine pharmacotherapy also has been associated with severe skin reactions, such as Stevens-Johnson syndrome and Lyell's syndrome. Discontinue carbamazepine pharmacotherapy immediately if signs and symptoms suggesting a severe skin reaction are noted. The management of carbamazepine pharmacotherapy generally requires collaboration with the patient's family physician or other specialists (e.g., dermatologist, hematologist, internist, nephrologist) because of the possible occurrence of the noted potentially serious ADRs.

Discontinuing Carbamazepine Pharmacotherapy Discontinue carbamazepine pharmacotherapy gradually. Abrupt discontinuation may result in seizures.

AVAILABLE DOSAGE FORMS, STORAGE, AND COMPATIBILITY

Suspension, oral: 100 mg/5 ml (citrus-vanilla flavored)
Tablets, oral: 200 mg
Tablets, oral chewable: 100, 200 mg
Tablets, oral extended-release: 100, 200, 400 mg

Notes

Carbamazepine extended-release tablets provide a lower average maximal blood concentration without a reduction in the average minimal concentration. Thus, carbamazepine pharmacotherapy with extended-release tablets helps to ensure that the blood concentrations remain largely stable throughout the day and allows twice-daily dosing. It also results in a lower incidence of intermittent concentration-dependent ADRs.

General Instructions for Patients Instruct patients who are receiving carbamazepine pharmacotherapy to

- shake the carbamazepine oral suspension well before measuring each dose to help to evenly disperse the suspension and, thus, assure an accurate dose is measured and ingested.
- thoroughly chew or dissolve in the mouth before swallowing each dose of the carbamazepine chewable tablets.
- safely store carbamazepine oral dosage forms out of the reach of children in tightly closed child- and light-resistant containers at controlled room temperature (15° to 30°C; 59° to 86°F).
- obtain an available patient information sheet regarding carbamazepine pharmacotherapy from their pharmacist at the time that their prescription is dispensed. Encourage patients to clarify any questions that they may have concerning carbamazepine pharmacotherapy with their pharmacist or, if needed, to consult their prescribing psychologist.

PROPOSED MECHANISM OF ACTION

The exact mechanism of carbamazepine's antimanic action has not been fully determined. It appears to be related to decreased neurochemical activity in the nucleus ventralis of the thalamus and decreased summation of temporal stimulation leading to neuronal discharge.

PHARMACOKINETICS/PHARMACODYNAMICS

Carbamazepine is slowly, but well absorbed (over 70%) following oral ingestion. Peak blood levels are generally obtained within 4 to 24 hours. There are no clinically significant differences in bioavailability among the oral dosage forms (e.g., oral chewable tablets, oral extended-release tablets, oral suspension, oral tablets). In addition, the ingestion of food has no significant effect on either the rate or extent of absorption, regardless of the oral dosage form. Carbamazepine is extensively metabolized primarily in the liver, with less than 3% eliminated in unchanged form in the urine. It is moderately plasma protein-bound (~75%) and has an apparent volume of distribution of 1 to 2 L/kg. Mean total body clearance is 100 ml/minute (range from 50 to

125 ml/minute). The mean half-life of elimination is approximately 36 hours following a single oral dose. However, repeated doses over two to four weeks result in autoinduction of hepatic enzymes and a reduction in half-life to 16 to 24 hours.

Therapeutic Drug Monitoring

Dosage must be determined by individual patient response and *not* by carbamazepine blood concentrations. A correlation between carbamazepine blood concentrations and the prophylactic or symptomatic management of bipolar disorder has not been clearly established. However, carbamazepine blood concentrations may be useful for monitoring either the patient's ability to manage carbamazepine pharmacotherapy or possible overdosage. For therapeutic drug monitoring, it is generally recommended to sample from trough concentrations just prior to the next dose. However, in cases of suspected overdosages, sampling can be done at any time. The therapeutic blood concentration range for the management of *seizure disorders* is generally estimated as 17 to 50 μmol/L (4 to 12 μg/ml). This therapeutic blood concentration range has no relevance for managing carbamazepine pharmacotherapy for the prophylactic or symptomatic management of bipolar (manic depressive) disorder.

RELATIVE CONTRAINDICATIONS

Atrioventricular block
Blood disorders, severe
Bone marrow depression
Hypersensitivity to carbamazepine or to TCAs (e.g., amitriptyline, imipramine, trimipramine) or their analogues or metabolites. Carbamazepine has a similar chemical structure to these drugs and chemicals.
Liver dysfunction
MAOI pharmacotherapy, concurrent or within 14 days
Porphyria, acute intermittent

CAUTIONS AND COMMENTS

Prescribe carbamazepine pharmacotherapy cautiously to patients who

- have histories of adverse hematological reactions to other pharmacotherapy. Baseline assessment and periodic monitoring for signs and symptoms of bone marrow depression are required for these patients. Discontinue carbamazepine pharmacotherapy immediately if such signs and symptoms are identified.
- have histories of interrupted courses of pharmacotherapy with carbamazepine.
- have histories of kidney dysfunction. Baseline assessment and periodic monitoring of kidney function are required. Discontinue carbamazepine pharmacotherapy immediately if signs and symptoms of kidney dysfunction are identified.
- have histories of liver dysfunction. Baseline assessment and periodic monitoring of liver function are required, particularly for elderly, frail, or debilitated patients and those who have histories of liver disease, including alcoholic cirrhosis. Discontinue carbamazepine pharmacotherapy immediately if signs and symptoms of aggravated liver dysfunction or active liver disease are identified.

• have received MAOI pharmacotherapy within 14 days. Do *not* prescribe carbamazepine pharmacotherapy immediately before, concurrently with, or immediately after MAOI pharmacotherapy. When carbamazepine pharmacotherapy is required for these patients, assure a drug-free interval for as long as clinically possible before initiating carbamazepine pharmacotherapy. In no case should this interval be less than 14 days. Initially prescribe a lower dosage of carbamazepine, and increase the dosage gradually according to individual patient response. See Relative Contraindications.

Caution patients who are receiving carbamazepine pharmacotherapy in regard to the need to immediately report the early signs and symptoms of potentially serious ADRs, particularly blood, kidney, liver, and skin reactions. The onset of such potentially serious ADRs may be rapid. Advise patients to immediately inform their prescribing psychologist if they develop such early signs and symptoms of these reactions as a fever, sore throat, rash, ulcers in the mouth, or easy bruising.

CLINICALLY SIGNIFICANT DRUG INTERACTIONS

Concurrent carbamazepine pharmacotherapy and the following may result in clinically significant drug interactions:

Pharmacotherapy With Drugs That Inhibit Hepatic Microsomal Enzymes

The hepatic metabolism of carbamazepine may be inhibited and its actions increased significantly by concurrent cimetidine (Tagamet®), diltiazem (Cardizem®), erythromycin (E-Mycin®), isoniazid (INH®), ketoconazole (Nizoral®), propoxyphene (Darvon®), troleandomycin (TAO®), or verapamil (Calan®) pharmacotherapy. For patients receiving carbamazepine pharmacotherapy, the clinical response should be closely monitored when pharmacotherapy with these drugs is initiated and discontinued, or when adjustments are made to their dosages.

Pharmacotherapy With Drugs That Are Primarily Metabolized by the Liver

Carbamazepine, a hepatic microsomal enzyme inducer, may increase the hepatic metabolism of benzodiazepines, corticosteroids, ethosuximide (Zarontin®), oral anticoagulants (e.g., warfarin [Coumadin®]), oral contraceptives (the reliability of oral contraceptives may be adversely affected by carbamazepine), theophylline (Theo-Dur®), thyroid hormones, valproic acid (Depakene®), and other drugs that are primarily metabolized by the liver. When concurrent pharmacotherapy is required, collaboration with other prescribers may be necessary to help to assure optimal pharmacotherapy.

ADVERSE DRUG REACTIONS

Carbamazepine has moderate anticholinergic actions. Tolerance may develop to these actions after a few months of pharmacotherapy. Carbamazepine pharmacotherapy also has been associated with the following ADRs, listed according to body system:

Cardiovascular: suppression of ventricular automaticity (due to its membrane-depressant action, which is similar to that of the antidysrhythmics quinidine [Quinate®] and procainamide [Pronestyl®]). This ADR is associated with suppression of phase 4 depolarization of the heart muscle fiber.
CNS: dizziness, drowsiness, and headache
Cutaneous: skin reactions, severe (e.g., Stevens-Johnson syndrome, Lyell's syndrome)
Genitourinary: urinary retention
GI: nausea
Hematologic: blood disorders (potentially fatal), leukopenia, and thrombocytopenia
Hepatic: hepatocellular and cholestatic jaundice and hepatitis
Ocular: double vision (diplopia)
Renal: kidney dysfunction

OVERDOSAGE

Signs and symptoms of carbamazepine overdosage include impaired consciousness, irregular breathing, neuromuscular disturbances, tachycardia, and urinary retention. Carbamazepine overdosage requires emergency symptomatic medical support of body systems with attention to increasing carbamazepine elimination. There is no known antidote.

CHLORAL HYDRATE

(klor al hye'drate)

TRADE NAMES

Aquachloral Supprettes®
Noctec®
Novo-Chlorhydrate®

CLASSIFICATION

Sedative-hypnotic trichloroacetaldehyde (C-IV)

APPROVED INDICATIONS FOR PSYCHOLOGICAL DISORDERS

Adjunctive pharmacotherapy for the short-term symptomatic management of:

Sleep Disorders: Insomnia

USUAL DOSAGE AND ADMINISTRATION

Insomnia

Adults: 500 to 1000 mg orally or rectally 15 to 30 minutes before retiring for bed in the evening.

MAXIMUM: 2000 mg per single dose orally or rectally

Women who are, or who may become, pregnant: FDA Pregnancy Category "not established." Safety and efficacy of chloral hydrate pharmacotherapy for women who are pregnant have not been established. Chloral hydrate crosses the placenta, and long-term use during pregnancy can result in maternal addiction and habituation and signs and symptoms of the chloral hydrate withdrawal syndrome among neonates. Avoid prescribing chloral hydrate pharmacotherapy to women who are pregnant. If chloral hydrate pharmacotherapy is required, advise patients of potential benefits and possible risks to themselves and the embryo, fetus, or neonate. Collaboration with the patient's obstetrician is indicated.

Women who are breast-feeding: Safety and efficacy of chloral hydrate pharmacotherapy for women who are breast-feeding and their neonates and infants have not been established. However, both chloral hydrate and its active metabolite, trichloroethanol, are excreted in significant concentrations in breast milk and may cause drowsiness or addiction among breast-fed neonates and infants. Avoid prescribing chloral hydrate pharmacotherapy to women who are breast-feeding. If chloral hydrate pharmacotherapy is required, breast-feeding probably should be discontinued. If desired, lactation may be maintained and breast-feeding resumed following the discontinuation of short-term chloral hydrate pharmacotherapy. Collaboration with the patient's pediatrician is indicated.

Elderly, frail, or debilitated patients: Initially, 250 mg orally or rectally 15 to 30 minutes before retiring for bed in the evening. Increase the dosage gradually, if needed, according to individual patient response. Generally prescribe lower dosages for elderly, frail, or debilitated patients. These patients may be more sensitive to the pharmacologic actions of chloral hydrate than are younger or healthier adult patients.

Children: 25 to 50 mg/kg orally or rectally as a single dose 15 to 30 minutes before bedtime.

MAXIMUM: 1000 mg per single dose orally or rectally

Notes, Insomnia

Drowsiness occurs within 10 to 15 minutes following a hypnotic dose. Sleep occurs usually within 30 to 60 minutes and lasts approximately 4 to 8 hours. Chloral hydrate provides mild cerebral depression and quiet, deep sleep with little or no residual "hangover" effects. It also decreases sleep latency and nighttime awakenings, with minimal effects on REM sleep. Thus, the discontinuation of chloral hydrate pharmacotherapy is not associated with REM rebound. However, chloral hydrate's effects on sleep generally diminish significantly after approximately two weeks of nightly use.

Prescribe chloral hydrate only for short-term pharmacotherapy. Long-term pharmacotherapy is *not* recommended and may produce addiction and habituation. Abrupt discontinuation of long-term chloral hydrate pharmacotherapy may result in signs and symptoms similar to alcoholic delirium tremens, including hallucinations, and may be fatal. Discontinue long-term chloral hydrate pharmacotherapy gradually.

AVAILABLE DOSAGE FORMS, STORAGE, AND COMPATIBILITY

Capsules, oral: 250, 500 mg
Suppositories, rectal: 325, 500, 650 mg
Syrup, oral: 250, 500 mg/5 ml

Notes

Doses for oral ingestion and rectal insertion are equivalent. If required, oral capsules may be inserted rectally after moistening with water. Alternatively, capsules may be dissolved in cottonseed oil, olive oil, or a hydrophilic polyethylene glycol base, and administered as a retention enema. Chloral hydrate is volatile and sensitive to light.

General Instructions for Patients　Instruct patients who are receiving chloral hydrate pharmacotherapy to

- dilute each dose of the chloral hydrate oral syrup in a small amount of water or juice (i.e., 80 to 120 ml) before ingestion. Diluting the syrup formulation before ingestion will help to minimize associated irritation to the oral, esophageal, and gastric mucosa.
- ingest each dose of the chloral hydrate capsules with a full (i.e., 160 to 240 ml) glass of water, milk, fruit juice, or ginger ale. Instruct patients to swallow each capsule whole and to avoid breaking or chewing them. These instructions will help to ensure optimal therapeutic benefit while minimizing associated gastrointestinal irritation.
- safely store chloral hydrate oral dosage forms out of the reach of children in air-tight, child- and light-resistant containers at controlled room temperature (15° to 30°C; 59° to 86°F).
- obtain an available patient information sheet regarding chloral hydrate pharmacotherapy from their pharmacist at the time that their prescription is dispensed. Encourage patients to clarify any questions that they may have concerning chloral hydrate pharmacotherapy with their pharmacist or, if needed, to consult their prescribing psychologist.

PROPOSED MECHANISM OF ACTION

The CNS depressant action of chloral hydrate is due to its active metabolite, trichloroethanol. The mechanism of action appears to be similar to that for alcohol. However, the exact mechanism of action has not yet been clearly established.

PHARMACOKINETICS/PHARMACODYNAMICS

Chloral hydrate is rapidly and well absorbed (approximately 100%) from the gastrointestinal tract following oral or rectal administration. It is 70% to 80% plasma protein-bound and has an apparent volume of distribution of approximately 0.6 L/kg. Chloral hydrate is rapidly and extensively metabolized in the liver and erythrocytes by alcohol dehydrogenase to its active metabolite, trichloroethanol. It is widely distributed to all body tissues, including the placenta. It is found in cerebral spinal fluid and breast milk. Trichloroethanol has a mean half-life of elimination of 8 hours (range 4 to 12 hours). Trichloroethanol is variably metabolized, primarily in the liver, but also in the kidneys, to trichloracetic acid (an inactive metabolite). The half-life of trichloroethanol is prolonged among pre-term neonates (37 hours) and children (10 hours).

RELATIVE CONTRAINDICATIONS

Cardiovascular disorders, severe
Gastric or duodenal ulcers, severe or untreated
Hypersensitivity to chloral hydrate
Kidney dysfunction, severe
Liver dysfunction, severe
Respiratory dysfunction, acute

CAUTIONS AND COMMENTS

Prescribe chloral hydrate pharmacotherapy cautiously to patients who

- are receiving oral anticoagulant pharmacotherapy because of the associated difficulty stabilizing prothrombin times. See Clinically Significant Drug Interactions.
- have cardiac dysfunction (severe). Chloral hydrate pharmacotherapy, especially high-dosage pharmacotherapy, has been associated with cardiac dysrhythmias and hypotension.
- have CNS dysfunction. Chloral hydrate pharmacotherapy may exacerbate CNS dysfunction.
- have depression, with or without suicidal ideation. Chloral hydrate pharmacotherapy may exacerbate depression.
- have histories of esophagitis, gastritis, gastric or duodenal ulcers, proctitis, or colitis. Oral dosage forms of chloral hydrate are irritating to the esophageal and gastric mucosa. Also avoid rectal use among patients who have proctitis or colitis because of its irritant effects to the intestinal and rectal mucosa.
- have histories of problematic patterns of abusable psychotropic use. Chloral hydrate is addicting and habituating.
- have kidney failure (severe). Although a dosage adjustment is not generally required for patients who have mild kidney dysfunction, it may be required for patients who have severe kidney dysfunction. Collaboration with the patient's family physician or nephrologist is indicated.
- have liver dysfunction (severe)
- have obstructive sleep apnea. Chloral hydrate may exacerbate this condition.
- have pain disorders. Chloral hydrate has little analgesic action and may produce excitement or delirium among these patients, particularly if their pain is ineffectively managed.

Caution patients who are receiving chloral hydrate pharmacotherapy against performing activities that require alertness, judgment, and physical coordination (e.g., driving an automobile, operating dangerous equipment, supervising children) until their response to chloral hydrate is known. Chloral hydrate pharmacotherapy may adversely affect these mental and physical functions.

CLINICALLY SIGNIFICANT DRUG INTERACTIONS

Concurrent chloral hydrate pharmacotherapy and the following may result in clinically significant drug interactions:

Alcohol Use

Concurrent use of alcohol and chloral hydrate produces additive and possibly synergistic CNS depression. A vasodilation reaction also may occur when alcohol and chloral hydrate are ingested concurrently. Caution patients regarding these interactions and advise them to avoid, or limit, their use of alcohol while receiving chloral hydrate pharmacotherapy.

Anticoagulant (Oral) Pharmacotherapy

Chloral hydrate may displace oral anticoagulants (e.g., warfarin [Coumadin®]) from plasma protein binding sites. This interaction may result in increased anticoagulant action and excessive bleeding. When chloral hydrate pharmacotherapy is initiated or discontinued, or when dosage changes are made, frequent prothrombin time determinations are required. Collaboration with the prescriber of the anticoagulant is indicated.

Furosemide Pharmacotherapy

Concurrent chloral hydrate and intravenous furosemide (Lasix®) pharmacotherapy has been associated with blood pressure variations, flushing, profuse sweating (diaphoresis), and uneasiness. The mechanism of this interaction is unknown. Caution is required when furosemide is intravenously injected within 24 hours of chloral hydrate use. Collaboration with the prescriber of the furosemide is indicated.

Pharmacotherapy With Central Nervous System Depressants and Other Drugs That Produce Central Nervous System Depression

Concurrent chloral hydrate pharmacotherapy with opiate analgesics, other sedative-hypnotics, or other drugs that produce CNS depression (e.g., antihistamines, phenothiazines, TCAs) may result in additive CNS depression.

ADVERSE DRUG REACTIONS

Chloral hydrate pharmacotherapy is generally well tolerated. However, pharmacotherapy with the oral syrup formulation has been frequently associated with an unpleasant taste, flatulence, gastrointestinal irritation, diarrhea, nausea, stomach pain, and vomiting. Gastrointestinal reactions have been rarely associated with the oral capsules. Toxicity associated with long-term regular use may produce signs of gastritis, hypotension, kidney damage, myocardial depression, peripheral vasodilation, and skin rash. Chloral hydrate pharmacotherapy also has been associated with the following ADRs, listed according to body system:

Cardiovascular: Higher dosages of chloral hydrate reportedly may produce atrial and ventricular dysrhythmias, depression of myocardial contractility, hypotension, shortening of the refractory period, and torsade de pointes (i.e., rapid ventricular tachycardia characterized by a gradually changing QRS complex in the ECG that may result in ventricular fibrillation). Patients who have histories of cardiovascular dysfunction are highly susceptible to toxicity.

CNS: Chloral hydrate's CNS depressant action has been associated with such ADRs as confusion, drowsiness, headaches, incoordination (ataxia), lightheadedness, malaise, nightmares, and vertigo. Although a hangover effect may occur, it occurs less commonly than with barbiturate or some benzodiazepine pharmacotherapy. Chloral hydrate pharmacotherapy also has been rarely associated with idiosyncratic and paradoxical reactions. These reactions include delirium, disorientation, excitement (unusual), hallucinations, incoherence, and paranoia.

Cutaneous: Although uncommon, cutaneous reactions may include angioedema, bullous lesions, eczematoid dermatitis, erythema multiforme, erythematous rash, hives (urticaria), nonthrombocytopenic purpura, and scarlatiniform exanthema. Some cutaneous reactions are accompanied by fever. Chloral hydrate also is an irritant of the skin and mucous membranes. Avoid direct skin contact with the oral syrup.

GI: A case of ileus involving an infant has been reported.

Hematologic: Eosinophilia and leukopenia have been reported.

Metabolic/Endocrine: Chloral hydrate has precipitated attacks of acute intermittent porphyria. Ketonuria rarely has been reported.

Ocular: Chloral hydrate pharmacotherapy may cause oculo-toxicities with allergic conjunctivitis or keratoconjunctivitis and ptosis (drooping eyelid).

Otic: Increased middle ear pressure among infants and children has been reported.

Respiratory: Life-threatening respiratory obstruction has been reported among young children. However, therapeutic dosages of chloral hydrate have little effect on respirations and blood pressure. Higher dosages may cause depression of respiratory and vasomotor centers.

OVERDOSAGE

Signs and symptoms of acute chloral hydrate overdosage resemble barbiturate overdosage. These signs and symptoms include CNS depression and deep coma, respiratory depression, hypotension, and cardiac dysrhythmias. Cardiac dysrhythmias account for most overdosage fatalities. Gastritis, nausea, and vomiting are common. Gastric necrosis, perforation, GI hemorrhage, and esophageal stricture also have been reported. Other signs and symptoms may include abnormal contraction of the pupils or pinpoint pupils (miosis), cyanosis, hypothermia, kidney damage with albuminuria, liver damage with jaundice, muscle flaccidity, and pulmonary edema. The usual lethal dose is 10 grams. However, fatalities have been reported with overdosages of as little as 4 grams. Survival has been documented with overdosages of as much as 30 grams. Chloral hydrate overdosage requires emergency symptomatic medical support of body systems with attention to increasing chloral hydrate elimination. There is no known antidote.

CHLORDIAZEPOXIDE

(klor dye az e pox'ide)

TRADE NAMES

Librium®
Novo-Poxide®

CLASSIFICATION

Sedative-Hypnotic (Benzodiazepine) (C-IV)

See also Benzodiazepines General Monograph

APPROVED INDICATIONS FOR PSYCHOLOGICAL DISORDERS

Adjunctive pharmacotherapy for the short-term symptomatic management of:

- Anxiety Disorders, Other Than Panic Disorder. Chlordiazepoxide pharmacotherapy is *not* indicated for the symptomatic management of panic disorder nor is it indicated for the symptomatic management of everyday anxiety or tension, or for anxiety that can be managed with psychotherapy alone. Chlordiazepoxide pharmacotherapy also is *not* recommended for the management of anxiety associated with depression because it has the potential to exacerbate the depression while alleviating the anxiety. The depression associated with anxiety generally resolves with appropriate adjunctive pharmacotherapy (i.e., antidepressant pharmacotherapy) and psychotherapy.
- Substance-Related Disorders: Alcohol Withdrawal Syndrome

USUAL DOSAGE AND ADMINISTRATION

Anxiety Disorders, Other Than Panic Disorder

Adults:　Dosage is determined by the signs and symptoms of anxiety and individual patient response.

MILD OR MODERATE ANXIETY:　15 to 40 mg daily orally in three or four divided doses, as needed

SEVERE ANXIETY:　Initially, 50 to 100 mg intramuscularly or intravenously; then 75 to 150 mg daily orally in three or four divided doses, as needed

MAXIMUM:　300 mg daily intramuscularly, intravenously, or orally

Women who are, or who may become, pregnant: FDA Pregnancy Category D. Safety and efficacy of chlordiazepoxide pharmacotherapy for women who are pregnant have not been established. Chlordiazepoxide readily crosses the placental barrier. Fetal blood concentrations are approximately equal to maternal blood concentrations. Chlordiazepoxide appears to be relatively safe for the developing embryo and fetus when prescribed during pregnancy. However, some studies have suggested an increased risk for congenital malformations (i.e., birth defects) for several benzodiazepines, including chlordiazepoxide, when prescribed during the first three months (first trimester) of pregnancy.

Maternal use of benzodiazepines during pregnancy also may result in the neonatal benzodiazepine withdrawal syndrome. This syndrome is characterized by crying, insomnia, irritability, and poor breast-feeding among newborns. Avoid prescribing chlordiazepoxide pharmacotherapy to women who are pregnant. If chlordiazepoxide pharmacotherapy is required, advise patients of potential benefits and possible risks to themselves and the embryo, fetus, and neonate. Collaboration with the patient's obstetrician is indicated.

Women who are breast-feeding: Safety and efficacy of chlordiazepoxide pharmacotherapy for women who are breast-feeding and their neonates and infants have not been established. Chlordiazepoxide is excreted into breast milk. Breast-fed neonates and infants may display drowsiness or lethargy. They also may become addicted. Avoid prescribing chlordiazepoxide pharmacotherapy to women who are breast-feeding. If chlordiazepoxide pharmacotherapy is required, breast-feeding probably should be discontinued. If desired, lactation may be maintained and breast-feeding resumed following the discontinuation of short-term chlordiazepoxide pharmacotherapy. Collaboration with the patient's pediatrician is indicated.

Elderly, frail, or debilitated patients: Initially, 10 to 20 mg daily orally in two to four divided doses. Increase the dosage gradually, if needed, according to individual patient response. Generally prescribe lower dosages for elderly, frail, or debilitated patients. These patients may be more sensitive to the pharmacologic actions of chlordiazepoxide than are younger or healthier adult patients. Initially, prescribe the lowest effective dosage that does not cause incoordination (ataxia) or over-sedation.

Children 6 years of age and older: Initially, 10 to 40 mg daily orally in two to four divided doses, as needed. Increase the dosage to 60 mg daily in two to four divided doses, as needed.

Notes, Anxiety Disorders Other Than Panic Disorder

The optimal dosage varies in regard to the signs and symptoms of the psychological disorder being treated and individual patient response. Prescribe the lowest effective dosage adjusted to individual patient response. Periodic blood counts and liver function tests are recommended for patients who require long-term chlordiazepoxide pharmacotherapy. Chlordiazepoxide is addicting and habituating. Avoid abrupt discontinuation of long-term chlordiazepoxide pharmacotherapy because of the possibility of precipitating the benzodiazepine withdrawal syndrome. To discontinue chlordiazepoxide pharmacotherapy, reduce the dosage gradually, and monitor individual patient response carefully.

Injectable Pharmacotherapy   The maximum recommended injectable dosage is 300 mg daily in divided doses. Generally, the acute signs and symptoms of anxiety (or alcohol withdrawal) may be rapidly controlled by intramuscular or intravenous chlordiazepoxide pharmacotherapy. Replace injectable pharmacotherapy with oral pharmacotherapy as soon as possible. Injectable pharmacotherapy has occasionally produced mild transitory fluctuations in blood pressure. This action has not been generally clinically problematic, and emergency supportive medical management has not been required. Some patients may become drowsy or unsteady following the injection of chlordiazepoxide. Thus, patients should lie down for injectable chlordiazepoxide pharmacotherapy and remain lying down for 30 to 60 minutes following the injection.

INTRAMUSCULAR PHARMACOTHERAPY   For intramuscular injection, reconstitute injectable immediately before injection. Add the diluent supplied with the injectable formulation that is labeled for intramuscular use only, according to the manufacturer's directions. Do not use the diluent if the solution is cloudy. Once the diluent is added to the dry drug, agitate gently until a clear solution is obtained. Inject intramuscularly into a healthy muscle site (e.g., dorsogluteal or ventrogluteal sites). Do *not* inject intravenously because air bubbles are formed when the injectable is reconstituted for intramuscular use. Thus, intravenous injection of this intramuscular injectable formulation may result in an air embolism. Discard any unused drug appropriately.

INTRAVENOUS PHARMACOTHERAPY   Intravenous pharmacotherapy is indicated for the symptomatic management of acute agitation and hyperactivity associated with acute anxiety disorders. It also is indicated for the management of the alcohol withdrawal syndrome when rapid action is required and oral ingestion or intramuscular injection is not feasible. For intravenous injection, dilute 100 mg with 5 ml sterile water or isotonic sodium chloride (i.e., normal saline) for injection. Agitate gently. Do *not* add to intravenous fluids or mix with any other drugs. Do not dilute further. Inject intravenously slowly into a large lumen vein over one minute. Inject patients cautiously for whom a drop in blood pressure may lead to cardiac complications. The dosage may need to be reduced for patients who have liver dysfunction. Do *not* inject intramuscularly because the intravenous solution diluted with normal saline or sterile water for injection may cause significant pain upon intramuscular injection. Discard any unused drug appropriately.

Alcohol Withdrawal Syndrome

Adults: Initially, 50 to 100 mg intramuscularly, intravenously, or orally. Repeat every two to four hours, as needed, to a maximum of 300 mg daily. Initially, injectable pharmacotherapy is usually required for the management of the signs and symptoms associated with acute alcohol withdrawal.

MAXIMUM: 300 mg daily intramuscularly, intravenously, or orally

Women who are, or who may become, pregnant: FDA Pregnancy Category D. Safety and efficacy of chlordiazepoxide pharmacotherapy for women who are pregnant have not been established (see Usual Dosage and Administration, Anxiety Disorders). However, short-term pharmacotherapy associated with this indication (i.e., generally three to five days) would not be expected to pose a significant risk for the embryo, fetus, or neonate. Collaboration with the patient's obstetrician is indicated.

Women who are breast-feeding: Safety and efficacy of chlordiazepoxide pharmacotherapy for women who are breast-feeding and their neonates and infants have not been established. Chlordiazepoxide is excreted into breast milk. Breast-fed neonates and infants may display drowsiness or lethargy. They also may become addicted. Avoid prescribing chlordiazepoxide pharmacotherapy to women who are breast-feeding. If chlordiazepoxide pharmacotherapy is required, breast-feeding probably should be discontinued. If desired, lactation may be maintained and breast-feeding resumed following the discontinuation of short-term chlordiazepoxide pharmacotherapy. Collaboration with the patient's pediatrician is indicated.

Elderly, frail, or debilitated patients and those who have liver dysfunction: 25 to 50 mg intramuscularly, intravenously, or orally. Repeat every two to four hours, as needed, to a maximum of 150 mg daily. Initially prescribe lower dosages according to individual patient response. Elderly, frail, or debilitated patients and those who have liver dysfunction usually require one-half the recommended adult dosage because they may be more sensitive to chlordiazepoxide's CNS depressant action. Initially prescribe the lowest effective dosage that does not cause incoordination (ataxia) or over-sedation. Increase the dosage gradually, if needed, according to individual patient response.

MAXIMUM: 150 mg daily intramuscularly, intravenously, or orally

Children 12 years of age and younger: Safety and efficacy of chlordiazepoxide pharmacotherapy for the symptomatic management of the alcohol withdrawal syndrome for children 12 years of age and younger have not been established. Chlordiazepoxide pharmacotherapy for this indication is *not* recommended for this age group.

Adolescents 13 years of age and older: Initially, 25 to 50 mg intramuscularly, intravenously, or orally. Repeat the initial dose every two to four hours, as needed, to a maximum of 150 mg daily. Initially prescribe lower dosages for adolescents. Increase the dosage gradually according to individual patient response. Adolescents require usually one-half the recommended adult dosage.

MAXIMUM: 150 mg daily intramuscularly, intravenously, or orally

Notes, Alcohol Withdrawal Syndrome

See Notes, Anxiety Disorders Other Than Panic Disorder

AVAILABLE DOSAGE FORMS, STORAGE, AND COMPATIBILITY

Capsules, oral: 5, 10, 25 mg
Injectable, intramuscular or intravenous duplex pack: 100 mg. The duplex pack consists of one ampule of dry drug and one 2 ml ampule of special diluent for intramuscular injection. The dry drug also can be reconstituted with 5 ml of normal saline or sterile water for intravenous injection.
Tablets, oral: 5, 10, 25 mg

Notes

Store chlordiazepoxide capsules and tablets in tightly closed child- and light-resistant containers at controlled room temperature (15° to 30°C; 59° to 86°F). Store the duplex pack diluent at 2° to 8°C (36° to 46°F). Do not freeze. Do not use the diluent if the diluent is cloudy. Return the diluent to the dispensing pharmacy or manufacturer for safe and appropriate disposal. The dry drug supplied in the duplex pack may be stored at 15° to 30°C (59° to 86°F).

General Instructions for Patients   Instruct patients who are receiving chlordiazepoxide pharmacotherapy to

- safely store chlordiazepoxide capsules and tablets out of the reach of children in tightly closed child- and light-resistant containers at controlled room temperature (15° to 30°C; 59° to 86°F).
- obtain an available patient information sheet regarding chlordiazepoxide pharmacotherapy from their pharmacist at the time that their prescription is dispensed. Advise patients to clarify any questions that they may have concerning chlordiazepoxide pharmacotherapy with their pharmacist or, if needed, to consult their prescribing psychologist.

PROPOSED MECHANISM OF ACTION

Chlordiazepoxide has sedative, hypnotic, and muscle relaxant actions. The exact mechanisms of chlordiazepoxide's actions have not been fully determined. However, they appear to be mediated by the actions of the inhibitory neurotransmitter GABA. Chlordiazepoxide acts selectively on polysynaptic neuronal pathways and may inhibit, or augment, neuronal transmission, depending on the endogenous function of GABA.

See also Benzodiazepines General Monograph

PHARMACOKINETICS/PHARMACODYNAMICS

Chlordiazepoxide is completely absorbed (100%) following oral ingestion. Intramuscular absorption is generally slow and erratic. Following oral ingestion, chlordiazepoxide appears in the bloodstream in 30 to 60 minutes. Peak blood levels occur in 2 to 4 hours. After intramuscular injection, effects appear within 15 to 30 minutes and following intravenous injection, effects appear within 3 to 30 minutes. Chlordiazepoxide is highly plasma protein-bound (95% to 98%) and has an apparent volume of distribution of approximately 0.3 L/kg. Chlordiazepoxide is extensively metabolized primarily in the liver. Less than 2% is excreted in unchanged form in the urine. Chlordiazepoxide has several active metabolites, including desmethyldiazepam and oxazepam. The mean half-life of elimination is approximately 10 hours (range 5 to 30 hours). The mean total body clearance is ~ 35 ml/minute.

RELATIVE CONTRAINDICATIONS

Coma
Glaucoma, acute narrow-angle
Hypersensitivity to chlordiazepoxide or other benzodiazepines
Myasthenia gravis
Shock, acute

CAUTIONS AND COMMENTS

Long-term chlordiazepoxide pharmacotherapy, or regular personal use, may result in addiction and habituation. Addiction and habituation have been rarely associated with the use of recommended dosages of chlordiazepoxide. Abrupt discontinuation of long-term chlordiazepoxide pharmacotherapy, or regular personal use, may result in the chlordiazepoxide withdrawal syndrome.

See Benzodiazepines General Monograph

Prescribe chlordiazepoxide pharmacotherapy cautiously for patients who

- are elderly, frail, or debilitated. These patients may be more susceptible to the CNS depressant actions of chlordiazepoxide.
- have histories of problematic patterns of alcohol or other abusable psychotropic use. These patients may be at risk for developing problematic patterns of chlordiazepoxide use.
- have liver or kidney dysfunction (severe).

Caution patients who are receiving chlordiazepoxide pharmacotherapy against

- drinking alcohol while receiving chlordiazepoxide pharmacotherapy. Alcohol can increase the CNS depressant action of chlordiazepoxide significantly.
- performing activities that require alertness, judgment, and physical coordination (e.g., driving an automobile, operating dangerous equipment, supervising children). Chlordiazepoxide's CNS depressant actions may adversely affect these mental and physical functions.

In addition to these general precautions for patients, caution women to inform their prescribing psychologist if they become, or intend to become, pregnant while receiving chlordiazepoxide pharmacotherapy, so that their pharmacotherapy can be safely discontinued.

CLINICALLY SIGNIFICANT DRUG INTERACTIONS

Concurrent chlordiazepoxide pharmacotherapy and the following may result in clinically significant drug interactions:

Alcohol Use

Concurrent alcohol use may increase the CNS depressant action of chlordiazepoxide. Advise patients to avoid, or limit, their use of alcohol while receiving chlordiazepoxide pharmacotherapy.

Pharmacotherapy With Central Nervous System Depressants and Other Drugs That Produce Central Nervous System Depression

Concurrent chlordiazepoxide pharmacotherapy with opiate analgesics, other sedative-hypnotics, or other drugs that produce CNS depression (e.g., antihistamines, phenothiazines, TCAs) may result in additive CNS depression.

See also Benzodiazepines General Monograph

ADVERSE DRUG REACTIONS

Chlordiazepoxide pharmacotherapy has been associated with the following ADRs, listed according to body system. Most ADRs occur infrequently and can be generally managed by reducing the dosage.

> **Cardiovascular:** fainting (syncope)
> **CNS:** confusion; drowsiness; extrapyramidal reactions; EEG pattern alterations (e.g., low voltage, fast activity), which may appear during or following chlordiazepoxide pharmacotherapy; incoordination (ataxia); and paradoxical reactions (e.g., elevation of mood, rage, unusual excitement), particularly among patients who have histories of psychoses or children who are hyperactive and aggressive. These paradoxical reactions may be secondary to the relief of the signs and symptoms of anxiety. Monitor patients for these reactions, particularly during initial pharmacotherapy.
> **Cutaneous:** edema and skin eruptions
> **Genitourinary:** rarely, changes in sex drive (increase or decrease)
> **GI:** constipation and nausea
> **Hematologic:** blood disorders, including leukopenia and agranulocytosis (rare)
> **Hepatic:** jaundice and liver dysfunction (occasionally)

See also Benzodiazepines General Monograph

OVERDOSAGE

Signs and symptoms of chlordiazepoxide overdosage include confusion, diminished reflexes, drowsiness, incoordination (ataxia), and coma. Depression of the cardiovascular and respiratory centers may occur. Chlordiazepoxide overdosage requires emergency symptomatic medical support of body systems with attention to increasing chlordiazepoxide elimination. Flumazenil (Anexate®, Romazicon®), the benzodiazepine antagonist, may be required.

CHLORMEZANONE*

(klor'mez a none)

TRADE NAME

Trancopal®

CLASSIFICATION

Sedative (nonhypnotic)

APPROVED INDICATIONS FOR PSYCHOLOGICAL DISORDERS

Adjunctive pharmacotherapy for the short-term symptomatic management of:

> Anxiety Disorders. Chlormezanone pharmacotherapy is *not* indicated for the management of the signs and symptoms of everyday anxiety or tension, or for anxiety that can be managed with psychotherapy alone. Chlormezanone pharmacotherapy also is *not* recommended for the management of anxiety associated with depression because it has the potential to exacerbate the depression while alleviating the anxiety. The anxiety associated with depression generally remits with appropriate adjunctive antidepressant pharmacotherapy and psychotherapy.

USUAL DOSAGE AND ADMINISTRATION

Anxiety Disorders

Adults: 300 to 800 mg daily orally in three or four divided doses, as needed

Women who are, or who may become, pregnant: FDA Pregnancy Category "not established." Safety and efficacy of chlormezanone pharmacotherapy for women who are pregnant have not been established. Avoid prescribing chlormezanone pharmacotherapy to women who are pregnant. If chlormezanone pharmacotherapy is required, advise patients of potential benefits and possible risks to themselves and the embryo, fetus, or neonate. Collaboration with the patient's obstetrician is required.

Women who are breast-feeding: Safety and efficacy of chlormezanone pharmacotherapy for women who are breast-feeding and their infants have not been established. Avoid prescribing chlormezanone pharmacotherapy to women who are breast-feeding. If chlormezanone is required, breast-feeding probably should be discontinued. If desired, lactation may be maintained and breast-feeding resumed following the discontinuation of short-term chlormezanone pharmacotherapy. Collaboration with the patient's pediatrician may be indicated.

Elderly, frail, or debilitated patients: Generally prescribe lower dosages for elderly, frail, or debilitated patients. Increase the dosage gradually, if needed, according to individual patient response. These patients may be more sensitive to the pharmacologic actions of chlormezanone than are younger or healthier adult patients.

Children younger than 5 years of age: Safety and efficacy of chlormezanone pharmacotherapy for children younger than 5 years of age have not been established. Chlormezanone pharmacotherapy is *not* recommended for this age group.

Children 5 to 12 years of age: 150 to 400 mg daily orally in three or four divided doses, as needed

Notes, Anxiety Disorders

Initiate pharmacotherapy with the lowest recommended dosage and increase the dosage gradually, as needed, according to individual patient response. Individual response to sedative pharmacotherapy varies among patients, particularly children and elderly, frail, or debilitated patients. The management of the signs and symptoms of mild anxiety is often apparent within 15 to 30 minutes and may last for up to 6 hours or longer. Abrupt discontinuation of long-term chlormezanone pharmacotherapy, or regular personal use, may result in REM sleep rebound and sleep disturbance. Safety and efficacy of chlormezanone pharmacotherapy for longer than 4 months have not been established. Reevaluate patients who appear to require chlormezanone pharmacotherapy for longer than 4 months.

AVAILABLE DOSAGE FORMS, STORAGE, AND COMPATIBILITY

Tablets, oral caplets: 100, 200 mg

Notes

General Instructions to Patients Instruct patients who are receiving chlormezanone pharmacotherapy to

- safely store chlormezanone tablets out of the reach of children in child-resistant containers at controlled room temperature (15° to 30°C; 59° to 86°F).
- obtain an available patient information sheet regarding chlormezanone pharmacotherapy from their pharmacist at the time that their prescription is dispensed. Encourage patients to clarify any questions that they may have concerning chlormezanone pharmacotherapy with their pharmacist or, if needed, to consult their prescribing psychologist.

PROPOSED MECHANISM OF ACTION

Chlormezanone, a nonhypnotic sedative, provides symptomatic management of mild anxiety and tension. Its exact mechanism of action has not yet been fully determined.

PHARMACOKINETICS/PHARMACODYNAMICS

Chlormezanone is well absorbed following oral ingestion. Its onset of action is generally within 30 minutes and lasts for up to 6 hours. Additional data are unavailable.

RELATIVE CONTRAINDICATIONS

Hypersensitivity to chlormezanone

CAUTIONS AND COMMENTS

Caution patients who are receiving chlormezanone pharmacotherapy against

- drinking alcohol or using other drugs that produce CNS depression. Drinking alcohol or using other drugs that produce CNS depression during chlormezanone pharmacotherapy may result in excessive CNS depression.

- performing activities that require alertness, judgment, and physical coordination (e.g., driving an automobile, operating dangerous equipment, supervising children) until their response to chlormezanone is known. Chlormezanone's CNS depressant actions may adversely affect these mental and physical functions.

CLINICALLY SIGNIFICANT DRUG INTERACTIONS

Concurrent chlormezanone pharmacotherapy and the following may result in clinically significant drug interactions:

Alcohol Use

Concurrent alcohol use may increase the CNS depressant action of chlormezanone. Advise patients to avoid, or limit, their use of alcohol while receiving chlormezanone pharmacotherapy.

Pharmacotherapy With Central Nervous System Depressants and Other Drugs That Produce Central Nervous System Depression

Concurrent chlormezanone pharmacotherapy with opiate analgesics, other sedative-hypnotics, or other drugs that produce CNS depression (e.g., antihistamines, phenothiazines, TCAs) may result in additive CNS depression.

ADVERSE DRUG REACTIONS

Chlormezanone pharmacotherapy may require an adjustment in dosage or discontinuation if the patient exhibits any of the following ADRs, listed according to body system:

CNS: confusion, depression, dizziness, drowsiness, headache, and unusual excitement
Cutaneous: edema, erythema multiforme, flushing, rash, Stevens-Johnson syndrome (rare), and toxic epidermal necrolysis (rare)
Genitourinary: difficulty urinating
GI: nausea
Hepatic: cholestatic jaundice (rare and usually reversible with discontinuation of pharmacotherapy)
Musculoskeletal: tremor and weakness

OVERDOSAGE

Signs and symptoms of chlormezanone overdosage include absent reflexes, flaccidity, hypotension, and coma. These signs and symptoms have been observed following the ingestion of 7 grams of chlormezanone. Overdosage involving larger amounts of chlormezanone may result in alternation between coma and excitement. Chlormezanone overdosage requires emergency symptomatic medical support of body systems with attention to increasing chlormezanone elimination. There is no known antidote.

CHLORPROMAZINE

(klor proe'ma zeen)

TRADE NAMES

Chlorpromanyl®
Largactil®
Thorazine®

CLASSIFICATION

Antipsychotic (phenothiazine, propylamino derivative)

See also Phenothiazines General Monograph

APPROVED INDICATIONS FOR PSYCHOLOGICAL DISORDERS

Adjunctive pharmacotherapy for the symptomatic management of:

- Psychotic Disorders: Schizophrenia and Other Psychotic Disorders
- Severe Behavioral Disorders Among Children Characterized by Inappropriate Combativeness and Explosive Hyperexcitable Behavior

USUAL DOSAGE AND ADMINISTRATION

Schizophrenia and Other Psychotic Disorders

Adults: For prompt control of severe symptoms, 25 mg intramuscularly. Repeat dose in one hour, if needed. Replace injectable chlorpromazine pharmacotherapy with oral pharmacotherapy as soon as feasible. For less severe symptoms, initially, 30 to 75 mg daily orally in three divided doses. Increase the dosage gradually until signs and symptoms are managed. Maximal improvement may not be seen for several weeks or months. Continue the optimum daily chlorpromazine dosage for two weeks. Reduce the dosage gradually to the lowest effective maintenance dosage according to individual patient response.

MAINTENANCE: Generally, 30 to 1000 mg daily intramuscularly or orally in three to six divided doses. A daily dosage of 200 mg is not unusual. Some patients may require higher dosages. Patients who have been discharged from mental hospitals may require 800 mg daily. Stabilized patients may benefit from a single daily dose 30 minutes before retiring for bed in the evening.

MAXIMUM: 1000 mg daily intramuscularly or orally. Dosages exceeding 1000 mg daily generally have been associated with an increase in the frequency or severity of ADRs without a significant increase in therapeutic benefit.

Women who are, or who may become, pregnant: FDA Pregnancy Category C. Avoid prescribing chlorpromazine pharmacotherapy to women who are pregnant. Safety and efficacy of chlorpromazine pharmacotherapy for women who are pregnant have not been established. Conflicting data have been reported. Maternal chlorpromazine pharmacotherapy immediately before delivery has been associated with neonatal CNS depression and extrapyramidal reactions. If chlorpromazine pharmacotherapy is required, advise patients, or their legal guardians in regard to the patient, of potential benefits and possible risks to themselves and the embryo, fetus, or neonate. Collaboration with the patient's obstetrician is indicated.

Women who are breast-feeding: Avoid prescribing chlorpromazine pharmacotherapy to women who are breast-feeding. Safety and efficacy of chlorpromazine pharmacotherapy for women who are breast-feeding and their neonates and infants have not been established. Chlorpromazine is excreted in breast milk and may cause drowsiness and lethargy among breast-fed neonates and infants. If chlorpromazine pharmacotherapy is required, breast-feeding probably should be discontinued. Collaboration with the patient's pediatrician is indicated.

Elderly, frail, or debilitated patients and those who have liver dysfunction: Initiate chlorpromazine pharmacotherapy with lower dosages, and increase the dosage gradually until signs and symptoms are controlled. Generally, lower dosages are sufficient to control signs and symptoms of schizophrenia or other psychotic disorders among elderly, frail, or debilitated patients. Adjust dosage according to individual patient response. Patients who have liver dysfunction also may require lower dosages. After signs and symptoms have been controlled for a reasonable period of time, reduce the dosage gradually to the lowest effective maintenance dosage.

Children: Safety and efficacy of chlorpromazine pharmacotherapy for the symptomatic management of schizophrenia and other psychotic disorders among children have not been established. Chlorpromazine pharmacotherapy for these indications is *not* recommended for this age group.

Notes, Schizophrenia and Other Psychotic Disorders

Initiating and Maintaining Chlorpromazine Pharmacotherapy Prescribe the dosage according to the severity of the signs and symptoms of schizophrenia or other psychotic disorders. Adjust the dosage gradually according to individual patient response. Recognize that the milligram-for-milligram potency relationship among all dosage forms has not been established precisely clinically.

Prescribe chlorpromazine pharmacotherapy cautiously with attention to its potential to produce tardive dyskinesia. Prescribe long-term chlorpromazine pharmacotherapy only for patients who are known to benefit from antipsychotic pharmacotherapy and for whom alternative and equally effective and potentially less harmful pharmacotherapy is unavailable or inappropriate. Prescribe the lowest effective dosage for the shortest period of time. Reevaluate at regular intervals the need to adjust the maintenance dosage or discontinue chlorpromazine pharmacotherapy. If signs and symptoms of tardive dyskinesia are observed, discontinue chlorpromazine pharmacotherapy, whenever possible. Some patients may require continued chlorpromazine pharmacotherapy despite the presence of tardive dyskinesia.

INJECTABLE PHARMACOTHERAPY   Inject intramuscularly, slowly and deeply into large, healthy muscle sites. Rotate injection sites to avoid tissue irritation. Patients should lie down for injections and remain lying down for 30 to 60 minutes following injections because of associated postural hypotension. Increase the injectable dosage only for patients who do not experience associated postural hypotension. Avoid subcutaneous injection of chlorpromazine because of its potential to cause significant tissue irritation and serious tissue damage.

Discontinuing Chlorpromazine Pharmacotherapy   Although chlorpromazine pharmacotherapy has not been associated with the development of addiction and habituation, some signs and symptoms resembling those of physical withdrawal (e.g., dizziness, gastritis, nausea, tremors, vomiting) may occur following the abrupt discontinuation of high-dosage, long-term pharmacotherapy. These signs and symptoms can usually be avoided or minimized by gradually reducing the dosage. Anti-parkinsonian pharmacotherapy may be required for several weeks following the discontinuation of chlorpromazine pharmacotherapy.

Severe Behavioral Disorders Among Children

Children (hospitalized):   Prescribe the most appropriate method of administration and dosage according to the child's general age and severity of signs and symptoms. Generally initiate chlorpromazine pharmacotherapy with lower dosages. Increase the dosage gradually according to individual patient response.

INTRAMUSCULAR: For children who are younger than 5 years of age (or up to 50 lbs; 23 kg), do *not* exceed 40 mg daily; for children 5 to 12 years of age (or 50 to 100 lbs; 23 to 46 kg), do *not* exceed 75 mg daily, except for children who are otherwise unmanageable.

ORAL: Younger children may require 50 to 100 mg daily. Older children may require 200 mg or more daily. There is little evidence that improvement in behavior among severely disturbed mentally retarded children is further improved by daily dosages exceeding 500 mg.

Children (non-hospitalized):   Prescribe the most appropriate method of administration and dosage according to the child's body weight and severity of the signs and symptoms. Increase the dosage gradually according to individual patient response:

INTRAMUSCULAR: 0.25 mg/lb (0.55 mg/kg) every six to eight hours, as needed

ORAL: 0.25 mg/lb (0.55 mg/kg) every four to six hours, as needed

RECTAL: 0.5 mg/lb (1.1 mg/kg) every six to eight hours, as needed

Notes, Severe Behavioral Disorders Among Children

See Notes, Schizophrenia and Other Psychotic Disorders

AVAILABLE DOSAGE FORMS, STORAGE, AND COMPATIBILITY

Capsules, oral extended-release: 30, 75, 150, 200, 300 mg
Injectable, intramuscular: 25 mg/ml (ampules and multidose vials)
Concentrated solution, oral (Chlorpromazine Intensol®): 20, 30, 40, 100 mg/ml (for hospital
   and residential care) (contains 0.07% alcohol) (custard or peppermint flavored)
Suppositories, rectal: 25, 100 mg
Syrup, oral: 10, 50 mg/5 ml (orange-custard flavor)
Tablets, oral: 10, 25, 50, 100, 200 mg

Notes

Injectable Chlorpromazine Formulations   Inspect injectable solutions carefully for discoloration prior to use. Pink or otherwise discolored injectable solutions should be returned to
the dispensing pharmacy or manufacturer for safe and appropriate disposal. A slight yellowing
will not alter potency. However, do not use markedly discolored dark yellow solutions, and discard them appropriately. Avoid getting the injectable solution on the hands or clothing because
of associated contact dermatitis.

Chlorpromazine ampules and multidose vials contain benzyl alcohol, sodium bisulfite, and
sodium sulfite. Sulfites have been associated with hypersensitivity reactions, including anaphylactic signs and symptoms and life-threatening or less severe asthmatic episodes, among susceptible patients. Sulfite sensitivity is more frequently observed among patients who have asthma.

Oral Chlorpromazine Formulations

ORAL CONCENTRATED SOLUTION   To increase palatability, the oral concentrate can
be diluted in 60 to 120 ml (2 to 4 fluid ounces) of water or a compatible beverage (e.g., tomato
or fruit juice, milk, simple syrup, orange syrup, carbonated beverages, coffee, tea) just prior
to ingestion. The oral concentrate also can be gently mixed into a small amount of cold, soft
food (e.g., puddings or pureed foods). A precipitate will form if the oral concentrate is diluted
with beverages that do not have a pH between 4 and 5. Advise patients to avoid getting the oral
concentrate on the hands or clothing because of associated contact dermatitis.

The oral concentrate (e.g., Chlorpromanyl®) may contain sodium metabisulfite and sodium
sulfite. These sulfites have been associated with hypersensitivity reactions, including anaphylactic signs and symptoms and life-threatening or less severe asthmatic episodes, among susceptible patients. Sulfite sensitivity is more frequently observed among patients who have asthma.
The oral concentrate (e.g., Chlorpromanyl®) may also contain tartrazine (FD&C Yellow No. 5).
Tartrazine has been associated with hypersensitivity reactions (e.g., bronchial asthma) among
susceptible patients, particularly those who have a hypersensitivity to aspirin.

ORAL EXTENDED-RELEASE CAPSULES (SPANSULES®)   Patients who have been
stabilized on oral tablet or syrup dosage formulations may benefit from pharmacotherapy with the
oral extended-release capsule formulation. The daily dosage for the oral tablet and syrup dosage
forms of chlorpromazine can generally be applied to the Spansule® extended-release capsule
dosage form on the basis of total daily dosage in milligrams. The Spansule® is formulated so
that the initial dose is released promptly and the remaining dose is released over a prolonged
period.

ORAL SYRUP   The oral syrup is light sensitive and is dispensed in amber glass bottles. The oral syrup is custard flavored and may be preferred by some patients.

ORAL TABLETS   The 100 mg and 200 mg tablets are generally prescribed for patients who require high dosages for the symptomatic management of severe psychotic disorders.

Rectal Formulations (suppositories)   Refrigerate suppositories between 2° and 8°C (36° and 46°F).

General Instructions for Patients   Instruct patients who are receiving chlorpromazine pharmacotherapy (or their legal guardians in regard to the patient) to

- protect the chlorpromazine oral dosage forms from light.
- safely store the chlorpromazine oral dosage forms out of the reach of children in child-resistant containers at controlled room temperature (15° to 30°C; 59° to 86°F). Oral dosage forms do not require refrigeration.
- safely store the chlorpromazine rectal suppositories under refrigeration between 2° and 8°C (36° and 46°F) and out of the reach of children.
- obtain an available patient information sheet regarding chlorpromazine pharmacotherapy from their pharmacist at the time that their prescription is dispensed. Encourage patients to clarify any questions that they may have concerning chlorpromazine pharmacotherapy with their pharmacist or, if needed, to consult their prescribing psychologist.

PROPOSED MECHANISM OF ACTION

The exact mechanism of action by which chlorpromazine exerts its antipsychotic action is complex and has not yet been fully determined. Although chlorpromazine's principal therapeutic actions are for the management of psychotic disorders, it also exerts sedative and antiemetic activity. Chlorpromazine acts at all levels of the CNS, but primarily at the subcortical levels. It also acts on multiple body organ systems. Chlorpromazine has strong antiadrenergic and weak peripheral anticholinergic activity. Its ganglionic blocking action is relatively slight, as is its antihistamine and antiserotonin activity. Its antipsychotic activity appears to be primarily related to its interaction with dopamine-containing neurons. Specifically, chlorpromazine appears to block dopamine receptors both pre- and post-synaptically, particularly in the mesolimbic system.

See also the Phenothiazines General Monograph

PHARMACOKINETICS/PHARMACODYNAMICS

Chlorpromazine is readily absorbed following oral ingestion. However, it has limited oral bioavailability (i.e., approximately 33%) because of its significant first-pass hepatic metabolism. Chlorpromazine is highly plasma protein-bound (92% to 96%) and is widely distributed throughout the body. Its apparent volume of distribution is approximately 20 L/kg. Chlorpromazine is extensively metabolized in the liver, with less than 1% excreted in unchanged form in the urine. The mean half-life of elimination is approximately 30 hours (range 18 to 31 hours). The mean total body clearance is ∼630 ml/minute. Additional data are unavailable.

RELATIVE CONTRAINDICATIONS

Blood disorders

CNS depressant (e.g., alcohol, opiate analgesic, sedative-hypnotic) intoxication (severe) or overdosage

Coma

Heart disease, severe

Hypersensitivity to chlorpromazine or other phenothiazines. The injectable formulation contains benzyl alcohol and sulfites. The former is contraindicated among patients who are receiving disulfiram pharmacotherapy. The latter is contraindicated for patients who have histories of asthma.

Liver dysfunction

Parkinson's disease

CAUTIONS AND COMMENTS

Prescribe chlorpromazine pharmacotherapy cautiously to patients who

- have bone marrow depression or histories of hypersensitivity reactions (e.g., blood disorders) associated with previous chlorpromazine or other pharmacotherapy. If chlorpromazine pharmacotherapy is required for these patients, potential benefits must be weighed against possible risks.
- have cardiovascular dysfunction. See Adverse Drug Reactions.
- have exposure to extremely warm environmental temperatures, exposure to organophosphorous insecticides, or are receiving atropine or related drugs that can affect body temperature regulation
- have glaucoma. Chlorpromazine has anticholinergic actions that may exacerbate this condition.
- have histories of prolactin-dependent cancer. Antipsychotic drugs increase prolactin levels. Increased prolactin levels persist during long-term pharmacotherapy. Collaboration with the patient's oncologist may be indicated.
- have histories of seizure disorders. Chlorpromazine may lower the seizure threshold. Prescribe chlorpromazine with extreme caution for patients who have epilepsy or other seizure disorders. Patients who are concurrently receiving anticonvulsant pharmacotherapy may require dosage adjustments. Collaboration with the prescriber of the anticonvulsant is indicated.
- have kidney dysfunction
- have liver dysfunction. Patients who have histories of hepatic encephalopathy due to cirrhosis may have increased sensitivity to the CNS actions of chlorpromazine (e.g., impaired cerebration and abnormal slowing of the EEG). See also Adverse Drug Reactions.
- have medical disorders for which the antiemetic action of chlorpromazine may mask changes in their clinical conditions (e.g., the signs and symptoms of overdosage of other drugs; diagnosis and treatment of head injuries, brain tumors, or other medical disorders associated with increased intracranial pressure; intestinal obstruction; or Reye's syndrome). When prescribed for patients who are receiving cancer chemotherapy, vomiting as a sign of the toxicity associated with chemotherapy may be obscured by the antiemetic action of chlorpromazine.
- have respiratory dysfunction (e.g., severe asthma, emphysema, acute respiratory infections, particularly among children), because of its CNS depressant actions. Chlorpromazine can suppress the cough reflex. Aspiration of vomitus is possible.

Caution patients who are receiving chlorpromazine pharmacotherapy (or their legal guardians in regard to the patient) against

- direct skin contact with the oral concentrate and injectable solutions. Inadvertent skin contact with these dosage formulations has been associated with contact dermatitis.
- drinking alcohol or using other drugs that have CNS depressant actions. Concurrent use of alcohol or other drugs that produce CNS depression may result in excessive CNS depression and hypotension.
- performing activities that require alertness, judgment, and physical coordination (e.g., driving an automobile, operating dangerous equipment, supervising children). Chlorpromazine may adversely affect these mental and physical functions, especially during the first few days of pharmacotherapy.

In addition to these general precautions, caution patients in regard to the association between chlorpromazine pharmacotherapy and the possible development of tardive dyskinesia, particularly when long-term pharmacotherapy is being considered. Whenever possible, patients, or their legal guardians, should receive full information about this risk. The decision to inform patients and their guardians should take into consideration the clinical circumstances and the competency of the patient to understand the information provided.

CLINICALLY SIGNIFICANT DRUG INTERACTIONS

Concurrent chlorpromazine pharmacotherapy and the following may result in clinically significant drug interactions:

Alcohol Use

Concurrent alcohol use may increase the CNS depressant action of chlorpromazine. Advise patients to avoid, or limit, their use of alcohol while receiving chlorpromazine pharmacotherapy.

Anticoagulant (Oral) Pharmacotherapy

Chlorpromazine diminishes the action of oral anticoagulants (i.e., warfarin [Coumadin®]).

Anticonvulsant Pharmacotherapy

Chlorpromazine and other phenothiazines decrease the seizure threshold. Thus, an increase in the dosage of the anticonvulsant may be required. In addition, chlorpromazine interferes with the metabolism of phenytoin (Dilantin®). This interaction may result in phenytoin toxicity. However, chlorpromazine does not potentiate the anticonvulsant action of barbiturates. The barbiturate anticonvulsant dosage should not be reduced if chlorpromazine pharmacotherapy is initiated. Rather, chlorpromazine pharmacotherapy should be initiated at lower dosages and gradually increased, as needed, according to individual patient response. Collaboration with the prescriber of the anticonvulsant is indicated.

Guanethidine Pharmacotherapy

Chlorpromazine may decrease the neuronal uptake of guanethidine (Ismelin®) and, thus, decrease its hypotensive action. An adjustment in the guanethidine dosage may be required. To help to assure appropriate management of the patient's hypertension, collaboration with the prescriber of the guanethidine is indicated.

Pharmacotherapy With Anticholinergics and Other Drugs That Produce Anticholinergic Actions

Concurrent chlorpromazine pharmacotherapy with anticholinergics (e.g., atropine) or other drugs that produce anticholinergic actions (e.g., TCAs) may result in additive anticholinergic actions.

Pharmacotherapy With Central Nervous System Depressants and Other Drugs That Produce Central Nervous System Depression

Concurrent chlorpromazine pharmacotherapy with opiate analgesics, sedative-hypnotics, or other drugs that produce CNS depression (e.g., antihistamines, TCAs) may result in additive CNS depression. Chlorpromazine prolongs and intensifies the actions of these drugs. If concurrent pharmacotherapy is required, prescribe one-fourth to one-half the usual dosage of these drugs. Whenever possible, discontinue pharmacotherapy with other CNS depressants before initiating chlorpromazine pharmacotherapy. If necessary, the CNS depressant pharmacotherapy can be reinstituted at lower dosages and increased gradually, as needed.

Propranolol Pharmacotherapy

Concurrent chlorpromazine and propranolol (Inderal®) pharmacotherapy may result in the increased blood levels of both drugs.

Sympathomimetic Pharmacotherapy

The actions of sympathomimetics (e.g., amphetamines, ephedrine) may be blocked by chlorpromazine. Phenothiazines can produce alpha-adrenergic blockade and resultant effects including hypotension and nasal congestion.

Thiazide Diuretic Pharmacotherapy

Thiazide diuretics (e.g., hydrochlorothiazide [HydroDIURIL®]) may accentuate the postural hypotension associated with chlorpromazine and other phenothiazine pharmacotherapy.
See also Phenothiazines General Monograph

ADVERSE DRUG REACTIONS

Chlorpromazine pharmacotherapy has been commonly associated with anticholinergic ADRs (e.g., blurred vision; drowsiness; dry mouth; urinary retention). The following ADRs, listed according to body system, also have been associated with chlorpromazine pharmacotherapy. Some of these ADRs may be more likely to occur, or occur with a greater intensity, among patients who have concurrent medical disorders (e.g., patients who have mitral insufficiency or pheochromocytoma have experienced severe hypotension following recommended dosages of chlorpromazine).

Cardiovascular

Nonspecific ECG changes and Q-T wave distortions, usually reversible, have been reported among some patients receiving phenothiazine pharmacotherapy, including chlorpromazine. Sudden death, apparently due to cardiac arrest, has been reported.

Injectable chlorpromazine pharmacotherapy also has been associated with various cardiovascular ADRs. Postural hypotension, tachycardia, momentary fainting, and dizziness may occur after the first injection and occasionally with subsequent injections. Recovery is usually spontaneous within 1/2 to 2 hours. Occasionally, a more severe and prolonged shock-like condition may occur. To minimize postural hypotension following chlorpromazine injections, patients should be lying down for injections and should remain lying down for at least 30 minutes. To manage associated hypotension, keep the patient lying down in a head-low position with the legs raised. A vasoconstrictor may be required. Thus, initial injectable pharmacotherapy probably should be reserved for those situations where appropriate medical treatment for severe hypotensive reactions is readily available.

Central Nervous System

Mild to moderate drowsiness may occur, particularly during the first or second week of chlorpromazine pharmacotherapy. The drowsiness usually resolves with continued pharmacotherapy. If troublesome, reduce the dosage. Other ADRs affecting the CNS include catatonia (rare), cerebral edema, and petit mal and grand mal seizures, particularly among patients who have EEG abnormalities or a history of seizure disorders.

Chlorpromazine pharmacotherapy also is associated with the occurrence of two potentially serious clinical syndromes: (1) extrapyramidal reactions, including tardive dyskinesia; and (2) the NMS. The diagnosis and management of these syndromes may require collaboration with the patient's family physician or a specialist (e.g., neurologist).

Extrapyramidal Reactions   Extrapyramidal reactions include dystonias, motor restlessness, pseudoparkinsonism, and tardive dyskinesia. The EPRs associated with chlorpromazine pharmacotherapy appear to be dose related. If chlorpromazine pharmacotherapy is required for patients who have histories of EPRs associated with previous pharmacotherapy, reinstitute pharmacotherapy at lower dosages. However, do not reinstitute pharmacotherapy for children or pregnant women.

DYSTONIA: Signs and symptoms of dystonias may include spasm of the neck muscles progressing to acute, reversible torticollis; extensor rigidity of the back muscles, sometimes progressing to opisthotonos (i.e., head and heels are bent backward and the body is bowed forward); spasms of the wrist and foot (carpopedal spasm); clonic contraction of the muscles used for chewing (trismus); swallowing difficulty; oculogyric crisis (i.e., involuntary deviation and fixation of the eyeballs, usually upward, lasting for minutes or hours); and protrusion of the tongue. These reactions usually subside within a few hours after the discontinuation of chlorpromazine pharmacotherapy and almost always subside within 24 to 48 hours.

In mild cases, psychological support is often sufficient. In moderate cases, barbiturate pharmacotherapy may be required for the rapid relief of these ADRs. In more severe cases, an antiparkinsonian drug, other than levodopa, may be required for the rapid reversal of signs and symptoms. For children, these ADRs can be usually managed with psychological support and barbiturate pharmacotherapy. Injectable diphenhydramine pharmacotherapy also may be helpful. If these countermeasures are ineffective, reevaluate the diagnosis. Collaboration with the patient's family physician or a specialist (e.g., neurologist) may be required.

MOTOR RESTLESSNESS: Signs and symptoms of motor restlessness may include agitation, insomnia, jitteriness, or signs and symptoms similar to the patient's original signs and symptoms of psychosis. Motor restlessness often disappears spontaneously with continued pharmacotherapy. Dosage should be increased until these ADRs have subsided. If too troublesome, they can usually be managed by a reduction of dosage, changing the patient's antipsychotic pharmacotherapy, or prescribing additional pharmacotherapy with an anti-parkinsonian, benzodiazepine, or beta-adrenergic blocker (e.g., propranolol). Collaboration with the patient's family physician or a specialist (e.g., neurologist) may be required.

PSEUDOPARKINSONISM: Signs and symptoms of pseudoparkinsonism may include cogwheel rigidity and shuffling gait, drooling, mask-like facies, pill-rolling motion of the hands, and tremors. In most cases, these signs and symptoms can be managed with concurrent anti-parkinsonian pharmacotherapy (other than levodopa) for a few weeks to two or three months. (*Note:* Levodopa pharmacotherapy has *not* been found effective for managing phenothiazine-induced pseudoparkinsonism.) After this time, patients should be reevaluated to determine their need for continued anti-parkinsonian pharmacotherapy. Some patients may require a reduction in their chlorpromazine dosage or discontinuation of their chlorpromazine pharmacotherapy. Anti-parkinsonian pharmacotherapy should only be used when required.

TARDIVE DYSKINESIA: Signs and symptoms of TD may include rhythmical involuntary movements of the face, jaw, mouth, and tongue (e.g., puffing of cheeks, chewing movements, puckering of mouth, protruding tongue). Sometimes these signs and symptoms may be accompanied by involuntary movements of the extremities. Involuntary movements are rarely the only signs and symptoms of tardive dyskinesia. A variant of tardive dyskinesia, tardive dystonia, has also been described.

Tardive dyskinesia is usually associated with long-term chlorpromazine pharmacotherapy but also may occur, although less frequently, after relatively brief periods of low-dosage chlorpromazine pharmacotherapy or after chlorpromazine pharmacotherapy has been discontinued. Tardive dyskinesia may occur among patients of all ages. However, it appears most commonly among elderly patients, especially elderly women. Unfortunately, it is impossible to predict which patients will develop TD. It is important to identify early signs and symptoms of the syndrome because TD is persistent and, for some patients, may be irreversible. An early sign of the syndrome is fine vermicular movements of the tongue. If chlorpromazine pharmacotherapy is immediately discontinued when fine vermicular movements of the tongue are first noted, the development of the full syndrome may be prevented.

If other signs and symptoms are identified, discontinue chlorpromazine pharmacotherapy and all other antipsychotic pharmacotherapy. Unfortunately, some patients may require reinstitution of chlorpromazine pharmacotherapy. An increase in the dosage, or a change to another antipsychotic drug, may mask the syndrome. There is no known effective treatment for TD. Anti-parkinsonian pharmacotherapy does *not* alleviate its signs and symptoms.

Neuroleptic Malignant Syndrome   The NMS is a potentially fatal syndrome associated with chlorpromazine and other antipsychotic pharmacotherapy. Signs and symptoms of NMS may include altered mental states, autonomic nervous system instability (e.g., cardiac dysrhythmias, diaphoresis, irregular pulse, fluctuation of blood pressure, tachycardia), hyperpyrexia, and muscle rigidity. The diagnosis of NMS requires the identification of concurrent untreated or unresponsive EPRs and serious medical disorders (e.g., pneumonia, systemic infection). Thus, collaboration with the patient's family physician is required. Other signs and symptoms important for the differential diagnosis of NMS include central anticholinergic toxicity, drug fever, heat stroke, and primary CNS pathology.

The management of NMS includes (1) immediate discontinuation of chlorpromazine pharmacotherapy and any other antipsychotic or nonessential pharmacotherapy, (2) intensive symptomatic medical treatment of diagnosed medical disorders, and (3) aggressive symptomatic medical treatment of other signs and symptoms of the NMS. There is no general consensus regarding the specific pharmacotherapy for the management of uncomplicated NMS. Patients who require the reinstitution of antipsychotic pharmacotherapy after their recovery from NMS require a cautious reintroduction of their pharmacotherapy and careful monitoring for the recurrence of NMS.

Cutaneous

Chlorpromazine concentrated oral solution and the injectable formulation are irritating to the skin. Avoid skin contact, and advise patients to avoid skin contact. Also advise patients to dilute each dose of the oral concentrate before ingestion to avoid irritating the mucous membranes of the mouth and throat. A mild urticarial type of photosensitivity has also been reported. Advise patients to avoid undue exposure to sunlight. More severe reactions, including exfoliative dermatitis, have also occasionally been reported.

Long-term high-dosage chlorpromazine pharmacotherapy has been rarely associated with skin pigmentation (see also Ocular). This ADR has been observed among hospitalized patients, particularly women, who have received chlorpromazine pharmacotherapy for three years or longer with dosages ranging from 500 to 1500 mg daily. The pigmentary changes, restricted to exposed skin areas, range from an almost imperceptible darkening of the skin to a slate gray discoloration of the skin, sometimes with a violet hue. Histology reveals a pigment, chiefly in the dermis, which is probably a melanin-like complex. The pigmentation may fade following the discontinuation of chlorpromazine pharmacotherapy.

Gastrointestinal

Chlorpromazine pharmacotherapy has been associated with adynamic ileus, atonic colon, constipation, dry mouth, nausea, and obstipation (extreme constipation).

Genitourinary

Chlorpromazine pharmacotherapy has been associated with ejaculatory disorders, impotence, priapism, and urinary retention. Chlorpromazine may discolor urine pink or red-brown. Warn patients of this possible color change of the urine to prevent undue concern.

Hematologic

Chlorpromazine pharmacotherapy has been associated with the development of several blood disorders, including agranulocytosis, eosinophilia, leukopenia, hemolytic anemia, aplastic anemia, thrombocytopenia, purpura, and pancytopenia.

Agranulocytosis: Most cases of agranulocytosis (deficit or absolute lack of granulocytic white blood cells, i.e., basophils, eosinophils, and neutrophils) have occurred between one and three months of pharmacotherapy. Monitor patients closely, and periodically obtain blood counts during this time period. Also monitor patients and periodically obtain blood counts during the course of long-term chlorpromazine pharmacotherapy. Advise patients to immediately report the sudden appearance of a sore throat or other signs and symptoms of infection. Collaboration with the patient's family physician or a specialist (e.g., hematologist) may be required. If white blood cell and differential counts indicate cellular depression, discontinue chlorpromazine pharmacotherapy immediately. Antibiotic pharmacotherapy or other suitable medical treatment may be required. Moderate suppression of white blood cells without signs and symptoms of infection does not usually require discontinuation of chlorpromazine pharmacotherapy.

Hepatic

Chlorpromazine pharmacotherapy has been associated with a low incidence of jaundice. Considered to be a hypersensitivity reaction, the jaundice occurs most commonly between the second and fourth weeks of pharmacotherapy. The reaction resembles infectious hepatitis. However, laboratory features of obstructive jaundice, rather than those of parenchymal damage, are characteristic. Although the jaundice is usually promptly reversible with the discontinuation of chlorpromazine pharmacotherapy, chronic jaundice also has been reported.

There is no evidence that preexisting liver dysfunction predisposes patients to jaundice. Patients who have histories of alcoholism with cirrhosis have been successfully treated with chlorpromazine for their psychotic disorders without hepatic ADRs. However, caution is required when chlorpromazine pharmacotherapy is prescribed to patients who have histories of liver dysfunction. Patients who have a history of jaundice associated with previous chlorpromazine or other phenothiazine pharmacotherapy should not, if possible, be reexposed to phenothiazines.

If fever with grippe-like signs and symptoms occurs, appropriate liver function studies should be obtained. If tests indicate abnormality, chlorpromazine pharmacotherapy should be discontinued. Collaboration with a the patient's family physician or a specialist (e.g., internist) is required.

Ocular

In addition to miosis or mydriasis (abnormal contraction or dilation of the pupils, respectively), several ADRs affecting the ocular system have been associated with chlorpromazine pharmacotherapy. Ocular changes have occurred more frequently than skin pigmentation changes (see Cutaneous). These changes have been reported more commonly among patients who have received chlorpromazine pharmacotherapy for two years or longer and with daily dosages of 300 mg or more.

The ocular changes are characterized by the deposition of fine particulate matter in the lens and cornea. In more advanced cases, star-shaped opacities have also been reported in the anterior portion of the lens. The nature of the ocular deposits has not yet been determined. Severe ocular changes with visual impairment have occurred among a small number of patients. In addition to corneal and lenticular changes, epithelial keratopathy and pigmentary retinopathy have been reported.

These ocular changes may remit after chlorpromazine pharmacotherapy is discontinued. However, it is recommended that patients who are receiving long-term moderate- to high-dosage chlorpromazine pharmacotherapy have periodic eye examinations. The ocular changes may also be associated with exposure to light. Thus, these patients should be cautioned to protect their eyes from excessive sunlight. In the event that ocular changes are noted, the benefits of continued chlorpromazine pharmacotherapy should be weighed against the possible risks for irreversible ocular damage. Depending on the individual patient, a decision to continue, lower the dosage of, or discontinue chlorpromazine pharmacotherapy may be required. Collaboration with the patient's family physician or ophthalmologist is required.

Respiratory

Asthma, laryngeal edema, and nasal congestion

Miscellaneous

Mild fever may occur after large intramuscular doses. Angioneurotic edema, anaphylactic reactions, hyperpyrexia, increased appetite with weight gain, peripheral edema, and a systemic lupus erythematosus-like syndrome have been reported.

Note: There have been occasional reports of sudden death among patients receiving phenothiazine pharmacotherapy. In some cases, the cause appears to have been cardiac arrest or asphyxia due to failure of the cough reflex.

See also Phenothiazines General Monograph

OVERDOSAGE

Signs and symptoms of chlorpromazine overdosage include agitation and restlessness, anticholinergic reactions (e.g., cardiac dysrhythmias, including ECG changes; dry mouth; fever; hypotension; ileus), coma, convulsions, and somnolence. Chlorpromazine overdosage requires emergency symptomatic medical support of body systems with attention to increasing chlorpromazine elimination. There is no known antidote.

CLOMIPRAMINE

(kloe mi'pra meen)

TRADE NAMES

Anafranil®
Novo-Clopamine®

CLASSIFICATION

Antidepressant (tricyclic)

See also Tricyclic Antidepressants General Monograph

APPROVED INDICATIONS FOR PSYCHOLOGICAL DISORDERS

Adjunctive pharmacotherapy for the symptomatic management of:

- Anxiety Disorders: Obsessive-Compulsive Disorder. For a definitive diagnosis, obsessions and compulsions must cause marked distress, be time consuming, or significantly interfere with personal and social functioning, including occupational functioning.
- Mood Disorders, Depressive Disorders: Major Depressive Disorder

USUAL DOSAGE AND ADMINISTRATION

Major Depressive Disorder

Adults: Initially, 25 mg daily orally. May increase the daily dosage, according to individual patient response, by 25 mg increments at three to four day intervals to a total daily dosage of 150 mg by the end of two weeks. Thereafter, may increase the dosage gradually over a period of several weeks to 200 mg daily. Dosages exceeding 200 mg daily are not recommended for non-hospitalized patients. Occasionally, severely depressed hospitalized patients may require dosages up to 300 mg daily.

MAINTENANCE: Prescribe the lowest effective dosage. To minimize associated day time sedation, the total daily dosage may be prescribed as a single daily dose 30 minutes before retiring for bed in the evening. Continue maintenance pharmacotherapy for the expected duration of the depressive episode in order to minimize the possibility of relapse following clinical improvement.

Women who are, or who may become, pregnant: FDA Pregnancy Category C. Avoid prescribing clomipramine to women who are pregnant, particularly during the third trimester of pregnancy. Safety and efficacy of clomipramine pharmacotherapy for women who are pregnant have not been established. Signs and symptoms resembling a withdrawal syndrome, including tremors, convulsions, and respiratory depression, have been reported among neonates whose mothers received clomipramine pharmacotherapy during the third trimester of pregnancy. If clomipramine pharmacotherapy is required, advise patients of potential benefits and possible risks to themselves and the embryo, fetus, or neonate. Collaboration with the patient's obstetrician is indicated.

Women who are breast-feeding: Safety and efficacy of clomipramine pharmacotherapy for women who are breast-feeding and their neonates and infants have not been established. Clomipramine is excreted in breast milk. Avoid prescribing clomipramine pharmacotherapy to women who are breast-feeding. If clomipramine pharmacotherapy is required, breast-feeding probably should be discontinued. Collaboration with the patient's pediatrician may be required.

Elderly, frail, or debilitated patients: Initially, 20 to 30 mg daily orally in divided doses. Increase the daily dosage gradually by 10 mg increments according to individual patient response. Generally, lower dosages are recommended for elderly, frail, or debilitated patients. These patients may be more sensitive to the pharmacologic actions of clomipramine than are younger or healthier adult patients. Monitor blood pressure and cardiac rhythm regularly, particularly among patients who have unstable cardiovascular function. Collaboration with the patient's family physician or a specialist (e.g., cardiologist, gerontologist) is indicated.

MAINTENANCE: Prescribe the lowest effective dosage. To minimize day time sedation, the total daily dosage may be prescribed as a single daily dose 30 minutes before retiring for bed in the evening. Continue maintenance pharmacotherapy for the expected duration of the depressive episode in order to minimize the possibility of relapse following clinical improvement.

Children: Safety and efficacy of clomipramine pharmacotherapy for the symptomatic management of depression among children have not been established. Clomipramine pharmacotherapy for this indication is *not* recommended for this age group.

Notes, Major Depressive Disorder

Initiating Clomipramine Pharmacotherapy   Dosage should be individualized according to the patient's signs and symptoms and clinical response. Initiate clomipramine pharmacotherapy at the lowest recommended dosage, and increase the dosage gradually as recommended while monitoring individual patient response. During the initial dosage titration phase, the total daily dosage may be divided and ingested with meals to decrease associated GI irritation.

Steady-state plasma levels may not be achieved for two to three weeks after a dosage adjustment because of the long elimination half-life of clomipramine and its active metabolite, desmethylclomipramine. It may be advisable to wait two to three weeks after the initial dosage titration phase before attempting further dosage adjustments. A lag in therapeutic response usually occurs initially and may last for several days to a few weeks. Increasing the dosage does not usually shorten this latency period and may increase the incidence of ADRs.

Maintaining Clomipramine Pharmacotherapy   The safety and efficacy of long-term clomipramine pharmacotherapy (i.e., more than 10 weeks) have not been established. When long-term clomipramine pharmacotherapy is required, reevaluate the need for continued pharmacotherapy periodically.

Discontinuing Clomipramine Pharmacotherapy   A variety of signs and symptoms have been associated with the abrupt discontinuation of clomipramine pharmacotherapy. These signs and symptoms include dizziness, headache, hyperthermia, irritability, malaise, nausea, sleep disturbances, and vomiting. Patients also may experience a worsening of their psychological disorder. Although these effects have not been systematically evaluated, they have been frequently associated with the discontinuation of other related TCA pharmacotherapy. Discontinue clomipramine pharmacotherapy gradually while monitoring patient response.

Obsessive-Compulsive Disorder

Adults: Initially, 25 mg daily orally. May increase the daily dosage, according to individual patient response, by 25 mg increments at three or four day intervals to a total daily dosage of 100 to 150 mg by the end of two weeks. Thereafter, may increase the dosage gradually over a period of several weeks to 200 mg daily. Dosages exceeding 200 mg daily are not generally recommended for non-hospitalized patients. However, patients who have severe cases of obsessive-compulsive disorder may require dosages up to 250 mg daily.

MAINTENANCE: Adjunctive clomipramine pharmacotherapy for the symptomatic management of obsessive-compulsive disorder can be continued, if required, for up to one year without loss of efficacy. Dosage adjustments may be made to maintain patients at the lowest effective dosage. To minimize associated daytime sedation, the total daily dosage may be prescribed as a single daily dose 30 minutes before retiring for bed in the evening. If signs and symptoms of obsessive-compulsive disorder recur, increase the dosage until the signs and symptoms are controlled. Reevaluate long-term clomipramine pharmacotherapy periodically to determine the need for continued pharmacotherapy. To discontinue clomipramine pharmacotherapy, decrease the dosage gradually while monitoring patient response to avoid the associated withdrawal syndrome.

MAXIMUM: 250 mg daily orally

Women who are, or who may become, pregnant: FDA Pregnancy Category C. Safety and efficacy of clomipramine pharmacotherapy for women who are pregnant have not been established. Signs and symptoms resembling a withdrawal syndrome, including tremors, convulsions, and respiratory depression, have been reported among neonates whose mothers received clomipramine pharmacotherapy during the third trimester of pregnancy. Avoid prescribing clomipramine to women who are pregnant, particularly during the third trimester. If clomipramine pharmacotherapy is required, advise patients of potential benefits and possible risks to themselves and the embryo, fetus, or neonate. Collaboration with the patient's obstetrician is indicated.

Women who are breast-feeding: Safety and efficacy of clomipramine pharmacotherapy for women who are breast-feeding and their neonates and infants have not been established. Clomipramine is excreted in breast milk. Avoid prescribing clomipramine pharmacotherapy to women who are breast-feeding. If clomipramine pharmacotherapy is required, breast-feeding probably should be discontinued. Collaboration with the patient's pediatrician may be required.

Elderly, frail, or debilitated patients: Initially, 20 to 30 mg daily orally in divided doses. Increase the daily dosage gradually by 10 mg increments according to individual patient response. Generally, lower dosages are required for elderly, frail, or debilitated patients. These patients may be more sensitive to the pharmacologic actions of clomipramine than are younger or healthier adult patients. Monitor blood pressure and cardiac rhythm regularly, particularly among patients who have unstable cardiovascular function. Collaboration with the patient's family physician or a specialist (e.g., cardiologist, gerontologist) is indicated.

MAINTENANCE: Adjunctive clomipramine pharmacotherapy for the management of obsessive-compulsive disorder can be continued, if required, for up to one year without loss of efficacy. Dosage adjustments may be made to maintain patients at the lowest effective dosage. To minimize associated daytime sedation, the total daily dosage may be prescribed as a single daily dose 30 minutes before retiring for bed in the evening. If signs and symptoms of obsessive-compulsive disorder recur, increase the dosage until the signs and symptoms are controlled. Reevaluate long-term clomipramine pharmacotherapy periodically to determine the need for continued pharmacotherapy. To discontinue clomipramine pharmacotherapy, decrease the dosage gradually while monitoring patient response to avoid the associated withdrawal syndrome.

Children younger than 10 years of age: Safety and efficacy of clomipramine pharmacotherapy for the management of obsessive-compulsive disorder among children younger than

10 years of age have not been established. Clomipramine pharmacotherapy for this indication is *not* recommended for this age group.

Children and adolescents, 10 to 17 years of age: Initially, 25 mg daily orally. May increase the daily dosage, according to individual patient response, by 10 to 25 mg increments at three to four day intervals to a total daily dosage of 100 mg or 3 mg/kg, whichever dosage is lower, by the end of two weeks. Thereafter, increase the daily dosage gradually to 200 mg or 3 mg/kg, whichever dosage is lower.

MAXIMUM: 200 mg or 3 mg/kg daily, whichever dosage is lower

MAINTENANCE: Adjunctive clomipramine pharmacotherapy for the symptomatic management of obsessive-compulsive disorder can be continued, if required, for up to one year without loss of efficacy. Adjust dosage to maintain patients at the lowest effective dosage. To minimize associated daytime sedation, the total daily dosage may be prescribed as a single daily dose 30 minutes before bedtime. If signs and symptoms of obsessive-compulsive disorder recur, increase the dosage until the signs and symptoms are controlled. Reevaluate clomipramine pharmacotherapy periodically to determine the need for continued pharmacotherapy. To discontinue clomipramine pharmacotherapy, decrease the dosage gradually while monitoring patient response to avoid the associated withdrawal syndrome.

Notes, Obsessive-Compulsive Disorder

See Notes, Major Depressive Disorder

AVAILABLE DOSAGE FORMS, STORAGE, AND COMPATIBILITY

Capsules, oral: 25, 50, 100 mg
Tablets, oral: 10, 25, 50 mg

Notes

General Instructions for Patients   Instruct patients who are receiving clomipramine pharmacotherapy to

- safely store clomipramine capsules and tablets out of the reach of children in tightly closed child-resistant containers at temperatures below 30°C (86°F).
- obtain an available patient information sheet regarding clomipramine pharmacotherapy from their pharmacist at the time that their prescription is dispensed. Encourage patients to clarify any questions that they may have concerning clomipramine pharmacotherapy with their pharmacist or, if needed, to consult their prescribing psychologist.

PROPOSED MECHANISM OF ACTION

Clomipramine has both antidepressant and antiobsessional actions. These actions are related to its influence on serotonergic neurotransmission. The actual neurochemical mechanism is unknown. However, clomipramine's capacity to inhibit serotonin re-uptake is thought to be important. Like other TCAs, clomipramine inhibits norepinephrine and serotonin uptake into central nerve terminals, possibly by blocking the neuronal membrane-pump. This action is thought to increase the concentration of these transmitter monoamines in the synapses and, consequently, results in increased activity at the post-synaptic neuron receptor sites. Clomipramine also appears to have a mild sedative action. This action may be of benefit for managing the anxiety that often accompanies depression.

PHARMACOKINETICS/PHARMACODYNAMICS

Clomipramine is rapidly and completely absorbed following oral ingestion. Peak blood levels are generally achieved within 2 hours. Clomipramine is highly plasma protein-bound (approximately 97%) within the therapeutic range. It has an apparent volume of distribution of approximately 12 L/kg body weight. Clomipramine is extensively metabolized in the liver to several metabolites, including its major active metabolite desmethylclomipramine. Less than 2% of a dose is excreted in unchanged form in the urine. The mean half-life of elimination is approximately 21 hours. Elderly patients may require lower dosages of clomipramine than younger patients because of its lower blood clearance. Some data suggest that clomipramine follows nonlinear kinetics at daily dosages of 150 mg or higher (e.g., the reported mean half-life of elimination is approximately 32 hours at this dosage).

RELATIVE CONTRAINDICATIONS

Blood disorders, history of
Congestive heart failure, acute
Glaucoma. Clomipramine's anticholinergic action may aggravate this condition.
Hypersensitivity to clomipramine or other TCAs belonging to the dibenzazepine group
Kidney dysfunction
Liver dysfunction
MAOI pharmacotherapy, concurrent or within 14 days. Concurrent pharmacotherapy has resulted in hypertensive crises, hyperactivity, hyperpyrexia, spasticity, severe convulsions, coma, and death.
Myocardial infarction, acute recovery phase

CAUTIONS AND COMMENTS

Abrupt discontinuation of long-term clomipramine pharmacotherapy may occasionally produce abdominal pain, anxiety, diarrhea, headache, malaise, nausea, nervousness, and vomiting. Although these signs and symptoms resemble a withdrawal syndrome, clomipramine is not considered to be addicting.

Prescribe clomipramine pharmacotherapy cautiously to patients who

- exhibit agitation or hyperactivity. Agitated or hyperactive patients may become overstimulated.
- are hyperthyroid or are receiving thyroid pharmacotherapy. Transient cardiac dysrhythmias have rarely occurred among patients who are receiving concurrent TCA and thyroid pharmacotherapy.

- are elderly, frail, debilitated, or bedridden. Clomipramine pharmacotherapy may cause paralytic ileus among these patients. Promote normal bowel function and assure appropriate measures are taken if constipation occurs. Collaboration with the patient's advanced practice nurse, family physician or a specialist (e.g., gerontologist) may be indicated. Among elderly patients who are predisposed, TCA (and, hence, clomipramine) pharmacotherapy may, particularly at night, provoke pharmacogenic psychosis. This delirious psychosis usually remits within a few days of discontinuing TCA pharmacotherapy.
- have bipolar disorders. Patients who have bipolar disorders, or manic-depressive tendencies, may experience hypomanic or manic shifts.
- have depression or suicidal ideation. The risk for suicide is increased among depressed patients, including those who have obsessive-compulsive disorder. Monitor all patients during clomipramine pharmacotherapy for suicide risk. To minimize the risk for an intentional overdosage of clomipramine by a depressed and suicidal patient, prescribe the smallest possible quantity of clomipramine for dispensing and implement other suicide precautions as needed. Hospitalization or concomitant ECT also may be required.
- have histories of cardiovascular disorders, particularly conduction disorders and circulatory lability. Clomipramine's hypotensive action may be detrimental to these patients. Tricyclic antidepressants, particularly high dosages, may produce various cardiovascular reactions, including dysrhythmias (e.g., sinus tachycardia) and changes in conduction time. ECG abnormalities commonly include premature ventricular contractions (PVCs), T wave changes, and abnormalities involving intraventricular conduction. These abnormalities have been rarely associated with significant clinical signs and symptoms.

    Before initiating clomipramine pharmacotherapy, evaluate the patient's cardiovascular function, including blood pressure. Patients who have hypotension or a labile circulation may react to clomipramine pharmacotherapy with a fall in blood pressure. Evaluate blood pressure regularly for susceptible patients. For some patients, postural hypotension may be managed by reducing the dosage. Also monitor cardiac function, including ECG, for patients who require long-term pharmacotherapy. A gradual dosage titration is recommended. Collaboration with the patient's family physician or a specialist (e.g., cardiologist) is required.

    Unexpected death rarely has been reported among patients who have histories of cardiovascular disorders. Myocardial infarction and stroke have been implicated because of their association with TCA pharmacotherapy. Initiate clomipramine pharmacotherapy at lower dosages, and increase the dosage gradually, only if needed, according to individual patient response. Monitor cardiac function and ECG for these patients at all dosage levels. Collaboration with the patient's family physician or a specialist (e.g., cardiologist) is indicated.
- have histories of hypotensive episodes, increased intraocular pressure, or urinary retention, particularly when associated with prostatic hypertrophy. Clomipramine's anticholinergic action may exacerbate these conditions.
- have histories of seizure disorders and other predisposing factors (e.g., brain damage, alcoholism, concurrent pharmacotherapy with other drugs that lower the seizure threshold) that may increase their risk for seizures. Tricyclic antidepressants lower the seizure threshold. To minimize seizure risk, total daily dosages of clomipramine should not exceed the recommended total daily dosage.
- have liver dysfunction. Isolated cases of obstructive jaundice have been reported among patients who were receiving clomipramine pharmacotherapy. Clomipramine has also been occasionally associated with potentially clinically significant increases in AST and ALT (i.e., values greater than 3 times the upper limit of normal). In most cases, these enzyme increases were not associated with other clinical findings suggestive of liver damage. Caution is indicated when clomipramine pharmacotherapy is prescribed to patients who have known liver dysfunction. Monitoring of liver function is recommended. Collaboration with the patient's family physician or a specialist (e.g., internist) is indicated.

- require elective surgery. Withhold clomipramine pharmacotherapy before elective surgery for as long as clinically feasible. Little is known about the interaction between clomipramine and general anesthetics. Collaboration with the patient's surgeon or anesthesiologist is indicated.
- require ECT. Concurrent ECT may be hazardous, and should be used only when essential.
- have schizophrenia or other psychotic disorders. Clomipramine pharmacotherapy may activate latent schizophrenia or aggravate existing psychotic signs and symptoms among patients diagnosed with schizophrenia or other psychotic disorders. A reduction in the dose or discontinuation of clomipramine pharmacotherapy may be required.
- have tumors of the adrenal medulla (e.g., pheochromocytoma, neuroblastoma). Clomipramine pharmacotherapy may increase the risk among these patients for the occurrence of hypertensive crises. Collaboration with the patient's family physician or a specialist (e.g., internist, oncologist) is indicated.

Caution patients who are receiving clomipramine pharmacotherapy against

- drinking alcohol or using other drugs that produce CNS depression (e.g., antihistamines, opiate analgesics, sedative-hypnotics). Concurrent use of these drugs may result in excessive CNS depression.
- performing activities that require alertness, judgment, and physical coordination (e.g., driving an automobile, operating dangerous equipment, swimming, climbing). Clomipramine's anticholinergic action may produce sedation and adversely affect these mental and physical functions.

CLINICALLY SIGNIFICANT DRUG INTERACTIONS

Clomipramine pharmacotherapy and the following may result in clinically significant drug interactions:

Alcohol Use

Concurrent alcohol use may increase the CNS depressant action of clomipramine. Advise patients to avoid, or limit, their use of alcohol while receiving clomipramine pharmacotherapy.

Antidysrhythmic Pharmacotherapy

The TCAs should *not* be prescribed in combination with Type 1A and 1C antidysrhythmics (e.g., disopyramide [Norpace®]), procainamide [Pronestyl®], and quinidine [Biquin®]) and related drugs. Concurrent pharmacotherapy may increase the risk for dysrhythmias associated with QRS widening.

Antihypertensive Pharmacotherapy

Clomipramine may diminish or abolish the antihypertensive actions of clonidine (Catapres®), guanethidine (Ismelin®), methyldopa (Aldomet®), and reserpine (Serpasil®). Patients who require concurrent antihypertensive pharmacotherapy should probably be prescribed a different type of antihypertensive pharmacotherapy (e.g., beta-blockers, diuretic). Collaboration with the prescriber of the antihypertensive is indicated.

Antipsychotic Pharmacotherapy

Clomipramine pharmacotherapy rarely has been associated with hyperthermia when prescribed in combination with other drugs that affect body temperature regulation. Concurrent clomipramine and antipsychotic (e.g., phenothiazine, butyrophenone) pharmacotherapy has been associated with cases considered to be examples of the neuroleptic malignant syndrome. Phenothiazines, butyrophenones, and other antipsychotics may increase the plasma concentration of clomipramine.

Cimetidine Pharmacotherapy

Cimetidine (Tagamet®) inhibits the metabolism of clomipramine, resulting in clinically significant increases in plasma levels and possible toxicity.

Estrogen Pharmacotherapy

Concurrent clomipramine and estrogen pharmacotherapy can result in the inhibition of the metabolism of clomipramine. A reduction in clomipramine dosage may be required.

Fluoxetine Pharmacotherapy

Concurrent clomipramine and fluoxetine (Prozac®) pharmacotherapy may result in an increase in both the blood concentrations of clomipramine and the related pharmacologic activity.

Pharmacotherapy With Anticholinergics and Other Drugs That Produce Anticholinergic Actions

Concurrent clomipramine pharmacotherapy with anticholinergics (e.g., atropine) or other drugs that produce anticholinergic actions (e.g., biperiden [Akineton®], phenothiazines, TCAs) may result in exaggeration of anticholinergic actions. When TCAs are prescribed in combination with these drugs, delirium or hyperexcitation may occur. The exacerbation of glaucoma or paralytic ileus may also occur.

Pharmacotherapy With Drugs That Affect Hepatic Metabolism

Barbiturates, phenytoin (Dilantin®), nicotine, and other drugs that activate the hepatic mono-oxygenase enzyme system may lower plasma concentrations of clomipramine and reduce its antidepressant action.

Pharmacotherapy With Drugs That Are Highly Bound to Plasma Protein

Clomipramine is highly bound to plasma proteins. Thus, clomipramine may displace, or be displaced by, other highly plasma protein-bound drugs (e.g., digoxin [Lanoxin®], warfarin [Coumadin®]). This interaction may result in higher free drug blood concentrations and potential toxicity.

Phenytoin Pharmacotherapy

Concomitant clomipramine and phenytoin (Dilantin®) pharmacotherapy may result in increased phenytoin blood levels. An appropriate adjustment in phenytoin dosage may be required. Collaboration with the prescriber of the phenytoin is indicated.

Sympathomimetic Pharmacotherapy

Clomipramine may potentiate the cardiovascular actions of amphetamines, epinephrine or norepinephrine, methylphenidate (Ritalin®), or nonprescription cough and cold drug products (e.g., decongestant nasal sprays) that contain sympathomimetics.

See also Tricyclic Antidepressants General Monograph

ADVERSE DRUG REACTIONS

Clomipramine pharmacotherapy has been associated with the following ADRs, listed according to body system:

Cardiovascular: hypotension, particularly postural hypotension with associated sinus tachycardia, and palpitations. A quinidine-like reaction and other reversible ECG changes (e.g., flattening or inversion of T-waves, depressed S-T segments) among patients who have normal cardiac function have also been associated with clomipramine pharmacotherapy. Other ADRs affecting the cardiovascular system include conduction disorders (e.g., widening of QRS complex, PQ changes, bundle-branch block), dysrhythmias, hypertension, and syncope. Fibrillation, myocardial infarction, stroke, and unexpected death among patients who have cardiovascular disorders have been reported with TCA pharmacotherapy.

CNS: activation of latent psychosis, aggravated depression, aggressiveness, anxiety, agitation, confusion accompanied by disorientation (particularly among elderly patients and those who have Parkinson's disease), convulsions, delirium, delusions, depersonalization, disturbed concentration, dizziness, drowsiness, EEG changes, extrapyramidal reactions, fatigue, headache, hypomania or manic episodes, impaired memory, insomnia, nervousness, nightmares, sleep disturbances, slurred speech, somnolence, speech disorders, tremor, visual hallucinations, vertigo, and yawning

Cutaneous: allergic skin reactions, including hives (urticaria), photosensitivity, severe itching (pruritus) and skin rash, edema, drug fever, and hot flushes. Discontinue clomipramine pharmacotherapy if an allergic skin reaction is noted.

Genitourinary: change in sex drive, ejaculatory failure, impotence, urination disorders, and urinary retention

GI: abdominal pain, constipation, diarrhea, dry mouth, dyspepsia, increased appetite with weight gain, loss of appetite with weight loss (anorexia), nausea, paralytic ileus, taste perversion, and vomiting. Long-term TCA pharmacotherapy has been associated with an increased incidence of dental caries.

Hematologic: agranulocytosis, eosinophilia, leukopenia, purpura, and thrombocytopenia. A case of pancytopenia has been reported. Isolated cases of bone marrow depression with agranulocytosis also have been reported. Leukocyte and differential blood cell counts are recommended for patients who are receiving long-term clomipramine pharmacotherapy and should be obtained for patients who develop a fever, an influenza-like infection, or sore throat. Collaboration with the patient's family physician or a specialist (e.g., hematologist) may be required.

Hepatic: elevated transaminases, hepatitis with or without jaundice, and obstructive jaundice

Metabolic/Endocrine: clomipramine pharmacotherapy has been associated with an increased formation and excretion of porphyrin among susceptible patients.

Musculoskeletal: fatigue, incoordination (ataxia), muscle hypertonia, muscle weakness, numbness or tingling of the extremities (paresthesia), and twitching or muscle spasms (myoclonus). Peripheral neuropathy also has been associated with other TCA pharmacotherapy.

Ocular: abnormal dilation of the pupils (mydriasis), accommodation difficulty, glaucoma, and visual changes, such as blurred vision

Otic: ringing in the ears (tinnitus)

Renal: long-term clomipramine pharmacotherapy requires monitoring of kidney function.

Miscellaneous: hyperpyrexia (see also Cutaneous)

See also Tricyclic Antidepressants General Monograph

OVERDOSAGE

Children may be more sensitive than adults to acute clomipramine overdosage. Fatalities involving children have been reported. Accidental ingestion among children should be regarded as serious and potentially fatal. Signs and symptoms of clomipramine overdosage resemble those observed with other TCA overdosage. These signs and symptoms may vary according to the amount of drug absorbed, the interval between ingestion and overdosage treatment, age of patient, and other factors.

Generally, 30 minutes to 2 hours after ingestion of the overdosage, severe anticholinergic reactions occur, with drowsiness, stupor, ataxia, vomiting, hyperactive reflexes, muscle rigidity, athetoid and choreiform movements, and convulsions. Hyperpyrexia, mydriasis, bowel and bladder paralysis, and respiratory depression may occur. Initial hypertension with increasing hypotension may lead to shock. Serious cardiovascular disturbances frequently occur, including tachycardia, cardiac dysrhythmias (e.g., flutter, atriofibrillation, premature ventricular beats, ventricular tachycardia), impaired myocardial conduction, atrio-ventricular and intraventricular block, ECG abnormalities (e.g., widening QRS complexes and marked S-T shifts and signs of congestive heart failure) and cardiac arrest. Coma may ensue.

Suspected or actual clomipramine overdosage requires emergency symptomatic medical support of body systems with attention to increasing clomipramine elimination. There is no known antidote.

CLORAZEPATE

(klor az′e pate)

TRADE NAMES

Gen-Xene®
Novo-Clopate®
Tranxene®
Tranxene-SD®

CLASSIFICATION

Sedative-hypnotic (benzodiazepine) (C-IV)

See also Benzodiazepines General Monograph

APPROVED INDICATIONS FOR PSYCHOLOGICAL DISORDERS

Adjunctive pharmacotherapy for the short-term symptomatic management of:

- Anxiety Disorders. *Note:* Clorazepate is *not* indicated for the management of everyday anxiety or tension that can be managed with psychotherapy alone. Clorazepate also is *not* recommended for the management of anxiety associated with depression because it has the potential to exacerbate the depression while alleviating the anxiety. The depression associated with anxiety generally resolves with appropriate adjunctive pharmacotherapy (i.e., antidepressant pharmacotherapy) and psychotherapy.
- Substance-Related Disorders: Alcohol Withdrawal Syndrome (Acute)

USUAL DOSAGE AND ADMINISTRATION

Anxiety Disorders

Adults: Initially, 15 to 30 mg daily orally in two to four divided doses. Clorazepate also may be prescribed as a single daily dose 30 minutes before retiring for bed in the evening. Adjust the dosage gradually within the range of 15 to 60 mg daily according to individual patient response. The recommended initial dosage is 15 mg daily. The usual dosage is 30 mg daily.

MAXIMUM: 90 mg daily orally

Women who are, or who may become, pregnant: FDA Pregnancy Category C. An increased risk for congenital malformations (i.e., birth defects) has been associated with the use of benzodiazepines, such as chlordiazepoxide (Librium®) and diazepam (Valium®), during the first trimester of pregnancy. Clorazepate, a benzodiazepine derivative, has not been clearly associated with an increased risk. However, avoid prescribing clorazepate pharmacotherapy to women who are pregnant because of its similarity to these and other benzodiazepines. If clorazepate pharmacotherapy is required, advise patients of potential benefits and possible risks to themselves and the embryo, fetus, or neonate. Collaboration with the patient's obstetrician is indicated.

Women who are breast-feeding: Safety and efficacy of clorazepate pharmacotherapy for women who are breast-feeding and their neonates and infants have not been established. The active metabolite of clorazepate, nordiazepam, is excreted in breast milk. Drowsiness and lethargy may occur among breast-fed neonates and infants, who may also become addicted. Avoid prescribing clorazepate to women who are breast-feeding. If clorazepate pharmacotherapy is required, breast-feeding probably should be discontinued. If desired, lactation may be maintained and breast-feeding resumed following the discontinuation of short-term clorazepate pharmacotherapy. Collaboration with the patient's pediatrician is indicated.

Elderly, frail, or debilitated patients and those who have kidney or liver dysfunction: Initially, 7.5 to 15 mg daily orally in two to four divided doses. Increase the dosage gradually to 60 mg daily, as needed, according to individual patient response. Generally prescribe lower initial dosages for elderly, frail, or debilitated patients. Increase the dosage more gradually in order to avoid associated incoordination (ataxia) or excessive sedation. Also prescribe lower dosages for patients who have kidney or liver dysfunction.

Children younger than 9 years of age: Safety and efficacy of clorazepate pharmacotherapy for the management of anxiety disorders for children younger than 9 years of age have not been established. Clorazepate pharmacotherapy for this indication is *not* recommended for this age group.

Notes, Anxiety Disorders

Initiating and Maintaining Clorazepate Pharmacotherapy Drowsiness may occur upon the initiation of clorazepate pharmacotherapy and with incremental increases in dosage. The safety and efficacy of long-term (longer than 4 months) clorazepate pharmacotherapy for the symptomatic management of anxiety have not been established. Reevaluate patients who appear to require clorazepate pharmacotherapy for longer than 4 months. Monitor blood counts and liver function tests periodically for patients who require long-term clorazepate pharmacotherapy. Collaboration with the patient's family physician or a specialist (e.g., hematologist) may be indicated.

Discontinuing Clorazepate Pharmacotherapy Long-term clorazepate pharmacotherapy, or regular personal use, may lead to addiction and habituation. Abrupt discontinuation of long-term clorazepate pharmacotherapy, or regular personal use, may result in the clorazepate withdrawal syndrome. This syndrome may include seizures. Discontinue clorazepate pharmacotherapy gradually.

Alcohol Withdrawal Syndrome (Acute)

Adults: The following daily dosage schedule is recommended:

Day 1 (first 24 hours): Initially, 30 mg orally, then an additional 30 to 60 mg orally in two to four divided doses
Day 2 (second 24 hours): 45 to 90 mg orally in two to four divided doses
Day 3 (third 24 hours): 22.5 to 45 mg orally in two to four divided doses
Day 4 (fourth 24 hours): 15 to 30 mg orally in two to four divided doses
Day 5 and thereafter: reduce the daily dosage gradually to 7.5 to 15 mg. Discontinue clorazepate pharmacotherapy completely as soon as the patient's condition stabilizes.

MAXIMUM: 90 mg daily orally

Notes, Alcohol Withdrawal Syndrome (Acute)

To adequately manage the signs and symptoms of the acute alcohol withdrawal syndrome, avoid excessive reductions in the total daily dosage prescribed on successive days.

AVAILABLE DOSAGE FORMS, STORAGE, AND COMPATIBILITY

Capsules, oral: 3.75, 7.5, 15 mg
Tablets, oral: 3.75, 7.5, 11.25, 15 mg
Tablets, oral extended-release: 11.25, 22.5 mg

Notes

Oral Extended-Release Tablets Extended-release tablets are formulated for once-daily dosing for patients who have been stabilized on regular capsule or tablet formulations. Prescribe extended-release tablets, 11.25 mg or 22.5 mg, as a single daily dose for patients who have been stabilized on daily dosages of 3.75 mg or 7.5 mg three times a day, respectively. The extended-release tablets are intended as a convenient alternative for patients who are stabilized on clorazepate pharmacotherapy and prefer once daily dosing. Extended-release tablets are *not* intended for the initiation of clorazepate pharmacotherapy.

General Instructions for Patients Instruct patients who are receiving clorazepate pharmacotherapy to

- swallow each dose of the clorazepate extended-release tablets whole without crushing or chewing.
- safely store clorazepate oral dosage forms out of the reach of children in child-resistant containers at temperatures below 25°C (77°F).
- obtain an available patient information sheet regarding clorazepate pharmacotherapy from their pharmacist at the time that their prescription is dispensed. Encourage patients to clarify any questions that they may have concerning clorazepate pharmacotherapy with their pharmacist or, if needed, to consult their prescribing psychologist.

PROPOSED MECHANISM OF ACTION

Clorazepate has the chemical characteristics of the benzodiazepines and produces similar CNS depressant actions. The exact mechanism of action of clorazepate has not yet been fully determined. However, it appears to be mediated or to work in concert with the inhibitory neurotransmitter GABA.

See also the Benzodiazepines General Monograph

PHARMACOKINETICS/PHARMACODYNAMICS

Clorazepate is rapidly metabolized in the liver to its active major metabolite, nordiazepam (desmethyldiazepam). There is virtually no circulating parent drug in the blood. Nordiazepam is highly plasma protein-bound (~98%). It is further metabolized in the liver, and the metabolites are primarily excreted in the urine (less than 1% of nordiazepam is excreted in unchanged form in the urine). The mean half-life of elimination for nordiazepam is approximately three days. The mean total body clearance is ~1 ml/minute.

RELATIVE CONTRAINDICATIONS

Glaucoma, acute narrow-angle
Hypersensitivity to clorazepate or other benzodiazepines
Myasthenia gravis
Pain, severe uncontrolled

CAUTIONS AND COMMENTS

Clorazepate is addicting and habituating. A clorazepate withdrawal syndrome similar to the alcohol withdrawal syndrome has occurred following the abrupt discontinuation of long-term high-dosage clorazepate pharmacotherapy, or regular personal use. Signs and symptoms of the clorazepate withdrawal syndrome include diarrhea, hallucinations, insomnia, irritability, memory impairment, muscle aches, nervousness, and tremor. Monitor all patients for whom clorazepate pharmacotherapy is discontinued for signs and symptoms of withdrawal because abrupt discontinuation of other benzodiazepine pharmacotherapy, even prescribed therapeutic dosages for several months, has resulted in a benzodiazepine withdrawal syndrome.

Prescribe clorazepate pharmacotherapy cautiously to patients who

- have depression accompanied with anxiety and for whom suicide tendencies may be present. Prescribe the least amount of clorazepate feasible for dispensing to these patients. Other suicide precautions may be indicated.
- have histories of problematic patterns of alcohol or other abusable psychotropic use. Clorazepate is addicting and habituating. These patients may be more likely to develop problematic patterns of clorazepate use, including addiction and habituation.
- have kidney or liver dysfunction

Caution patients who are receiving clorazepate pharmacotherapy against

- drinking alcohol or using other drugs that cause CNS depression (e.g., antihistamines, barbiturates, opiate analgesics, phenothiazines). Excessive CNS depression may result.
- performing activities that require alertness, judgment, or physical coordination (e.g., driving an automobile, operating dangerous equipment, supervising children). Clorazepate pharmacotherapy may adversely affect these mental and physical functions, particularly during the first few days of pharmacotherapy because of its sedative action.

In addition to these general precautions for patients, caution women to inform their prescribing psychologist if they become, or intend to become, pregnant while receiving clorazepate pharmacotherapy, so that their pharmacotherapy can be safely discontinued.

CLINICALLY SIGNIFICANT DRUG INTERACTIONS

Concurrent clorazepate pharmacotherapy and the following may result in clinically significant drug interactions:

Alcohol Use

Concurrent alcohol use may significantly increase the CNS depressant action of clorazepate. Advise patients to avoid, or limit, their use of alcohol while receiving clorazepate pharmacotherapy.

Cimetidine Pharmacotherapy

Cimetidine (Tagamet®), a hepatic enzyme inhibitor, may decrease the hepatic clearance of clorazepate. This interaction may result in clorazepate toxicity.

Pharmacotherapy With Central Nervous System Depressants and Other Drugs That Produce Central Nervous System Depression

Concurrent clorazepate pharmacotherapy with opiate analgesics, other sedative-hypnotics, or other drugs that cause CNS depression (e.g., MAOIs, phenothiazines, TCAs) may result in additive CNS depression.

See also Benzodiazepines General Monograph

ADVERSE DRUG REACTIONS

Clorazepate pharmacotherapy has been associated with the following ADRs, listed according to body system:

Cardiovascular: rarely, decreased systolic blood pressure
CNS: depression, dizziness, drowsiness, fatigue, headache, insomnia, irritability, mental confusion, nervousness, and slurred speech
Cutaneous: transient skin rashes
GI: dry mouth
Hematologic: rarely, decreased hematocrit
Musculoskeletal: incoordination (ataxia) and tremor
Ocular: blurred vision and double vision (diplopia)

See also Benzodiazepines General Monograph

OVERDOSAGE

Signs and symptoms of clorazepate overdosage correspond to varying degrees of CNS depression, ranging from slight sedation to coma. Clorazepate overdosage requires emergency symptomatic medical support of body systems with attention to increasing clorazepate elimination. The benzodiazepine antagonist flumazenil (Anexate®, Romazicon®) may be required.

CLOZAPINE

(kloe′za peen)

TRADE NAME

Clozaril®

CLASSIFICATION

Antipsychotic (atypical, dibenzodiazepine)

APPROVED INDICATIONS FOR PSYCHOLOGICAL DISORDERS

Adjunctive pharmacotherapy for the symptomatic management of:

Psychotic Disorders: Schizophrenia and Other Psychotic Disorders. *Note:* Prescribe clozapine pharmacotherapy only for patients who have failed to respond adequately to pharmacotherapy with standard antipsychotics (e.g., butyrophenones such as haloperidol, or phenothiazines such as chlorpromazine) because of its associated significant risk for agranulocytosis and seizures.

USUAL DOSAGE AND ADMINISTRATION

Schizophrenia and Other Psychotic Disorders

Adults:　Initially, 12.5 to 25 mg daily orally in one single or two divided doses. Increase the
daily dosage, according to individual patient response, by 25 to 50 mg increments to a dosage of
350 to 400 mg daily by the end of the second week of clozapine pharmacotherapy. Subsequently,
increase the daily dosage once or twice weekly by increments of 25 to 100 mg, if needed, according to individual patient response.

MAXIMUM:　900 mg daily orally

Women who are, or who may become, pregnant:　FDA Pregnancy Category B. Safety
and efficacy of clozapine pharmacotherapy for women who are pregnant have not been established. Avoid prescribing clozapine pharmacotherapy to women who are pregnant. If clozapine
pharmacotherapy is required, advise patients of potential benefits and possible risks to themselves
and the embryo, fetus, or neonate. Collaboration with the patient's obstetrician is indicated.

Women who are breast-feeding:　Safety and efficacy of clozapine pharmacotherapy for
women who are breast-feeding and their neonates and infants have not been established. Clozapine is excreted in breast milk. Do *not* prescribe clozapine pharmacotherapy to women who are
breast-feeding. If clozapine pharmacotherapy is required, breast-feeding should be discontinued.
Collaboration with the patient's pediatrician is indicated.

Elderly, frail, or debilitated patients:　Generally prescribe lower dosages for elderly,
frail, or debilitated patients. Increase the dosage gradually, if needed, according to individual
patient response. These patients may be more sensitive to the pharmacologic actions of clozapine than are younger or healthier adult patients.

Children and adolescents younger than 16 years of age:　Safety and efficacy of clozapine pharmacotherapy for children and adolescents who are younger than 16 years of age have
not been established. Clozapine pharmacotherapy is *not* recommended for this age group.

Notes, Schizophrenia and Other Psychotic Disorders

Clozapine pharmacotherapy has been associated with serious ADRs, including agranulocytosis, hypotension, over-sedation, and seizures (see Adverse Drug Reactions). *Only* prescribe clozapine pharmacotherapy in conjunction with weekly WBC counts in order to monitor patients for agranulocytosis. Titrate the dosage, and monitor patients carefully for hypotension, oversedation, and seizures. Collaboration with the patient's family physician or a specialist (e.g., hematologist) may be required.

Initiating Clozapine Pharmacotherapy   *Before* initiating clozapine pharmacotherapy:

- assure that separate alternative pharmacotherapy with two different antipsychotics has been given adequate evaluation in regard to dosage, duration of pharmacotherapy, and management of associated ADRs. Clozapine pharmacotherapy is reserved for the symptomatic management of severe schizophrenia among patients for whom other antipsychotic pharmacotherapy has proved ineffective.
- obtain baseline WBC and differential counts. The commercial availability of clozapine is regulated through a distribution system that ensures weekly testing of WBC and differential counts prior to delivery of the following week's supply of clozapine. Do *not* initiate clozapine pharmacotherapy if the WBC count is less than 3,500/mm^3.
- instruct patients, or their legal guardians in regard to the patient, as appropriate, to immediately report fever, lethargy, sore throat, weakness, or any other signs of infection while receiving clozapine pharmacotherapy.

Maintaining and Discontinuing Clozapine Pharmacotherapy   *Monitor* weekly WBC and differential counts. *Repeat* WBC and differential counts if

- the total WBC count has dropped below 3,500/mm^3 or the WBC count has dropped substantially from baseline, even if above 3,500/mm^3. A substantial drop is defined as a single drop of 3,000 or more in the WBC count or a cumulative drop of 3,000 or more in three weeks.
- immature cells are reported.

Obtain twice weekly WBC and differential counts if

- subsequent WBC and differential counts reveal a total WBC count between 3,000 and 3,500/mm^3 and
- an ANC above 1,500/mm^3.

Interrupt clozapine pharmacotherapy, *obtain* daily WBC and differential counts, and *monitor* patients for flu-like signs and symptoms, or other signs and symptoms of infection, if

- the patient's total WBC count falls below 3,000/mm^3 *or*
- the ANC falls below 1,500/mm^3.

Resume clozapine pharmacotherapy and *obtain* twice weekly WBC and differential counts for patients, if

- no signs and symptoms of infection are present,
- the total WBC counts return to levels above 3,000/mm^3, *and*
- the ANC returns to levels above 1,500/mm^3.

Continue twice weekly WBC and differential counts until the total WBC count returns to levels above 3,500/mm^3.

Discontinue clozapine pharmacotherapy if

- the total WBC count falls below 2,000/mm^3.
- the ANC falls below 1,000/mm^3. A bone marrow aspiration to ascertain granulopioetic status is recommended. If granulopoiesis is found deficient, protective isolation with close medical monitoring may be required.
- infection is present. Culture and sensitivity tests should be obtained so that appropriate antibiotic pharmacotherapy can be initiated. Collaboration with the patient's family physician or a specialist (e.g., hematologist) is required for related medical diagnosis and treatment.

Continue monitoring and follow-up:

- obtain daily WBC and differential counts. Do *not* rechallenge these patients with clozapine. Patients who have agranulocytosis will again develop agranulocytosis upon rechallenge, often with a shorter latency of reexposure.
- reduce the risk for patients who have experienced significant bone marrow suppression during clozapine pharmacotherapy for the inadvertent prescription of clozapine pharmacotherapy, by recommending their listing in a confidential national master file established for this purpose.

AVAILABLE DOSAGE FORMS, STORAGE, AND COMPATIBILITY

Tablets, oral: 25, 100 mg

Notes

It is generally recommended that the number of clozapine tablets dispensed *not* exceed a one-week supply and that dispensing be contingent upon the satisfactory results of weekly WBC and differential counts. For further information and assistance with the management of clozapine pharmacotherapy, contact Novartis Pharmaceuticals at 1-888-669-6682 (United States) or 1-800-267-2726 (Canada).

General Instructions for Patients   Instruct patients who are receiving clozapine pharmacotherapy to

- safely store clozapine tablets out of the reach of children in child-resistant containers at controlled room temperature below 30°C (86°F).
- obtain an available patient information sheet regarding clozapine pharmacotherapy from their pharmacist at the time that their prescription is dispensed. Encourage patients to clarify any questions that they may have concerning clozapine pharmacotherapy with their pharmacist or, if needed, to consult their prescribing psychologist.

PROPOSED MECHANISM OF ACTION

Clozapine, a dibenzodiazepine derivative, is classified as an atypical antipsychotic because it does not significantly inhibit dopamine binding to the dopamine receptors (D-1 and D-2) as do the standard antipsychotics. Also in contrast to the standard antipsychotics, clozapine produces little or no increase in prolactin levels, increases delta and theta brain wave activity and slows dominant alpha frequencies, and significantly increases REM sleep. Its exact mechanism of antipsychotic action is complex and has not yet been fully determined. Clozapine appears to be more active at receptors in the limbic system rather than at receptors in the striatal region of the CNS. This proposed mechanism of action may help explain its generally lower associated incidence of extrapyramidal reactions. Clozapine also acts as an antagonist at adrenergic, cholinergic, histaminergic, and serotonergic receptors.

PHARMACOKINETICS/PHARMACODYNAMICS

Clozapine is moderately absorbed (~60%) following oral ingestion. Peak blood levels are generally achieved within 3 hours. Clozapine is highly plasma protein-bound (~97%) with a mean apparent volume of distribution of 5.5 L/kg. Clozapine is extensively metabolized in the liver with less than 1% excreted in unchanged form in the urine. The mean half-life of elimination is 12 hours. The mean total body clearance is 430 ml/minute.

Clozapine is primarily metabolized by the hepatic microsomal enzymes, specifically cytochrome P450 isoenzyme 2D6. Approximately 3% to 10% of the general population in North America has reduced activity of this enzyme. North Americans who comprise this portion of the general population are consequently referred to as "poor metabolizers" of clozapine and other drugs, such as dextromethorphan (Benylin DM®, Novahistine DM®), and TCAs. Prescribing usual recommended dosages of clozapine for patients who are poor metabolizers may result in higher than expected blood concentrations.

RELATIVE CONTRAINDICATIONS

Blood disorders
Clozapine-induced agranulocytosis or granulocytopenia, history of
CNS depression, severe
Coma (due to any cause)
Hypersensitivity to clozapine
Myeloproliferative disorders (e.g., aplastic anemia)
Ritonavir (Norvir®) pharmacotherapy, concurrent
Seizure disorders, uncontrolled

CAUTIONS AND COMMENTS

Although risk factors for the development of agranulocytosis associated with clozapine pharmacotherapy have not been established, the following factors may be related to increased risk:

- Clozapine pharmacotherapy for a period of four to ten weeks
- Jewish background

- Women, the elderly, and patients who are cachectic or have serious underlying medical disorders. Agranulocytosis associated with other antipsychotic pharmacotherapy has been reported to occur with greater frequency among these patients. These patients also may be at particular risk with clozapine pharmacotherapy. Prescribe clozapine pharmacotherapy cautiously to these patients.

Also prescribe clozapine pharmacotherapy cautiously to patients who

- have cardiovascular dysfunction. These patients are at increased risk for related cardiovascular ADRs, including ECG repolarization changes, hypotension, syncope, and tachycardia. Collaboration with the patient's family physician or cardiologist is indicated.
- have narrow-angle glaucoma, paralytic ileus, or prostatic enlargement. Clozapine has potent anticholinergic actions and can significantly adversely affect these conditions. Collaboration with the patient's family physician or advanced practice nurse is indicated.

Caution patients who are receiving clozapine pharmacotherapy against performing activities that require alertness, judgment, or physical coordination (e.g., driving an automobile, operating dangerous equipment, supervising children) until their response to clozapine pharmacotherapy is known. Clozapine has a sedative action that is generally most pronounced during the first few days of pharmacotherapy.

CLINICALLY SIGNIFICANT DRUG INTERACTIONS

Concurrent clozapine pharmacotherapy and the following may result in clinically significant drug interactions:

Alcohol Use

Concurrent alcohol use may increase the CNS depressant action of clozapine. Advise patients to avoid, or limit, their use of alcohol while receiving clozapine pharmacotherapy.

Fluoxetine and Related Selective-Serotonin Reuptake Inhibitor Pharmacotherapy

Fluoxetine (Prozac®) and related SSRI pharmacotherapy inhibit the hepatic cytochrome P450 microsomal enzyme system. This inhibition may significantly increase the blood concentrations of both clozapine and its metabolite, norclozapine. This interaction also has been clinically documented with sertraline (Zoloft®). For patients who are receiving clozapine, monitor clinical response carefully, and adjust the clozapine dosage as needed when SSRI pharmacotherapy is initiated, SSRI dosages are adjusted, or SSRI pharmacotherapy is discontinued.

Pharmacotherapy With Central Nervous System Depressants and Other Drugs That Produce Central Nervous System Depression

Concurrent clozapine pharmacotherapy with opiate analgesics, sedative-hypnotics, or other drugs that produce CNS depression (e.g., antihistamines, phenothiazines, TCAs) may result in additive CNS depression.

Pharmacotherapy With Drugs That Produce Myelosuppression

Concurrent clozapine pharmacotherapy with antineoplastics, phenothiazines, or other drugs that produce myelosuppression (e.g., cyclosporine [Sandimmune®]) place patients at increased risk for developing potentially fatal agranulocytosis. Clozapine pharmacotherapy is not generally recommended for patients who are concurrently receiving pharmacotherapy with other drugs that produce myelosuppression. This combination of pharmacotherapy may result in synergistic actions and an increase in the incidence and severity of bone marrow suppression.

Ritonavir Pharmacotherapy

Ritonavir (Norvir®), an antiretroviral drug indicated for the pharmacologic management of HIV infection, can significantly inhibit the hepatic microsomal enzyme metabolism of clozapine. This interaction may result in severe clozapine toxicity, including agranulocytosis and seizures. Concurrent clozapine and ritonavir pharmacotherapy is contraindicated. See Relative Contraindications.

ADVERSE DRUG REACTIONS

Clozapine pharmacotherapy has been associated with the development of agranulocytosis, postural hypotension, and seizures. These ADRs are serious and potentially life threatening. These ADRs also present a continuing risk over time. Patients who do not achieve therapeutic benefit following a reasonable period of clozapine pharmacotherapy require discontinuation of clozapine pharmacotherapy because of the significant risk for these ADRs. Patients who achieve therapeutic benefit also require periodic reevaluation of the need for continued pharmacotherapy because of the significant risk for the occurrence of these ADRs.

Agranulocytosis

Agranulocytosis, defined as an ANC less than $500/mm^3$, reportedly occurs in ~1.3% of patients receiving clozapine. The agranulocytosis, if not appropriately recognized and treated, may result in death. Therefore, WBC and differential counts are required before initiating clozapine pharmacotherapy, weekly during clozapine pharmacotherapy, and for four weeks following the discontinuation of clozapine pharmacotherapy.

Postural Hypotension

Postural (orthostatic) hypotension may occur and result in fainting (syncope). This ADR can be particularly hazardous for patients who are elderly, particularly elderly women who have osteoporosis. Postural hypotension can be profound (rarely) and can be accompanied by cardiac or respiratory arrest. Postural hypotension is more likely to occur during the first two days following the initiation of clozapine pharmacotherapy. It also has been associated with rapid increases in dosage.

In order to minimize the possible occurrence of postural hypotension, initiate pharmacotherapy with lower dosages (i.e., 12.5 mg daily), and increase the dosage gradually. Instruct patients to monitor for this effect and to carefully change positions (e.g., from lying in bed to standing) until they know their response to clozapine pharmacotherapy (i.e., how much of a postural hypotensive effect they may expect to experience).

Seizures

Seizures reportedly occur among ~5% of patients who are receiving clozapine pharmacotherapy. The incidence of seizures appears to be dose-related. A higher incidence of seizures has been reported among patients who are receiving higher dosages. Seizures may result in a loss of consciousness. Therefore, patients should be cautioned to avoid activities (e.g., driving an automobile, mountain climbing, operating dangerous equipment, supervising children, swimming) for which sudden unanticipated loss of consciousness could cause serious risk to themselves and others.

Other Adverse Drug Reactions

Clozapine pharmacotherapy has been commonly associated with constipation, dizziness, drowsiness, dry mouth, fainting (syncope), fever, headache, hypotension, nausea, salivation (excessive), sedation, sweating, tachycardia (with an average increase of 12 beats per minute, which may pose a risk for certain patients who have severely compromised cardiovascular function), tremor, vertigo, and visual disturbances (e.g., blurring of vision), and tachycardia. Clozapine also has been associated with the following ADRs, listed according to body system:

Cardiovascular: chest pain, deep vein thrombosis, hypertension, and pulmonary embolism
CNS: agitation, akinesia, confusion, fatigue, nightmares, restlessness and an inability to sit
   down (akathisia), rigidity, seizures, and sleep disturbances (see also Miscellaneous)
Cutaneous: skin rash
Genitourinary: incontinence, priapism (rare), urinary retention, and urinary urgency
GI: constipation (which, because of the potent anticholinergic activity of clozapine, can
   progress to paralytic ileus), diarrhea, dyspepsia, loss of appetite (anorexia), vomiting,
   and weight gain
Hematologic: eosinophilia (if the differential blood count reveals a total eosinophil count
   above 4,000/mm^3, then clozapine pharmacotherapy should be interrupted [withheld] until
   the eosinophil count falls below 3,000/mm^3), leukopenia, and neutropenia
Hepatic: cholestatic jaundice (rare) and hepatitis
Metabolic/Endocrine: hyperglycemia and weight gain
Musculoskeletal: muscle pain, muscle spasm, and muscle weakness (see also Miscellaneous)
Miscellaneous: NMS and TD

OVERDOSAGE

Signs and symptoms of clozapine overdosage commonly include agitation, areflexia, coma, confusion, delirium, drowsiness, heart block, hypotension, lethargy, respiratory depression, salivation (excessive), and tachycardia. Clozapine overdosage has been fatal in approximately 12% of cases. Clozapine overdosage requires emergency symptomatic medical support of body systems with attention to increasing clozapine elimination. There is no known antidote.

CODEINE (Methylmorphine)

(koe'deen)

TRADE NAMES

Codeine Contin®
Paveral®

CLASSIFICATION

Opiate analgesic (C-II)

See also Opiate Analgesics General Monograph

APPROVED INDICATIONS FOR PSYCHOLOGICAL DISORDERS

Adjunctive pharmacotherapy for the short-term symptomatic management of pain disorders:

- Acute Pain, Moderate
- Chronic Cancer Pain, Moderate. *Note:* The extended-release formulation Codeine Contin® is indicated for the long-term symptomatic management of moderate cancer pain.

USUAL DOSAGE AND ADMINISTRATION

Acute Pain, Moderate, and Chronic Cancer Pain, Moderate

Adults: 0.5 to 2 mg/kg intramuscularly, orally, or subcutaneously every four to six hours

MAXIMUM: For regular dosage formulations, 60 mg/dose; 300 mg daily. For the extended-release tablet, 600 mg daily orally in two equally divided doses at 12-hour intervals.

Women who are, or who may become, pregnant: FDA Pregnancy Category C. Safety and efficacy of codeine pharmacotherapy for women who are pregnant have not been established. Codeine pharmacotherapy is not generally recommended for women who are pregnant because codeine crosses the placenta. However, it is unlikely that codeine is a teratogen. If it is, its potency and incidence as a teratogen are extremely low. Codeine is widely used during pregnancy, particularly in combination analgesic and cough and cold products. Only a few cases of possible teratogenic effects (e.g., cleft lip and palate) have been reported in the literature. Maternal use near term can result in neonatal depression, which is associated with the expected actions of an opiate analgesic. Long-term maternal pharmacotherapy, or regular personal use, may result in the neonatal opiate withdrawal syndrome. Avoid prescribing codeine pharmacotherapy to women who are pregnant. If codeine pharmacotherapy is required, advise patients of potential benefits and possible risks to themselves and the embryo, fetus, or neonate. Collaboration with the patient's obstetrician is indicated.

Women who are breast-feeding: Safety and efficacy of codeine pharmacotherapy for women who are breast-feeding and their neonates and infants have not been established. The active metabolites of codeine (e.g., morphine) are excreted in low concentrations in breast milk. Neonatal respiratory depression following several days of breast-feeding has been reported among neonates. Drowsiness and lethargy may occur among breast-fed neonates and infants. These neonates and infants also may become addicted. Avoid prescribing codeine to women who are breast-feeding. If codeine pharmacotherapy is required, breast-feeding probably should be discontinued. If desired, lactation may be maintained and breast-feeding resumed following the discontinuation of short-term codeine pharmacotherapy. Collaboration with the patient's pediatrician may be indicated.

Elderly, frail, or debilitated patients and those who have kidney or liver dysfunction: Initially, prescribe lower dosages of codeine. Increase the dosage gradually, as needed, according to individual patient response. Elderly, frail, or debilitated patients may be more sensitive to the CNS or respiratory depressant actions of codeine than are younger or healthier adult patients. Also prescribe lower dosages for patients who have severe kidney or liver dysfunction.

Children: 0.5 to 1.0 mg/kg intramuscularly, orally, or subcutaneously every four to six hours, according to individual signs and symptoms of pain and clinical response.

MAXIMUM:　1.5 mg/kg/dose to a maximum of 60 mg/dose

Notes, Acute Pain, Moderate, and Chronic Cancer Pain, Moderate

In terms of analgesia, oral codeine pharmacotherapy is ~60% as potent as intramuscular codeine pharmacotherapy. The oral formulation of codeine phosphate is approximately one-tenth as potent as the oral formulation of morphine sulfate (i.e., 10 mg codeine ≈ 1 mg morphine). Avoid intravenous injection because of the associated release of histamine. Oral doses may be only two-thirds as effective as equal injectable doses because of differences in bioavailability.

The Approximate Opiate Analgesic Equivalents table provides a general guide for oral dosage equivalents and duration of analgesic action for several commonly prescribed opiate analgesics (see also Opiate Analgesics General Monograph). This table and a knowledge of the patient's current opiate analgesic requirements provide a useful guide for estimating a patient's total daily codeine dosage requirements. Prescribe an approximately 25% *lower* daily dosage. Dose one-half of the daily dosage every 12 hours. If breakthrough pain occurs toward the end of the dosing interval, increase the dosage gradually, as needed, according to individual patient response. Once pain relief has been achieved, reduce the dosage gradually to the lowest effective dosage. At regular intervals, reevaluate the patient's need for a further decrease or increase in dosage.

Approximate Opiate Analgesic Equivalents.[1]

Opiate Analgesic	Oral Dose (mg)	Duration of Action (hr)
codeine	200	3 to 4
anileridine	75	2 to 3
heroin	20	3 to 4
hydromorphone	7.5	2 to 4
levorphanol	4	4 to 8
meperidine	300	1 to 3
morphine	30	3 to 4
oxycodone	30	2 to 4
pentazocine	180	3 to 4
propoxyphene	100	2 to 4

[1]The sensation of pain and analgesia is the result of a complex interaction between both physiological and psychological variables. Thus, significant variation is noted among patients.

AVAILABLE DOSAGE FORMS, STORAGE, AND COMPATIBILITY

Elixir, oral: 10 mg/5 ml (contains 7% alcohol)
Injectables, intramuscular, subcutaneous: 15, 30, 60 mg/ml
Solution, oral: 15 mg/ml
Syrup, oral: 25 mg/5 ml
Tablets, oral: 15, 30, 60 mg
Tablets, oral extended-release: 100, 150, 200 mg

Notes

Injectable formulations: The injectable formulation of some manufacturers contains sodium bisulfite or sodium metabisulfite. Sulfites have been associated with hypersensitivity reactions, including anaphylactic reactions, among susceptible patients. Although relatively uncommon, these reactions appear to occur with a higher incidence among patients who have asthma.

Oral formulations: The oral extended-release tablets contain two codeine salts, codeine monohydrate and codeine sulfate trihydrate. However, the formulation is labeled and dosed in terms of anhydrous codeine. For example, the 100 mg extended-release tablet contains 53 mg of codeine monohydrate and 62.7 mg of codeine sulfate trihydrate. Each salt form is equivalent to 50 mg of anhydrous codeine.

*Extended-release codeine tablets are recommended **only** for cancer patients who have moderate pain and require long-term pharmacotherapy. They are **not** recommended for patients whose pain is adequately managed with 90 mg daily or less of codeine phosphate. See the Approximate Opiate Analgesic Equivalents table.*

General Instructions for Patients Instruct patients who require codeine pharmacotherapy to

- safely store codeine tablets out of the reach of children in tightly closed child- and light-resistant containers at controlled room temperature (15° to 25°C; 59° to 77°F).

- swallow each dose of the codeine extended-release tablets whole without breaking, chewing, or crushing, with adequate liquid chaser (60 to 120 ml). These tablets are scored and, if required, can be halved for dosage adjustment or to facilitate swallowing.
- obtain an available patient information sheet regarding codeine pharmacotherapy from their pharmacist at the time that their prescription is dispensed. Encourage patients to clarify any questions that they may have concerning their codeine pharmacotherapy with their pharmacist or, if needed, to consult their prescribing psychologist.

PROPOSED MECHANISM OF ACTION

Codeine appears to elicit its analgesic action primarily by binding to the endorphin receptors in the CNS. This binding to receptors is thought to result in the inhibition of neurotransmission in the ascending pain pathways and diminished pain perception. However, the exact mechanism of action has not yet been fully determined.

Similar to other opiate analgesics, codeine produces other actions in addition to analgesia. These actions are mediated by both central and peripheral mechanisms of action and include: cough reduction associated with suppression of the central cough center, constipation associated with decreased gastrointestinal motility, nausea and vomiting associated with stimulation of the CTZ in the medulla, and respiratory depression associated with decreased responsiveness of the central respiratory center to stimulation by carbon dioxide.

See also Opiate Analgesics General Monograph

PHARMACOKINETICS/PHARMACODYNAMICS

The oral availability of codeine varies (i.e., 40% to 70%; mean = 53%). It is only slightly (7%) bound to plasma protein and has an apparent volume of distribution of 2 to 3 L/kg. The onset of action is generally within 30 minutes after oral ingestion or intramuscular or subcutaneous injection. The duration of action is 4 to 6 hours and is extended to ~12 hours for the extended-release formulation. Codeine is metabolized in the liver to several active metabolites, including ~10% of which is morphine (see Morphine Monograph). Less than 5% is excreted in unchanged form in the urine. The mean half-life of elimination is approximately 3 hours. The total body clearance is ~800 ml/minute.

RELATIVE CONTRAINDICATIONS

Alcoholism, acute
CNS depression, severe
Cor pulmonale
Hypersensitivity to codeine or other opiate analgesics
Liver dysfunction, severe
Respiratory depression, severe

CAUTIONS AND COMMENTS

Long-term high-dosage pharmacotherapy, or regular personal use, may result in addiction and habituation.

Prescribe codeine pharmacotherapy cautiously to patients

- who are children. The respiratory center of young children is particularly sensitive to the CNS depressant action of codeine.
- have obstructive airway disorders, such as sleep apnea. Codeine's depressant action on respiratory drive may significantly exacerbate these conditions and may exacerbate the apnea.
- have respiratory dysfunction, including asthma and emphysema. Codeine's drying action on airway secretions and its depressant action on the cough reflex may aggravate these conditions.
- have traumatic head injury, brain tumors, or other conditions associated with increased intracranial pressure. Codeine pharmacotherapy may exacerbate these clinical conditions because of its ability to increase cerebrospinal fluid pressure. It also may mask the clinical course of these patients.

Caution patients who are receiving codeine pharmacotherapy against performing activities that require alertness, judgment, or physical coordination (e.g., driving an automobile, operating dangerous equipment, supervising children). Codeine may cause marked sedation and adversely affect these mental and physical functions.

CLINICALLY SIGNIFICANT DRUG INTERACTIONS

Concurrent codeine pharmacotherapy and the following may result in clinically significant drug interactions:

Alcohol Use

Concurrent alcohol use may increase the CNS depressant action of codeine. Advise patients to avoid, or limit, their use of alcohol while receiving codeine pharmacotherapy (see Relative Contraindications).

Pharmacotherapy With Central Nervous System Depressants and Other Drugs That Produce Central Nervous System Depression

Concurrent codeine pharmacotherapy with other opiate analgesics, sedative-hypnotics, or other drugs that produce CNS depression (e.g., antihistamines, phenothiazines, TCAs) may result in additive CNS depression. It also is important to note that codeine is one of the most common opiates found in prescription and nonprescription cough products.

See also Opiate Analgesics General Monograph

ADVERSE DRUG REACTIONS

Codeine pharmacotherapy has been commonly associated with constipation, dizziness, light-headedness, nausea, sedation, sweating (excessive), and vomiting. Codeine pharmacotherapy also has been associated with the following ADRs, listed according to body system:

CNS: depression, drowsiness, and headache
Cutaneous: flushing

Genitourinary: urinary retention

GI: cramps, dry mouth, and loss of appetite (anorexia)

Ocular: abnormal contraction of the pupils (miosis); blurred vision; constant, involuntary cyclical movement of the eyeball (nystagmus); and double vision (diplopia)

Respiratory: bronchospasm and laryngospasm (generally related to hypersensitivity reactions)

Miscellaneous: chills

See also Opiate Analgesics General Monograph

OVERDOSAGE

See Opiate Analgesics General Monograph

DESIPRAMINE (Desmethylimipramine)

(dess ip′ra meen)

TRADE NAMES

Norpramin®
Pertofrane®

CLASSIFICATION

Antidepressant (tricyclic)

See also Tricyclic Antidepressants General Monograph

APPROVED INDICATIONS FOR PSYCHOLOGICAL DISORDERS

Adjunctive pharmacotherapy for the symptomatic management of mood disorders:

Depressive disorders: Major depressive disorder

USUAL DOSAGE AND ADMINISTRATION

Depressive Disorders: Major Depressive Disorder

Adults: Initially, 100 to 200 mg daily orally in a single dose or divided doses. Generally prescribe lower dosages, and increase the dosage gradually according to individual patient response. For more severely depressed patients, prescribe 300 mg daily, if needed. Pharmacotherapy for patients who require higher daily dosages generally should be initiated in the hospital, where appropriate monitoring and emergency equipment and personnel are immediately available (see Overdosage).

MAINTENANCE: 50 to 100 mg daily orally as a single daily dose. Once the desired therapeutic response is achieved, which usually requires two to three weeks, maintenance pharmacotherapy may be initiated.

MAXIMUM: 300 mg daily orally

Women who are, or who may become, pregnant: FDA Pregnancy Category C. Safety and efficacy of desipramine pharmacotherapy for women who are pregnant have not been established. Maternal desipramine pharmacotherapy near term has been associated with neonatal urinary retention and a neonatal distress syndrome, which includes clonus, hypertonia, respiratory distress, and tremor. Avoid prescribing desipramine pharmacotherapy to women who are pregnant, particularly near term. If desipramine pharmacotherapy is required, advise patients of potential benefits and possible risks to themselves and the embryo, fetus, or neonate. Collaboration with the patient's obstetrician is indicated.

Women who are breast-feeding: Safety and efficacy of desipramine pharmacotherapy for women who are breast-feeding and their neonates and infants have not been established. Desipramine is excreted in breast milk. Breast milk concentrations of desipramine are approximately 30% higher than maternal serum concentrations. Avoid prescribing desipramine pharmacotherapy to women who are breast-feeding. If desipramine pharmacotherapy is required, breast-feeding should be discontinued. Collaboration with the patient's pediatrician may be indicated.

Elderly, frail, or debilitated patients: Initially, orally 25 to 50 mg daily as a single or divided dose. Increase the dosage gradually to 100 mg daily according to individual patient response. Elderly patients who have severe depression may require 150 mg daily. Dosages exceeding 150 mg daily generally are not recommended for elderly, frail, or debilitated patients.

MAINTENANCE: After an optimal desipramine dosage has been established, which usually requires two to three weeks, the daily maintenance dosage may be prescribed as a single daily dose for patient convenience.

MAXIMUM: 150 mg daily orally

Adolescents: Initially, 25 to 50 mg daily orally as a single or divided dose. Increase the dosage gradually to 100 mg daily according to individual patient response. Patients who have severe depression may require 150 mg daily.

MAINTENANCE: After an optimal desipramine dosage has been established, which usually requires two to three weeks, the daily maintenance dosage may be prescribed as a single daily dose for patient convenience.

MAXIMUM: 150 mg daily orally

Children: Safety and efficacy of adjunctive desipramine pharmacotherapy for the symptomatic management of depression have not been established for children. Desipramine pharmacotherapy for this indication is *not* recommended for this age group.

Notes, Depressive Disorders: Major Depressive Disorder

Prescribe for dispensing the smallest quantity of desipramine feasible (generally a two-week supply) because of the risk for suicide among depressed patients. It is recommended that in no case should the dispensed amount exceed a 30-day supply because of desipramine's relatively low therapeutic index. Other suicide precautions may be indicated.

AVAILABLE DOSAGE FORMS, STORAGE, AND COMPATIBILITY

Capsules, oral: 25, 50 mg
Tablets, oral: 10, 25, 50, 75, 100, 150 mg

Notes

General Instructions to Patients Instruct patients who are receiving desipramine pharmacotherapy to

- safely store desipramine tablets out of the reach of children in tightly closed child-resistant containers at room temperature, preferably below 30°C (86°F).
- obtain an available patient information sheet regarding desipramine pharmacotherapy from their pharmacist at the time that their prescription is dispensed. Encourage patients to clarify any questions that they may have concerning their desipramine pharmacotherapy with their pharmacist or, if needed, to consult their prescribing psychologist.

PROPOSED MECHANISM OF ACTION

Desipramine appears to produce its antidepressant action primarily by potentiating the actions of the CNS biogenic amines, specifically norepinephrine and serotonin, by blocking their re-uptake at the presynaptic nerve terminals. This inhibition of re-uptake increases the amount of norepinephrine and serotonin in the synapses and, consequently, results in increased activity at the post-synaptic neuron receptor sites. Evidence suggests that desipramine may block the re-uptake of norepinephrine to a greater extent than serotonin.

See also the Tricyclic Antidepressants General Monograph

PHARMACOKINETICS/PHARMACODYNAMICS

Desipramine is variably absorbed (mean ~40%) following oral ingestion. Up to a 36-fold difference in blood levels may be observed among patients who ingest equal oral doses of desipramine. It is highly plasma protein-bound (~90%) and has an apparent volume of distribution of 20 L/kg. Desipramine is extensively metabolized in the liver and has an active metabolite, 2-hydroxydesipramine. Approximately 2% of an ingested dose is excreted in the urine in unchanged form. The mean half-life of elimination is 22 hours (range 12 to 60 hours). Although therapeutic benefit may occasionally be seen as early as five days after the initiation of desipramine pharmacotherapy, full benefit usually requires two to three weeks of pharmacotherapy.

Therapeutic Drug Monitoring

Dosage must be determined by individual patient response and not desipramine blood levels because it is difficult to correlate blood levels with therapeutic response and ADRs. Absorption and distribution in body fluids vary. However, blood levels may be useful for monitoring the patient's ability to manage his or her pharmacotherapy or for confirming possible overdosage. It is generally recommended to sample from trough concentrations approximately 12 hours after the last dose. However, in cases of suspected overdosage, sampling can be done at anytime. The usual therapeutic blood concentration range is from 430 to 675 nmol/L.

RELATIVE CONTRAINDICATIONS

Hypersensitivity to desipramine or other TCAs
MAOI pharmacotherapy, concurrent or within 14 days

Myocardial infarction, acute recovery phase
Narrow-angle glaucoma, acute

CAUTIONS AND COMMENTS

Prescribe desipramine pharmacotherapy cautiously to patients who

- have bipolar (manic-depressive) disorders. Desipramine pharmacotherapy may induce hypomania after termination of the depressive phase.
- have cardiovascular dysfunction. These patients are at increased risk for cardiac conduction defects, dysrhythmias, myocardial infarction (acute), strokes, and tachycardia. Hypertensive episodes also have been reported among patients who were receiving desipramine pharmacotherapy.
- have diabetes mellitus. Changes in blood sugar levels (i.e., decrease, increase) have been associated with desipramine pharmacotherapy.
- have glaucoma. Desipramine's anticholinergic action may exacerbate this condition.
- have histories of seizure disorders. Desipramine may lower the seizure threshold.
- require elective surgery. Discontinue desipramine pharmacotherapy as soon as possible before elective surgery because of the risk for adverse cardiovascular effects. Collaboration with the patient's surgeon or anesthesiologist is indicated.
- require ECT. If concurrent desipramine pharmacotherapy is required, potential benefits should be weighed against possible risks.
- have schizophrenia or other psychotic disorders. Desipramine pharmacotherapy may exacerbate psychosis among these patients.
- have thyroid disease or are receiving thyroid pharmacotherapy. The risk for cardiovascular toxicity, including dysrhythmias, is increased among these patients.
- have urinary retention. Desipramine's anticholinergic action may exacerbate this condition.

Caution patients who are receiving desipramine pharmacotherapy against

- drinking alcohol. Excessive alcohol use may increase suicide risk among depressed patients. Concurrent alcohol use with desipramine pharmacotherapy may potentiate the CNS depressant action of both alcohol and desipramine.
- performing activities that require alertness, judgment, and physical coordination (e.g., driving an automobile, operating dangerous equipment, supervising children). Desipramine may impair these mental and physical functions.

CLINICALLY SIGNIFICANT DRUG INTERACTIONS

Concurrent desipramine pharmacotherapy and the following may result in clinically significant drug interactions:

Alcohol Use

Concurrent alcohol use may increase the CNS depressant action of desipramine. Advise patients to avoid, or limit, their use of alcohol while receiving desipramine pharmacotherapy.

Clonidine Pharmacotherapy

Concurrent desipramine pharmacotherapy may decrease the antihypertensive action of clonidine (Catapres®).

Guanethidine Pharmacotherapy

Concurrent desipramine pharmacotherapy may decrease the neuronal uptake of guanethidine (Ismelin®) and, thus, decrease its antihypertensive action.

Monoamine Oxidase Inhibitor Pharmacotherapy

Desipramine and MAOI pharmacotherapy, concurrent or within 14 days, may result in hypertensive crises, including severe convulsions and death. When MAOI pharmacotherapy is replaced with desipramine pharmacotherapy, allow at least 14 days to elapse before initiating desipramine pharmacotherapy. Initiate desipramine pharmacotherapy cautiously, and increase the dosage gradually with careful monitoring of individual patient response. See Relative Contraindications.

Pharmacotherapy With Anticholinergics and Other Drugs That Produce Anticholinergic Actions

Concurrent desipramine pharmacotherapy with anticholinergics (e.g., atropine) or other drugs that produce anticholinergic actions (e.g., phenothiazines), may result in additive anticholinergic actions.

Pharmacotherapy With Central Nervous System Depressants and Other Drugs That Produce Central Nervous System Depression

Concurrent desipramine pharmacotherapy with opiate analgesics, sedative-hypnotics, or other drugs that produce CNS depression (e.g., antihistamines; phenothiazines) may result in additive CNS depression.

See also Tricyclic Antidepressants General Monograph

ADVERSE DRUG REACTIONS

Desipramine pharmacotherapy has been associated with an unpleasant taste in the mouth, drowsiness, and fever. Desipramine pharmacotherapy rarely has been associated with serious blood disorders. Monitor patients for signs and symptoms of blood disorders, including flu-like signs and symptoms. Obtain leukocyte and differential counts for patients who develop a fever or sore throat during desipramine pharmacotherapy. Collaboration with the patient's physician or a specialist (e.g., hematologist) may be required. The pharmacologic similarities among the TCAs require that the general ADRs associated with this class of drugs be considered when desipramine pharmacotherapy is prescribed.

See also Tricyclic Antidepressants General Monograph

OVERDOSAGE

There are no specific early signs and symptoms of desipramine overdosage. Serious sequelae are frequently associated with blood levels exceeding 1,000 ng/ml. Overdosages of 10 to 30 times the usual recommended daily dosage are considered to be within the lethal range for adults. The lethal overdosage for children and elderly, frail, or debilitated patients is significantly lower.

Blood levels are not generally helpful for the diagnosis and treatment of desipramine overdosage. CNS effects, respiratory depression, and cardiac dysrhythmias may suddenly occur. Desipramine overdosage requires emergency symptomatic medical support of body systems with attention to increasing desipramine elimination. Hospitalization and close monitoring are generally advisable in cases of suspected overdosage even when the amount ingested is thought to be small and the initial signs and symptoms appear slight or moderate. Low blood desipramine levels are generally obtained after overdosage because of its large volume of distribution, which also explains the ineffectiveness of forced diuresis and hemodialysis in the emergency medical management of overdosage. There is no specific antidote for desipramine overdosage.

DEXFENFLURAMINE[1] ★

(dex fen flure'a meen)

TRADE NAME

Redux®

CLASSIFICATION

Anorexiant (CNS stimulant, amphetamine derivative) (C-IV)

See also Amphetamines General Monograph

APPROVED INDICATIONS FOR PSYCHOLOGICAL DISORDERS

Adjunctive pharmacotherapy for the symptomatic management of:

Eating Disorders: Exogenous Obesity

Dexfenfluramine pharmacotherapy should be prescribed in conjunction with appropriate psychotherapy and a weight-reducing program that includes strategies to suppress appetite and

---

[1] On September 15, 1997, at the request of the FDA, the pharmaceutical manufacturers of dexfenfluramine (Redux®) and fenfluramine (Pondimin®) voluntarily withdrew these two drugs from the market. This action was predicated on the documentation of a significant risk for the development of valvular heart disease among women treated for obesity with a combination of phentermine and fenfluramine (commonly known as "phen-fen") or dexfenfluramine with or without phentermine. For additional discussion, see Adverse Drug Reactions.

reduce caloric intake among patients who have exogenous obesity. The loss of weight among patients who have received anorexiant pharmacotherapy is generally only moderately greater than that obtained by those who have received weight-reducing programs alone. Weight loss is generally significantly greater during initial pharmacotherapy. Unfortunately, the rate of weight loss tends to decrease with continued anorexiant pharmacotherapy because of the development of tolerance to the anorexiant action of these drugs. When weight loss is critical, such as in emergency situations (e.g., preparation for non-elective surgery), pharmacotherapy may be used as an adjunct to dietary measures for as long as, but not beyond, the period of continuous active weight loss. More data are needed regarding the role of psychotherapy alone, or in combination with, anorexiant pharmacotherapy and caloric restriction for the management of exogenous obesity. Safety and efficacy of dexfenfluramine pharmacotherapy beyond twelve months duration have not yet been determined.

USUAL DOSAGE AND ADMINISTRATION

Exogenous Obesity

Adults: 30 mg daily orally in two divided doses

MAXIMUM: 30 mg daily orally

Women who are, or who may become, pregnant: FDA Pregnancy Category C. Safety and efficacy of dexfenfluramine pharmacotherapy for women who are pregnant have not been established. Avoid prescribing dexfenfluramine pharmacotherapy to women who are pregnant. If dexfenfluramine pharmacotherapy is required, advise patients of potential benefits and possible risks to themselves and the embryo, fetus, or neonate. Collaboration with the patient's obstetrician is indicated.

Women who are breast-feeding: Safety and efficacy of dexfenfluramine pharmacotherapy for women who are breast-feeding and their neonates and infants have not been established. Avoid prescribing dexfenfluramine pharmacotherapy to women who are breast-feeding. If dexfenfluramine pharmacotherapy is required, breast-feeding probably should be discontinued. Collaboration with the patient's pediatrician may be indicated.

Elderly, frail, or debilitated patients: Generally prescribe lower dosages for elderly, frail, or debilitated patients. Increase the dosage gradually, if needed, according to individual patient response. These patients may be more sensitive to the pharmacologic actions of dexfenfluramine than are younger or healthier patients.

Children: Safety and efficacy of dexfenfluramine pharmacotherapy for the symptomatic management of eating disorders (exogenous obesity) for children have not been established. Dexfenfluramine pharmacotherapy is *not* recommended for this age group.

Notes, Exogenous Obesity

As for other anorexiant pharmacotherapy, exclude organic causes of obesity (e.g., hypothyroidism) before prescribing dexfenfluramine pharmacotherapy. If patients do not lose at least

4 pounds (1.7 kg) within the first month of pharmacotherapy, reevaluate the need for continued dexfenfluramine pharmacotherapy. Discontinue dexfenfluramine pharmacotherapy when tolerance to its anorexiant action occurs. Weight regain is common after discontinuation of anorexiant pharmacotherapy.

AVAILABLE DOSAGE FORMS, STORAGE, AND COMPATIBILITY

Capsules, oral extended-release: 15 mg

Notes

General Instructions for Patients   Instruct patients who are receiving dexfenfluramine to

- safely store dexfenfluramine capsules out of the reach of children in tightly closed child-resistant containers at controlled room temperature (15° to 30°C; 59° to 86°F).
- obtain an available patient information sheet regarding dexfenfluramine pharmacotherapy from their pharmacist at the time that their prescription is dispensed. Encourage patients to clarify any questions that they may have concerning dexfenfluramine pharmacotherapy with their pharmacist or, if needed, to consult their prescribing psychologist.

PROPOSED MECHANISM OF ACTION

Dexfenfluramine is a sympathomimetic amine with anorexiant action. The exact mechanism of dexfenfluramine's anorexiant action has not yet been fully determined. However, it appears to be associated with increased serotonin levels and increased glucose utilization.

PHARMACOKINETICS/PHARMACODYNAMICS

Dexfenfluramine is completely absorbed following oral ingestion. However, it has a systemic bioavailability of ~68% due to hepatic first-pass metabolism. Dexfenfluramine is lipid soluble and widely distributed in most body tissues with an apparent volume of distribution of 12 L/kg. It is extensively metabolized in the liver to several active and inactive metabolites, including fenfluramine, its de-ethylated metabolite norfenfluramine, and the final metabolite m-trifluoromethyl-hippuric acid, all of which are excreted in the urine. Its mean half-life of elimination is approximately 20 hours, and its mean total body clearance is ~690 ml/minute. The extent of metabolism and urinary excretion is affected by the pH of the urine. Excretion is more rapid in acidic urine than in alkaline urine (e.g., the half-life of elimination can be reduced to 10 hours).

RELATIVE CONTRAINDICATIONS

Glaucoma
Hypersensitivity to dexfenfluramine or fenfluramine
Hypertension, severe
MAOI pharmacotherapy, concurrent or within 14 days

Pulmonary hypertension
Valvular heart disease

CAUTIONS AND COMMENTS

When compared to other anorexiants that have amphetamine-like actions, long-term dexfenfluramine pharmacotherapy has not been as strongly associated with addiction and habituation. Although dexfenfluramine shares common features with the amphetamines, its clinical use reportedly has not resulted in significant problematic patterns of use.

Prescribe dexfenfluramine pharmacotherapy cautiously to patients who

- have histories of mental depression. The discontinuation of dexfenfluramine pharmacotherapy has been associated with depression. Avoid the abrupt discontinuation of dexfenfluramine pharmacotherapy. Gradually reduce the dosage before completely discontinuing pharmacotherapy, and monitor these patients for depression.
- have histories of problematic patterns of abusable psychotropic use. Dexfenfluramine pharmacotherapy may result in addiction and habituation among patients who have a predisposition to problematic patterns of abusable psychotropic use. Monitor these patients closely for the development of problematic patterns of use.
- have hypertension. Dexfenfluramine pharmacotherapy has been associated with hypertension. When prescribed for these patients, monitor for changes in blood pressure carefully. Collaboration with the patient's advanced practice nurse, family physician, or a specialist (e.g., cardiologist) is indicated.

Caution patients who are receiving dexfenfluramine pharmacotherapy against

- performing activities that require alertness, judgment, or physical coordination (e.g., driving an automobile, operating dangerous equipment, supervising children) until their response to dexfenfluramine is known. Dexfenfluramine has a sedative action that may produce mild to moderate drowsiness.

In addition to this general precaution, caution patients to immediately report any deterioration in exercise tolerance (e.g., shortness of breath on exertion). The possible occurrence of primary pulmonary hypertension, a potentially fatal condition, among these patients should be investigated. Collaboration with the patient's family physician or a respiratory specialist is indicated. Primary pulmonary hypertension rarely has been reported and is usually reversible upon discontinuation of dexfenfluramine pharmacotherapy.

CLINICALLY SIGNIFICANT DRUG INTERACTIONS

Concurrent dexfenfluramine pharmacotherapy and the following may result in clinically significant drug interactions:

Antihypertensive Pharmacotherapy

Concurrent dexfenfluramine and antihypertensive pharmacotherapy may require an adjustment in the dosage of the antihypertensive. Collaboration with the prescriber of the antihypertensive is required.

Monoamine Oxidase Inhibitor Pharmacotherapy

Dexfenfluramine may interact with MAOIs (e.g., phenelzine [Nardil®]) and cause the release of large amounts of catecholamines and associated pharmacologic effects (e.g., headache, hypertension), culminating in hypertensive crises. Concurrent dexfenfluramine and MAOI pharmacotherapy is contraindicated.

See also Amphetamines General Monograph

ADVERSE DRUG REACTIONS

Special Warning: As noted at the beginning of this monograph, dexfenfluramine was withdrawn from the market on September 15, 1997, because of the significant risk of developing aortic or mitral valvular regurgitation. The overall estimate from all available studies of related absolute risk is approximately 30%. In comparison to the expected rate in the general population, this risk represents a 15-fold increased risk for valvular dysfunction. In addition to this serious ADR, dexfenfluramine pharmacotherapy has been commonly associated with diarrhea, drowsiness, and dry mouth. Other ADRs associated with dexfenfluramine pharmacotherapy, listed according to body system, include:

Cardiovascular: angina pectoris, edema, heart block (rarely), hypertension, palpitations, valvular heart disease (see *Special Warning*, above), and vasodilation

CNS: agitation, anxiety, confusion, elevated mood, hostility, insomnia, irritability, migraine, and nervousness

Cutaneous: hives, itching, loss of hair (alopecia), rash, and sweating (excessive)

Genitourinary: increased sex drive, painful menses (dysmenorrhea), polyuria, and urinary frequency

GI: abdominal pain, constipation, dyspepsia, flatulence, gastritis, increased appetite, nausea, and thirst (excessive)

Hematologic: anemia

Metabolic/Endocrine: breast pain, diabetes mellitus, goiter, and low blood sugar (hypoglycemia)

Musculoskeletal: arthritis, arthralgia, gout, hypertonia, myalgia, paresthesias, and tremor

Ocular: abnormal reduction or dimness of vision (amblyopia), blurred vision, conjunctivitis, eye irritation, and glaucoma

Respiratory: asthma, bronchitis, inflammation of the sinuses (sinusitis), pulmonary hypertension (see Cautions and Comments), and runny nose (rhinitis)

Miscellaneous: back pain, chills, and fever

See also Amphetamines General Monograph

OVERDOSAGE

Fatal dexfenfluramine overdosages have occurred but reportedly are relatively rare. Signs and symptoms of dexfenfluramine overdosage include abnormal dilation of the pupils (mydriasis), agitation, drowsiness, nausea, sweating (excessive), and vomiting. Dexfenfluramine overdosage requires emergency symptomatic medical support of body systems with attention to increasing dexfenfluramine elimination. There is no known antidote.

DEXTROAMPHETAMINE
(Dexamphetamine)

(dex troe am fet'a meen)

TRADE NAME

Dexedrine®

CLASSIFICATION

CNS stimulant (amphetamine) (C-II)

See also Amphetamines General Monograph

APPROVED INDICATIONS FOR PSYCHOLOGICAL DISORDERS

Adjunctive pharmacotherapy for the symptomatic management of:

- Attention-Deficit/Hyperactivity Disorder
- Sleep Disorders: Narcolepsy

USUAL DOSAGE AND ADMINISTRATION

Attention-Deficit/Hyperactivity Disorder

Adults: Initially, 5 mg daily orally in a single morning dose. Increase the daily dosage weekly by increments of 5 mg until optimal therapeutic response is achieved. Avoid prescribing late afternoon or evening doses because of associated insomnia.

MAXIMUM: 40 mg daily orally

Women who are, or who may become, pregnant: FDA Pregnancy Category C. Safety and efficacy of dextroamphetamine pharmacotherapy for women who are pregnant have not been established. Studies to date on the use of dextroamphetamine during the first trimester of pregnancy have provided mixed results in relation to congenital malformations (i.e., birth defects) and, thus, are inconclusive. Neonates born to mothers who are addicted to amphetamines have an increased risk for premature delivery and low birth weight. During the neonatal period, they also may display signs and symptoms of the amphetamine withdrawal syndrome, including agitation and lassitude. Avoid prescribing dextroamphetamine pharmacotherapy to women who are pregnant. If dextroamphetamine pharmacotherapy is required, advise patients of potential benefits and possible risks to themselves and the embryo, fetus, or neonate. Collaboration with the patient's obstetrician is indicated.

Women who are breast-feeding: Safety and efficacy of dextroamphetamine pharma-cotherapy for women who are breast-feeding and their neonates and infants have not been es-tablished. Amphetamines are excreted in breast milk. Expected pharmacologic actions may be observed among breast-fed neonates and infants, who also may become addicted. Avoid pre-scribing dextroamphetamine pharmacotherapy to women who are breast-feeding. If dextroam-phetamine pharmacotherapy is required, breast-feeding probably should be discontinued. Col-laboration with the patient's pediatrician may be indicated.

Children 3 to 5 years of age: Initially, 2.5 mg daily orally in a single morning dose. Increase the daily dosage weekly by increments of 2.5 mg until optimal therapeutic response is achieved. Avoid prescribing late afternoon or evening doses because of associated insomnia.

MAXIMUM: 40 mg daily orally

Children 6 years of age and older: Initially, 5 mg daily orally in a single morning dose. Increase the daily dosage weekly by increments of 5 mg until optimal therapeutic response is achieved. Avoid prescribing late afternoon or evening doses because of associated insomnia.

MAXIMUM: 40 mg daily orally

Notes, Attention-Deficit/Hyperactivity Disorder

Adjunctive dextroamphetamine pharmacotherapy is not indicated for all adults and children who are diagnosed with A-D/HD. Adjunctive pharmacotherapy should only be considered after a comprehensive psychological assessment has been completed. For children, collaboration with the parents, pediatrician, and teachers is indicated. In addition to appropriate adjunctive phar-macotherapy, a comprehensive multidisciplinary (e.g., psychological, educational, and social) therapeutic program is generally required. This program should be guided by the goal of achiev-ing optimal symptomatic management of A-D/HD among children 3 years of age and older.

Decrements in predicted growth (i.e., height, weight) have been associated with long-term dextroamphetamine pharmacotherapy among children. Monitor children closely who require long-term pharmacotherapy. Whenever possible, interrupt dextroamphetamine pharmacotherapy occasionally to reevaluate the need for continued pharmacotherapy.

Narcolepsy

Adults: 5 to 60 mg daily orally in a single dose or two or three divided doses

Women who are, or who may become, pregnant: FDA Pregnancy Category C. Safety and efficacy of dextroamphetamine pharmacotherapy for women who are pregnant have not been established. Studies to date on the use of dextroamphetamine during the first trimester of preg-nancy have provided mixed results in relation to congenital malformations (i.e., birth defects) and, thus, are inconclusive. Neonates born to mothers who are addicted to amphetamines have an increased risk for premature delivery and low birth weight. During the neonatal period, they also may display signs and symptoms of the amphetamine withdrawal syndrome, including agi-tation and lassitude. Avoid prescribing dextroamphetamine pharmacotherapy to women who are pregnant. If dextroamphetamine pharmacotherapy is required, advise patients of potential ben-efits and possible risks to themselves and the embryo, fetus, or neonate. Collaboration with the patient's obstetrician is indicated.

Women who are breast-feeding: Safety and efficacy of dextroamphetamine pharmacotherapy for women who are breast-feeding and their neonates and infants have not been established. Amphetamines are excreted in breast milk. Expected pharmacologic actions may be observed among breast-fed neonates and infants, who also may become addicted. Avoid prescribing dextroamphetamine pharmacotherapy to women who are breast-feeding. If dextroamphetamine pharmacotherapy is required, breast-feeding probably should be discontinued. Collaboration with the patient's pediatrician may be indicated.

Elderly, frail, or debilitated patients: Generally prescribe lower dosages for elderly, frail, or debilitated patients. Increase the dosage gradually, if needed, according to individual patient response. These patients may be more sensitive to the pharmacologic actions of dextroamphetamine than are younger or healthier adult patients.

Children 6 to 12 years of age: Initially, 5 mg daily orally in a single dose upon awakening in the morning. Increase the daily dosage weekly by increments of 5 mg until optimal therapeutic response is achieved. Narcolepsy seldom occurs among children who are younger than 12 years of age.

MAXIMUM: 60 mg daily orally

Children 12 years of age and older: Initially, 10 mg daily orally in a single dose upon awakening in the morning. Increase the daily dosage weekly by increments of 10 mg until optimal therapeutic response is achieved.

MAXIMUM: 60 mg daily orally

Notes, Narcolepsy

Prescribe the lowest effective dosage. Adjust the dosage according to individual patient response. Late evening doses should be avoided because of associated insomnia. Dexedrine® capsules (Spansules®) are designed to provide extended drug release into the GI tract and sustained therapeutic action for ten to twelve hours. Prescribe these capsules for once daily dosing, when appropriate.

AVAILABLE DOSAGE FORMS, STORAGE, AND COMPATIBILITY

Capsules, oral extended-release: 5, 10, 15 mg
Tablets, oral: 5, 10 mg

Notes

Some oral dosage forms (e.g., Dexedrine® capsules and tablets) contain tartrazine (FD&C Yellow No. 5). Tartrazine has been associated with hypersensitivity reactions (e.g., bronchial asthma) among susceptible patients, particularly those who have a hypersensitivity to aspirin.

General Instructions for Patients   Instruct patients who are receiving dextroamphetamine pharmacotherapy to

- safely store dextroamphetamine capsules and tablets out of the reach of children in tightly closed child- and light-resistant containers at controlled room temperature (15° to 30°C; 59° to 86°F).
- obtain an available patient information sheet regarding dextroamphetamine pharmacotherapy from their pharmacist at the time that their prescription is dispensed. Encourage patients to clarify any questions that they may have concerning dextroamphetamine pharmacotherapy with their pharmacist or, if needed, to consult their prescribing psychologist.

PROPOSED MECHANISM OF ACTION

Dextroamphetamine is a member of the amphetamine group of sympathomimetic amines that have CNS stimulant action. Peripheral actions include elevation of systolic and diastolic blood pressures and weak bronchodilator and respiratory stimulant actions. Dextroamphetamine appears to elicit its stimulant action primarily by increasing the release of norepinephrine from presynaptic storage vesicles in adrenergic neurons. A direct effect on α- and β-adrenergic receptors, inhibition of the enzyme amine oxidase, and the release of dopamine also may be involved. However, the exact mechanism of action has not yet been fully determined.

PHARMACOKINETICS/PHARMACODYNAMICS

Dextroamphetamine appears to be fairly well absorbed following oral ingestion. Peak blood concentrations occur within ~2 hours. The mean half-life of elimination is 10 hours. Additional data are unavailable.

RELATIVE CONTRAINDICATIONS

Addiction and habituation to amphetamines or other abusable psychotropics, history of
Agitation
Arteriosclerosis, advanced
Glaucoma
Heart disease, symptomatic
Hypersensitivity to amphetamines or sympathomimetic amines
Hypertension, moderate to severe
Hyperthyroidism
MAOI pharmacotherapy, concurrent or within 14 days. Hypertensive crisis may result.

CAUTIONS AND COMMENTS

Amphetamines have a high potential for addiction and habituation. Thus, they should be prescribed as adjunctive pharmacotherapy cautiously for the symptomatic management of A-D/HD and narcolepsy. Long-term amphetamine pharmacotherapy, or regular personal use, may lead to addiction and habituation. Thus, attention must be given to the possibility that some patients may become addicted or habituated to dextroamphetamine as a result of their pharmacotherapy. Attention also must be given to the possibility that some patients may seek dextroamphetamine prescriptions to support their addiction or habituation to dextroamphetamines. Prescribe small quantities of dextroamphetamine, and monitor pharmacotherapy closely. Limit prescriptions to the smallest amount that is feasible for dispensing at one time in order to minimize the possible development of problematic patterns of use.

Prescribe dextroamphetamine pharmacotherapy cautiously to patients who

- have cardiovascular disorders, including mild hypertension. Amphetamine pharmacotherapy has been associated with cardiac dysrhythmias and hypertension among these patients.
- have histories of schizophrenia or other psychotic disorders. Amphetamine pharmacotherapy for children who have psychotic disorders may exacerbate signs and symptoms of behavior disturbance and thought disorder. Amphetamines reportedly exacerbate motor and phonic tics and Tourette's disorder (Gilles de la Tourette's syndrome). Clinical assessment of children for tics and Gilles de la Tourette's syndrome should precede prescription of dextroamphetamine pharmacotherapy.

Caution patients who are receiving dextroamphetamine pharmacotherapy against performing activities that require alertness, judgment, and physical coordination (e.g., driving an automobile, operating dangerous equipment, supervising children) until their response to dextroamphetamine pharmacotherapy is known. Dextroamphetamine's CNS stimulant action may adversely affect these mental and physical functions.

See also Amphetamines General Monograph

CLINICALLY SIGNIFICANT DRUG INTERACTIONS

Concurrent dextroamphetamine pharmacotherapy and the following may result in clinically significant drug interactions:

Antipsychotic Pharmacotherapy

Chlorpromazine (Largactil®, Thorazine®), haloperidol (Haldol®), and presumably, other antipsychotics antagonize the CNS stimulatory actions of the amphetamines (see Overdosage).

Guanethidine Pharmacotherapy

Dextroamphetamine pharmacotherapy may decrease the neuronal uptake of guanethidine (Ismelin®) and, thus, decrease its antihypertensive action. A dosage adjustment may be necessary. Collaboration with the prescriber of the guanethidine is required.

Insulin Pharmacotherapy

Dextroamphetamine pharmacotherapy may alter insulin requirements among patients who have insulin-dependent diabetes mellitus. Collaboration with the prescriber of the insulin is required.

Monoamine Oxidase Inhibitor Pharmacotherapy

Dextroamphetamine may interact with MAOIs (e.g., phenelzine [Nardil®]) and cause the release of large amounts of catecholamines. Hypertensive crisis characterized by severe headache and hypertension may result. Dextroamphetamine pharmacotherapy, concurrent or within 14 days of MAOI pharmacotherapy, is *contraindicated*. See Relative Contraindications.

Pharmacotherapy With Drugs That Acidify the Urine

Drugs that acidify the urine (e.g., ammonium chloride) increase the urinary excretion of dextroamphetamine.

Pharmacotherapy With Drugs That Alkalinize the Urine

Drugs that alkalinize the urine (e.g., acetazolamide, sodium bicarbonate) decrease the urinary excretion of dextroamphetamine.

Tricyclic Antidepressant Pharmacotherapy

Concurrent dextroamphetamine and TCA pharmacotherapy (as with other amphetamine or sympathomimetic pharmacotherapy) may result in additive actions. Monitor patients closely and adjust the dosage carefully of both drugs when concurrent pharmacotherapy is prescribed. Both drugs tend to enhance the pharmacologic actions of each other.

See also Amphetamines General Monograph

ADVERSE DRUG REACTIONS

Dextroamphetamine pharmacotherapy has been associated with the following ADRs, listed according to body system:

Cardiovascular: increased blood pressure, palpitations, and tachycardia
CNS: dizziness, dysphoria, euphoria, headache, insomnia, and overstimulation. Psychotic episodes and Gilles de la Tourette's syndrome rarely have been reported at recommended dosages.
Cutaneous: hives (urticaria)
Genitourinary: changes in sex drive and impotence
GI: constipation, diarrhea, dry mouth, gastrointestinal complaints, loss of appetite (anorexia), weight loss, and unpleasant taste
Metabolic/Endocrine: see Genitourinary
Musculoskeletal: restlessness and tremor. Suppression of growth also has been reported among children who have received long-term dextroamphetamine pharmacotherapy

See also Amphetamines General Monograph

OVERDOSAGE

Signs and symptoms of acute dextroamphetamine overdosage, include assaultiveness, cardiovascular reactions (e.g., dysrhythmias, hypertension or hypotension, and circulatory collapse), confusion, gastrointestinal complaints (e.g., abdominal cramps, diarrhea, nausea, and vomiting), dilated and reactive pupils, hallucinations, hyperpyrexia, hyperreflexia, panic, rapid respirations, restlessness, rhabdomyolysis, and tremor. Depression and fatigue usually follow the central stimulation. Fatal poisoning usually terminates in convulsions and coma.

Dextroamphetamine overdosage requires emergency symptomatic medical support of body systems with attention to increasing amphetamine elimination. There is no known antidote. However, the antipsychotics, chlorpromazine and haloperidol, block dopamine and norepinephrine re-uptake and, thus, inhibit the central stimulant actions of dextroamphetamine.

DEZOCINE *

(dez'oh seen)

TRADE NAME

Dalgan®

CLASSIFICATION

Opiate analgesic (mixed agonist/antagonist)

See also Opiate Analgesics General Monograph

APPROVED INDICATIONS FOR PSYCHOLOGICAL DISORDERS

Adjunctive pharmacotherapy for the symptomatic management of:

Pain Disorders: Acute or Chronic Pain, Moderate to Severe

USUAL DOSAGE AND ADMINISTRATION

Acute or Chronic Pain, Moderate to Severe

Adults: 5 to 20 mg intramuscularly every three to six hours; or 2.5 to 10 mg intravenously every two to four hours

MAXIMUM: 20 mg/dose intramuscularly; 120 mg daily intramuscularly

Women who are, or who may become, pregnant: FDA Pregnancy Category C. Safety and efficacy of dezocine pharmacotherapy for women who are pregnant have not been established. Avoid prescribing dezocine pharmacotherapy to women who are pregnant. If dezocine pharmacotherapy is required, advise patients of potential benefits and possible risks to themselves and the embryo, fetus, or neonate. Collaboration with the patient's obstetrician is indicated.

Women who are breast-feeding: Safety and efficacy of dezocine pharmacotherapy for women who are breast-feeding and their neonates and infants have not been established. Avoid prescribing dezocine pharmacotherapy to women who are breast-feeding. If dezocine pharmacotherapy is required, breast-feeding probably should be discontinued. If desired, lactation may be maintained and breast-feeding resumed following the discontinuation of short-term dezocine pharmacotherapy.

Elderly, frail, or debilitated patients: Generally prescribe lower dosages for elderly, frail, or debilitated patients. Increase the dosage gradually, if needed, according to individual patient response. These patients may be more sensitive to the pharmacologic actions of dezocine than are younger or healthier adult patients.

Children and adolescents younger than 18 years of age: Safety and efficacy of dezocine pharmacotherapy for children and adolescents have not been established. Dezocine pharmacotherapy is *not* recommended for this age group.

Notes, Acute or Chronic Pain, Moderate to Severe

Note the differences between the recommended dosages for intramuscular and intravenous injections. Subcutaneous injection is irritating, and should be avoided.

AVAILABLE DOSAGE FORMS, STORAGE, AND COMPATIBILITY

Injectable, intramuscular, intravenous: 5, 10, 15 mg/ml

Notes

The injectable formulation contains sodium metabisulfite. Sulfites have been associated with hypersensitivity reactions, including anaphylactic reactions, among susceptible patients. Although relatively uncommon, these reactions appear to occur with a higher incidence among patients who have asthma.

Store the dezocine injectable safely protected from light at room temperature below 30°C (86°F). Inspect the injectable prior to use for a precipitate. If a precipitate is noted, do not use the injectable formulation. Return the product to the dispensing pharmacy or manufacturer for safe and appropriate disposal.

PROPOSED MECHANISM OF ACTION

Dezocine elicits its analgesic, CNS depressant, and respiratory depressant actions primarily by binding to the endorphin receptors in the CNS. However, the exact mechanism of action has not yet been fully determined.

See also Opiate Analgesics General Monograph

PHARMACOKINETICS/PHARMACODYNAMICS

Dezocine is rapidly and completely absorbed (F = 1) following intramuscular injection. The mean apparent volume of distribution is 10 L/kg. Dezocine is extensively metabolized in the liver, with less than 1% excreted in unchanged form in the urine. The mean half-life of elimination is 2.5 hours (range 1 to 7 hours), and the mean total body clearance is 3 L/hour.

RELATIVE CONTRAINDICATIONS

Hypersensitivity to dezocine

CAUTIONS AND COMMENTS

Dezocine is addicting and habituating. Long-term dezocine pharmacotherapy, or regular personal use, may result in addiction and habituation. Abrupt discontinuation after long-term pharmacotherapy, or regular personal use, may result in a reportedly mild form of the opiate withdrawal syndrome.

See Opiate Analgesics General Monograph

Prescribe dezocine pharmacotherapy cautiously for patients who

- have acute cholecystitis or pancreatitis or will be undergoing surgery of the biliary tract. Opiate agonist analgesics generally increase biliary tract pressure. Although dezocine reportedly may cause little or no elevation of biliary pressure, caution is advised.
- are receiving long-term opiate agonist analgesic (e.g., morphine) pharmacotherapy. Dezocine pharmacotherapy may cause the opiate withdrawal syndrome among these patients because it has mixed opiate agonist/antagonist analgesic properties.
- have head injuries, intracranial lesions, or other conditions associated with increased intracranial pressure. The respiratory depressant action associated with dezocine and its potential for elevating cerebrospinal fluid pressure may markedly exaggerate intracranial pressure among these patients. Dezocine's analgesic and sedative actions may also obscure the clinical course of these patients.
- have histories of addiction and habituation to opiate agonist analgesics (e.g., heroin, morphine). Patients who are addicted and habituated to opiate agonist analgesics may experience the signs and symptoms of the opiate analgesic withdrawal syndrome. Dezocine, a mixed opiate agonist/antagonist analgesic, has weak opiate antagonist action.
- have liver dysfunction. Serious liver dysfunction appears to predispose patients to a higher incidence of ADRs (e.g., anxiety, dizziness, drowsiness, marked apprehension) even when usual recommended dosages are prescribed. These ADRs may be the result of decreased dezocine metabolism by the liver and resultant accumulation and toxicity.
- have respiratory depression, limited respiratory function (e.g., severely limited respiratory reserve, severe bronchial asthma, other obstructive respiratory conditions, such as sleep apnea), or cyanosis. The respiratory depressant action of dezocine may further compromise the respiratory function of these patients.

Caution patients who are receiving dezocine pharmacotherapy against performing activities that require alertness, judgment, and physical coordination (e.g., driving an automobile, operating dangerous equipment, supervising children). The CNS depressant action of dezocine may adversely affect these mental and physical functions.

CLINICALLY SIGNIFICANT DRUG INTERACTIONS

Concurrent dezocine pharmacotherapy and the following may result in clinically significant drug interactions:

Alcohol Use

Concurrent alcohol use may increase the CNS depressant action of dezocine. Advise patients to avoid, or limit, their use of alcohol while receiving dezocine pharmacotherapy.

Pharmacotherapy With Central Nervous System Depressants and Other Drugs That Produce Central Nervous System Depression

Concurrent dezocine pharmacotherapy with other opiate analgesics, sedative-hypnotics, or other drugs that produce CNS depression (e.g., antihistamines, phenothiazines, TCAs) may result in additive CNS depression.

See also Opiate Analgesics General Monograph

ADVERSE DRUG REACTIONS

Dezocine pharmacotherapy commonly has been associated with nausea, sedation, and vomiting. Dezocine pharmacotherapy also has been associated with the following ADRs, listed according to body system:

Cardiovascular: hypotension
CNS: anxiety, confusion, depression, dizziness, and headache
Cutaneous: edema, itching, local irritation at the injection site, rash, and redness of the skin
GI: constipation and dry mouth
Hematologic: low hemoglobin (anemia)
Musculoskeletal: cramps and muscle pain
Ocular: blurred vision and double vision (diplopia)
Otic: congestion in the ears and ringing in the ears (tinnitus)
Respiratory: respiratory depression

See also Opiate Analgesics General Monograph

OVERDOSAGE

Signs and symptoms of dezocine overdosage are similar to the signs and symptoms associated with other opiate analgesic overdosage (e.g., acute respiratory depression, cardiovascular compromise, and delirium). Dezocine overdosage requires emergency symptomatic medical support of body systems with attention to increasing dezocine elimination. Naloxone (Narcan®) is a specific and effective antidote.

DIAZEPAM

(dye az'e pam)

TRADE NAMES

Diazemuls®
Dizac®
Novo-Dipam®
Valium®
Vivol®

CLASSIFICATION

Sedative-hypnotic (benzodiazepine) (C-IV)

See also Benzodiazepines General Monograph

APPROVED INDICATIONS FOR PSYCHOLOGICAL DISORDERS

Adjunctive pharmacotherapy for the short-term symptomatic management of:

- Anxiety Disorders. Diazepam pharmacotherapy is *not* indicated for the management of everyday anxiety or tension, or anxiety that can be managed with psychotherapy alone. Diazepam also is *not* recommended for the management of anxiety associated with depression because it has the potential to exacerbate the depression while alleviating the anxiety. The depression associated with anxiety generally resolves with appropriate adjunctive pharmacotherapy (i.e., antidepressant pharmacotherapy) and psychotherapy.
- Substance-Related Disorders: Alcohol Withdrawal Syndrome (Acute). Diazepam pharmacotherapy has been found to be of benefit for the symptomatic management of the acute agitation, tremor, impending or acute delirium tremens, and hallucinations associated with the acute alcohol withdrawal syndrome.

USUAL DOSAGE AND ADMINISTRATION

Anxiety Disorders

Adults: Initially, 4 to 40 mg daily orally in two to four divided doses according to the severity of the signs and symptoms of anxiety. Injectable pharmacotherapy may be required for the symptomatic management of moderate and severe anxiety.

MODERATE ANXIETY: 2 to 5 mg intramuscularly or intravenously. Repeat the dose in three to four hours, if needed, according to individual patient response.

SEVERE ANXIETY: 5 to 10 mg intramuscularly or intravenously. Repeat the dose in three to four hours, if needed, according to individual patient response.

Women who are, or who may become, pregnant: FDA Pregnancy Category D. An increased risk for congenital malformations (e.g., cleft lip and palate, limb and digit malformations) has been associated with diazepam pharmacotherapy during the first trimester of pregnancy. However, data are inconclusive. Maternal use near term has been associated with expected pharmacologic actions among neonates, including hypotonia, low Apgar scores, poor feeding, and signs and symptoms of diazepam withdrawal. Avoid prescribing diazepam pharmacotherapy to women who are pregnant. If diazepam pharmacotherapy is required, advise patients of potential benefits and possible risks to themselves and the embryo, fetus, or neonate. Collaboration with the patient's obstetrician is indicated.

Women who are breast-feeding: Safety and efficacy of diazepam pharmacotherapy for women who are breast-feeding and their neonates and infants have not been established. Diazepam is excreted in breast milk in sufficient quantities to cause sedation and addiction among breast-fed neonates and infants. Avoid prescribing diazepam pharmacotherapy to women who are breast-feeding. If diazepam pharmacotherapy is required, breast-feeding should be discontinued. If desired, lactation may be maintained and breast-feeding resumed following the discontinuation of short-term diazepam pharmacotherapy. Collaboration with the patient's pediatrician is indicated.

Elderly, frail, or debilitated patients and those who have cardiovascular or respiratory dysfunction: Initially, 2 to 5 mg daily orally in a single or two divided doses. Generally prescribe lower dosages for elderly, frail, or debilitated patients. Increase the dosage gradually, if needed, according to individual patient response. These patients may be more sensitive to the pharmacologic actions of diazepam than are younger or healthier patients. When injectable diazepam pharmacotherapy is required, also prescribe lower dosages. Inject diazepam intravenously with extreme caution among these patients and those who have cardiovascular or respiratory dysfunction. These patients are at particular risk for apnea and cardiac arrest. Resuscitative equipment and emergency medical personnel should be readily available when intravenous diazepam pharmacotherapy is administered.

Children: Initially, 3 to 10 mg daily orally in three or four divided doses. Generally prescribe lower dosages for children. Increase the dosage gradually, as needed, according to individual patient response. When injectable diazepam pharmacotherapy is required, inject diazepam intravenously at a slow rate over a three-minute period. Do *not* exceed 0.25 mg/kg. After an interval of 15 to 30 minutes, the initial dose may be safely repeated, if needed, according to individual patient response. However, if the signs and symptoms of anxiety are not managed after a third injection, other adjunctive therapy appropriate for the symptomatic management of anxiety is recommended. These recommendations for injectable diazepam pharmacotherapy using lower dosages of the drug will help to assure maximal therapeutic benefit with a minimal risk for serious ADRs (e.g., apnea or prolonged periods of somnolence).

MAXIMUM: 10 mg/dose intravenously; 20 mg/dose orally (all regular oral dosage forms); 30 mg/dose orally (extended-release capsules)

Notes, Anxiety Disorders

Adjust dosage according to individual patient response for optimal therapeutic benefit. While most patients will benefit from usual recommended dosages, some patients may require higher dosages. Increase the dosage gradually for these patients to avoid associated ADRs. Patients who are stabilized on dosages of 5 or 10 mg three times daily may benefit from once daily dosing with the extended-release formulation. Prescribe one 15 or 30 mg extended-release capsule orally daily for these patients, respectively.

Periodic blood counts and liver function tests are advised for patients who require long-term (i.e., periods up to 4 months) diazepam pharmacotherapy. Long-term diazepam pharmacotherapy rarely has been associated with jaundice and neutropenia. Collaboration with the patient's family physician or a specialist (e.g., hematologist) is indicated.

The safety and efficacy of long-term diazepam pharmacotherapy (longer than four months) have not been established. Reevaluate patients who appear to require diazepam pharmacotherapy for longer than four months. A benzodiazepine withdrawal syndrome similar to the alcohol withdrawal syndrome may occur after discontinuation of long-term diazepam pharmacotherapy.

Injectable diazepam pharmacotherapy: The usual recommended dosage for injectable diazepam pharmacotherapy for children and adults ranges from 2 to 20 mg intramuscularly or intravenously. The dosage prescribed depends on the indication for diazepam pharmacotherapy and the severity of the patient's signs and symptoms. Injectable diazepam pharmacotherapy is contraindicated for patients who are in shock, are comatose, are acutely intoxicated with alcohol, or have cardiovascular or respiratory depression. Patients should be lying down for injectable pharmacotherapy. Monitor patients carefully following injectable diazepam pharmacotherapy until complete alertness and psychomotor functions are restored. Do not mix or dilute diazepam injectable with other drugs in the same syringe or intravenous solution.

Lower dosages (usually 2 to 5 mg) and a gradual increase in dosage are recommended for elderly, frail, or debilitated patients. Lower dosages also are recommended for patients who are receiving concurrent pharmacotherapy with other drugs that produce CNS and respiratory depression (e.g., opiate analgesics). Concurrent diazepam pharmacotherapy with drugs that produce CNS and respiratory depression may increase respiratory depression and the risk for apnea. Although some patients may not continue to require concurrent CNS and respiratory depressant pharmacotherapy, when concurrent pharmacotherapy is required, gradually reduce the daily dosage of the drug that produces CNS or respiratory depression by at least one-third, and dose through the day in small increments. Once the acute signs and symptoms of anxiety have been appropriately managed with injectable diazepam pharmacotherapy, replace the injectable pharmacotherapy with oral diazepam pharmacotherapy, if further pharmacotherapy is required.

INTRAMUSCULAR PHARMACOTHERAPY.   Inject diazepam intramuscularly deep into healthy muscle sites. Rotate injection sites carefully when more than one injection is required.

INTRAVENOUS PHARMACOTHERAPY.   Intravenous diazepam pharmacotherapy requires the immediate availability of facilities and personnel for emergency medical support of respiratory function because of the increased risk for apnea. Venous thrombosis, phlebitis, local irritation, and swelling also have been associated with the intravenous injection of diazepam. To avoid or minimize these ADRs, slowly inject each dose of diazepam, taking at least one minute for each 5 mg (1 ml) injected. Avoid injecting the small veins on the back of the hand or near the wrist. Assure correct placement of the needle or catheter in the vein before injection, and use extreme care to avoid intra-arterial injection or extravasation. If it is not feasible to slowly inject diazepam directly into a vein, inject diazepam slowly through the tubing of a patent continuous intravenous infusion as close as possible to the vein insertion site.

Alcohol Withdrawal Syndrome, Acute

Adults: Initially, 30 to 40 mg orally during the first 24 hours in three or four divided doses. Depending on the severity of the patient's signs and symptoms, reduce the dosage to 15 to 20 mg daily orally in three or four divided doses, as needed. Initially, some patients may require 10 mg intramuscularly or intravenously. This dose may be followed by an additional dose of 5 to 10 mg intramuscularly or intravenously in three to four hours, if needed.

Women who are, or who may become, pregnant: See Usual Dosage and Administration, Anxiety Disorders

Women who are breast-feeding: See Usual Dosage and Administration, Anxiety Disorders

Elderly, frail, or debilitated patients: Initially, 15 mg daily orally in three divided doses. Increase the dosage gradually, if needed, according to individual patient response. Generally prescribe lower dosages for elderly, frail, or debilitated patients. These patients may be more sensitive to the pharmacologic actions of diazepam than are younger or healthier adult patients.

Children: Safety and efficacy of diazepam pharmacotherapy for the symptomatic management of the acute alcohol withdrawal syndrome among children have not been established. Diazepam pharmacotherapy is *not* recommended for this indication for this age group.

Notes, Alcohol Withdrawal Syndrome, Acute

See Notes, Anxiety Disorders

AVAILABLE DOSAGE FORMS, STORAGE, AND COMPATIBILITY

Capsules, oral extended-release (Valrelease®): 15 mg
Injectable, intravenous (Dizac®): 5 mg/ml
Injectable, intramuscular and intravenous (Diazemuls®): 5 mg/ml (oil/water emulsion)
Injectable, Tel-E-Ject® disposable syringe: 5 mg/ml
Solution, oral: 1 mg/ml
Solution, oral concentrate (Diazepam Intensol®): 5 mg/ml (contains 19% alcohol)
Tablets, oral: 2, 5, 10 mg

Notes

Injectable Dosage Formulations Injectable diazepam emulsion (Diazemuls®) is for intramuscular and intravenous use. Diazemuls® is incompatible with morphine and glycopyrrolate (Robinul®). For intravenous injection, do *not* administer with intravenous infusion sets containing PVC. Use glass, polyethylene, or polyethylene/polypropylene syringes and infusion sets.

Injectable diazepam (Dizac®, Zetran®) contains both benzyl alcohol and propylene glycol and is for intravenous injection *only*. Store Dizac® and Zetran® safely protected from light at room temperature below 25°C (77°F), and avoid freezing. Dizac® and Zetran® are incompatible with morphine and glycopyrrolate (Robinul®).

Oral Dosage Formulations Do not confuse the oral solution with the concentrated oral solution. Serious overdosage may result.

General Instructions for Patients Instruct patients who are receiving diazepam pharmacotherapy to

- safely store diazepam tablets out of the reach of children in child- and light-resistant containers at controlled room temperature (15° to 30°C; 59° to 86°F).
- obtain an available patient information sheet regarding diazepam pharmacotherapy from their pharmacist at the time that their prescription is dispensed. Encourage patients to clarify any questions that they may have concerning diazepam pharmacotherapy with their pharmacist or, if needed, to consult their prescribing psychologist.

PROPOSED MECHANISM OF ACTION

The exact mechanism of action of diazepam has not yet been fully determined. However, it appears to be primarily mediated by, or to work in concert with, the inhibitory neurotransmitter GABA. Thus, diazepam appears to act by binding to the benzodiazepine receptors within the GABA complex.

See also Benzodiazepines General Monograph

PHARMACOKINETICS/PHARMACODYNAMICS

Diazepam is virtually completely absorbed following oral ingestion (F ~ 1) and achieves peak blood concentrations within 1 to 2 hours. Following intravenous injection, peak blood concentrations are achieved within 15 minutes. Although absorption following intramuscular injection may be erratic, depending on blood flow to the muscle, peak absorption usually occurs within 2 hours. Once absorbed, diazepam is highly plasma protein-bound (approximately 98%) and has an apparent volume of distribution of ~1 L/kg. It is extensively metabolized in the liver to both active (e.g., desmethyldiazepam, oxazepam) and inactive metabolites. Less than 1% of diazepam is excreted in unchanged form in the urine. The mean half-life of elimination is 43 hours, and the mean total body clearance is 28 ml/minute.

RELATIVE CONTRAINDICATIONS

Glaucoma, acute narrow-angle. Diazepam pharmacotherapy may be prescribed to patients who have open-angle glaucoma and are receiving appropriate pharmacotherapy. Collaboration with the patient's ophthalmologist is indicated.

Hypersensitivity to diazepam or other benzodiazepines

CAUTIONS AND COMMENTS

Long-term diazepam pharmacotherapy, or regular personal use, may result in addiction and habituation. Abrupt discontinuation of long-term high-dosage pharmacotherapy, or regular personal use, has been associated with a diazepam withdrawal syndrome similar to the alcohol withdrawal syndrome. Signs and symptoms of the diazepam withdrawal syndrome include abdominal and muscle cramps, convulsions, tremor, vomiting, and sweating. Milder withdrawal signs and symptoms, such as dysphoria and insomnia, have been associated with the abrupt discontinuation of benzodiazepine pharmacotherapy among patients who have used recommended dosages over several months. Avoid discontinuing diazepam pharmacotherapy abruptly, particularly when pharmacotherapy has been extended over several months. A gradual tapering of the dosage is recommended.

Prescribe diazepam pharmacotherapy cautiously to patients who have

- histories of problematic patterns of alcohol or other abusable psychotropic use. Diazepam can produce addiction and habituation. Monitor patients closely for signs and symptoms of problematic patterns of use.
- kidney or liver dysfunction
- severe or latent depression

Caution patients who are receiving diazepam pharmacotherapy against

- drinking alcohol or using other drugs that produce CNS depression. The use of alcohol or other drugs that produce CNS depression may result in excessive CNS and respiratory depression.
- increasing their prescribed dosage of diazepam, using their diazepam more often than prescribed, or abruptly discontinuing their diazepam pharmacotherapy without first consulting with their prescribing psychologist. Diazepam is addicting and habituating, and a withdrawal syndrome has been associated with abruptly discontinuing use.
- performing activities that require alertness, judgment, or physical coordination (e.g., driving an automobile, operating dangerous equipment, supervising children). Diazepam's associated CNS depressant action may adversely affect these mental and physical functions.

In addition to these general precautions for patients, caution women to inform their prescribing psychologist if they become, or intend to become, pregnant while receiving diazepam pharmacotherapy, so that their pharmacotherapy can be safely discontinued.

CLINICALLY SIGNIFICANT DRUG INTERACTIONS

Concurrent diazepam pharmacotherapy and the following may result in clinically significant drug interactions:

Alcohol Use

Concurrent alcohol use may increase the CNS depressant action of diazepam. Advise patients to avoid, or limit, their use of alcohol while receiving diazepam pharmacotherapy.

Cimetidine Pharmacotherapy

Concurrent diazepam and cimetidine (Tagamet®) pharmacotherapy may result in the delayed or decreased elimination of diazepam. The clinical significance of this interaction is unclear.

Pharmacotherapy With Central Nervous System Depressants and Other Drugs That Produce Central Nervous System Depression

Concurrent diazepam pharmacotherapy with opiate analgesics, other sedative-hypnotics, or other drugs that produce CNS depression (e.g., antihistamines, phenothiazines, TCAs) may result in additive CNS depression.

See also Benzodiazepines General Monograph

ADVERSE DRUG REACTIONS

Diazepam pharmacotherapy commonly has been associated with drowsiness, fatigue, and incoordination (ataxia). Hypotension and muscular weakness have been associated with injectable diazepam pharmacotherapy, particularly among patients who were using alcohol or were concurrently receiving barbiturate or opiate analgesic pharmacotherapy. Adverse drug reactions associated with the intravenous injection of diazepam include phlebitis and venous thrombosis at the injection site. Other ADRs associated with diazepam pharmacotherapy, listed according to body system, include:

Cardiovascular: bradycardia, cardiovascular collapse, fainting (syncope), and hypotension
CNS: confusion, depression, headache, hypoactivity, slurred speech, tremor, and vertigo. Paradoxical reactions, including anxiety (acute), hyper-excited states, hallucinations, insomnia, rage, sleep disturbances, and over-stimulation, have been reported. If these ADRs are observed, discontinue diazepam pharmacotherapy. Minor changes in EEG pattern, usually low-voltage fast activity, have been observed among patients during and following diazepam pharmacotherapy. These changes are of no known clinical significance.
Cutaneous: hives (urticaria) and skin rash
Genitourinary: changes in sex drive, urinary incontinence, and urinary retention
GI: changes in salivation, constipation, fecal incontinence, hiccups, and nausea
Hematologic: decreased neutrophils (neutropenia)
Hepatic: jaundice
Musculoskeletal: difficult and defective speech due to impairment of the tongue or other muscles essential to speech (dysarthria), muscle spasms, and tremor
Ocular: blurred vision; constant, involuntary, cyclical movement of the eyeball (nystagmus); and double vision (diplopia)

See also Benzodiazepines General Monograph

OVERDOSAGE

Signs and symptoms of diazepam overdosage include confusion, somnolence, coma, and diminished reflexes. Diazepam overdosage requires emergency symptomatic medical support of body systems with attention to increasing diazepam elimination. Flumazenil (Anexate®, Romazicon®), the benzodiazepine antagonist, may be required.

DIETHYLPROPION (Amfepramone)

(dye eth il proe'pee on)

TRADE NAMES

Tenuate®
Tenuate Dospan®

CLASSIFICATION

Anorexiant (CNS stimulant, amphetamine derivative) (C-IV)

See also Amphetamines General Monograph

APPROVED INDICATIONS FOR PSYCHOLOGICAL DISORDERS

Adjunctive pharmacotherapy for the short-term symptomatic management of:

Eating Disorders: Exogenous Obesity

USUAL DOSAGE AND ADMINISTRATION

Exogenous Obesity

Adults: 75 mg daily orally in three divided doses one hour before meals; or 75 mg extended-release tablet daily orally in the mid-morning. If required, an additional 25 mg oral dose may be prescribed for the mid-evening to overcome hunger during the night. Tolerance to diethylpropion's anorexiant action usually develops within a few weeks. When tolerance to the anorexiant action is noted, discontinue diethylpropion pharmacotherapy. Do *not* exceed the recommended dosage in an attempt to maintain diethylpropion's anorexiant action.

Women who are, or who may become, pregnant: FDA Pregnancy Category "not established." Safety and efficacy of diethylpropion pharmacotherapy for women who are pregnant have not been established. Avoid prescribing diethylpropion pharmacotherapy to women who are pregnant. If diethylpropion pharmacotherapy is required, advise patients of potential benefits and possible risks to themselves and the embryo, fetus, or neonate. Collaboration with the patient's obstetrician is indicated.

Women who are breast-feeding: Safety and efficacy of diethylpropion pharmacotherapy for women who are breast-feeding and their neonates and infants have not been established. Avoid prescribing diethylpropion pharmacotherapy to women who are breast-feeding. If diethylpropion pharmacotherapy is required, breast-feeding probably should be discontinued. If desired, lactation may be maintained and breast-feeding resumed following the discontinuation of short-term diethylpropion pharmacotherapy. Collaboration with the patient's pediatrician may be indicated.

Children younger than 12 years of age: The safety and efficacy of diethylpropion pharmacotherapy for children younger than 12 years of age have not been established. Diethylpropion pharmacotherapy is *not* recommended for this age group.

Notes, Exogenous Obesity

Diethylpropion is indicated only for short-term adjunctive pharmacotherapy (a maximum of 12 weeks) for weight loss among obese patients who also are receiving appropriate psychotherapy, caloric restriction, and other appropriate treatment (e.g., supervised exercise program). The reportedly limited therapeutic effectiveness of diethylpropion pharmacotherapy for these patients must be weighed against potential risks, including addiction and habituation (see Adverse Drug Reactions).

AVAILABLE DOSAGE FORMS, STORAGE, AND COMPATIBILITY

Tablets, oral: 25 mg
Tablets, oral extended-release: 75 mg

Notes

General Instructions for Patients Instruct patients who are receiving diethylpropion pharmacotherapy to

- swallow whole, without breaking, crushing, or chewing, each dose of the diethylpropion extended-release tablets with adequate water or compatible liquid chaser (60 to 120 ml).
- safely store diethylpropion oral dosage forms out of the reach of children in tightly closed child-resistant containers at controlled room temperature (15° to 30°C; 59° to 86°F).
- obtain an available patient information sheet regarding diethylpropion pharmacotherapy from their pharmacist at the time that their prescription is dispensed. Encourage patients to clarify any questions that they may have concerning diethylpropion pharmacotherapy with their pharmacist or, if needed, to consult their prescribing psychologist.

PROPOSED MECHANISM OF ACTION

Diethylpropion is a CNS stimulant sympathomimetic amine pharmacologically derived from the amphetamines. Actions include CNS stimulation and elevation of blood pressure. Diethylpropion also has been associated with tachyphylaxis and tolerance. The exact mechanism of the anorexiant action of diethylpropion, including appetite suppression, has not yet been fully determined. However, diethylpropion appears to stimulate the CNS directly. Metabolic or other actions also may be involved.

PHARMACOKINETICS/PHARMACODYNAMICS

Data are unavailable.

RELATIVE CONTRAINDICATIONS

Agitation
Arteriosclerosis, advanced
Glaucoma
Hypersensitivity to diethylpropion or sympathomimetic amines
Hyperthyroidism
MAOI pharmacotherapy, concurrent or within 14 days. Concurrent diethylpropion and
  MAOI pharmacotherapy may result in hypertensive crises.
Problematic patterns of diethylpropion, amphetamine, or other abusable psychotropic use,
  history of

CAUTIONS AND COMMENTS

Long-term diethylpropion pharmacotherapy, or regular personal use, may result in addiction and
habituation. Diethylpropion is chemically and pharmacologically related to the amphetamines,
which have high abuse potential. Patients may try to increase their dosages to many times those
recommended or use their diethylpropion more often than recommended. Monitor patients for
such signs and symptoms of problematic patterns of use as hyperactivity, irritability, insomnia,
personality changes, and severe dermatoses. Psychosis also has been associated with problematic patterns of use. It is often clinically indistinguishable from schizophrenia. Prescribe the least
amount of diethylpropion feasible for dispensing at one time to minimize the possible development of problematic patterns of use.

The abrupt discontinuation of long-term diethylpropion pharmacotherapy, or regular personal use, has been associated with an amphetamine-like withdrawal syndrome. This syndrome
includes signs and symptoms of extreme fatigue and mental depression. Changes also have been
reported on EEGs. Avoid discontinuing long-term diethylpropion pharmacotherapy or regular
personal use abruptly. A gradual tapering of dosage is recommended.

Prescribe diethylpropion pharmacotherapy cautiously to patients who

- have insulin-dependent diabetes mellitus. Diethylpropion, particularly when prescribed
  with concurrent caloric restrictions or an exercise program, may alter insulin requirements.
- have severe cardiovascular disorders, including severe hypertension. Diethylpropion may
  increase blood pressure.

Caution patients who are receiving diethylpropion pharmacotherapy against performing activities that require alertness, judgment, and physical coordination (e.g., driving an automobile,
operating dangerous equipment, supervising children) until their response to diethylpropion pharmacotherapy is known. Diethylpropion's CNS stimulant actions may adversely affect these mental and physical functions.

CLINICALLY SIGNIFICANT DRUG INTERACTIONS

Concurrent diethylpropion pharmacotherapy and the following may result in clinically significant
drug interactions:

Guanethidine Pharmacotherapy

Diethylpropion may decrease the neuronal uptake of guanethidine (Ismelin®) and, thus, decrease its antihypertensive action. An adjustment in the guanethidine dosage may be required. Collaboration with the prescriber of the guanethidine is indicated.

Monoamine Oxidase Inhibitor Pharmacotherapy

Diethylpropion may interact with MAOIs (e.g., phenelzine [Nardil®]). This interaction may cause the release of large amounts of catecholamines and result in hypertensive crisis characterized by a severe headache and hypertension. Concurrent diethylpropion and MAOI pharmacotherapy is *contraindicated*.

See also Amphetamines General Monograph

ADVERSE DRUG REACTIONS

Diethylpropion pharmacotherapy has been associated with the following ADRs, listed according to body system:

Cardiovascular: hypertension, palpitations, and tachycardia
CNS: anxiety, dizziness, euphoria, insomnia, jitteriness, and nervousness
Cutaneous: hives (urticaria), rash, and redness of the skin (erythema)
Genitourinary: decreased sex drive, impotence, menstrual irregularities, and excessive urination (polyuria)
GI: abdominal discomfort, constipation, diarrhea, dry mouth, dyspepsia, nausea, and vomiting
Metabolic/Endocrine: see Genitourinary
Musculoskeletal: muscle pain

See also Amphetamines General Monograph

OVERDOSAGE

Signs and symptoms of acute diethylpropion overdosage include convulsions, drowsiness, exhaustion, insomnia, irritability, nervousness, and tachycardia. Diethylpropion overdosage requires emergency symptomatic medical support of body systems with attention to increasing diethylpropion elimination. There is no known antidote.

DISULFIRAM

(dye sul'fi ram)

TRADE NAME

Antabuse®

CLASSIFICATION

Anti-alcoholic (alcohol dehydrogenase inhibitor)

APPROVED INDICATIONS FOR PSYCHOLOGICAL DISORDERS

Adjunctive pharmacotherapy for the behavioral management of chronic alcoholism:

Alcohol Abstinence Maintenance. Disulfiram pharmacotherapy is *not* a cure for alcoholism. Prescribed alone, without appropriate psychotherapy or other supportive treatment (e.g., Alcoholics Anonymous), it is unlikely that disulfiram pharmacotherapy will have more than a brief positive effect on the patient's established drinking pattern.

USUAL DOSAGE AND ADMINISTRATION

Alcohol Abstinence Maintenance

Adults: Initially, 500 mg daily orally in a single dose, preferably ingested in the morning, for one to two weeks. Patients who experience sedation may ingest their daily dose 30 minutes before retiring for bed in the evening. Some patients may require a decrease in dosage.

MAINTENANCE: 125 to 500 mg daily orally as a single dose in the morning or 30 minutes before retiring for bed in the evening. Therapeutic benefit for most patients may be achieved with a dosage of 250 mg daily.

MAXIMUM: 500 mg daily orally

Women who are, or who may become, pregnant: FDA Pregnancy Category X. Safety and efficacy of disulfiram pharmacotherapy for women who are pregnant have not been established. Although the potential for congenital malformations (i.e., birth defects) is inconclusive, limb reduction anomalies among neonates born to mothers who received disulfiram pharmacotherapy during pregnancy have been reported. Do *not* prescribe disulfiram pharmacotherapy to woman who are pregnant.

Women who are breast-feeding: Safety and efficacy of disulfiram pharmacotherapy for women who are breast-feeding and their neonates and infants have not been established. It is unknown whether disulfiram is excreted in breast milk. Avoid prescribing disulfiram pharmacotherapy to women who are breast-feeding. If disulfiram pharmacotherapy is required, breast-feeding should be discontinued. Collaboration with the patient's pediatrician is indicated.

Children: Safety and efficacy of disulfiram pharmacotherapy for the behavioral management of chronic alcoholism among children have not been established. Disulfiram pharmacotherapy is *not* recommended for this age group.

Notes, Alcohol Abstinence Maintenance

Initiating Disulfiram Pharmacotherapy Before initiating disulfiram pharmacotherapy, assure that patients have abstained from the use of alcohol for at least 12 hours. Advise patients fully about the disulfiram-alcohol reaction and caution them against surreptitious drinking during disulfiram pharmacotherapy. In this regard, assure, as much as possible, their understanding of the consequences of drinking any alcohol while receiving disulfiram pharmacotherapy. Patients must understand the potential seriousness of the disulfiram-alcohol reaction.

Advise patients that if they ingest alcoholic beverages, alcohol-containing foods (sauces and vinegars), cough and cold products, aftershave lotions, or liniments that contain alcohol, they will experience the "disulfiram reaction" (i.e., alcohol challenge reaction). This reaction may result in cardiovascular collapse, convulsions, facial flushing, gastrointestinal distress (acute), headache, palpitations, respiratory depression, or death.

Obtain transaminase tests upon the initiation of disulfiram pharmacotherapy, and within 10 to 14 days, to detect any liver dysfunction that may be associated with disulfiram pharmacotherapy. Also obtain a complete blood count and a sequential multiple analysis-12 test (SMA 12) every six months for patients who are receiving long-term disulfiram pharmacotherapy. Collaboration with the patient's family physician is indicated.

Maintaining Disulfiram Pharmacotherapy Daily disulfiram pharmacotherapy must be continued uninterrupted until patients are able to establish alternative means for remaining abstinent from alcohol (e.g., cognitive skills training). Some patients may require disulfiram maintenance pharmacotherapy for months or years. The possibility of these patients initiating a new addiction or habituation (e.g., substituting another abusable psychotropic for their alcohol, such as a benzodiazepine) requires careful consideration and appropriate monitoring.

Patients who report unaffected drinking behavior in relation to their prescribed disulfiram pharmacotherapy may not be correctly following their prescribed pharmacotherapy. Some patients may be disposing of their tablets without ingesting them. Correct use must be confirmed for these patients. For these patients, crush the oral tablet and mix it well with a compatible liquid or soft food for ingestion with supervision. Supervised ingestion will help to confirm noncompliance or the reported lack of efficacy associated with the prescribed disulfiram pharmacotherapy.

Discontinuing Disulfiram Pharmacotherapy After a patient has maintained abstinence for a satisfactory period, disulfiram pharmacotherapy may be discontinued. Advise patients to maintain abstinence because the disulfiram reaction may occur for up to 14 days following the discontinuation of disulfiram pharmacotherapy. Some patients may continue to require disulfiram pharmacotherapy for those situations where they are at increased risk for relapse (e.g., traveling away from home and staying in a hotel room where alcohol may be readily available).

AVAILABLE DOSAGE FORMS, STORAGE, AND COMPATIBILITY

Tablets, oral: 250, 500 mg

Notes

General Instructions for Patients   Instruct patients who are receiving disulfiram pharmacotherapy to

- safely store their disulfiram tablets out of the reach of children in tightly closed child- and light-resistant containers at controlled room temperature (15° to 30°C; 59° to 86°F).
- obtain an available patient information sheet regarding disulfiram pharmacotherapy from their pharmacist at the time that their prescription is dispensed. Encourage patients to clarify any questions that they may have concerning disulfiram pharmacotherapy with their pharmacist or, if needed, to consult their prescribing psychologist.

PROPOSED MECHANISM OF ACTION

Disulfiram blocks the metabolism (oxidation) of alcohol at the acetaldehyde stage by inhibiting the enzyme acetaldehyde dehydrogenase. This action produces blood concentrations of acetaldehyde 5 to 10 times higher than those concentrations produced when the same amount of alcohol is metabolized alone. Accumulation of acetaldehyde in the blood produces a constellation of unpleasant signs and symptoms referred to as the disulfiram-alcohol-reaction, or "disulfiram flush."

The signs and symptoms of the disulfiram-alcohol-reaction include blurred vision, chest pain, confusion, dyspnea, fainting (syncope), flushing, hyperventilation, hypotension, marked uneasiness, tachycardia, throbbing headache, vertigo, vomiting (copious), and weakness. Severe reactions have been associated with respiratory depression, cardiovascular collapse, dysrhythmias, myocardial infarction, acute congestive heart failure, unconsciousness, convulsions, and death. The disulfiram-alcohol-reaction, the intensity of which may vary among patients, is proportional to both the dosage of disulfiram and the amount of alcohol ingested. The reaction will persist as long as alcohol is available for metabolism in the body. Disulfiram does not appear to influence the rate of the elimination of alcohol.

Mild reactions may occur among sensitive patients when their blood alcohol concentrations are increased as little as 5 to 10 mg/100 ml (5 to 10 mg%). The signs and symptoms usually associated with the reaction are fully developed at blood alcohol concentrations of 50 mg/100 ml. When blood alcohol concentrations reach 125 to 150 mg/100 ml, unconsciousness may occur.

Mild cases of the disulfiram reaction generally last for 30 to 60 minutes. More severe cases may last for hours, depending on the presence of alcohol in the blood. Severe reactions require emergency symptomatic medical support of body systems with attention to restoring blood pressure and treating shock. Some patients may require chlorpromazine pharmacotherapy to inhibit the disulfiram reaction.

The possible occurrence of this unpleasant, and perhaps life threatening, reaction enables selected patients who have histories of chronic alcoholism to remain in a state of "enforced sobriety." This enforced sobriety also encourages them to focus on their psychotherapy and other supportive treatments (Alcoholics Anonymous) and to learn non-pharmacologic strategies (e.g., cognitive skills training) that may help them to maintain continued abstinence from the use of alcohol.

PHARMACOKINETICS/PHARMACODYNAMICS

The pharmacokinetics of disulfiram have not been well studied. Disulfiram is well absorbed (80% to 95%), although slowly, following oral ingestion. It is rapidly distributed to body fluids and tissues. Disulfiram is metabolized to diethyldithiocarbamate or mixed disulfides, an end product of which is carbon disulfide. Disulfiram is eliminated slowly from the body by excretion in the urine, feces, and breath. Thus, the duration of the alcohol-disulfiram-reaction varies and can last from 30 minutes to several hours. The reaction also may occur when alcohol is ingested up to two weeks following the discontinuation of disulfiram pharmacotherapy. Long-term disulfiram pharmacotherapy does not produce tolerance. The longer patients remain on disulfiram pharmacotherapy, the more sensitive they become to alcohol. Additional data are unavailable.

RELATIVE CONTRAINDICATIONS

Alcohol intoxication or use within 12 hours
Cardiovascular dysfunction, severe
Cerebral injury or dysfunction
Diabetes mellitus
Epilepsy or other seizure disorders
Hepatic cirrhosis or liver dysfunction
Hypersensitivity to disulfiram
Hypothyroidism
Nephritis, acute and chronic
Paraldehyde pharmacotherapy
Pregnancy
Psychosis

CAUTIONS AND COMMENTS

Prescribe disulfiram pharmacotherapy cautiously to patients who have histories of industrial contact dermatitis or who currently work, or previously worked, in the rubber industry. These patients should be evaluated for hypersensitivity to disulfiram before disulfiram pharmacotherapy is initiated. Patients exposed to organic solvents, which may contain alcohol, acetaldehyde, paraldehyde, or structural analogues, are at risk for experiencing the disulfiram reaction. Exposure to these products should be eliminated prior to the initiation of disulfiram pharmacotherapy.

Caution patients who are receiving disulfiram pharmacotherapy against performing activities that require alertness, judgment, and physical coordination (e.g., driving an automobile, operating dangerous equipment, supervising children) until their response to disulfiram is known. Disulfiram's CNS sedative action may adversely affect these mental and physical functions.

In addition to this general precaution, caution patients to carry an identification card stating that they are currently receiving disulfiram pharmacotherapy. The card should identify the name and telephone number of the prescribing psychologist and other people (e.g., family member) who should be contacted in case of an emergency (cards may be obtained from the manufacturer, Wyeth-Ayerst, upon request).

In addition to these general precautions for patients, caution women to inform their prescribing psychologist if they become, or intend to become, pregnant while receiving disulfiram pharmacotherapy, so that their pharmacotherapy can be safely discontinued.

CLINICALLY SIGNIFICANT DRUG INTERACTIONS

Concurrent disulfiram pharmacotherapy and the following may result in clinically significant drug interactions:

Anticoagulant (Oral) Pharmacotherapy

Concurrent disulfiram pharmacotherapy may increase the pharmacologic action of warfarin (Coumadin®). An adjustment to the dosage of the oral anticoagulant may be needed. Collaboration with the prescriber of the oral anticoagulant is required.

Isoniazid and Metronidazole Pharmacotherapy

Concurrent disulfiram and isoniazid (INH® [antitubercular]) or metronidazole (Flagyl® [antiprotozoal]) pharmacotherapy may result in confusion or psychosis. Disulfiram inhibits enzyme induction and, thus, may interfere with the metabolism of isoniazid and metronidazole. Disulfiram pharmacotherapy should be discontinued among patients who are receiving isoniazid pharmacotherapy if an unsteady gait or marked changes in their mental status are noted.

Phenytoin Pharmacotherapy

Concurrent disulfiram pharmacotherapy may inhibit the metabolism of phenytoin (Dilantin®) and, thus, increase its pharmacologic action. For patients who are receiving phenytoin pharmacotherapy, a baseline phenytoin blood concentration should be obtained before disulfiram pharmacotherapy is initiated. Following the initiation of disulfiram pharmacotherapy, phenytoin blood concentrations should be reevaluated on different days for evidence of an increase or continuing rise in blood concentrations. Appropriate dosage adjustment should be made if elevated phenytoin blood concentrations are found. Collaboration with the prescriber of the phenytoin is required.

ADVERSE DRUG REACTIONS

Disulfiram pharmacotherapy commonly has been associated with drowsiness. It also has been associated with the following ADRs, listed according to body system. These ADRs usually remit with continued pharmacotherapy or generally can be managed with a reduction in dosage.

> **CNS:** headache. Psychotic reactions also have been reported among some patients receiving disulfiram pharmacotherapy. These reactions have been attributed to the use of high dosages of disulfiram, toxicity of concurrent pharmacotherapy (e.g., metronidazole [antiprotozoal] or isoniazid [antitubercular] pharmacotherapy), or the unmasking of psychoses associated with the alcohol withdrawal syndrome.
> **Cutaneous:** acneiform eruptions, allergic dermatitis, skin eruptions, and rashes
> **Genitourinary:** impotence
> **GI:** gastrointestinal complaints
> **Hepatic:** cholestatic and fulminant hepatitis and, rarely, liver toxicity
> **Musculoskeletal:** fatigue, peripheral neuritis, and polyneuritis
> **Ocular:** optic neuritis
> **Miscellaneous:** garlic- or metallic-like aftertaste, breath, and body odor, especially during the first two weeks of pharmacotherapy

OVERDOSAGE

Several severe cases of disulfiram overdosage involving accidental ingestion by children have been reported. Within a few hours of ingestion of a large quantity of disulfiram, drowsiness may occur, accompanied by persistent nausea, vomiting, aggressive and psychotic behavior, ascending flaccid paralysis, which can affect the cranial nerves, and coma. Disulfiram overdosage requires emergency symptomatic medical support of body systems with attention to increasing disulfiram elimination. There is no known antidote.

DOXEPIN

(dox'e pin)

TRADE NAMES

Adapin®
Sinequan®

CLASSIFICATION

Antidepressant (tricyclic)

See also Tricyclic Antidepressants General Monograph

APPROVED INDICATIONS FOR PSYCHOLOGICAL DISORDERS

Adjunctive pharmacotherapy for the symptomatic management of:

Mood Disorders: Depressive Disorders, including Depression with Anxiety

USUAL DOSAGE AND ADMINISTRATION

Depressive Disorders

Adults: Initially, 75 mg daily orally in three divided doses. Increase the dosage by 25 mg increments at appropriate intervals until optimal therapeutic benefit is achieved. The usual optimal dosage range is 75 to 150 mg daily. Some patients may require up to 300 mg daily. However, there rarely is any benefit associated with exceeding this dosage. Once optimal therapeutic response has been achieved, reduce the dosage to the lowest effective dosage.

MAINTENANCE: 50 to 150 mg daily orally in a single dose, preferably 30 minutes before retiring for bed in the evening

MAXIMUM: 300 mg daily orally

Women who are, or who may become, pregnant: FDA Pregnancy Category C. Safety and efficacy of doxepin pharmacotherapy for women who are pregnant have not been established. Avoid prescribing doxepin pharmacotherapy to women who are pregnant. If doxepin pharmacotherapy is required, advise patients of potential benefits and possible risks to themselves and the embryo, fetus, or neonate. Collaboration with the patient's obstetrician is indicated.

Women who are breast-feeding: Safety and efficacy of doxepin pharmacotherapy for women who are breast-feeding and their neonates and infants have not been established. Doxepin is excreted in low concentrations is breast milk. If doxepin pharmacotherapy is required, breast-feeding probably should be discontinued. Collaboration with the patient's pediatrician is indicated.

Elderly, frail, or debilitated patients: Initiate doxepin pharmacotherapy with lower dosages. Increase the dosage gradually according to individual patient response. Generally prescribe lower dosages for elderly, frail, or debilitated patients. These patients may be more sensitive to the pharmacologic actions of doxepin than are younger or healthier adult patients.

Children younger than 12 years of age: Safety and efficacy of doxepin pharmacotherapy for the symptomatic management of depression among children younger than 12 years of age have not been established. Doxepin pharmacotherapy for this indication is *not* recommended for this age group.

Notes, Depressive Disorders

The optimum daily dosage of doxepin depends on the severity of the patient's signs and symptoms and individual response to adjunctive pharmacotherapy. Therapeutic benefit may be prompt or require up to two weeks or longer of doxepin pharmacotherapy.

AVAILABLE DOSAGE FORMS, STORAGE, AND COMPATIBILITY

Capsules, oral: 10, 25, 50, 75, 100, 150 mg
Concentrate, oral solution: 10 mg/ml (peppermint flavored)

Notes

The 150 mg capsule is only intended for maintenance doxepin pharmacotherapy. It is not recommended for initiating doxepin pharmacotherapy. Prescribe the 150 mg capsule only after the patient's daily dosage has been stabilized.

General Instructions for Patients   Instruct patients who are receiving doxepin pharmacotherapy to

- dilute each dose of the doxepin oral concentrate with 120 ml (4 ounces) of milk, water, or fruit or tomato juice before ingestion. Advise patients *not* to dilute their doses with carbonated beverages because of physical incompatibility.

- safely store doxepin capsules or oral concentrate out of the reach of children in tightly closed child- and light-resistant containers at controlled room temperature (15° to 30°C; 59° to 86°F).
- obtain an available patient information sheet regarding doxepin pharmacotherapy from their pharmacist at the time that their prescription is dispensed. Encourage patients to clarify any questions that they may have concerning doxepin pharmacotherapy with their pharmacist or, if needed, to consult their prescribing psychologist.

PROPOSED MECHANISM OF ACTION

Doxepin has antidepressant, sedative, and anticholinergic actions. At higher dosages, it has peripheral adrenergic blocking actions. Doxepin's exact mechanism of action has not yet been fully determined. Its antidepressant action appears to be primarily associated with its ability to block the re-uptake of CNS biogenic amines, specifically norepinephrine and serotonin, at the presynaptic nerve terminals. This inhibition of re-uptake increases the amount of norepinephrine and serotonin in the synapses and, consequently, results in increased activity at the post-synaptic neuron receptor sites.

See also the Tricyclic Antidepressants General Monograph

PHARMACOKINETICS/PHARMACODYNAMICS

Doxepin is moderately absorbed following oral ingestion (mean bioavailability of 30%). It is 80% to 85% bound to plasma proteins, and its mean apparent volume of distribution is 20 L/kg. Maximal antidepressant action generally does not become apparent for at least two weeks following the initiation of doxepin pharmacotherapy. Doxepin is metabolized extensively in the liver to both active (e.g., desmethyldoxepin) and inactive metabolites. The mean half-life of elimination is 15 hours, and the total body clearance is ~1 L/minute.

RELATIVE CONTRAINDICATIONS

Blood disorders
Glaucoma, narrow angle
Hypersensitivity to doxepin or other TCAs
MAOI pharmacotherapy, concurrent or within 14 days
Urinary retention

CAUTIONS AND COMMENTS

Prescribe doxepin pharmacotherapy cautiously for patients who

- have cardiovascular dysfunction
- have histories of blood disorders. If sore throat or fever occur, obtain leukocyte and differential counts and liver function studies to rule out agranulocytosis, particularly when patients are receiving long-term high-dosage doxepin pharmacotherapy. Collaboration with the patient's family physician or a specialist (e.g., hematologist) is indicated.
- have histories of liver dysfunction
- have histories of seizure disorders

CLINICALLY SIGNIFICANT DRUG INTERACTIONS

Concurrent doxepin pharmacotherapy and the following may result in clinically significant drug interactions:

Clonidine Pharmacotherapy

Concurrent doxepin pharmacotherapy may decrease the antihypertensive action of clonidine (Catapres®). Collaboration with the prescriber of the clonidine is required.

Guanethidine Pharmacotherapy

Concurrent doxepin pharmacotherapy may decrease the neuronal uptake of guanethidine (Ismelin®) and, thus, decrease its antihypertensive action. An adjustment in the guanethidine dosage may be required. Collaboration with the prescriber of the guanethidine is indicated.

Monoamine Oxidase Inhibitors Pharmacotherapy

Concurrent doxepin and MAOI pharmacotherapy may result in an increase in the therapeutic and toxic effects of both drugs. Concurrent doxepin and MAOI pharmacotherapy is contraindicated.

Pharmacotherapy With Anticholinergics or Other Drugs That Produce Anticholinergic Actions

Concurrent doxepin pharmacotherapy and pharmacotherapy with anticholinergics (e.g., atropine) or other drugs that produce anticholinergic actions (e.g., phenothiazines) may result in additive anticholinergic actions. Monitor patients closely who require concurrent pharmacotherapy, and adjust dosages, as required, according to individual patient response. Collaboration with the prescriber of the anticholinergic may be required.

See also Tricyclic Antidepressants General Monograph

ADVERSE DRUG REACTIONS

Doxepin pharmacotherapy has been associated with the following ADRs, listed according to body system. The chemical pharmacological similarities among the TCAs require that the ADRs generally associated with this class of drugs also be considered when doxepin pharmacotherapy is prescribed.

Cardiovascular: hypotension and palpitations
CNS: drowsiness, sedation, and seizures
Genitourinary: urinary retention
GI: dry mouth and gastrointestinal complaints

See also Tricyclic Antidepressants General Monograph

OVERDOSAGE

Early signs and symptoms of doxepin overdosage may include excessive drowsiness with minor alterations in consciousness and non-responsiveness. Other signs and symptoms include increased psychomotor agitation and convulsions with apnea and coma. Changes in ECG (e.g., broadening of QRS and T-wave abnormalities) may occur as a late finding and are not always accompanied by cardiovascular changes. Doxepin overdosage requires emergency symptomatic medical support of body systems with attention to increasing doxepin elimination. There is no known antidote.

ESTAZOLAM *

(es ta'zoe lam)

TRADE NAME

ProSom®

CLASSIFICATION

Sedative-hypnotic (benzodiazepine) (C-IV)

See also Benzodiazepines General Monograph

APPROVED INDICATIONS FOR PSYCHOLOGICAL DISORDERS

Adjunctive pharmacotherapy for the short-term symptomatic management of:

Sleep Disorders: Difficulty falling asleep, frequent nocturnal awakenings, and/or early morning awakenings

USUAL DOSAGE AND ADMINISTRATION

Difficulty Falling Asleep, Frequent Nocturnal Awakenings, and/or Early Morning Awakenings

Adults: Initially, 1 mg daily orally 30 minutes before retiring for bed in the evening

MAXIMUM: 2 mg daily orally

Women who are, or who may become, pregnant: FDA Pregnancy Category X. Safety and efficacy of estazolam pharmacotherapy for women who are pregnant have not been established. However, based upon animal studies and the noted teratogenic effects associated with other benzodiazepines, estazolam pharmacotherapy is *contraindicated* during pregnancy.
See the Benzodiazepines General Monograph

Women who are breast-feeding: Safety and efficacy of estazolam pharmacotherapy for women who are breast-feeding and their neonates and infants have not been established. Avoid prescribing estazolam pharmacotherapy to women who are breast-feeding. If estazolam pharmacotherapy is required, breast-feeding probably should be discontinued. If desired, lactation may be maintained and breast-feeding resumed following the discontinuation of short-term estazolam pharmacotherapy. Collaboration with the patient's pediatrician may be indicated.

Elderly, frail, or debilitated patients: Initially, 0.5 mg daily orally 30 minutes before retiring for bed in the evening. Initiate estazolam pharmacotherapy with the lowest dosage to avoid associated incoordination (ataxia) or over-sedation among these patients. Increase the dosage gradually, if required, according to individual patient response. Do *not* exceed 2 mg per dose for elderly, frail, or debilitated patients.

Children and adolescents younger than 18 years of age: Safety and efficacy of estazolam pharmacotherapy for children and adolescents younger than 18 years of age have not been established. Estazolam pharmacotherapy is *not* recommended for this age group.

Notes, Difficulty Falling Asleep, Frequent Nocturnal Awakenings, and/or Early Morning Awakenings

Adjust dosage according to individual patient response for optimal therapeutic benefit. Although usual recommended dosages will meet the needs of most patients, some patients may require higher dosages. Increase the dosage gradually for these patients to avoid or minimize the occurrence of associated ADRs.

The safety and efficacy of long-term estazolam pharmacotherapy (longer than four months) have not been established. Reevaluate patients who appear to require estazolam pharmacotherapy for longer than four months. A benzodiazepine withdrawal syndrome similar to the alcohol withdrawal syndrome may occur after discontinuation of long-term estazolam pharmacotherapy, or regular personal use.

AVAILABLE DOSAGE FORMS, STORAGE, AND COMPATIBILITY

Tablets, oral: 1, 2 mg

Notes

General Instructions for Patients Instruct patients who are receiving estazolam pharmacotherapy to

- safely store estazolam oral tablets out of the reach of children in child-resistant containers at controlled room temperature (15° to 30°C; 59° to 86°F).
- obtain an available patient information sheet regarding estazolam pharmacotherapy from their pharmacist at the time that their prescription is dispensed. Encourage patients to clarify any questions that they may have concerning estazolam pharmacotherapy with their pharmacist or, if needed, to consult their prescribing psychologist.

PROPOSED MECHANISM OF ACTION

Estazolam is a benzodiazepine with hypnotic action. The exact mechanism of action of estazolam has not yet been fully determined. Estazolam's hypnotic action appears to be mediated by, or work in concert with, the inhibitory neurotransmitter GABA. Thus, its action appears to be accomplished by binding to benzodiazepine receptors within the GABA complex.

See also Benzodiazepines General Monograph

PHARMACOKINETICS/PHARMACODYNAMICS

Estazolam is well and extensively absorbed following oral ingestion (F > 0.9). Peak blood levels generally are achieved within two hours. Estazolam is ~93% bound to plasma proteins and is widely distributed in body tissue and fluids. It is extensively metabolized in the liver. Estazolam and its metabolites primarily are excreted in the urine. Less than 5% of estazolam is excreted in unchanged form in the urine. The mean half-life of elimination is ~18 hours (range 13 to 35 hours).

RELATIVE CONTRAINDICATIONS

Acute narrow-angle glaucoma. Estazolam pharmacotherapy may be prescribed to patients who have open-angle glaucoma and are receiving appropriate pharmacotherapy. Collaboration with the patient's ophthalmologist is indicated.
Hypersensitivity to estazolam or other benzodiazepines
Myasthenia gravis
Pregnancy
Sleep apnea syndrome

CAUTIONS AND COMMENTS

Short- or long-term estazolam pharmacotherapy may result in addiction and habituation. Abrupt discontinuation of pharmacotherapy, or regular personal use, has been associated with a withdrawal syndrome similar to the alcohol withdrawal syndrome. Signs and symptoms of the benzodiazepine withdrawal syndrome include abdominal and muscle cramps, convulsions, sweating, tremor, and vomiting. Signs and symptoms of mild withdrawal include dysphoria and insomnia. These signs and symptoms have been observed among patients following the abrupt discontinuation of benzodiazepine pharmacotherapy when that pharmacotherapy consisted of recommended dosages over several months. Signs and symptoms of severe withdrawal have been associated with the discontinuation of long-term high dosage pharmacotherapy, or regular personal use. Avoid abruptly discontinuing estazolam pharmacotherapy, particularly when pharmacotherapy has been extended over several months. Reduce the dosage gradually, and monitor individual patient response carefully.

Prescribe estazolam pharmacotherapy cautiously to patients who

- have depression, severe or latent. Benzodiazepine pharmacotherapy may exacerbate depression among these patients. Monitor these patients carefully for increased risk for suicide. Suicidal precautions are indicated.
- have histories of problematic patterns of abusable psychotropic use, including alcohol, or other abusable psychotropic use. If estazolam pharmacotherapy is required, monitor these patients closely for signs and symptoms of problematic patterns of use.
- have kidney or liver dysfunction. The half-life of elimination may be increased significantly among these patients.

Caution patients who are receiving estazolam pharmacotherapy against

- drinking alcohol or using other drugs that produce CNS depression. Concurrent use of alcohol or other drugs that produce CNS depression may result in excessive CNS depression.

- increasing their prescribed dosages or abruptly discontinuing their pharmacotherapy without first consulting with their prescribing psychologist. Estazolam can produce addiction and habituation. Abrupt discontinuation of use may result in the benzodiazepine withdrawal syndrome.
- performing activities that require mental alertness, judgment, or physical coordination (e.g., driving an automobile, operating dangerous equipment, supervising children). Estazolam's associated CNS depressant action may adversely affect these mental and physical functions.

In addition to these general precautions for patients, caution women to inform their prescribing psychologist if they become, or intend to become, pregnant while receiving estazolam pharmacotherapy, so that their pharmacotherapy can be safely discontinued.

CLINICALLY SIGNIFICANT DRUG INTERACTIONS

Concurrent estazolam pharmacotherapy and the following may result in clinically significant drug interactions:

Alcohol Use

Concurrent alcohol use may increase the CNS depressant action of estazolam. Advise patients to avoid, or limit, their use of alcohol while receiving estazolam pharmacotherapy.

Pharmacotherapy With Cimetidine or Other Drugs That Inhibit Cytochrome P450-Mediated Hepatic Metabolism

Concurrent estazolam and cimetidine (Tagamet®) pharmacotherapy, or pharmacotherapy with other drugs that inhibit cytochrome P450-mediated hepatic metabolism, may result in the delayed or decreased elimination of estazolam. The clinical significance of this interaction is unclear.

Pharmacotherapy With Central Nervous System Depressants and Other Drugs That Produce Central Nervous System Depression

Concurrent estazolam pharmacotherapy with opiate analgesics, other sedative-hypnotics, or other drugs that produce CNS depression (e.g., antihistamines, phenothiazines, TCAs) may result in additive CNS depression.

See also Benzodiazepines General Monograph

ADVERSE DRUG REACTIONS

Estazolam pharmacotherapy commonly has been associated with dizziness, drowsiness, fatigue, and incoordination (ataxia). Other ADRs associated with estazolam pharmacotherapy are listed according to body system. The chemical and pharmacological similarities among the benzodiazepines require that the ADRs generally associated with this class of drugs also be considered when estazolam pharmacotherapy is prescribed.

Cardiovascular: palpitations (infrequent)
CNS: confusion and depression. Paradoxical reactions, including anxiety (acute), also have been reported. If these ADRs are observed, discontinue estazolam pharmacotherapy.
Cutaneous: hives (urticaria), severe itching (pruritus), and skin rash
Genitourinary: rarely, involuntary urination (urinary incontinence)
GI: constipation, dry mouth, and nausea
Hematologic: rarely, agranulocytosis

See also Benzodiazepines General Monograph

OVERDOSAGE

Signs and symptoms of estazolam overdosage include confusion, somnolence, coma, and diminished reflexes. Estazolam overdosage requires emergency symptomatic medical support of body systems with attention to increasing estazolam elimination. Flumazenil (Anexate®; Romazicon®), the benzodiazepine antagonist, may be required.

ETHCHLORVYNOL

(eth klor vi'nole)

TRADE NAME

Placidyl®

CLASSIFICATION

Sedative-hypnotic (chlorinated tertiary acetylenic carbinol) (C-IV)

APPROVED INDICATIONS FOR PSYCHOLOGICAL DISORDERS

Adjunctive pharmacotherapy for the short-term (one week) symptomatic management of:

Sleep Disorders: Insomnia

USUAL DOSAGE AND ADMINISTRATION

Sleep Disorders: Insomnia

Adults: 500 to 1000 mg orally 30 minutes before retiring for bed in the evening, depending on the severity of insomnia

Women who are, or who may become, pregnant: FDA Pregnancy Category C. Safety and efficacy of ethchlorvynol pharmacotherapy for women who are pregnant have not been established. Avoid prescribing ethchlorvynol pharmacotherapy to women who are pregnant. If ethchlorvynol pharmacotherapy is required, advise patients of potential benefits and possible risks to themselves and the embryo, fetus, or neonate. Collaboration with the patient's obstetrician is indicated.

Women who are breast-feeding: Safety and efficacy of ethchlorvynol pharmacotherapy for women who are breast-feeding and their neonates and infants have not been established. Avoid prescribing ethchlorvynol to women who are breast-feeding. If ethchlorvynol pharmacotherapy is required, breast-feeding probably should be discontinued. If desired, lactation may be maintained and breast-feeding resumed following the discontinuation of short-term ethchlorvynol pharmacotherapy. Collaboration with the patient's pediatrician is indicated.

Elderly, frail, or debilitated patients and those who have kidney or liver dysfunction: Generally prescribe lower dosages for elderly, frail, or debilitated patients. Increase the dosage gradually, if needed, according to individual patient response. These patients may be more sensitive to the pharmacologic actions of ethchlorvynol than are younger or healthier adult patients. Also prescribe lower dosages for patients who have kidney or liver dysfunction.

Children: Safety and efficacy of ethchlorvynol pharmacotherapy for the symptomatic management of sleep disorders among children have not been established. Ethchlorvynol pharmacotherapy for this indication is *not* recommended for this age group.

Notes, Sleep Disorders: Insomnia

A supplemental dose of 200 mg orally upon awakening has been recommended by the manufacturer to reinstate sleep among adult patients who awake during the early morning hours. However, concerns have been raised regarding the possible aspiration of the ethchlorvynol capsule or consumption of the wrong dose because of associated patient drowsiness and confusion upon awakening. Thus, rather than prescribing a supplemental dose, it is recommended that ethchlorvynol pharmacotherapy be replaced with a different, longer-acting sedative-hypnotic for these patients.

Prescribe ethchlorvynol pharmacotherapy for no longer than one week. Reevaluate patients who appear to require longer ethchlorvinyl pharmacotherapy.

AVAILABLE DOSAGE FORMS, STORAGE, AND COMPATIBILITY

Capsules, oral soluble elastic: 100, 200, 300, 500, 750 mg

Notes

The 750 mg capsules (Placidyl®) contain tartrazine (FD&C Yellow No. 5). Tartrazine has been associated with hypersensitivity reactions, including bronchial asthma, among susceptible patients, particularly those who are hypersensitive to aspirin.

General Instructions for Patients   Instruct patients who are receiving ethchlorvynol pharmacotherapy to

- ingest each dose of ethchlorvynol with food or milk to decrease its rapid GI absorption and associated ADRs (e.g., incoordination [ataxia], lightheadedness, stomach upset) (see Adverse Drug Reactions).
- avoid chewing or biting the ethchlorvynol soluble elastic capsule.
- safely store ethchlorvynol capsules out of the reach of children in tightly closed child- and light-resistant containers at controlled room temperature (15° to 30°C; 59° to 86°F).
- obtain an available patient information sheet regarding ethchlorvynol pharmacotherapy from their pharmacist at the time that their prescription is dispensed. Encourage patients to clarify any questions that they may have concerning ethchlorvynol pharmacotherapy with their pharmacist or, if needed, to consult their prescribing psychologist.

PROPOSED MECHANISM OF ACTION

The mechanism of action of ethchlorvynol has not yet been determined.

PHARMACOKINETICS/PHARMACODYNAMICS

Ethchlorvynol has a short latency to onset and short duration of action. It has adequate bioavailability following oral ingestion and produces sleep within 15 to 60 minutes. Peak blood concentrations are achieved within 1 to 1.5 hours. Ethchlorvynol is 35% to 50% bound to plasma proteins and has an apparent volume of distribution of 3 to 4 L/kg. Ethchlorvynol is metabolized in the liver. Both ethchlorvynol and its metabolites undergo extensive enterohepatic recirculation. Its half-life of elimination has a range of 10 to 32 hours. Additional data are unavailable.

RELATIVE CONTRAINDICATIONS

Hypersensitivity to ethchlorvynol
Porphyria, latent or active

CAUTIONS AND COMMENTS

Long-term ethchlorvynol pharmacotherapy, or regular personal use, may result in addiction and habituation. Avoid long-term ethchlorvynol pharmacotherapy. Reevaluate patients who appear to require pharmacotherapy exceeding one week. Abrupt discontinuation of long-term ethchlorvynol pharmacotherapy, or regular personal use, may result in the ethchlorvynol withdrawal syndrome. This withdrawal syndrome is characterized by signs and symptoms similar to those associated with the alcohol and barbiturate withdrawal syndromes. Abrupt discontinuation of ethchlorvynol pharmacotherapy consisting of dosages as low as 1,000 mg daily has been associated with a severe ethchlorvynol withdrawal syndrome, including convulsions and delirium.

Prescribe ethchlorvynol pharmacotherapy cautiously to patients who

- have depression or suicidal tendencies. Ethchlorvynol pharmacotherapy may exacerbate depression among these patients. Monitor these patients carefully for suicidal risk. Do not prescribe more than a one-week supply of ethchlorvynol for these patients. Other suicidal precautions may be required.

- have histories of paradoxic excitement associated with barbiturate pharmacotherapy. These patients may have a similar response to ethchlorvynol pharmacotherapy.
- have histories of problematic patterns of alcohol or other abusable psychotropic use. If ethchlorvynol pharmacotherapy is required, monitor these patients closely for signs and symptoms of problematic patterns of use.

CLINICALLY SIGNIFICANT DRUG INTERACTIONS

Concurrent ethchlorvynol pharmacotherapy and the following may result in clinically significant drug interactions:

Alcohol Use

Concurrent alcohol use may increase the CNS depressant action of ethchlorvynol. Advise patients to avoid, or limit, their use of alcohol while receiving ethchlorvynol pharmacotherapy.

Anticoagulant (Oral) Pharmacotherapy

Ethchlorvynol reportedly decreases the prothrombin time response among patients receiving oral anticoagulants (e.g., warfarin [Coumadin®]). An adjustment of the anticoagulant dosage may be needed. Collaboration with the prescriber of the anticoagulant is required.

Pharmacotherapy With Central Nervous System Depressants and Other Drugs That Produce Central Nervous System Depression

Concurrent ethchlorvynol pharmacotherapy with drugs that produce CNS depression (e.g., antihistamines, phenothiazines, other sedative-hypnotics, TCAs) may result in exaggerated CNS depression.

ADVERSE DRUG REACTIONS

Ethchlorvynol pharmacotherapy has been generally associated with gastrointestinal complaints. Other ADRs associated with ethchlorvynol pharmacotherapy, listed according to body system, include the following:

Cardiovascular: rarely, fainting (syncope). The fainting is usually not associated with marked hypotension and is thought to be an unusual hypersensitivity reaction to ethchlorvynol.

CNS: dizziness, facial numbness, and mild "hangover" effects. Rarely, excitement, hysteria, prolonged hypnosis, and vertigo. Ethchlorvynol absorption may be more rapid among some patients, resulting in giddiness and incoordination (ataxia). These ADRs may be avoided by instructing patients to ingest each subsequent dose with a small amount of food or milk.

Cutaneous: hives (urticaria)

GI: after taste, nausea, and vomiting

Hepatic: cholestatic jaundice

Musculoskeletal: rarely, profound muscular weakness

Ocular: a reversible reduction or dimness of vision (amblyopia) and blurred vision

OVERDOSAGE

Signs and symptoms of ethchlorvynol overdosage include increasing sedation and coma. Some patients have recovered from overdosages involving 1,000 to 6,000 mg of ethchlorvynol following a period of coma lasting approximately one week. Although fatal blood concentrations usually range from 20 to 50 μg/ml, blood concentrations of approximately 14 μg/ml (i.e., 10 times the maximal concentration attained after the ingestion of 1,000 mg) have been fatal. Ethchlorvynol overdosage requires emergency symptomatic medical support of body systems with attention to increasing ethchlorvynol elimination. There is no known antidote.

FENFLURAMINE[1] ★

(fen flure'a meen)

TRADE NAMES

Ponderal®
Pondimin®

CLASSIFICATION

CNS stimulant (anorexiant, amphetamine congener) (C-IV)

See also Amphetamines General Monograph

APPROVED INDICATIONS FOR PSYCHOLOGICAL DISORDERS

Adjunctive pharmacotherapy for the short-term symptomatic management of:

Eating Disorders: Exogenous Obesity

Fenfluramine pharmacotherapy may be prescribed as an adjunct to appropriate psychotherapy, which includes strategies to suppress appetite and reduce the excessive ingestion of calories, among patients who have exogenous obesity. Adjunctive pharmacotherapy for the management of exogenous obesity is strictly limited to a few weeks duration. The loss of weight among patients who have received anorexiant pharmacotherapy is only moderately greater than that obtained by those who have received weight-reducing programs alone. Unfortunately, the rate of weight loss among these patients tends to decrease within a few weeks of anorexiant pharmacotherapy. The development of tolerance to the anorexiant action of fenfluramine and other related drugs is the limiting factor. When weight loss is critical, such as in emergency situations (e.g., preparation for non-elective surgery), pharmacotherapy may be used as an adjunct to psychotherapy and dietary measures as long as, but not exceeding, the period of continuous active weight loss. More data are needed regarding the role of psychotherapy alone, or in combination with, anorexiant pharmacotherapy and other measures, including caloric restriction and exercise, for the management of exogenous obesity.

---

[1]On September 15, 1997, at the request of the FDA, the pharmaceutical manufacturers of dexfenfluramine (Redux®) and fenfluramine (Pondimin®) voluntarily withdrew these two drugs from the U.S. market. This action was predicated on documentation of a significant risk for the development of valvular heart disease among women treated for obesity with a combination of phentermine and fenfluramine (known commonly as "phen-fen") or dexfenfluramine with or without phentermine. For additional discussion, see Adverse Drug Reactions.

USUAL DOSAGE AND ADMINISTRATION

Exogenous Obesity

Adults: Initially, 60 mg daily orally in three divided doses one hour before meals. If satisfactory therapeutic benefit is not achieved, increase the daily dosage weekly by 20 mg, as needed, to a maximum of 120 mg daily orally in three divided doses before meals. Adjust dosage to individual patient response. Some patients may prefer to dose their fenfluramine pharmacotherapy in the early evening to manage nocturnal eating. Fenfluramine also has sedative action that may be of benefit to patients when dosed in the evening.

If single daily dosing is preferred, prescribe a 60 mg extended-release capsule daily orally in the morning. May increase dosage to 120 mg (two 60 mg extended-release capsules) daily orally in the morning, if needed, according to individual patient response.

MAXIMUM: 120 mg daily orally

Women who are, or who may become, pregnant: FDA Pregnancy Category C. Safety and efficacy of fenfluramine pharmacotherapy for women who are pregnant have not been established. Avoid prescribing fenfluramine pharmacotherapy to women who are pregnant. If fenfluramine pharmacotherapy is required, advise patients of potential benefits and possible risks to themselves and the embryo, fetus, or neonate. Collaboration with the patient's obstetrician is indicated.

Women who are breast-feeding: Safety and efficacy of fenfluramine pharmacotherapy for women who are breast-feeding and their neonates and infants have not been established. Avoid prescribing fenfluramine pharmacotherapy to women who are breast-feeding. If fenfluramine pharmacotherapy is required, breast-feeding probably should be discontinued. If desired, lactation may be maintained and breast-feeding resumed following the discontinuation of short-term fenfluramine pharmacotherapy. Collaboration with the patient's pediatrician is indicated.

Elderly patients: Safety and efficacy of fenfluramine pharmacotherapy for the symptomatic management of eating disorders among elderly patients have not been established. Fenfluramine pharmacotherapy for this indication is *not* recommended for this age group.

Children younger than 12 years of age: Safety and efficacy of fenfluramine pharmacotherapy for the symptomatic management of eating disorders among children younger than 12 years of age have not been established. Fenfluramine pharmacotherapy for this indication is *not* recommended for this age group.

Notes, Exogenous Obesity

As with other anorexiants, exclude organic causes of obesity before prescribing fenfluramine pharmacotherapy. Collaboration with the patient's family physician is required. As occurs with other anorexiant drugs (e.g., methamphetamine), tolerance develops rapidly to the appetite suppressant action of fenfluramine. Discontinue fenfluramine pharmacotherapy when tolerance to its anorexiant action occurs. Prolonged use may result in severe addiction and habituation. Weight regain is common after pharmacotherapy is discontinued.

AVAILABLE DOSAGE FORMS, STORAGE, AND COMPATIBILITY

Capsules, oral extended-release: 60 mg
Tablets, oral: 20 mg

Notes

General Instructions for Patients   Instruct patients who are receiving fenfluramine pharmacotherapy to

- safely store their fenfluramine oral tablets or capsules out of the reach of children in tightly closed child-resistant containers at controlled room temperature (20° to 25°C; 68° to 77°F).
- obtain an available patient information sheet regarding fenfluramine pharmacotherapy from their pharmacist at the time that their prescription is dispensed. Encourage patients to clarify any questions that they may have concerning fenfluramine pharmacotherapy with their pharmacist or, if needed, to consult their prescribing psychologist.

PROPOSED MECHANISM OF ACTION

Fenfluramine is a sympathomimetic amine amphetamine congener with anorexiant action. The exact mechanism of fenfluramine's anorexiant action has not yet been fully determined. However, it appears to be associated with its ability to increase serotonin levels and glucose utilization, particularly within the ventromedial nucleus of the hypothalamus.

PHARMACOKINETICS/PHARMACODYNAMICS

Fenfluramine is absorbed readily following oral ingestion. The onset of action is generally within 1 to 2 hours. The duration of anorexiant activity is ~4 to 6 hours. Steady-state blood concentrations generally are achieved within three to four days. Fenfluramine is lipid soluble and widely distributed to most body tissues. It is metabolized in the liver. Fenfluramine, its de-ethylated metabolite norfenfluramine, and its final metabolite m-trifluoromethyl-hippuric acid are primarily excreted in the urine. Its mean half-life of elimination is ~20 hours. The extent of fenfluramine's metabolism and urinary excretion is affected by the pH of the urine. Excretion is more rapid in acidic urine than in alkaline urine (e.g., the half-life of elimination can be reduced to 10 hours among patients who have acidic urine). Additional data are unavailable.

RELATIVE CONTRAINDICATIONS

Alcoholism
Cardiovascular dysfunction, severe
General anesthesia
Glaucoma
Hypersensitivity to fenfluramine or other amphetamines
Hypertension, severe
MAOI pharmacotherapy, concurrent or within 14 days

Schizophrenia
Valvular heart disease

CAUTIONS AND COMMENTS

When compared to other anorexiants that have amphetamine-like actions, fenfluramine has not been as strongly associated with addiction and habituation. Although fenfluramine shares common features with the amphetamines, its clinical use has not been associated with significant problematic patterns of use.

Prescribe fenfluramine pharmacotherapy cautiously to patients who

- have depression or a history of depression. Depression has been associated with fenfluramine pharmacotherapy and its discontinuation. Monitor these patients for any exacerbation of depression and avoid abrupt discontinuation of fenfluramine pharmacotherapy. Reduce the dosage gradually before completely discontinuing fenfluramine pharmacotherapy.
- have diabetes mellitus. Fenfluramine pharmacotherapy may increase the pharmacologic actions of insulin and oral antihyperglycemics (i.e., sulfonylureas), resulting in hypoglycemia. When prescribed to these patients, monitor individual patient response carefully. Dosage adjustment of the antidiabetics may be required. Collaboration with the patient's family physician is indicated.
- have hypertension. A pressor effect is uncommon at recommended anorexiant dosages. Fenfluramine may be of therapeutic benefit to patients who require an anorexiant and have hypertension. When prescribed for these patients, monitor individual patient response carefully with attention to the effect of fenfluramine pharmacotherapy on blood pressure.
- have histories of problematic patterns of CNS stimulant or other abusable psychotropic use. Fenfluramine pharmacotherapy may result in addiction and habituation among patients who have a predisposition to problematic patterns of abusable psychotropic use. Monitor these patients for problematic patterns of fenfluramine use.

Caution patients who are receiving fenfluramine against performing activities that require alertness, judgment, or physical coordination (e.g., driving an automobile, operating dangerous equipment, supervising children) until their response to fenfluramine is known. Fenfluramine has a sedative action that may produce mild to moderate drowsiness and, thus, adversely affect these mental and physical functions.

In addition to this general precaution, caution patients to

immediately report any deterioration in exercise tolerance (e.g., shortness of breath on exertion). The possible occurrence of primary pulmonary hypertension, a potentially fatal condition, should be investigated among patients who report exercise intolerance. Collaboration with the patient's family physician or a respiratory specialist is indicated. Primary pulmonary hypertension rarely has been reported and is usually reversible upon discontinuation of fenfluramine pharmacotherapy.

CLINICALLY SIGNIFICANT DRUG INTERACTIONS

Concurrent fenfluramine pharmacotherapy and the following may result in clinically significant drug interactions:

Alcohol Use

Concurrent alcohol use may increase the CNS depressant action of fenfluramine. Advise patients to avoid, or limit, their use of alcohol while receiving fenfluramine pharmacotherapy.

Antidiabetic (Insulin and Oral Antihyperglycemic) Pharmacotherapy

Concurrent fenfluramine pharmacotherapy may increase the pharmacologic actions of insulin and the sulfonylureas (e.g., chlorpropamide [Diabinese®]). Dosage adjustment of these antidiabetics may be required. Collaboration with the prescriber of the antidiabetics is indicated.

Antihypertensive Pharmacotherapy

Concurrent fenfluramine and antihypertensive pharmacotherapy may require an adjustment in the dosage of the antihypertensive. Collaboration with the prescriber of the antihypertensive is required (see also Guanethidine Pharmacotherapy).

Guanethidine Pharmacotherapy

Fenfluramine may decrease the neuronal uptake of guanethidine (Ismelin®) and, thus, decrease its antihypertensive action. An adjustment in the dosage of the antihypertensive may be required. Collaboration with the prescriber of the guanethidine is indicated.

Monoamine Oxidase Inhibitor Pharmacotherapy

Fenfluramine may interact with MAOIs (e.g., phenelzine [Nardil®]). This interaction may cause the release of large amounts of catecholamines and associated pharmacologic actions, including hypertensive crisis. Hypertensive crisis is characterized by severe headache and hypertension. Concurrent fenfluramine and MAOI pharmacotherapy is *contraindicated*.

Pharmacotherapy With Central Nervous System Depressants and Other Drugs That Produce Central Nervous System Depression

Concurrent fenfluramine pharmacotherapy and pharmacotherapy with opiate analgesics, sedative-hypnotics, or other drugs that produce CNS depression (e.g., antihistamines, phenothiazines, TCAs) may result in excessive CNS depression.

See also Amphetamines General Monograph

ADVERSE DRUG REACTIONS

Special Warning: As noted at the beginning of this monograph, fenfluramine was withdrawn from the market on September 15, 1997, because of the significant risk for developing aortic or mitral valvular regurgitation. The overall estimate from all available studies of related absolute risk is approximately 30%. In comparison to the expected rate in the general population, this estimate represents a 15-fold increased risk for valvular dysfunction.

Fenfluramine pharmacotherapy also has been commonly associated with diarrhea, dizziness, drowsiness, dry mouth, nausea, and urinary frequency. Although fenfluramine is associated with less CNS stimulation than the amphetamines, it is associated with more CNS depression. An elevated mood with an impaired ability to concentrate and a depression of mood following the discontinuation of fenfluramine pharmacotherapy also have been reported. Higher dosages have been associated with signs and symptoms resembling psychosis (i.e., psychotomimetic effects). Other ADRs associated with fenfluramine pharmacotherapy, listed according to body system, include:

Cardiovascular: fainting (syncope), hypertension or hypotension, palpitations, and valvular heart disease (see *Special Warning*)
CNS: agitation, anxiety, confusion, depression, elevated mood, fatigue, headache, incoordination (ataxia), insomnia, irritability, lethargy, nervousness, and tension
Cutaneous: burning sensation, hives (urticaria), rash, swelling, and sweating (excessive)
Genitourinary: impotence, increased sex drive, and painful urination (dysuria)
GI: abdominal pain, unpleasant taste in the mouth, and constipation
Musculoskeletal: difficult and defective speech associated with impairment of the tongue or other muscles essential to speech (dysarthria), and weakness
Ocular: blurred vision and eye irritation
Respiratory: pulmonary hypertension
Miscellaneous: chest pain, chills, and fever

See also Amphetamines General Monograph

OVERDOSAGE

Fatal fenfluramine overdosages have been associated with the ingestion of 140 to 1,800 mg of fenfluramine. The highest reported nonfatal adult overdosage was with 1,800 mg of fenfluramine. Signs and symptoms of fenfluramine overdosage include agitation, confusion, dilated nonreactive pupils, drowsiness, flushing, fever, hyperthermia, hyperventilation, nausea, pain (abnormal), rotary nystagmus, sweating, tremors (or shivering), and vomiting. Reflexes may be exaggerated or depressed. EEG changes resemble those observed with mild amphetamine overdosage or the amphetamine withdrawal syndrome. Coma, ventricular extrasystoles, and ventricular fibrillation may occur with overdosages involving large amounts of fenfluramine. Fenfluramine overdosage requires emergency symptomatic medical support of body systems with attention to increasing fenfluramine elimination. There is no known antidote.

FENTANYL

(fen'ta nil)

TRADE NAMES

Duragesic®
Fentanyl Oralet®

CLASSIFICATION

Opiate analgesic (C-II)

See also Opiate Analgesics General Monograph

APPROVED INDICATIONS FOR PSYCHOLOGICAL DISORDERS

Adjunctive pharmacotherapy for the symptomatic management of:

Pain Disorders: Severe Pain

USUAL DOSAGE AND ADMINISTRATION

Severe Pain

Adults: 50 to 100 μg intramuscularly for the management of post-operative pain. Repeat dose, if needed, in one to two hours according to individual patient response. Individualize dosage with attention to age, body weight, general physical health, severity of pain, degree of opiate tolerance, and concurrent pharmacotherapy. For transdermal dosage, see Notes, Severe Pain.

Women who are, or who may become, pregnant: FDA Pregnancy Category C. Safety and efficacy of fentanyl pharmacotherapy for women who are pregnant have not been established (see Opiate Analgesics General Monograph). Avoid prescribing fentanyl pharmacotherapy to women who are pregnant. If fentanyl pharmacotherapy is required, advise patients of potential benefits and possible risks to themselves and the embryo, fetus, or neonate. Collaboration with the patient's obstetrician is indicated.

Women who are breast-feeding: Safety and efficacy of fentanyl pharmacotherapy for women who are breast-feeding and their neonates and infants have not been established. Fentanyl is excreted in breast milk. Pharmacologic effects (e.g., drowsiness, lethargy) may be expected among breast-fed neonates and infants, who also may become addicted. Avoid prescribing fentanyl pharmacotherapy to women who are breast-feeding. If fentanyl pharmacotherapy is required, breast-feeding probably should be discontinued. If desired, lactation may be maintained and breast-feeding resumed following the discontinuation of short-term fentanyl pharmacotherapy. Collaboration with the patient's pediatrician is indicated.

Elderly, frail, or debilitated patients: Initially, prescribe lower dosages of fentanyl. Dosage may be as low as one-fourth to one-third the usual recommended adult dosage. For transdermal fentanyl dosage, see Notes, Severe Pain. Higher dosages are associated with a prolonged duration of action and respiratory depression, particularly among elderly patients. Consider the total dosage of all opiate analgesics composing a patient's pharmacotherapy before prescribing fentanyl. Increase the dosage gradually according to individual patient response.

Children younger than 2 years of age: Safety and efficacy of fentanyl pharmacotherapy for children younger than 2 years of age have not been established. Fentanyl injectable or transdermal pharmacotherapy is *not* recommended for this age group.

Children 2 years of age and older: 2 to 3 μg/kg intramuscularly. Repeat the dose, if needed, in one to two hours according to individual patient response. The safety and efficacy of transdermal fentanyl for children younger than 18 years of age have not been established. Transdermal fentanyl pharmacotherapy is *not* recommended for this age group.

Notes, Severe Pain

Concurrent pharmacotherapy with other CNS depressants will generally necessitate a reduction in the dosage of fentanyl by 25% to 75%. Adjust the dosage cautiously according to individual patient response. When moderate or high doses of fentanyl are required, assure that resuscitative equipment and adequately prepared medical personnel are available immediately for monitoring and maintaining the patient's respiratory and cardiovascular function until the patient's response to fentanyl pharmacotherapy is known. The opiate antagonist naloxone (Narcan®) also should be available immediately. Emergency symptomatic medical support of body systems, particularly the respiratory system, may be required.

Injectable Fentanyl Pharmacotherapy Injectable fentanyl pharmacotherapy is used primarily for patients during or immediately following surgery (e.g., to enhance anesthesia, to provide short-acting analgesia during anesthesia, and to provide analgesia immediately following surgery).

INTRAVENOUS FENTANYL PHARMACOTHERAPY Intravenous fentanyl pharmacotherapy has been associated with muscle rigidity, particularly involving the muscles of respiration. This ADR appears to be related to the rate by which fentanyl is injected intravenously. To avoid this ADR, administer fentanyl by slow intravenous injection. Intravenous fentanyl pharmacotherapy also has been associated with abnormal contraction of the pupils (miosis), bronchospasm, bradycardia, and euphoria. Inject fentanyl intravenously only in the hospital setting, where airway maintenance (i.e., intubation), resuscitative equipment, and adequately prepared personnel are available immediately if emergency symptomatic medical support of body systems, including assisted or controlled respiration, is required. The opiate antagonist naloxone (Narcan®) also should be available immediately for emergency use.

Transdermal Fentanyl Pharmacotherapy

INITIATING AND MAINTAINING TRANSDERMAL FENTANYL PHARMACOTHERAPY The safety and efficacy of transdermal fentanyl pharmacotherapy for the *initial* management of chronic, moderate to severe pain have not been established. Thus, although initial dosages have been suggested and used clinically, transdermal fentanyl pharmacotherapy generally should be reserved for patients who have chronic, severe pain (e.g., patients who have terminal cancer) and whose pain has been adequately managed with another opiate analgesic. The advantages of transdermal fentanyl pharmacotherapy for these patients, include more consistent opiate blood levels and, therefore, analgesia; less frequent dosing; and more convenient and less painful (compared to intramuscular injection) opiate analgesic administration. See the following table for approximate dosage equivalents for patients who are receiving oral morphine pharmacotherapy.

Approximate Transdermal Fentanyl Dosage Equivalents for Patients Who Are Receiving Oral Morphine.[2]

Oral Morphine (mg/day)	Transdermal Fentanyl (μg/hour)
45 to 134	25
135 to 224	50
225 to 314	75
315 to 404	100
405 to 494	125
495 to 584	150
585 to 674	175
675 to 764	200
765 to 854	225
855 to 944	250
945 to 1034	275
1035 to 1124	300

[2]See the Opiate Analgesics General Monograph for "morphine dosage equivalents" for injectable morphine pharmacotherapy or *other* opiate analgesic pharmacotherapy.

The equivalent dosages listed in the table generally are conservative. Many patients may, therefore, require dose adjustments. The maximal analgesic action of the fentanyl transdermal system generally is not apparent for at least 24 hours after its initial application. Initially prescribe supplemental doses of a different short-acting opiate analgesic (see Opiate Analgesics General Monograph), based on individual patient response, to prevent breakthrough pain. After three days, an appropriate increase in the fentanyl transdermal dosage can be made, based upon the amount of supplemental opiate analgesia required during this transition period. For this calculation, the recommended ratio is 90 mg daily of oral morphine (or equivalent) to each 25 μg/hour increase for the fentanyl transdermal system.

Although pain may be managed adequately for most patients with the application of a fresh transdermal system every 72 hours, a small percentage of patients may require more frequent application (i.e., every 48 hours). Always prescribe the lowest effective dosage and longest effective dosing interval.

DISCONTINUING FENTANYL TRANSDERMAL PHARMACOTHERAPY   If fentanyl transdermal pharmacotherapy requires discontinuation, remove the system, and monitor patient response carefully. Up to 20 hours may be required for fentanyl blood levels to decrease by 50%. If transdermal pharmacotherapy is being replaced with other opiate analgesic pharmacotherapy, remove the system, and titrate the dosage of the replacement opiate analgesic according to individual patient response. During this time, monitor patients for adequate pain management and signs and symptoms of toxicity.

AVAILABLE DOSAGE FORMS, STORAGE, AND COMPATIBILITY

Injectable, intramuscular or intravenous: 50 μg/ml (2 and 5 ml ampules)
Transdermal drug delivery systems, 72 hour: 25, 50, 75, or 100 μg/hour
Transmucosal (buccal) lozenge (Fentanyl Oralet®): 200, 300, 400 μg

Notes

The fentanyl dosage is prescribed in micrograms: 1 microgram (μg) = 0.001 mg.

Injectables   Store fentanyl injectables safely protected from light at controlled room temperature (15° to 30°C; 59° to 86°F).

Transdermal Drug Delivery Systems   The 50, 75, and 100 μg/hour fentanyl transdermal systems are *only* recommended for patients who are opiate tolerant. Return the transdermal system to the manufacturer or dispensing pharmacy for appropriate disposal if it is outdated or if the package seal has been broken.

Transmucosal Drug Delivery System   A buccal lozenge form of fentanyl (Fentanyl Oralet®) also is available to provide fentanyl pharmacotherapy without the need for injection. However, the use of this fentanyl formulation generally is indicated for preoperative sedation or as an adjunct to anesthesia.

General Instructions for Patients   Instruct patients who are receiving fentanyl pharmacotherapy to

- safely store fentanyl transdermal drug delivery systems out of the reach of children and pets at controlled room temperature below 25°C (77°F).
- apply each fentanyl transdermal drug delivery system immediately after removal from its individual sealed pouch.
- remove each used fentanyl transdermal system from the skin, and place it in its original pouch for disposal. The used system should be disposed of immediately to prevent inadvertent access by children or pets.
- never apply more than one transdermal system at a time. Serious toxicity may occur.
- never cut the transdermal system to alter the dosage. Destroying the system by cutting may result in excessive drug absorption and toxicity. If a change in dosage is required, patients should consult their prescribing psychologist.
- obtain an available patient information sheet regarding fentanyl pharmacotherapy from their pharmacist at the time that their prescription is dispensed. Encourage patients to clarify any questions that they may have concerning fentanyl pharmacotherapy with their pharmacist or, if needed, to consult their prescribing psychologist.

PROPOSED MECHANISM OF ACTION

Fentanyl is an opiate analgesic that has actions similar to those of morphine and meperidine. A 100 μg dose of fentanyl approximately is equivalent in analgesic action to 10 mg of morphine or 75 mg of meperidine. Fentanyl elicits its analgesic, CNS depressant, and respiratory depressant actions primarily by binding to the endorphin receptors in the CNS. The exact mechanism of action has not yet been fully determined. See also Opiate Analgesics General Monograph.

PHARMACOKINETICS/PHARMACODYNAMICS

Fentanyl's onset of action is almost immediate following intravenous injection. However, its maximal analgesic and respiratory depressant actions may not occur for several minutes. The usual duration of analgesia is 30 to 60 minutes after a single intravenous dose of up to 100 μg. Following intramuscular injection, the onset of action is from 7 to 8 minutes and the duration of action is 1 to 2 hours. Fentanyl is ~85% plasma protein-bound. Its mean apparent volume of distribution is approximately 4 L/kg. Less than 10% is excreted in unchanged form in the urine. The mean half-life of elimination is ~4 hours. The mean total body clearance is ~1 L/minute.

Similar to other opiate analgesics, the alterations in respiratory rate and alveolar ventilation associated with fentanyl may last longer than its analgesic action. As the dosage is increased, pulmonary exchange becomes decreased. Although fentanyl preserves cardiac stability and decreases stress-related hormonal changes, apnea may occur with higher dosages. Fentanyl does not display cardiovascular actions even when injected intravenously at dosages of 0.7 μg/kg. It has less emetic action than other opiate analgesics. Fentanyl is most often used as an intravenous analgesic during surgery because of its short duration of action (i.e., 20 to 40 minutes after intravenous injection). It also may be used intramuscularly as a premedication for surgery (duration of action after intramuscular injection is 1 to 2 hours).

RELATIVE CONTRAINDICATIONS

Hypersensitivity to fentanyl

CAUTIONS AND COMMENTS

Fentanyl is addicting and habituating. See Opiate Analgesics General Monograph.
Prescribe fentanyl pharmacotherapy cautiously to patients who

- have cardiac bradydysrhythmias. Fentanyl can produce additional bradycardia among these patients.
- have chronic obstructive lung disease, decreased respiratory reserve, and potentially compromised respiration. Fentanyl may produce a further decrease in respiratory drive and increase airway resistance among these patients.
- have kidney or liver dysfunction. Kidney or liver dysfunction may affect fentanyl metabolism and excretion.
- have particular susceptibility to respiratory depression, such as patients who are comatose or have brain tumors, head injuries, or other medical disorders that are associated with increased intracranial pressure. Fentanyl pharmacotherapy also may obscure the clinical course of these patients.

Caution patients who are receiving fentanyl pharmacotherapy against performing activities that require alertness, judgment, and physical coordination (e.g., driving an automobile, operating dangerous equipment, supervising children) until their response to fentanyl is known. Fentanyl's CNS depressant action may adversely affect these mental and physical functions.

In addition to this general precaution, caution patients to inform their prescribing psychologist if they begin or discontinue any other pharmacotherapy while receiving fentanyl pharmacotherapy.

CLINICALLY SIGNIFICANT DRUG INTERACTIONS

Concurrent fentanyl pharmacotherapy and the following may result in clinically significant drug interactions:

Alcohol Use

Concurrent alcohol use may increase the CNS depressant action of fentanyl. Advise patients to avoid, or limit, their use of alcohol while receiving fentanyl pharmacotherapy.

Droperidol and Other Antipsychotic Pharmacotherapy

Concurrent fentanyl and droperidol (Inapsine®), or other antipsychotic, pharmacotherapy requires an understanding of the widely differing durations of action of these drugs. Concurrent pharmacotherapy also requires the immediate availability of adequately prepared medical personnel and facilities for the emergency symptomatic medical support of body systems, including attention to the management of hypertension. When concurrent fentanyl and droperidol or other antipsychotic pharmacotherapy is required, monitor patients cautiously for the following signs and symptoms listed according to body system:

Cardiovascular: elevated blood pressure, with or without preexisting hypertension. The hypertension may be related to unexplained alterations in sympathetic nervous system activity associated with high dosages or other clinical factors.

CNS: drowsiness; hallucinatory episodes, which may be associated with transient periods of mental depression; and restlessness. Extrapyramidal signs and symptoms include akathisia, dystonia, and oculogyric crisis.

Miscellaneous: chills and shivering

Monoamine Oxidase Inhibitor Pharmacotherapy

The safety and efficacy of concurrent fentanyl and MAOI pharmacotherapy have not been established. Concurrent fentanyl and MAOI pharmacotherapy may result in severe and unpredictable potentiation of MAOI actions. Fentanyl pharmacotherapy for patients who are receiving MAOI pharmacotherapy concurrently, or within 14 days, is *not* recommended.

Pharmacotherapy With Central Nervous System Depressants and Other Drugs That Produce Central Nervous System Depression

Concurrent fentanyl pharmacotherapy with other opiate analgesics, sedative-hypnotics, or other drugs that produce CNS depression (e.g., antihistamines, phenothiazines, TCAs) may result in additive CNS depression. When concurrent pharmacotherapy is required, the fentanyl dosage should be lower than usually recommended. Reduce the dosage of other CNS depressants when prescribed for patients who are receiving fentanyl pharmacotherapy.

See also Opiate Analgesics General Monograph

ADVERSE DRUG REACTIONS

As with other opiate analgesics, the most common serious ADRs associated with fentanyl pharmacotherapy are apnea, bradycardia, muscular rigidity, and respiratory depression. If untreated, these ADRs may result in respiratory arrest, circulatory depression, and cardiac arrest. Like other opiate analgesics, fentanyl can produce addiction and habituation. Other ADRs, listed according to body system, include:

Cardiovascular: hypotension
CNS: dizziness
GI: nausea and vomiting
Musculoskeletal: laryngospasm
Ocular: blurred vision
Respiratory: respiratory depression
Miscellaneous: sweating (excessive)

See also Opiate Analgesics General Monograph

OVERDOSAGE

Signs and symptoms of fentanyl overdosage vary. Generally, they are an extension of its CNS and respiratory depressant actions. Fentanyl overdosage requires emergency symptomatic medical support of body systems with attention to increasing fentanyl elimination. The opiate antagonist naloxone (Narcan®) is usually required to manage the severe respiratory depression associated with fentanyl overdosage. The duration of respiratory depression associated with fentanyl overdosage may be longer than the duration of action for the opiate antagonist. Thus, the opiate antagonist may require re-administration.

FLUMAZENIL (Flumazepil)

(floo′may ze nil)

TRADE NAMES

Anexate®
Romazicon®

CLASSIFICATION

Benzodiazepine receptor antagonist (imidazobenzodiazepine)

APPROVED INDICATIONS FOR PSYCHOLOGICAL DISORDERS

Diagnosis or symptomatic management of:

Substance-Related Disorders: Benzodiazepine Overdosage

USUAL DOSAGE AND ADMINISTRATION

Benzodiazepine Overdosage

Adults: Initially, 0.3 mg injected intravenously over 30 seconds. Repeat at 1 minute intervals until the patient clearly responds or the maximum recommended dosage of 3 mg is reached. If drowsiness recurs, repeat dosage at 20 minute intervals. If preferred, prescribe 0.1 to 0.4 mg/hour by continuous intravenous infusion. Adjust the rate individually according to the level of desired patient arousal.

MAXIMUM: 5 mg intravenously (total dosage)

Women who are, or who may become, pregnant: FDA Pregnancy Category C. Safety and efficacy of flumazenil pharmacotherapy for women who are pregnant have not been established. Avoid prescribing flumazenil pharmacotherapy to women who are pregnant. If flumazenil pharmacotherapy is required, patients (or their family members in regard to the patient, as appropriate, in the event of severe overdosage) should be advised of the importance of the use of the antidote and any possible risks to themselves and the embryo, fetus, or neonate. Collaboration with the patient's obstetrician is indicated.

Women who are breast-feeding: Safety and efficacy of flumazenil pharmacotherapy for women who are breast-feeding and their neonates and infants have not been established. If flumazenil pharmacotherapy is required, breast-feeding should be discontinued for at least 24 hours, lactation maintained, and breast-feeding resumed following treatment of benzodiazepine overdosage.

Elderly, frail, or debilitated patients: No special precautions or dosage restrictions generally are required for elderly, frail, or debilitated patients.

Children and adolescents younger than 18 years of age: Safety and efficacy of flumazenil pharmacotherapy for children and adolescents have *not* been established. However, in cases of benzodiazepine overdosage, prescribing psychologists may consider recommending the following suggested dosages: 0.01 mg/kg/dose intravenously over 30 seconds. Repeat, as indicated, or follow by a continuous intravenous infusion of 0.005 to 0.01 mg/kg/hour until the patient responds or the maximum recommended dosage of 2 mg is reached.

MAXIMUM: For children and adolescents weighing 30 kg (67 lb) or less, maximum is 2 mg intravenously (total dosage). For children and adolescents weighing *over* 30 kg (67 lb), maximum is the recommended adult dosage (see Adults). Limited data are available regarding flumazenil pharmacotherapy for the symptomatic management of benzodiazepine overdosage among children and adolescents.

Notes, Benzodiazepine Overdosage

The manufacturer recommends that flumazenil be administered intravenously by a physician who has experience in anesthesiology and that patients have an established airway and intravenous access before intravenous flumazenil pharmacotherapy is initiated. Flumazenil pharmacotherapy always should be administered with concurrent emergency symptomatic medical treatment for acute overdosage.

Flumazenil has a relatively short duration of action ($T_{1/2} = 1$ hour). Therefore, overdosages involving long-acting benzodiazepines require continued monitoring *after* initial therapeutic benefit has been achieved. If drowsiness recurs, a continuous intravenous infusion may be initiated (see Usual Dosage and Administration).

AVAILABLE DOSAGE FORMS, STORAGE, AND COMPATIBILITY

Injectable, intravenous: 0.1 mg/ml

Notes

The flumazenil injectable formulation is compatible for 24 hours with 5% dextrose in water, lactated Ringer's, and normal saline intravenous solutions. It should be stored safely at controlled room temperature (15° to 30°C; 59° to 86°F).

PROPOSED MECHANISM OF ACTION

Flumazenil is a benzodiazepine antagonist that acts at the benzodiazepine receptors by means of competitive inhibition (i.e., blocking the benzodiazepines from binding to their receptors and eliciting their pharmacologic action). The efficacy of flumazenil for reversing the sedation and respiratory depression associated with benzodiazepine overdosage is greatest in relation to sedation but may be limited or incomplete in relation to respiratory depression. Flumazenil also appears to possess weak anticonvulsant (i.e., benzodiazepine agonist) activity. However, this action does not appear to be of any therapeutic significance.

PHARMACOKINETICS/PHARMACODYNAMICS

Flumazenil is moderately bound to plasma proteins (~50%). It has a mean apparent volume of distribution of 1 L/kg. Flumazenil is metabolized extensively by the liver with less than 1% excreted in unchanged form in the urine. The mean half-life of elimination is 1 hour and the mean total body clearance is ~70 L/hour. The onset of the reversal of the signs and symptoms of benzodiazepine overdosage generally occurs within two minutes of the intravenous injection of flumazenil.

RELATIVE CONTRAINDICATIONS

Cyclic antidepressant overdosage (see Cautions and Comments)
Head injuries. Flumazenil may precipitate seizures among these patients.
Hypersensitivity to flumazenil or the benzodiazepines
Seizure disorders, including epilepsy. Flumazenil may precipitate seizures among these patients.

CAUTIONS AND COMMENTS

Excessive or rapid administration of flumazenil to patients who are addicted to benzodiazepines may induce the benzodiazepine withdrawal syndrome. Signs and symptoms of the benzodiazepine withdrawal syndrome include, depending upon the severity of addiction and habituation, anxiety, dizziness, excessive sweating, seizures, and tachycardia. Cardiac dysrhythmias and seizures also have been observed, particularly among patients whose overdosage has involved the benzodiazepines and cyclic antidepressants.

Recommend the cautious prescription of flumazenil pharmacotherapy for patients who

- have histories of panic disorder. Flumazenil pharmacotherapy may precipitate a panic attack among these patients.
- have histories of severe liver dysfunction. The clearance of flumazenil may be reduced by up to two-thirds among these patients. Although a lower initial flumazenil dose generally is not required, subsequent dosages may need to be reduced for these patients.

CLINICALLY SIGNIFICANT DRUG INTERACTIONS

Concurrent flumazenil pharmacotherapy and the following may result in clinically significant drug interactions:

Zopiclone Pharmacotherapy

Zopiclone (Imovane®, Rhovane®), a non-benzodiazepine sedative-hypnotic, acts by binding to the benzodiazepine receptor. Thus, flumazenil will block its actions and may be of benefit for the symptomatic management of zopiclone overdosage.

ADVERSE DRUG REACTIONS

Flumazenil pharmacotherapy generally has been well tolerated. Slight pain and irritation are noted occasionally at the injection site. Other ADRs associated with flumazenil pharmacotherapy (e.g., agitation, anxiety, crying, seizures) are most likely signs and symptoms of the benzodiazepine withdrawal syndrome.

OVERDOSAGE

Flumazenil overdosage has not been reported. Dosages of up to 100 mg intravenously failed to produce signs and symptoms of overdosage among healthy volunteers.

FLUOXETINE

(floo ox'e teen)

TRADE NAME

Prozac®

CLASSIFICATION

Antidepressant (SSRI)

See also SSRI General Monograph

APPROVED INDICATIONS FOR PSYCHOLOGICAL DISORDERS

Adjunctive pharmacotherapy for the symptomatic management of:

- Anxiety Disorders: Obsessive-Compulsive Disorder
- Eating Disorders: Bulimia Nervosa. Fluoxetine has been demonstrated to be of significant benefit for decreasing both binge-eating and purging behaviors.
- Mood Disorders, Depressive Disorders: Major Depressive Disorder

USUAL DOSAGE AND ADMINISTRATION

Obsessive-Compulsive Disorder

Adults: Initially, 20 mg daily orally in a single morning dose. Increase the dosage gradually according to individual patient response (see also Notes, Obsessive-Compulsive Disorder).

MAXIMUM: 80 mg daily orally

Women who are, or who may become, pregnant: See Usual Dosage and Administration, Mood Disorders, Depressive Disorders: Major Depressive Disorder

Women who are breast-feeding: See Usual Dosage and Administration, Mood Disorders, Depressive Disorders: Major Depressive Disorder

Elderly, frail, or debilitated patients and those who have liver dysfunction: See Usual Dosage and Administration, Mood Disorders, Depressive Disorders: Major Depressive Disorder

Children and adolescents younger than 19 years of age: See Usual Dosage and Administration, Mood Disorders, Depressive Disorders: Major Depressive Disorder

Notes, Obsessive-Compulsive Disorder

See Notes, Mood Disorders, Depressive Disorders: Major Depressive Disorder

Eating Disorders: Bulimia Nervosa

Adults: 60 mg daily orally in a single morning dose

Women who are, or who may become, pregnant: See Usual Dosage and Administration, Major Depressive Disorder

Women who are breast-feeding: See Usual Dosage and Administration, Major Depressive Disorder

Elderly patients and those who have liver dysfunction: See Usual Dosage and Administration, Major Depressive Disorder

Children and adolescents younger than 19 years of age: See Usual Dosage and Administration, Major Depressive Disorder

Notes, Eating Disorders: Bulimia Nervosa

See Notes, Major Depressive Disorder

Mood Disorders, Depressive Disorders: Major Depressive Disorder

Adults: Initially, 20 mg daily orally in a single morning dose. Gradually increase the dosage according to individual patient response (see also Notes, Major Depressive Disorder). Patients who require daily dosages exceeding 20 mg may benefit from a single daily dose or two divided doses, morning and noon.

MAXIMUM: 80 mg daily orally

Women who are, or who may become, pregnant: FDA Pregnancy Category B. Safety and efficacy of fluoxetine pharmacotherapy for women who are pregnant have not been established. Available data do not associate fluoxetine pharmacotherapy with congenital malformations (i.e., birth defects). However, risk for miscarriage may be significantly increased. In addition, signs and symptoms of possible fluoxetine toxicity (i.e., jitteriness, seizures, and tremor) have been reported among neonates whose mothers received fluoxetine pharmacotherapy during their pregnancies. Avoid prescribing fluoxetine pharmacotherapy to women who are pregnant. If fluoxetine pharmacotherapy is required, advise patients of potential benefits and possible risks to themselves and the embryo, fetus, or neonate. Collaboration with the patient's obstetrician is indicated.

Women who are breast-feeding: Safety and efficacy of fluoxetine pharmacotherapy for women who are breast-feeding and their neonates and infants have not been established. Fluoxetine generally is excreted in breast milk in concentrations equivalent to 25% to 50% of the maternal blood concentration. Avoid prescribing fluoxetine pharmacotherapy to women who are breast-feeding. If fluoxetine pharmacotherapy is required, breast-feeding probably should be discontinued. Collaboration with the patient's pediatrician is indicated.

Elderly, frail, or debilitated patients and those who have liver dysfunction: Initially, 10 to 20 mg daily orally in a single dose. Increase the dosage gradually, if needed, according to individual patient response. Generally prescribe lower dosages for elderly, frail, or debilitated patients or those who have liver dysfunction. These patients may be more sensitive to the pharmacologic actions of fluoxetine than are younger or healthier adult patients.

MAXIMUM: 20 mg daily orally. Safety and efficacy of higher dosages of fluoxetine for elderly, frail, or debilitated patients and those who have liver dysfunction have not been established.

Children and adolescents younger than 19 years of age: Safety and efficacy of fluoxetine pharmacotherapy for children and adolescents have not been established. Fluoxetine pharmacotherapy is *not* recommended for this age group.

Notes, Mood Disorders, Depressive Disorders: Major Depressive Disorder

Four or five weeks of fluoxetine pharmacotherapy may be required to reach steady state because of the long half-life of elimination of both fluoxetine and its active metabolite norfluoxetine. Therefore, allow sufficient time for the achievement of steady state before gradually increasing the dosage, if needed. Monitoring patient response in regard to steady-state fluoxetine blood concentrations will help to avoid higher than required dosages and the associated increased incidence and severity of ADRs.

AVAILABLE DOSAGE FORMS, STORAGE, AND COMPATIBILITY

Capsules, oral: 10, 20 mg
Solution, oral: 20 mg/5 ml (contains 0.23% alcohol, mint flavored)
Syrup, oral: 20 mg/5 ml (mint odor)

Notes

General Instructions for Patients Instruct patients who are receiving fluoxetine pharmacotherapy to

- safely store their oral dosage forms of fluoxetine out of the reach of children in tightly closed child-resistant containers at controlled room temperature (15° to 30°C; 59° to 86°F).
- obtain an available patient information sheet regarding fluoxetine pharmacotherapy from their pharmacist at the time that their prescription is dispensed. Encourage patients to clarify any questions that they may have concerning fluoxetine pharmacotherapy with their pharmacist or, if needed, to consult their prescribing psychologist.

PROPOSED MECHANISM OF ACTION

The exact mechanism of antidepressant, anti-obsessional, and other related actions of fluoxetine has not yet been fully determined. These actions appear to be directly related to the ability of fluoxetine to inhibit selectively the neuronal re-uptake of serotonin.

See also the Selective Serotonin Re-Uptake Inhibitors General Monograph

PHARMACOKINETICS/PHARMACODYNAMICS

Fluoxetine is relatively well absorbed (over 60%) following oral ingestion. Peak concentrations are achieved within 6 to 8 hours. The concurrent ingestion of food does not significantly affect the bioavailability of fluoxetine. Fluoxetine is highly plasma protein-bound (~94%), and its mean apparent volume of distribution is 35 L/kg. Fluoxetine is metabolized extensively in the liver to several metabolites, including the principal active metabolite norfluoxetine. The mean half-life of elimination is 2 days (range 1 to 3 days), and the mean total body clearance is ~700 ml/minute. The mean half-life of elimination of the principal active metabolite norfluoxetine is 9 days. Less than 5% of fluoxetine is excreted in unchanged form in the urine.

RELATIVE CONTRAINDICATIONS

Hypersensitivity to fluoxetine

MAOI pharmacotherapy, concurrent, within 14 days of discontinuing MAOI pharmacotherapy, or within 5 weeks of discontinuing fluoxetine pharmacotherapy. Concurrent use may result in the development of the serotonin syndrome.

See Selective Serotonin Re-Uptake Inhibitors General Monograph

CAUTIONS AND COMMENTS

Prescribe fluoxetine pharmacotherapy cautiously to patients who

- have anorexia nervosa, cachexia, or are underweight. Fluoxetine pharmacotherapy has been associated with anorexia and weight loss and may exacerbate these conditions.
- have anxiety, insomnia, or nervousness. Fluoxetine pharmacotherapy may exacerbate these conditions. Up to 20% of patients receiving fluoxetine pharmacotherapy have experienced anxiety, insomnia, or nervousness. These ADRs have been significant enough to warrant discontinuation of fluoxetine pharmacotherapy among approximately one-quarter of these patients.
- are receiving ECT. Although data are limited, an increase in the incidence and duration of seizures has been reported among these patients.
- have body fluid volume depletion related to diuretic pharmacotherapy or other causes. Fluoxetine may induce hyponatremia, possibly in association with the Syndrome of Inappropriate Antidiuretic Hormone Secretion (SIADH).
- have diabetes mellitus. Fluoxetine may cause hypoglycemia. In addition, the discontinuation of fluoxetine pharmacotherapy has been associated with hyperglycemia.
- have histories of bipolar disorder. Fluoxetine pharmacotherapy may induce mania in ~20% of patients who have bipolar disorders. It also may induce mania in patients who have unipolar disorders, but the incidence would be a much smaller percentage.
- have histories of seizure disorders. Fluoxetine may increase seizure activity among these patients.

Caution patients who are receiving fluoxetine pharmacotherapy against performing activities that require alertness, judgment, and physical coordination (e.g., driving an automobile, operating dangerous equipment, supervising children) until their response to fluoxetine pharmacotherapy is known.

In addition to this general precaution, caution patients to inform their prescribing psychologist if they begin or discontinue any other pharmacotherapy while receiving fluoxetine pharmacotherapy.

In addition to these general precautions, caution women to inform their prescribing psychologist if they become, or intend to become, pregnant while receiving fluoxetine pharmacotherapy, so that their pharmacotherapy can be safely discontinued.

CLINICALLY SIGNIFICANT DRUG INTERACTIONS

Concurrent fluoxetine pharmacotherapy and the following may result in clinically significant drug interactions:

Drugs That Are Highly Bound to Plasma Proteins

Fluoxetine may displace from their binding sites other drugs that are highly bound to plasma proteins (e.g., digitoxin [Crystodigin®], warfarin [Coumadin®]). This interaction results in significantly higher concentrations of free drug and associated actions, including ADRs. Conversely, fluoxetine may be displaced by other drugs, depending upon their affinity for the plasma protein binding sites.

Lithium Pharmacotherapy

Concurrent fluoxetine and lithium (Duralith®, Lithane®) pharmacotherapy has been associated with both decreases and increases in lithium blood concentrations and an associated lack of clinical response and toxicity, respectively. When concurrent pharmacotherapy is required, monitor lithium blood concentrations (see Lithium Monograph). Also monitor lithium blood concentrations following the discontinuation of fluoxetine pharmacotherapy.

Pharmacotherapy With Drugs That Are Metabolized by the Hepatic Cytochrome P450 Enzyme System, Particularly Isoenzyme CYP2D6

Fluoxetine inhibits the CYP2D6 hepatic isoenzyme and, consequently, reduces the rate and extent of metabolism of a number of different drugs that are metabolized by this system, including amitriptyline (Elavil®), clomipramine (Anafranil®), clozapine (Clozaril®), codeine, desipramine (Pertofrane®), diazepam (Valium®), flecainide (Tambocor®), haloperidol (Haldol®), imipramine (Tofranil®), nortriptyline (Aventyl®), paroxetine (Paxil®), perphenazine (Trilafon®), propafenone (Rythmol®), propranolol (Inderal®), risperidone (Risperdal®), sertraline (Zoloft®), thioridazine (Mellaril®), and venlafaxine (Effexor®). Concurrent fluoxetine pharmacotherapy and pharmacotherapy with drugs that are metabolized by the P450 enzyme system, particularly by the CYP2D6 isoenzyme, may result in toxicity associated with the latter. Dosage adjustments for these hepatically metabolized drugs may be needed. Collaboration with other prescribers may be required.

Phenytoin Pharmacotherapy

The initiation of fluoxetine pharmacotherapy for patients who have been stabilized on phenytoin (Dilantin®) has resulted in significantly increased phenytoin blood concentrations and associated signs and symptoms of toxicity (e.g., incoordination [ataxia], double vision [diplopia], CNS depression, and constant, involuntary, cyclical movement of the eyeball [nystagmus]).

See also Selective Serotonin Re-Uptake Inhibitors General Monograph

ADVERSE DRUG REACTIONS

Fluoxetine pharmacotherapy is commonly associated with anxiety, asthenia, diarrhea, dizziness, drowsiness, dry mouth, fatigue, headache, insomnia, lightheadedness, loss of appetite (anorexia), nausea, nervousness, sweating (excessive), and tremor. Other ADRs associated with fluoxetine pharmacotherapy, listed according to body system, include:

Cardiovascular: chest pain, fainting (syncope), hypotension, and tachycardia

CNS: abnormal dreams, agitation, and migraine

Cutaneous: acne, dry skin, edema, itching (severe), loss of hair (alopecia), and rash. Rash may be the first indication of a potentially serious hypersensitivity reaction. Approximately one-third of the 5% of patients who develop a rash discontinue fluoxetine pharmacotherapy because of related signs and symptoms of hypersensitivity. These signs and symptoms include edema, carpal tunnel syndrome, difficult or labored breathing, fever, leukocytosis, lymphadenopathy, protein in the urine (proteinuria), respiratory distress, and vasculitis. Refer patients who develop a rash to their family physician or advanced practice nurse for assessment and evaluation. Collaboration may be required in regard to the decision to continue fluoxetine pharmacotherapy.

Genitourinary: decreased sex drive (decreased libido), impotence, painful menstruation, and urinary incontinence

GI: dyspepsia and vomiting

Hematologic: anemia, hemorrhage, and lymphadenopathy

Metabolic/Endocrine: breast pain (see also Genitourinary)

Musculoskeletal: arthritis, back pain, joint pain (arthralgia), and muscle pain (myalgia)

Ocular: blurred vision, conjunctivitis, eye pain, and reduction or dimness of vision (amblyopia)

Respiratory: asthma, bronchitis, difficult or labored breathing (dyspnea), runny nose (rhinitis), and yawning (excessive)

Miscellaneous: chills, malaise, and weight loss

See also Selective Serotonin Re-Uptake Inhibitors General Monograph

OVERDOSAGE

Signs and symptoms of fluoxetine overdosage include agitation, hypomania, nausea, seizures, and vomiting. Fluoxetine overdosage requires emergency symptomatic medical support of body systems with attention to increasing fluoxetine elimination. There is no known antidote.

FLUPENTHIXOL

(floo pen thix′ole)

TRADE NAME

Fluanxol®

CLASSIFICATION

Antipsychotic (Thioxanthene)

APPROVED INDICATIONS FOR PSYCHOLOGICAL DISORDERS

Adjunctive pharmacotherapy for the symptomatic management of:

Psychotic Disorders: Schizophrenia and Other Psychotic Disorders *Not* Associated With Agitation, Excitement, or Hyperactivity

USUAL DOSAGE AND ADMINISTRATION

Schizophrenia and Other Psychotic Disorders Not Associated With Agitation, Excitement, or Hyperactivity

Adults: Initially, 3 mg daily orally in three divided doses. Increase the dosage by 1 mg every two to three days until signs and symptoms of psychosis are managed.

MAINTENANCE: oral formulation, 3 to 6 mg daily orally in divided doses; or long-acting depot formulation, 20 to 40 mg intramuscularly every two to three weeks. Some patients who are receiving daily oral flupenthixol pharmacotherapy may require dosages of 12 mg daily or more. For patients who require intramuscular flupenthixol pharmacotherapy, inject intramuscularly into a large, healthy muscle site, preferably the dorsogluteal site. Aspirate carefully before injecting to avoid inadvertent intravascular injection. Do *not* inject intravenously. The long-acting depot formulation has an oily base that, if injected intravenously, may cause lipid emboli.

MAXIMUM: 12 mg daily orally; or 80 mg/dose intramuscularly of the long-acting depot formulation

Women who are, or who may become, pregnant: FDA Pregnancy Category "not established." Safety and efficacy of flupenthixol pharmacotherapy for women who are pregnant have not been established. Avoid prescribing flupenthixol to women who are pregnant. If flupenthixol pharmacotherapy is required, advise patients (or their legal guardians in regard to the patient) of the potential benefits and possible risks to themselves and the embryo, fetus, or neonate. Collaboration with the patient's obstetrician is indicated.

Women who are breast-feeding:　Safety and efficacy of flupenthixol pharmacotherapy for women who are breast-feeding and their neonates and infants have not been established. Avoid prescribing flupenthixol pharmacotherapy to women who are breast-feeding. If flupenthixol pharmacotherapy is required, breast-feeding probably should be discontinued. Collaboration with the patient's pediatrician is indicated.

Elderly, frail, or debilitated patients:　Generally prescribe lower dosages for elderly, frail, or debilitated patients. Increase the dosage gradually, if needed, according to individual patient response. These patients may be more sensitive to the pharmacologic actions of flupenthixol than are younger or healthier adult patients. See also Available Dosage Forms, Storage, and Compatibility, Notes.

Children:　Safety and efficacy of flupenthixol pharmacotherapy for children have not been established. Flupenthixol pharmacotherapy is *not* recommended for this age group.

Notes, Schizophrenia and Other Psychotic Disorders Not Associated With Agitation, Excitement, or Hyperactivity

Long-term flupenthixol pharmacotherapy has been associated with irreversible tardive dyskinesia.

Initiating and Maintaining Short-Acting Oral and Long-Acting Injectable Flupenthixol Pharmacotherapy

SHORT-ACTING ORAL PHARMACOTHERAPY　Sleep disturbances may occur initially during short-acting oral flupenthixol pharmacotherapy. Patients who previously have received pharmacotherapy with antipsychotics that are associated with a marked sedative action appear to be particularly at risk for this ADR. If troublesome, the evening dose may be reduced. Following the management of the signs and symptoms of the psychotic disorder, replace the short-acting oral flupenthixol pharmacotherapy with the long-acting intramuscular depot formulation.

LONG-ACTING INJECTABLE PHARMACOTHERAPY　The injectable form of flupenthixol is a long-acting depot formulation that appears useful for maintenance pharmacotherapy for patients who have been stabilized with the oral flupenthixol formulation and would benefit from dosing every two to three weeks with the long-acting formulation. In order to maintain optimal clinical response when replacing short-acting oral flupenthixol pharmacotherapy with long-acting injectable flupenthixol pharmacotherapy, gradually proceed according to the following general recommendations while carefully monitoring individual patient response. Careful monitoring is required during the period of dosage adjustment to minimize the risk for overdosage or inadequate management of psychotic signs and symptoms between injections. There is no reliable dosage equivalent for the short-acting and long-acting formulations of flupenthixol.

Patients who previously have not received long-acting depot antipsychotic pharmacotherapy　Patients who previously have not received pharmacotherapy with long-acting depot antipsychotic pharmacotherapy, such as flupenthixol pharmacotherapy, should be given an initial test dose of 5 to 20 mg. Test doses usually are well tolerated. However, a 5-mg test dose is recommended for patients who are elderly, frail, or debilitated and for those who have family histories suggesting a predisposition to extrapyramidal reactions. During the subsequent five days, monitor patients for continued management of their signs and symptoms of psychosis. Also monitor patients for extrapyramidal reactions. Short-acting oral flupenthixol pharmacotherapy may be continued at a lower dosage while being replaced with the long-acting depot formulation.

Patients who previously have received long-acting depot antipsychotic pharmacotherapy Patients who have had a positive response to previous long-acting depot antipsychotic pharmacotherapy may be prescribed an initial dose of 20 to 40 mg. Except for particularly sensitive patients, a second dose of 20 to 40 mg may be injected four to ten days after the initial injection. Subsequent doses and the frequency of dosing must be determined for each patient according to their individual response. Psychotic signs and symptoms for most patients can be managed with 20 to 40 mg of flupenthixol (2%) every 2 to 3 weeks. However, the optimal dose and frequency of dosing vary among patients and must be guided by clinical circumstance and individual patient response. Doses exceeding 80 mg usually are unnecessary. However, some patients may require higher doses. Although therapeutic benefit following a single injection usually lasts for two to three weeks, for some patients it may last for four weeks or longer.

The amount of a dose should *not* be increased to prolong the interval between injections because of the associated risk for extrapyramidal reactions and other ADRs. The action of flupenthixol also may vary more when higher doses are prescribed. Thus, it is recommended that increases not exceed 20 mg per injection. After an appropriate dosage is achieved, monitor patient response at regular intervals so that further dosage adjustments can be made, if needed. For maintenance pharmacotherapy, prescribe the lowest effective dose and the longest effective dosing interval to avoid troublesome ADRs.

Discontinuing Long-Term Flupenthixol Pharmacotherapy Although abrupt discontinuation of short-term flupenthixol, or other antipsychotic pharmacotherapy, does not generally pose problems for patients, transient dyskinetic signs and symptoms, or withdrawal emergent neurological signs (WENS), may be experienced by some patients upon abrupt discontinuation of long-term maintenance pharmacotherapy. The signs and symptoms of transient dyskinesia are similar to those for tardive dyskinesia, except for their duration. Although it is unknown whether gradual discontinuation of flupenthixol pharmacotherapy will decrease the incidence of WENS, gradual discontinuation of pharmacotherapy is recommended.

AVAILABLE DOSAGE FORMS, STORAGE, AND COMPATIBILITY

Injectables, intramuscular: 2% (20 mg/ml), 10% (100 mg/ml)
Tablets, oral: 0.5, 3, 5 mg

Notes

Store injectables safely protected from light at controlled room temperature (15° to 30°C; 59° to 86°F).

General Instructions for Patients Instruct patients who are receiving flupenthixol pharmacotherapy to

- safely store flupenthixol oral tablets in child-resistant containers, out of the reach of children, protected from light at controlled room temperature (15° to 30°C; 59° to 86°F).

- obtain an available patient information sheet regarding flupenthixol pharmacotherapy from their pharmacist at the time that their prescription is dispensed. Encourage patients to clarify any questions that they may have concerning flupenthixol pharmacotherapy with their pharmacist or, if needed, to consult their prescribing psychologist.

PROPOSED MECHANISM OF ACTION

The exact mechanism of action of flupenthixol for the symptomatic management of schizophrenia and other psychotic disorders has not been determined. Its actions are similar to those of the phenothiazine antipsychotics. Flupenthixol is a thioxanthene antipsychotic that produces less sedation and hypotension than the phenothiazines. However, it has a greater propensity for producing extrapyramidal reactions.

See also Phenothiazines General Monograph

PHARMACOKINETICS/PHARMACODYNAMICS

The short-acting oral formulation of flupenthixol (dihydrochloride) is well absorbed following oral ingestion and achieves maximum blood concentrations within 3 to 8 hours. The long-acting injectable formulation is the decanoate ester of flupenthixol. The esterification of flupenthixol allows its slow release from the injection site and associated prolonged duration of action. The onset of action usually occurs between 24 and 72 hours after intramuscular injection. Pharmacokinetic studies indicate that peak blood concentrations of the long-acting flupenthixol injectable formulations occur within one week following intramuscular injection of 40 mg of flupenthixol (2% or 10% formulation). Although there is considerable variation among patients in regard to their individual response to long-acting flupenthixol pharmacotherapy, the duration of action for the symptomatic management of psychoses can be expected to continue for two to four weeks. Flupenthixol is excreted mainly in the feces. Small amounts also are excreted in the urine. Additional data are unavailable.

RELATIVE CONTRAINDICATIONS

Blood disorders
Cardiovascular dysfunction, severe
Cerebrovascular dysfunction
CNS depression
Coma
Kidney dysfunction
Liver dysfunction
Hypersensitivity to flupenthixol or other thioxanthenes. The possibility of cross-sensitivity between the thioxanthenes and phenothiazine derivatives should be considered.
Parkinsonism
Pheochromocytoma
Pregnancy
Subcortical brain damage, suspected or established

CAUTIONS AND COMMENTS

Prescribe flupenthixol pharmacotherapy cautiously to patients who

- are undergoing surgery, particularly those patients who have been prescribed high dosages of flupenthixol. These patients require careful monitoring for possible hypotension. The anesthetic or other CNS depressant drugs required for surgery may require a reduction in dosage. Collaboration with the patient's surgeon and anesthesiologist is indicated.
- have glaucoma, known or suspected. Flupenthixol's anticholinergic action, although relatively weak, may exacerbate this condition.
- have histories of head injury, brain tumors, or other medical disorders for which the signs and symptoms may be obscured by flupenthixol's action (see also next comment concerning seizure disorders).
- have histories of seizure disorders. Flupenthixol may lower the seizure threshold. In addition, although not directly associated with flupenthixol pharmacotherapy, sudden unexpected and unexplained deaths have been associated occasionally with phenothiazine antipsychotic pharmacotherapy. A history of previous brain injury or seizure disorders may be a predisposing factor. Avoid prescribing high dosages of flupenthixol to patients who have histories of brain injury or seizure disorders. Several patients have shown a recurrence of psychotic behavior shortly before death. Autopsy findings usually have revealed acute fulminating pneumonia or pneumonitis, aspiration of gastric contents, or intramyocardial lesions.
- may be exposed to extreme heat or organic phosphorous insecticides and those who are receiving pharmacotherapy with atropine or related drugs (e.g., TCAs). Flupenthixol's anticholinergic action, although weak, may affect the patient's ability to control body temperature, particularly if the patient is receiving concurrent pharmacotherapy with anticholinergics or other drugs that produce anticholinergic actions.
- have propensity for developing defects in cardiac conduction. Flupenthixol may produce cardiac conduction defects among these patients.

Caution patients who are receiving flupenthixol pharmacotherapy to inform their prescribing psychologist if they begin or discontinue any other pharmacotherapy while receiving flupenthixol pharmacotherapy.

CLINICALLY SIGNIFICANT DRUG INTERACTIONS

Concurrent flupenthixol pharmacotherapy and the following may result in clinically significant drug interactions:

Alcohol Use

Concurrent flupenthixol pharmacotherapy and alcohol use may result in additive CNS depression. Advise patients to avoid, or limit, their use of alcohol while receiving flupenthixol pharmacotherapy.

Pharmacotherapy With Anticholinergics or Other Drugs That Produce Anticholinergic Actions

Flupenthixol may potentiate the action of anticholinergics (e.g., atropine) or other drugs that produce anticholinergic actions (e.g., TCAs). Paralytic ileus has occasionally been reported, particularly among elderly patients who were receiving concurrent pharmacotherapy with several other drugs that produce anticholinergic actions.

Pharmacotherapy With Central Nervous System Depressants and Other Drugs That Produce Central Nervous System Depression

Concurrent flupenthixol pharmacotherapy with opiate analgesics, sedative-hypnotics, or other drugs that produce CNS depression (e.g., antihistamines, other phenothiazines, TCAs) may result in additive CNS depression.

See also Phenothiazines General Monograph

ADVERSE DRUG REACTIONS

Flupenthixol pharmacotherapy commonly has been associated with extrapyramidal reactions, including tardive dyskinesia. Other ADRs follow, listed according to body system. Flupenthixol shares many of the chemical and pharmacological properties of other thioxanthenes and the phenothiazines. Therefore, attention to the known ADRs associated with these antipsychotics is required when flupenthixol pharmacotherapy is prescribed.

See also Phenothiazines General Monograph

Extrapyramidal Reactions

Extrapyramidal reactions, if they occur, usually appear within the first few days of flupenthixol pharmacotherapy. These reactions, including TD and hypokinesis or hyperkinesis, reportedly have occurred among up to 30% of patients. The risk for EPRs seems to be greater among elderly patients who are receiving high-dosage flupenthixol pharmacotherapy, especially women. The signs and symptoms associated with EPRs are persistent and, in some patients, appear to be irreversible. The EPRs are characterized by rhythmical involuntary movements of the face, jaw, mouth, or tongue (e.g., puffing of cheeks, chewing movements, puckering of mouth, protrusion of tongue). Sometimes these signs and symptoms may be accompanied by involuntary movements of the extremities. Extrapyramidal reactions usually may be avoided or managed by reducing the dosage and prescribing standard anticholinergic anti-parkinsonian pharmacotherapy. The incidence of EPRs appears to be more frequent with the first few injections of the long-acting flupenthixol formulation. They appear to diminish thereafter. In these cases, prophylactic anti-parkinsonian pharmacotherapy is *not* recommended.

Tardive dyskinesia may occur during long-term flupenthixol pharmacotherapy or after its discontinuation. There is no known effective treatment for TD. Anti-parkinsonian pharmacotherapy usually does not alleviate the signs and symptoms of this syndrome. It is suggested that all flupenthixol and other antipsychotics be discontinued if the signs and symptoms of TD appear. For patients who require reinstitution of flupenthixol pharmacotherapy, increase the dosage or replace flupenthixol pharmacotherapy with a different antipsychotic drug. Although the patient may appear to benefit from prescribed antipsychotic pharmacotherapy, the syndrome may be masked. Extrapyramidal reactions may be alarming to patients. Warn them of the possible occurrence of these signs and symptoms, and provide them with appropriate psychologic support, as needed.

Prescribing psychologists may be able to reduce the risk for EPRs by prescribing antipsychotics only when necessary, reducing the dosage, if required, or discontinuing the drug, if possible, when signs and symptoms of this syndrome are first recognized, particularly among patients over fifty years of age. Reportedly, fine vermicular movements of the tongue may be an early sign of the syndrome. If antipsychotic pharmacotherapy is discontinued at this time, the full syndrome may not develop.

Other ADRs

Cardiovascular: fainting (syncope), palpitations, cardiac dysrhythmias, fluctuations in blood pressure, and ECG changes (nonspecific). If hypotension occurs, *epinephrine should not be used* for its pressor action because a paradoxical further lowering of blood pressure may result.

CNS: akathisia, anergy, depression, dizziness, drowsiness, dystonia, epileptiform seizures, fatigue, headache, hypomania, insomnia, over-activity, pseudo-parkinsonism, psychomotor agitation, restlessness, and somnolence

Cutaneous: contact dermatitis, eczema, exfoliative dermatitis, hives (urticaria), rash, redness of the skin (erythema), severe itching (pruritus), and sweating (excessive)

Genitourinary: impotence, loss of sex drive, and sexual excitement

GI: constipation, dry mouth, nausea, and salivation (excessive)

Hematologic: eosinophilia. Pharmacotherapy with other antipsychotic drugs has been associated with agranulocytosis, hemolytic anemia, leukopenia, nonthrombocytopenic purpura, pancytopenia, and thrombocytopenic purpura. Monitor patients for complaints of soreness of the mouth, gums, or throat. Also monitor for signs and symptoms of upper respiratory infection or any other signs and symptoms that may suggest a diminished resistance to infection associated with lowered blood cell counts. Obtain leukocyte counts to confirm cellular depression, which requires discontinuation of flupenthixol pharmacotherapy. Collaboration with the patient's family physician or a specialist (e.g., hematologist) is indicated for the confirmation of blood disorders and their medical management.

Hepatic: jaundice

Metabolic/Endocrine: abnormal lactation (galactorrhea), increased serum prolactin levels, and weight change. Other antipsychotic pharmacotherapy has been associated with abnormal breast enlargement (gynecomastia), false positive pregnancy tests, high or low blood sugar levels (hypoglycemia and hyperglycemia), menstrual irregularities, peripheral edema, and sugar in the urine (glycosuria).

Musculoskeletal: hyperreflexia, hypertonia, opisthotonos, and tremors (see also CNS)

Ocular: blurred vision, glaucoma, and oculogyric crisis

Miscellaneous: hypersensitivity reactions, including anaphylaxis, among susceptible patients

OVERDOSAGE

Signs and symptoms of flupenthixol overdosage frequently are preceded by extreme agitation, excitement, and confusion. Extrapyramidal reactions and respiratory and circulatory collapse may occur. Flupenthixol overdosage requires emergency symptomatic medical support of body systems with attention to increasing flupenthixol elimination. There is no known antidote.

FLUPHENAZINE

(floo fen'a zeen)

TRADE NAMES

Modecate®
Moditen®
Permitil®
Prolixin®

CLASSIFICATION

Antipsychotic (phenothiazine, propylpiperazine derivative)

See also Phenothiazines General Monograph

APPROVED INDICATIONS FOR PSYCHOLOGICAL DISORDERS

Adjunctive pharmacotherapy for the symptomatic management of:

Psychotic Disorders: Schizophrenia and Other Psychotic Disorders

USUAL DOSAGE AND ADMINISTRATION

Schizophrenia and Other Psychotic Disorders

Adults: Initially, 2.5 to 10 mg daily orally in three or four divided doses. Dosage is determined by the severity and duration of signs and symptoms and individual patient response.

MAINTENANCE: 1 to 5 mg daily, often as a single oral dose

MAXIMUM: 20 mg daily orally. A catatonic-like state has been associated with dosages exceeding the maximum recommended dosage.

Women who are, or who may become, pregnant: FDA Pregnancy Category C. Safety and efficacy of fluphenazine pharmacotherapy for women who are pregnant have not been established. Avoid prescribing fluphenazine pharmacotherapy to women who are pregnant. If fluphenazine pharmacotherapy is required, advise patients (or their legal guardians in regard to the patient) of potential benefits and possible risks to themselves and the embryo, fetus, or neonate. Collaboration with the patient's obstetrician is indicated.

Women who are breast-feeding: The safety and efficacy of fluphenazine pharmacotherapy for women who are breast-feeding and their neonates and infants have not been established. Avoid prescribing fluphenazine pharmacotherapy to women who are breast-feeding. If fluphenazine pharmacotherapy is required, breast-feeding probably should be discontinued. Collaboration with the patient's pediatrician is indicated.

Elderly, frail, or debilitated patients: Initially, 1 to 2.5 mg daily orally in divided doses. Generally prescribe lower dosages for elderly, frail, or debilitated patients. Increase the dosage gradually, if needed, according to individual patient response. These patients may be more sensitive to the pharmacologic actions of fluphenazine than are younger or healthier adult patients.

MAXIMUM: 10 mg daily orally

Children younger than 12 years of age: The safety and efficacy of fluphenazine pharmacotherapy for children younger than 12 years of age have not been established. Fluphenazine pharmacotherapy is *not* recommended for this age group.

Notes, Schizophrenia and Other Psychotic Disorders

Fluphenazine is a potent antipsychotic. The lowest effective dosage that will manage psychotic signs and symptoms must be carefully determined for each patient. The optimal dosage varies among patients. Prescribe a lower dosage initially, and increase the dosage gradually, as needed, according to individual patient response. Cautiously prescribe oral dosages exceeding 10 mg daily. Injectable dosages of fluphenazine generally are approximately one-third to one-half the oral dosage. For patients who have known hypersensitivity to phenothiazines, or who have disorders that predispose them to ADRs, initiate fluphenazine pharmacotherapy cautiously using the oral or injectable fluphenazine hydrochloride formulation.

Initiating Injectable Fluphenazine Pharmacotherapy for the Control of Acute Signs and Symptoms Initially severely agitated patients may require the rapid-acting formulation of injectable fluphenazine hydrochloride. When signs and symptoms are managed, oral maintenance fluphenazine pharmacotherapy may be initiated, often with single daily dosing.

Maintaining Fluphenazine Pharmacotherapy Prescribe oral or injectable maintenance fluphenazine pharmacotherapy according to individual patient requirements.

ORAL MAINTENANCE FLUPHENAZINE PHARMACOTHERAPY Generally, the oral dosage is approximately two to three times the injectable dosage of fluphenazine hydrochloride. When signs and symptoms of psychosis are managed, reduce the dosage gradually to daily maintenance dosages of 1 to 5 mg. The daily maintenance dosage may be prescribed as a single daily dose. Further adjustments to the dosage may be necessary during the course of maintenance pharmacotherapy to meet the needs of individual patients. Patients whose psychotic symptomatology is inadequately controlled may require a gradual increase in dosage. Oral dosages of up to 40 mg daily may be required for some patients. However, the safety and efficacy of long-term high-dosage fluphenazine pharmacotherapy have not been established.

INJECTABLE (DECANOATE, ENANTHATE) MAINTENANCE FLUPHENAZINE PHARMACOTHERAPY   The long-acting injectable decanoate formulations are indicated for patients who have been stabilized on a fixed oral daily dosage of fluphenazine and require long-term fluphenazine pharmacotherapy (e.g., patients who have chronic schizophrenia). *Caution:* when prescribing intramuscular fluphenazine pharmacotherapy, note which salt form of fluphenazine is being prescribed, the hydrochloride formulation or the decanoate or enanthate formulations. The hydrochloride formulation should not exceed 10 mg daily by intramuscular injection. The decanoate and enanthate formulations are long-acting formulations generally prescribed as a 25 to 100 mg (maximum) single intramuscular injection at two- to four-week intervals. The decanoate and enanthate formulations are *not* formulated for intravenous injection. *Fluphenazine decanoate or enanthate formulations should be injected only under the direct supervision of a clinician who is experienced in the clinical use of antipsychotics, particularly phenothiazines.*

Injections of fluphenazine decanoate or enanthate are extremely well tolerated. Local tissue reactions only rarely occur. Muscle rigidity, sometimes accompanied by hyperthermia, has been reported following pharmacotherapy with fluphenazine decanoate. A catatonic-like state has been associated with fluphenazine dosages exceeding the recommended maximum dosage.

Decanoate formulation   The decanoate formulation may be injected intramuscularly or subcutaneously. Use a dry sterile needle and syringe to prepare injections because moisture will cause solutions to become cloudy or to precipitate. Use at least a 21-gauge needle. Generally, initiate injectable decanoate pharmacotherapy with a dose of 12.5 to 25 mg. The onset of action generally occurs between 24 and 72 hours after injection. The management of the signs and symptoms of psychoses become significant within 48 to 96 hours. Subsequent injections, and the dosage interval, are determined by individual patient response. When prescribed for maintenance pharmacotherapy, a single injection may be effective for managing the presenting signs and symptoms of psychoses for up to four weeks or longer. The response to a single dose has been found to last as long as six weeks for some patients who are receiving maintenance pharmacotherapy.

For patients who have no history of phenothiazine pharmacotherapy, initially prescribe short-acting formulations of fluphenazine before initiating decanoate pharmacotherapy. Prescribing first the short-acting formulation will allow evaluation of individual patient response to fluphenazine and appropriate dosage adjustment. For patients who have been stabilized on a fixed daily dosage of an oral formulation, the replacement of the short-acting oral formulation with the long-acting injectable decanoate formulation can be attempted. Appropriate dosages of the injectable decanoate formulation should be individualized for each patient, and individual response carefully monitored. Although a precise formula for conversion generally is not available, a recommended approximate conversion ratio is 12.5 mg of the decanoate formulation every three weeks for every 10 mg of the oral fluphenazine hydrochloride formulation daily. Once the oral formulation has been replaced with the long-acting formulation, monitor patients and adjust the dosage according to individual patient response. Adjustments can be made, as needed, at the time of each injection.

Enanthate formulation   When therapeutic benefit is achieved and an appropriate dosage of fluphenazine has been established, an equivalent dose of the injectable enanthate formulation may be prescribed. Adjust subsequent dosages according to individual patient response. Dosages may range as widely as 12.5 to 100 mg every one to three weeks. However, the usual dosage is 25 mg every two weeks. If doses exceeding 50 mg are required, subsequent doses should be increased cautiously by increments of 12.5 mg. The *maximal* dose should not exceed 100 mg. The response to a single dose may last for as long as six weeks for some patients receiving maintenance fluphenazine pharmacotherapy.

AVAILABLE DOSAGE FORMS, STORAGE, AND COMPATIBILITY

Concentrate, oral (hydrochloride salt with its own calibrated dropper): 5 mg/ml (contains 1% alcohol [Permitil®], 14% alcohol [Prolixin®])

Elixir, oral (hydrochloride salt with its own calibrated dropper): 0.5 mg/ml (contains 14% alcohol)

Injectable, intramuscular (hydrochloride salt): 2.5 mg/ml

Injectable, intramuscular or subcutaneous (decanoate salt in sesame oil): 25, 100 mg/ml. Available in single-dose preassembled syringes and vials.

Injectable, intramuscular or subcutaneous (enanthate salt in sesame oil): 25 mg/ml

Tablets, oral (hydrochloride salt): 0.25, 1, 2.5, 5, 10 mg

Notes

Injectable Fluphenazine Formulations   Inspect injectables visually prior to use for particulate matter and discoloration. Injectable solutions may vary in color, ranging from essentially colorless to light amber. Do *not* use solutions that are darkly discolored or that contain particulate matter. These injectables should be returned to the dispensing pharmacy or manufacturer for safe and appropriate disposal. Store injectable fluphenazine solutions safely at controlled room temperature (15° to 30°C; 59° to 86°F).

INJECTABLE (HYDROCHLORIDE SALT)   The injectable hydrochloride formulation of fluphenazine is for intramuscular pharmacotherapy for patients who require the immediate management of acute signs and symptoms of psychosis and are unable, or unwilling, to ingest oral formulations.

INJECTABLE (DECANOATE AND ENANTHATE SALTS)   Injectable decanoate and enanthate are highly potent, have a markedly extended duration of action, and can be injected intramuscularly or subcutaneously. They are *not* to be injected intravenously.

Oral Fluphenazine Formulations

ORAL CONCENTRATE   Each dose should be measured only with the calibrated measuring device provided by the manufacturer. To increase palatability and stability, dilute each dose of the oral concentrate in at least 60 ml (2 ounces) of a compatible beverage (such as tomato or fruit juice, milk, and uncaffeinated soft drinks) *just prior to ingestion*. The oral concentrate should *not* be diluted with beverages containing caffeine (coffee, cola), tanics (tea), or pectinates (apple juice) because of potential incompatibility.

ORAL ELIXIR   Inspect the elixir prior to use. Upon standing, a slight wispy precipitate or globular material may develop due to the flavoring oils separating from the solution. However, potency is unaffected, and gentle shaking redisperses the oils and clears the elixir. Do not use oral elixirs that do *not* become clear with gentle shaking.

ORAL TABLETS   The 2.5, 5, and 10 mg tablets (e.g., Moditen®) may contain tartrazine (FD&C Yellow No. 5). Tartrazine has been associated with hypersensitivity reactions, including bronchial asthma, among susceptible patients, particularly those who have a hypersensitivity to aspirin.

General Instructions for Patients   Instruct patients who are receiving fluphenazine pharmacotherapy to

- safely store fluphenazine oral dosage forms out of the reach of children in tightly closed child-resistant containers.
- appropriately measure and dilute each dose of the oral concentrate or elixir immediately before ingestion.
- ingest each dose of the tablet formulation with an adequate amount of liquid chaser (e.g., 60 to 120 ml [2 to 4 ounces]).
- obtain an available patient information sheet regarding fluphenazine pharmacotherapy from their pharmacist at the time that their prescription is dispensed. Encourage patients to clarify any questions that they may have concerning fluphenazine pharmacotherapy with their pharmacist or, if needed, to consult their prescribing psychologist.

PROPOSED MECHANISM OF ACTION

The exact mechanism of action of fluphenazine is complex and has not yet been fully determined. Its antipsychotic action appears to be related primarily to its interaction with dopamine-containing neurons, specifically the blockade of dopamine receptors (D1 and D2) both pre- and post-synaptically.

See also Phenothiazines General Monograph

PHARMACOKINETICS/PHARMACODYNAMICS

Fluphenazine hydrochloride is absorbed rapidly following intramuscular injection (peak blood concentrations are achieved within 1.5 to 2 hours) or oral ingestion (peak blood concentrations are achieved within 30 minutes). The onset of action is within 1 hour, and the duration of action is 6 to 8 hours for both oral ingestion and intramuscular injection. Fluphenazine is highly bound to plasma proteins. The mean half-life of elimination is ~15 hours. Additional data are unavailable.

Other than their durations of action, there appears to be no difference in antipsychotic action between the fluphenazine decanoate and enanthate salts when compared to the fluphenazine hydrochloride salt. The esterification of fluphenazine markedly prolongs its duration of action with little attenuation. The onset of action is delayed between 24 and 72 hours after injection, but the duration of action is prolonged up to 3 weeks.

RELATIVE CONTRAINDICATIONS

Blood disorders
Cardiac dysfunction, severe
Coma
Hypersensitivity to fluphenazine or other phenothiazines. Cross-sensitivity to phenothiazine derivatives may occur.
Subcortical brain damage

CAUTIONS AND COMMENTS

Prescribe fluphenazine pharmacotherapy cautiously to patients who

- are exposed to extreme heat or phosphorus insecticides.
- have histories of hypersensitivity reactions to phenothiazine pharmacotherapy, including cholestatic jaundice, dermatoses, or other reactions, because of the possibility of cross-sensitivity.
- have histories of seizure disorders. Grand mal seizures have been reported among these patients.
- have medical disorders, including mitral insufficiency or other cardiovascular disorders, and pheochromocytoma.
- require long-term fluphenazine pharmacotherapy. Monitor these patients regularly for the possibility of the development of irreversible dyskinesia, lenticular and corneal deposits, liver damage, pigmentary retinopathy, and "silent pneumonias." These ADRs rarely have been associated with long-term phenothiazine pharmacotherapy.

Caution patients who are receiving fluphenazine pharmacotherapy to inform their prescribing psychologist if they begin or discontinue any other pharmacotherapy while receiving fluphenazine pharmacotherapy.

See also Phenothiazines General Monograph

CLINICALLY SIGNIFICANT DRUG INTERACTIONS

Concurrent fluphenazine pharmacotherapy and the following may result in clinically significant drug interactions:

Alcohol Use

Concurrent alcohol use may increase the CNS depressant action of fluphenazine. Advise patients to avoid, or limit, their use of alcohol while receiving fluphenazine pharmacotherapy.

Guanethidine Pharmacotherapy

Fluphenazine may decrease the neuronal uptake of guanethidine (Ismelin®) and, thus, decrease its antihypertensive action. Collaboration with the prescriber of the guanethidine is indicated.

Pharmacotherapy With Anticholinergics and Other Drugs That Produce Anticholinergic Actions

The actions of anticholinergics (e.g., atropine) and other drugs that produce anticholinergic actions (e.g., other phenothiazines, TCAs) are increased by the anticholinergic action of fluphenazine. Concurrent pharmacotherapy may result in excessive anticholinergic actions, including paralytic ileus among susceptible patients (e.g., elderly or bedridden patients). Prescribe concurrent pharmacotherapy cautiously and monitor these patients for signs and symptoms of constipation.

Pharmacotherapy With Central Nervous System Depressants and Other Drugs That Produce Central Nervous System Depression

Although generally not associated with fluphenazine pharmacotherapy, concurrent fluphenazine pharmacotherapy with opiate analgesics, sedative-hypnotics, or other drugs that produce CNS depression (e.g., antihistamines, other phenothiazines, TCAs) may result in additive CNS depression.

See also Phenothiazines General Monograph

ADVERSE DRUG REACTIONS

Fluphenazine pharmacotherapy commonly has been associated with adverse anticholinergic drug reactions (e.g., dry mouth, decreased GI secretions, and urinary retention). It also has been associated with the occurrence of EPRs. A higher incidence of EPRs has been associated with fluphenazine, particularly the decanoate or enanthate salts, than with the less potent piperazine derivatives or straight-chain phenothiazines, such as chlorpromazine (Largactil®, Thorazine®). Other ADRs associated with fluphenazine pharmacotherapy, listed according to body system, include:

Cardiovascular: hypertension or hypotension
CNS: catatonic-like state (with high dosages), drowsiness, headache, lethargy, NMS (rare), and TD (particularly with high dosages among women)
Genitourinary: excessive urination (polyuria)
GI: constipation, dry mouth, loss of appetite (anorexia), and salivation (excessive)
Ocular: blurred vision

See also Phenothiazines General Monograph

OVERDOSAGE

Signs and symptoms of fluphenazine overdosage are extensions of its pharmacologic actions and include EPRs, hypotension, and sedation. Fluphenazine overdosage requires emergency symptomatic medical support of body systems with attention to increasing fluphenazine elimination. There is no known antidote.

FLURAZEPAM

(flure az'e pam)

TRADE NAMES

Dalmane®
Novo-Flupam®
Somnol®

CLASSIFICATION

Sedative-hypnotic (benzodiazepine) (C-IV)

See also the Benzodiazepines General Monograph

APPROVED INDICATIONS FOR PSYCHOLOGICAL DISORDERS

Adjunctive pharmacotherapy for the short-term symptomatic management of:

Sleep Disorders: Insomnia, particularly insomnia characterized by difficulty falling asleep, frequent nocturnal awakenings, and early morning awakenings

USUAL DOSAGE AND ADMINISTRATION

Insomnia

Adults: 15 or 30 mg orally 30 minutes before retiring for bed in the evening. Individualize dosage for maximal therapeutic benefit.

Women who are, or who may become, pregnant: FDA Pregnancy Category "not established." Flurazepam crosses the placenta. Neonatal depression has been reported among neonates of mothers who received flurazepam pharmacotherapy during the last trimester of pregnancy. A neonate whose mother received 30 mg of flurazepam every evening 10 days prior to delivery appeared hypotonic and inactive during the first four days of life. Flurazepam pharmacotherapy is *contraindicated* for women who are pregnant.

Women who are breast-feeding: Safety and efficacy of flurazepam pharmacotherapy for women who are breast-feeding and their neonates and infants have not been established. Flurazepam is excreted in breast milk. Avoid prescribing flurazepam pharmacotherapy to women who are breast-feeding. If flurazepam pharmacotherapy is required, breast-feeding should be discontinued. If desired, lactation can be maintained and breast-feeding resumed following the discontinuation of short-term flurazepam pharmacotherapy. Collaboration with the patient's pediatrician is indicated.
See also the Benzodiazepines General Monograph

Elderly, frail, or debilitated patients: 15 mg orally 30 minutes before retiring for bed in the evening. Elderly, frail, or debilitated patients may be overly sensitive to usual adult dosages. Avoid prescribing dosages exceeding 15 mg for these patients because of the increased associated risk for confusion, dizziness, incoordination (ataxia), and over-sedation.

Children and adolescents younger than 15 years of age: Safety and efficacy of flurazepam pharmacotherapy for children and adolescents younger than 15 years of age have not been established. Flurazepam pharmacotherapy is *not* recommended for this age group.

Notes, Insomnia

Avoid prescribing flurazepam pharmacotherapy for longer than 10 consecutive days. Reevaluate patients who appear to require a longer duration of pharmacotherapy (i.e., longer than 28 consecutive days).

Flurazepam's hypnotic action may be more pronounced after the second or third consecutive evening dose. Flurazepam does not interfere with REM sleep. Abrupt discontinuation of long-term flurazepam pharmacotherapy, or regular personal use, has been associated with rebound insomnia. It also has been associated with the benzodiazepine withdrawal syndrome. Discontinue flurazepam pharmacotherapy gradually for these patients.

AVAILABLE DOSAGE FORMS, STORAGE, AND COMPATIBILITY

Capsules, oral: 15, 30 mg

Notes

General Instructions for Patients   Instruct patients who are receiving flurazepam pharmacotherapy to

- safely store flurazepam capsules out of the reach of children in tightly closed child- and light-resistant containers at controlled room temperature (15° to 30°C; 59° to 86°F).
- obtain an available patient information sheet regarding flurazepam pharmacotherapy from their pharmacist at the time that their prescription is dispensed. Encourage patients to clarify any questions that they may have concerning flurazepam pharmacotherapy with their pharmacist or, if needed, to consult their prescribing psychologist.

PROPOSED MECHANISM OF ACTION

The exact mechanism of action of flurazepam has not yet been fully determined. However, flurazepam appears to act by, or work in concert with, the inhibitory neurotransmitter GABA. This action appears to be accomplished by binding to benzodiazepine receptors within the GABA complex.

See also Benzodiazepines General Monograph

PHARMACOKINETICS/PHARMACODYNAMICS

Flurazepam is rapidly absorbed following oral ingestion. Initially, it undergoes rapid and pronounced metabolism to two pharmacologically active metabolites, flurazepam aldehyde and hydroxyethylflurazepam. After ingestion of a single dose, peak plasma levels of these two metabolites are achieved within 60 minutes. The metabolites are highly plasma protein-bound (~97%) and have a mean apparent volume of distribution of 22 L/kg. They are rapidly further metabolized in the liver and are excreted primarily in the urine, with less than 1% in unchanged form. The mean half-life of elimination for these metabolites is approximately 2 hours.

Flurazepam appears to be increasingly effective on the second and third night of consecutive use because of the formulation and accumulation of active metabolites, including the final active and principal metabolite desalkylflurazepam. Desalkylflurazepam has a mean half-life of elimination of 74 hours (range 50 to 100 hours). Thus, after discontinuation of flurazepam pharmacotherapy, both sleep latency and total wake time may continue to be decreased for one or two nights.

RELATIVE CONTRAINDICATIONS

Hypersensitivity to flurazepam or other benzodiazepines
Pregnancy

CAUTIONS AND COMMENTS

Flurazepam is addicting and habituating. As recommended, do not prescribe for longer than 10 consecutive days.

Prescribe flurazepam pharmacotherapy cautiously to patients who

- are elderly, frail, or debilitated. Flurazepam pharmacotherapy commonly has been associated with dizziness, drowsiness, incoordination (ataxia), lightheadedness, and staggering, particularly among elderly, frail, or debilitated patients. These ADRs have been associated with falls and serious injuries (e.g., fractured femur [hip fracture]) among these patients.
- have histories of problematic patterns of alcohol or other abusable psychotropic use. Carefully monitor these patients for problematic patterns of use.
- have kidney or liver dysfunction. Flurazepam metabolism and elimination may be decreased among these patients and result in a prolonged CNS depressant action.
- have pulmonary dysfunction. Flurazepam pharmacotherapy may exacerbate the pulmonary dysfunction.

Caution patients who are receiving flurazepam pharmacotherapy against

- increasing their dosage or using their flurazepam more often than prescribed. Ensure that patients understand that increasing the dosage, or using flurazepam more often than prescribed, may result in toxicity or addiction and habituation.
- drinking alcohol during the day following the use of flurazepam for the promotion of nighttime sleep. Also caution patients to avoid alcohol use for several days following the discontinuation of flurazepam pharmacotherapy. The potential for additive CNS depression may continue during the day following evening use and for a few days following the discontinuation of flurazepam pharmacotherapy.
- performing activities that require alertness, judgment, and physical coordination (e.g., driving an automobile, operating dangerous equipment, supervising children), particularly during the day following flurazepam use for the promotion of nighttime sleep. Flurazepam's CNS depressant action may adversely affect these mental and physical functions.

In addition to these general precautions, caution patients to inform their prescribing psychologist if they begin or discontinue any other pharmacotherapy while receiving flurazepam pharmacotherapy.

CLINICALLY SIGNIFICANT DRUG INTERACTIONS

Concurrent flurazepam pharmacotherapy and the following may result in clinically significant drug interactions:

Alcohol Use

Concurrent alcohol use may increase the CNS depressant action of flurazepam. Advise patients to avoid, or limit, their use of alcohol while receiving flurazepam pharmacotherapy and for several days following its discontinuation.

Pharmacotherapy With Central Nervous System Depressants and Other Drugs That Produce Central Nervous System Depression

Concurrent flurazepam pharmacotherapy with opiate analgesics, other sedative-hypnotics, or other drugs that produce CNS depression (e.g., antihistamines, phenothiazines, TCAs) may result in additive CNS depression.

See also Benzodiazepines General Monograph

ADVERSE DRUG REACTIONS

The ADRs commonly associated with flurazepam pharmacotherapy include dizziness, drowsiness, and lightheadedness. Flurazepam pharmacotherapy also has been associated with the following ADRs, listed according to body system:

Cardiovascular: chest pain, fainting (syncope), hypotension, and palpitations
CNS: apprehension, confusion, depression, euphoria, hallucinations, headache, nervousness, restlessness, slurred speech, talkativeness, and weakness. Rarely, paradoxical reactions (e.g., excitement, hyperactivity, and overstimulation).
Cutaneous: flushing, severe itching (pruritus), skin rash, and sweating (excessive)
GI: bitter taste, constipation, diarrhea, dry mouth, GI pain, heartburn, loss of appetite (anorexia), nausea, salivation (excessive), and stomach upset
Hematologic: rarely, abnormal decrease of granulocytic white blood cells (i.e., basophils, eosinophils, and neutrophils) (agranulocytopenia) and abnormal decrease of white blood cells usually below 5,000/mm^3 (leukopenia)
Musculoskeletal: body and joint pain and incoordination (ataxia)
Ocular: blurred vision, burning eyes, and difficulty focusing
Respiratory: shortness of breath

See also Benzodiazepines General Monograph

OVERDOSAGE

Signs and symptoms of flurazepam overdosage, include confusion, disorientation, lethargy, severe sedation or somnolence, and coma. Flurazepam overdosage requires emergency symptomatic medical support of body systems with attention to increasing flurazepam elimination. The benzodiazepine antagonist flumazenil (Anexate®, Romazicon®) may be required.

FLUSPIRILENE

(floo speer'i leen)

TRADE NAMES

Imap®
Imap Forte®

CLASSIFICATION

Antipsychotic (diphenylbutylpiperidine)

APPROVED INDICATIONS FOR PSYCHOLOGICAL DISORDERS

Adjunctive pharmacotherapy for the symptomatic management of:

Psychotic Disorders: Schizophrenia and Other Psychotic Disorders. Fluspirilene pharmacotherapy is indicated for those patients whose symptomatology does *not* include agitation, depression, excitement, or hyperactivity. Fluspirilene pharmacotherapy also may be of benefit for non-agitated patients who have chronic schizophrenia and who have been stabilized with short-acting antipsychotic pharmacotherapy because of its longer duration of action.

USUAL DOSAGE AND ADMINISTRATION

Schizophrenia and Other Psychotic Disorders

Adults: 2 to 10 mg intramuscularly once weekly (see Notes, Schizophrenia and Other Psychotic Disorders)

MAXIMUM: 15 mg intramuscularly once weekly

Women who are, or who may become, pregnant: FDA Pregnancy Category "not established." Safety and efficacy of fluspirilene pharmacotherapy for women who are pregnant have not been established. Avoid prescribing fluspirilene pharmacotherapy for women who are pregnant. If fluspirilene pharmacotherapy is required, advise patients (or their legal guardians in regard to the patient) of potential benefits and possible risks to themselves and the embryo, fetus, or neonate. Collaboration with the patient's obstetrician is indicated.

Women who are breast-feeding: Safety and efficacy of fluspirilene pharmacotherapy for women who are breast-feeding and their neonates and infants have not been established. Avoid prescribing fluspirilene pharmacotherapy for women who are breast-feeding. If fluspirilene pharmacotherapy is required, breast-feeding probably should be discontinued. Collaboration with the patient's pediatrician is indicated.

Elderly, frail, or debilitated patients: Generally prescribe lower dosages for elderly, frail, or debilitated patients. Increase the dosage gradually, if needed, according to individual patient response. These patients may be more sensitive to the pharmacologic actions of fluspirilene than are younger or healthier adult patients.

Children younger than 12 years of age: Safety and efficacy of fluspirilene pharmacotherapy for children younger than 12 years of age have not been established. Fluspirilene pharmacotherapy is *not* recommended for this age group.

Notes, Schizophrenia and Other Psychotic Disorders

Long-acting fluspirilene pharmacotherapy may be prescribed to replace short-acting antipsychotic pharmacotherapy for selected non-agitated patients who have chronic schizophrenia. These patients must be well-stabilized on shorter-acting antipsychotic pharmacotherapy before it is replaced with fluspirilene pharmacotherapy. The goal of long-acting fluspirilene pharmacotherapy is the maintenance of therapeutic response similar to, or better than, that achieved with the short-acting antipsychotic.

Fluspirilene is only administered by intramuscular injection. Inject fluspirilene intramuscularly into large healthy muscle sites, such as the dorsogluteal site. Generally, a 5-cm (2-inch) 21-gauge needle is recommended for intramuscular injection. Obese patients may require a 6.5-cm (2¹/2-inch) needle in order to help to assure that the injection is made deeply into muscle and not subcutaneous fat. Do *not* inject fluspirilene intravenously. Rotate intramuscular injection sites with each injection to prevent or minimize local tissue irritation. The injectable formulation is microcrystalline and has been associated with the development of subcutaneous nodules, particularly among patients who have received long-term fluspirilene injectable pharmacotherapy. The nodules tend to resolve upon discontinuation of fluspirilene pharmacotherapy.

Although the average duration of action for fluspirilene is 7 days or 1 week, therapeutic response may wane in 5 to 6 days for some patients. Thus, when replacing short-acting fluspirilene pharmacotherapy with long-acting pharmacotherapy, individually adjust the fluspirilene dosage over a number of weeks. Extrapyramidal reactions and other ADRs commonly occur after the injection of fluspirilene. Insufficient management of psychotic symptomatology also may occur shortly before the next injection is due. Thus, the optimal dosage and frequency of intramuscular injections must be individually determined for each patient. Collaboration with another clinician experienced in prescribing fluspirilene pharmacotherapy may be indicated. Unfortunately, the replacement of short-acting antipsychotic pharmacotherapy with long-acting fluspirilene pharmacotherapy may not be successful for all patients. Do *not* exceed the recommended dosage for these patients in an attempt to obtain desired therapeutic benefit. Prescribing dosages exceeding those recommended may result in overdosage.

Initiating Long-Acting Fluspirilene Pharmacotherapy To replace short-acting antipsychotic pharmacotherapy with long-acting fluspirilene pharmacotherapy, initially prescribe 2 to 3 mg intramuscularly once a week. Depending on the severity of the patient's signs and symptoms of psychosis, and previous response to other antipsychotic pharmacotherapy, 3 to 4 mg intramuscularly once weekly may be needed. Patients who have severe symptomatology, or a history of inadequate therapeutic response to antipsychotic pharmacotherapy, may require 4 mg or more intramuscularly once weekly.

Monitor patients for a feeling of tiredness or malaise following initial injections. These ADRs usually remit with continued pharmacotherapy. Also monitor patients for akathisia (i.e., feelings of restlessness or an inability to sit down without severe anxiety) after their first dose of fluspirilene pharmacotherapy. If patients experience transient akathisia during the first few days following their injection, reduce the next dose. For patients who do not experience akathisia, increase the initial dosage by weekly increments of 1 to 2 mg according to individual patient response. Optimal weekly dosages range from 2 to 10 mg. Avoid prescribing weekly dosages exceeding 15 mg. Some patients may require a shorter dosing interval between fluspirilene injections (e.g., some patients may require one injection every five or six days rather than one injection every seven days).

For patients who require higher dosages of fluspirilene, prescribe injections of the more concentrated formulation. The use of this formulation allows smaller injection volumes, which have been associated with less tissue irritation and are generally better tolerated.

Maintaining Long-Term Fluspirilene Pharmacotherapy After several weeks of pharmacotherapy, patients may complain of ADRs that appear to be related to drug accumulation. These ADRs include mild akathisia beginning on the day following the injection. After a few months of fluspirilene pharmacotherapy, nausea, rigidity, salivation, tremors, and vomiting rarely may occur on the day after the injection. These ADRs usually can be managed by a slight reduction in dosage or by withholding one weekly injection. Some patients may benefit from antiparkinsonian pharmacotherapy during the first or second day following their injections. Also monitor patients for the possible development of silent pneumonias.

AVAILABLE DOSAGE FORMS, STORAGE, AND COMPATIBILITY

Injectables, intramuscular: 2, 10 mg/ml (micronized formulation, average particle size is less than 10 μm)

Notes

The injectable formulation is *for intramuscular injection only.* Do *not* inject intravenously.

PROPOSED MECHANISM OF ACTION

Fluspirilene appears to act by blocking impulse transmission mediated by dopamine in the dopaminergic neurons in the subcortical areas of the brain. It also increases norepinephrine turnover at higher dosages. Fluspirilene produces EPRs typical of potent antipsychotics. It also has cardiac, autonomic, and endocrine actions.

PHARMACOKINETICS/PHARMACODYNAMICS

Fluspirilene is well absorbed after intramuscular injection. Peak blood levels are achieved within 24 hours. The duration of action is generally about one week. A peak effect occurs usually by the second day following injection. Fluspirilene is metabolized by conjugation and N-dealkylation. After a single intramuscular dose, elimination is slow, with less than 50% being excreted in one week. Approximately 70% of fluspirilene and its metabolites are excreted by the end of the month. Additional data are unavailable.

RELATIVE CONTRAINDICATIONS

Blood disorders
CNS depression
Coma
Kidney dysfunction
Hypersensitivity to fluspirilene or other diphenylbutylpiperidines
Liver dysfunction
Parkinson's disease
Subcortical brain damage

CAUTIONS AND COMMENTS

Prescribe fluspirilene pharmacotherapy cautiously to patients who

- have cardiovascular disorders. ECG changes suggestive of myocardial ischemia (ST depression and T-wave changes) and postural hypotension have occurred among patients who were receiving fluspirilene pharmacotherapy. Postural hypotension reportedly is more pronounced among patients who have hypertension. Considering fluspirilene's peripheral autonomic actions, attention also should be given to the potential interaction of fluspirilene and antihypertensive drugs (see Clinically Significant Drug Interactions).
- have cerebrovascular disorders. Fluspirilene pharmacotherapy may exacerbate these medical disorders.
- have head injuries, increased intracranial pressure, or other medical disorders for which the suppression of nausea and vomiting might obscure the clinical course. Fluspirilene has antiemetic actions similar to those of other antipsychotics. Collaboration with the patient's family physician or neurologist may be indicated.
- have histories (or family histories) of breast cancer. Although data are inconclusive, long-term high-dosage antipsychotic pharmacotherapy may predispose patients to breast cancer and place these patients at increased risk for breast cancer.
- have organic brain syndrome. Fluspirilene pharmacotherapy may exacerbate this medical disorder.
- require long-term fluspirilene pharmacotherapy. Monitor blood counts and heart, liver, and kidney function regularly during fluspirilene pharmacotherapy. Collaboration with the patient's family physician or a specialist (e.g., hematologist) is indicated. Reduce the dosage or discontinue fluspirilene pharmacotherapy if signs and symptoms of TD are identified among patients receiving long-term pharmacotherapy.
- require surgery. These patients may require careful monitoring for possible hypotension. The action of atropine and other commonly prescribed drugs for patients who require surgery (e.g., anesthetics or other CNS depressants) may be potentiated and, thus, require dosage reductions. Collaboration with the patient's surgeon and anesthesiologist is indicated.
- have seizure disorders, including those patients who are receiving anticonvulsant pharmacotherapy. Fluspirilene may lower the seizure threshold. Collaboration with the prescriber of the anticonvulsant is indicated so that appropriate adjustments can be made to the patient's anticonvulsant dosage.

Caution patients who are receiving fluspirilene pharmacotherapy (or their legal guardians in regard to the patient) against performing activities that require alertness, judgment, and physical coordination (e.g., driving an automobile, operating dangerous equipment, supervising children) until their response to fluspirilene pharmacotherapy is known.

In addition to this general precaution, caution patients to

- advise their surgeon and anesthesiologist, in the event that surgery is required, that they are receiving long-term fluspirilene pharmacotherapy.
- inform their prescribing psychologist if they begin or discontinue any other pharmacotherapy while receiving fluspirilene pharmacotherapy.

CLINICALLY SIGNIFICANT DRUG INTERACTIONS

Concurrent fluspirilene pharmacotherapy and the following may result in clinically significant drug interactions:

Alcohol Use

Concurrent alcohol use may increase the CNS depressant action of fluspirilene. Advise patients to avoid, or limit, their use of alcohol while receiving long-term fluspirilene pharmacotherapy.

Dopamine Agonist Pharmacotherapy

Fluspirilene inhibits the action of dopamine agonists (e.g., bromocriptine [Parlodel®], levodopa [Dopar®]).

Pharmacotherapy With Anticholinergics or Other Drugs That Produce Anticholinergic Actions

Concurrent fluspirilene pharmacotherapy may potentiate the action of anticholinergics (e.g., atropine) or other drugs that produce anticholinergic actions (e.g., TCAs). This interaction may result in excessive anticholinergic actions, including paralytic ileus among susceptible patients (e.g., elderly or bedridden patients). Prescribe concurrent pharmacotherapy cautiously, and monitor patients for signs and symptoms of constipation.

Pharmacotherapy With Central Nervous System Depressants and Other Drugs That Produce Central Nervous System Depression

Concurrent fluspirilene pharmacotherapy with opiate analgesics, sedative-hypnotics, or other drugs that produce CNS depression (e.g., antihistamines, TCAs) may result in additive CNS depression (see also Cautions and Comments).

Pharmacotherapy With Drugs That Induce Hepatic Enzyme Metabolism

Concurrent fluspirilene pharmacotherapy with drugs that induce the hepatic microsomal enzyme system (e.g., carbamazepine [Tegretol®], phenobarbital [Luminal®], phenytoin [Dilantin®]) may result in the need to adjust the fluspirilene dosage.

ADVERSE DRUG REACTIONS

Long-term fluspirilene pharmacotherapy has been associated with the following ADRs, listed according to body system:

Cardiovascular

ECG changes, including dysrhythmias (e.g., ST depression and T-wave changes, tachycardia), hypertension, or hypotension. Hypotension may be more pronounced among patients who are elderly, frail, or debilitated or those who have histories of hypertension.

Central Nervous System

Aggressiveness, agitation, anxiety, catatonia, depression, dizziness, drowsiness, EEG changes, headache, hallucinations, hypomania, insomnia, lethargy, sadness, sedation, seizures, and toxic confusional states. Two of the most serious ADRs involving the CNS include the NMS and EPRs, particularly TD. Akathisia, uncontrolled restlessness, may be a sign of drug-induced EPRs and should be distinguished from restlessness associated with the signs and symptoms of the patient's psychotic disorder.

Neuroleptic (Antipsychotic) Malignant Syndrome   Similar to other antipsychotics, fluspirilene pharmacotherapy has been associated with NMS. This syndrome is characterized by hyperpyrexia; muscle rigidity; altered mental states, including catatonia; and signs and symptoms of autonomic instability, such as irregular pulse or blood pressure. The syndrome also may include myoglobinuria (rhabdomyolysis) and acute kidney failure. A potentially fatal syndrome, NMS requires immediate discontinuation of antipsychotic pharmacotherapy and emergency symptomatic medical support of body systems with attention to the treatment of associated medical disorders.

Extrapyramidal Reactions   Extrapyramidal Reactions commonly have been associated with fluspirilene pharmacotherapy. These reactions include akathisia, dyskinesia, dystonia, hyperreflexia, opisthotonos, and, occasionally, oculogyric crisis. EPRs tend to occur, or peak, during the first two days following an injection of fluspirilene. Often dose-related, EPRs tend to subside when the dosage is reduced or fluspirilene pharmacotherapy is temporarily withheld. Anti-parkinsonian pharmacotherapy may be required during the first two days after a fluspirilene injection to manage serious EPRs. Avoid prescribing higher dosages of fluspirilene, and monitor long-term pharmacotherapy cautiously because of the possibility of frequent and serious EPRs, including TD.

Tardive Dyskinesia   Tardive dyskinesia may occur among some patients during long-term fluspirilene pharmacotherapy or when pharmacotherapy is discontinued. Risk appears greater for elderly patients who are receiving high dosages of fluspirilene pharmacotherapy, especially women. The signs and symptoms of TD are persistent and may be irreversible among some patients. Monitor for rhythmical involuntary movements of the face, jaw, mouth, or tongue (e.g., puffing of cheeks, chewing movements, puckering of mouth, protrusion of tongue). Involuntary movements of the trunk and extremities also may be observed. Persistent TD is thought to result from pharmacologically overloading the extrapyramidal system.

There is no known effective pharmacotherapy for the treatment of TD. Anti-parkinsonian drugs do not alleviate the signs and symptoms. Discontinue fluspirilene pharmacotherapy immediately if signs and symptoms occur. If reinstitution of antipsychotic pharmacotherapy is required, the dosage should be increased or another antipsychotic drug selected. However, the benefits of resuming antipsychotic pharmacotherapy must be weighed against the potential risks. Antipsychotic pharmacotherapy may mask the signs and symptoms of TD.

Prescribing psychologists may decrease the incidence of this serious syndrome by only prescribing fluspirilene pharmacotherapy, or other antipsychotic pharmacotherapy, when necessary and by reducing the dosage, or discontinuing pharmacotherapy, if possible, when early signs and symptoms are first identified. Fine vermicular movements of the tongue may be an early sign of TD. Discontinuing fluspirilene or other antipsychotic pharmacotherapy immediately may prevent the development of other signs and symptoms of TD.

Cutaneous

Skin rashes and other cutaneous reactions, photosensitivity, and sweating (excessive)

Genitourinary

Impotence among men, increased sex drive among women, and urinary retention

Gastrointestinal

Changes in appetite and weight, particularly weight gain; dry mouth; fecal impaction; gastric hypersecretion; nausea; paralytic ileus; salivation (excessive); and vomiting

Hematologic

Mild and generally transient eosinophilia, leukopenia, and leukocytosis have been associated with long-term fluspirilene pharmacotherapy. Attention also should be given to the possible occurrence of other blood disorders because of the similarity between fluspirilene and other antipsychotics. These blood disorders include agranulocytopenia, granulocytopenia, and thrombocytopenic purpura. These blood disorders are generally associated with an increased risk for infection.

Monitor patients carefully for soreness of the mouth, gums, or throat and any other signs and symptoms of infection (i.e., flu-like signs and symptoms). Collaboration with the patient's family physician, or a specialist (e.g, hematologist), may be indicated for confirmation of bone marrow depression. For these patients, discontinue fluspirilene pharmacotherapy immediately, and refer them for appropriate medical evaluation and treatment of related medical disorders. Emergency symptomatic medical support of body systems may be required.

Hepatic

Cholestatic jaundice

Metabolic/Endocrine

False positive results on pregnancy tests; hormonal changes, including hyperprolactinemia that, for some patients, may lead to absence of menses (amenorrhea) or abnormal lactation (galactorrhea)

Ocular

Blurred vision

Respiratory

Nasal congestion

Miscellaneous

Anaphylactic reactions. Sudden unexplained deaths, usually associated with fulminating pneumonia or intramyocardial lesions, occasionally have been reported among patients who were receiving antipsychotic (i.e., phenothiazine) pharmacotherapy. Attention should be given to this possible ADR because of fluspirilene's chemical and pharmacological similarity to the phenothiazines.

OVERDOSAGE

Signs and symptoms of fluspirilene overdosage are generally extensions of its pharmacologic actions and are similar to those associated with other antipsychotics. These signs and symptoms include progressive impairment of consciousness from drowsiness to coma. These signs and symptoms may initially include agitation, confusion, convulsions, delirium, disorientation, and EPRs. Other signs and symptoms include ECG changes, disturbances in temperature regulation, hypotension, and tachycardia. As with other antipsychotic overdosages, late respiratory failure and prolonged shock may terminate in cardiac arrest and death. Fluspirilene overdosage requires emergency symptomatic medical support of body systems with attention to increasing fluspirilene elimination. There is no known antidote.

FLUVOXAMINE

(floov ox'a meen)

TRADE NAME

Luvox®

CLASSIFICATION

Antidepressant (SSRI)

See also Selective Serotonin Re-Uptake Inhibitors General Monograph

APPROVED INDICATIONS FOR PSYCHOLOGICAL DISORDERS

Adjunctive pharmacotherapy for the symptomatic management of:

- Anxiety Disorders: Obsessive-Compulsive Disorder
- Mood Disorders, Depressive Disorders: Major Depressive Disorder

USUAL DOSAGE AND ADMINISTRATION

Obsessive-Compulsive Disorder

Adults: Initially, 50 mg daily orally in a single dose 30 minutes before retiring for bed in the evening. Increase the daily dosage by 50 mg increments every four to seven days, according to individual patient response. Usual effective daily dosage is between 100 and 300 mg.

MAXIMUM: 300 mg daily orally

Women who are, or who may become, pregnant: FDA Pregnancy Category C. Safety and efficacy of fluvoxamine pharmacotherapy for women who are pregnant have not been established. Avoid prescribing fluvoxamine pharmacotherapy to women who are pregnant. If fluvoxamine pharmacotherapy is required, advise patients of potential benefits and possible risks to themselves and the embryo, fetus, or neonate. Collaboration with the patient's obstetrician is indicated.

Women who are breast-feeding: Safety and efficacy of fluvoxamine pharmacotherapy for women who are breast-feeding and their neonates and infants have not been established. Fluvoxamine is excreted into breast milk. Avoid prescribing fluvoxamine pharmacotherapy to women who are breast-feeding. If fluvoxamine pharmacotherapy is required, breast-feeding probably should be discontinued. Collaboration with the patient's pediatrician is indicated.

Elderly, frail, or debilitated patients and those who have liver dysfunction: Generally prescribe lower dosages for elderly, frail, or debilitated patients and those who have liver dysfunction. Increase the dosage gradually, if needed, according to individual patient response. These patients may be more sensitive to the pharmacologic actions of fluvoxamine than are younger or healthier patients.

Children 8 years of age and older: Initially, 25 mg daily orally in a single dose 30 minutes before bedtime in the evening. Increase the daily dosage by 25 mg increments every four to seven days, according to individual patient response. Usual effective daily dosage is between 50 and 200 mg.

MAXIMUM: 200 mg daily orally

Notes, Obsessive-Compulsive Disorder

Safety and efficacy of long-term fluvoxamine pharmacotherapy (i.e., longer than 12 weeks) have not been established. Patients who require pharmacotherapy for longer than this period of time require regular periodic reevaluation for the need for continued fluvoxamine pharmacotherapy.

Major Depressive Disorder

Adults: Initially, 50 mg daily orally in a single dose 30 minutes before retiring for bed in the evening. Increase the daily dosage by 50 mg increments every four to seven days according to individual patient response. The usual effective daily dosage is between 100 and 200 mg.

MAXIMUM: 300 mg daily orally

Women who are, or who may become, pregnant: FDA Pregnancy Category C. Safety and efficacy of fluvoxamine pharmacotherapy for women who are pregnant have not been established. Avoid prescribing fluvoxamine pharmacotherapy to women who are pregnant. If fluvoxamine pharmacotherapy is required, advise patients of potential benefits and possible risks to themselves and the embryo, fetus, or neonate. Collaboration with the patient's obstetrician is indicated.

Women who are breast-feeding: Safety and efficacy of fluvoxamine pharmacotherapy for women who are breast-feeding and their neonates and infants have not been established. Fluvoxamine is excreted into breast milk. Avoid prescribing fluvoxamine pharmacotherapy to women who are breast-feeding. If fluvoxamine pharmacotherapy is required, breast-feeding probably should be discontinued. Collaboration with the patient's pediatrician is indicated.

Elderly, frail, or debilitated patients and those who have liver dysfunction: Generally prescribe lower dosages for elderly, frail, or debilitated patients and those who have liver dysfunction. Increase the dosage gradually, if needed, according to individual patient response. These patients may be more sensitive to the pharmacologic actions of fluvoxamine than are younger or healthier patients.

Children and adolescents younger than 18 years of age: Safety and efficacy of fluvoxamine pharmacotherapy for the symptomatic management of depression among children and adolescents have not been established. Fluvoxamine pharmacotherapy is *not* recommended for this indication for this age group.

Notes, Major Depressive Disorder

Safety and efficacy of long-term fluvoxamine pharmacotherapy (i.e., longer than 12 weeks) have not been established. Patients who require pharmacotherapy for longer than this period of time require regular periodic reevaluation for the need for continued fluvoxamine pharmacotherapy.

AVAILABLE DOSAGE FORMS, STORAGE, AND COMPATIBILITY

Tablets, oral: 50, 100 mg

Notes

Prescribe dosages exceeding 150 mg daily in divided doses with a maximum dose of 150 mg orally 30 minutes before retiring for bed in the evening.

General Instructions for Patients   Instruct patients who are receiving fluvoxamine pharmacotherapy to

- swallow each dose of the fluvoxamine tablets whole without chewing, with an adequate amount (i.e., 60 to 120 ml [2 to 4 ounces]) of water or another compatible beverage.
- safely store fluvoxamine tablets out of the reach of children in tightly closed child-resistant containers at controlled room temperature (15° to 30°C; 59° to 86°F).
- obtain an available patient information sheet regarding fluvoxamine pharmacotherapy from their pharmacist at the time that their prescription is dispensed. Encourage patients to clarify any questions that they may have concerning fluvoxamine pharmacotherapy with their pharmacist or, if needed, to consult their prescribing psychologist.

PROPOSED MECHANISM OF ACTION

The exact mechanism of antidepressant, anti-obsessional, and other related actions of fluvoxamine has not yet been fully determined. These actions appear to be directly related to the ability of fluvoxamine to selectively inhibit the neuronal re-uptake of serotonin.

See also Selective Serotonin Re-Uptake Inhibitors General Monograph

PHARMACOKINETICS/PHARMACODYNAMICS

Fluvoxamine is moderately absorbed following oral ingestion ($F = 0.53$). Oral bioavailability is unaffected by ingestion with food. Peak concentrations are achieved within 2 to 8 hours. Fluvoxamine is only moderately plasma protein-bound (i.e., ~77%). Its mean apparent volume of distribution is 25 L/kg. Fluvoxamine is extensively metabolized by the liver to several inactive metabolites. Approximately 2% of fluvoxamine is excreted in unchanged form in the urine. Its mean half-life of elimination is ~15 hours.

RELATIVE CONTRAINDICATIONS

Astemizole, cisapride, or terfenadine pharmacotherapy. Concurrent fluvoxamine pharmacotherapy may inhibit the metabolism of these drugs. This interaction may result in significantly elevated blood levels and associated QT prolongation and potentially fatal torsades de pointes-type ventricular tachycardia (i.e., rapid ventricular tachycardia characterized by a gradual change in the QRS complex of the ECG).

Hypersensitivity to fluvoxamine

MAOI pharmacotherapy, concurrent or within 14 days. Concurrent pharmacotherapy may result in the serotonin syndrome.

See Selective Serotonin Re-Uptake Inhibitors General Monograph

CAUTIONS AND COMMENTS

Prescribe fluvoxamine pharmacotherapy cautiously to patients who

- are receiving ECT. An increased incidence and duration of seizures have been associated with ECT and concurrent pharmacotherapy with other SSRIs (e.g., fluoxetine). Thus, caution is indicated with concurrent fluvoxamine pharmacotherapy.
- have histories of bipolar disorders. Fluvoxamine pharmacotherapy may induce mania in ~1% of patients. This percentage may be significantly increased among patients who have bipolar disorders.
- have histories of seizure disorders. Seizures rarely have been reported among patients who were receiving fluvoxamine pharmacotherapy. In the event of seizures, discontinue fluvoxamine pharmacotherapy.

Caution patients who are receiving fluvoxamine pharmacotherapy against

- drinking alcohol. Fluvoxamine may potentiate the CNS depressant action of alcohol and, consequently, adversely affect psychomotor function.
- performing activities that require alertness, judgment, and physical coordination (e.g., driving an automobile, operating dangerous equipment, supervising children) until their response to fluvoxamine pharmacotherapy is known.

In addition to these general precautions, caution patients to inform their prescribing psychologist if they begin or discontinue any other pharmacotherapy while receiving fluvoxamine pharmacotherapy.

CLINICALLY SIGNIFICANT DRUG INTERACTIONS

Concurrent fluvoxamine pharmacotherapy and the following may result in clinically significant drug interactions:

Pharmacotherapy With Drugs That Are Metabolized by the Hepatic Cytochrome P450 Enzyme System, Particularly Isoenzymes CYP1A2, CYP2C19, and CYP3A3/4

Fluvoxamine inhibits these particular hepatic isoenzymes. Consequently, it reduces the rate and extent of metabolism of a number of different drugs, including alprazolam (Xanax®), astemizole (Hismanal®), caffeine, calcium channel blockers, carbamazepine (Tegretol®), cisparide (Propulsid®), clozapine (Clozaril®), corticosteroids, diazepam (Valium®), imipramine (Tofranil®), midazolam (Versed®), omeprazole (Prilosec®), propranolol (Inderal®), quinidine (Cardioquin®), terfenadine (Seldane® [removed from the U.S. market in 1998 at the request of the FDA]), theophylline (Theolair®), triazolam (Halcion®), verapamil (Isoptin®), and warfarin (Coumadin®). Significant increases in blood concentrations and resultant toxicity have been clearly documented with alprazolam (Xanax®), diazepam (Valium®), theophylline (Theo-Dur®), TCAs, and warfarin (Coumadin®). This interaction may require a dosage reduction of up to 50% for these drugs, depending upon individual patient factors (e.g., liver function). Collaboration with other prescribers may be required so that any necessary dosage adjustments can be made. See Relative Contraindications

See also Selective Serotonin Re-Uptake Inhibitors General Monograph

ADVERSE DRUG REACTIONS

Fluvoxamine pharmacotherapy is commonly associated with agitation, anorexia, asthenia, constipation, delayed ejaculation, diarrhea, dizziness, drowsiness, dry mouth, dyspepsia, insomnia, nausea, nervousness, and tremor. Other ADRs associated with fluvoxamine pharmacotherapy, listed according to body systems, include:

Cardiovascular: fainting (syncope), hypotension, palpitations, and tachycardia
CNS: abnormal dreams, abnormal thinking, headache, and migraine
Cutaneous: itching (severe), rash, and sweating (excessive)
Genitourinary: impotence, urinary frequency, and urinary incontinence
GI: belching (eructation), difficulty swallowing (dysphagia), and salivation (excessive)
Musculoskeletal: arthritis, joint pain (arthralgia), leg cramps, and muscle pain (myalgia)
Ocular: abnormal vision and a reduction or dimness of vision (amblyopia)
Respiratory: cough (increased), difficult or labored breathing (dyspnea), pharyngitis, and runny nose (rhinitis)
Miscellaneous: weight gain

See also Selective Serotonin Re-Uptake Inhibitors General Monograph

OVERDOSAGE

Signs and symptoms of fluvoxamine overdosage include bradycardia, coma, convulsions, diarrhea, dizziness, hypotension, nausea, somnolence, tachycardia, and vomiting. Fluvoxamine overdosage requires emergency symptomatic medical support of body systems with attention to increasing fluvoxamine elimination. There is no known antidote.

HALOPERIDOL

(ha loe per'i dole)

TRADE NAMES

Haldol®
Peridol®

CLASSIFICATION

Antipsychotic (butyrophenone)

APPROVED INDICATIONS FOR PSYCHOLOGICAL DISORDERS

Adjunctive pharmacotherapy for the symptomatic management of:

- Psychotic Disorders: Schizophrenia and Other Psychotic Disorders
- Severe Behavior Problems Among Children (e.g., combativeness; explosive hyperexcitability, which cannot be accounted for by immediate provocation). Haloperidol pharmacotherapy is indicated for these children only after they have failed to respond to psychotherapy alone or in combination with non-antipsychotic pharmacotherapy (e.g., methylphenidate [Ritalin®] pharmacotherapy).
- Tic Disorders, including Tourette's Disorder (Gilles de la Tourette's Syndrome)

USUAL DOSAGE AND ADMINISTRATION

Schizophrenia and Other Psychotic Disorders

Adults, Acute, Moderate, and Severe Symptomatology

ACUTE SYMPTOMATOLOGY   For prompt control of acute agitation, 2 to 5 mg (short-acting lactate salt) intramuscularly. Prescribe subsequent doses at four- to eight-hour intervals. If necessary, dose as often as every hour. Some patients may require higher dosages for the prompt control of severe signs and symptoms.

Replace the short-acting injectable haloperidol pharmacotherapy with oral pharmacotherapy as soon as practical. Depending on the patient's clinical response, generally initiate oral haloperidol pharmacotherapy within 12 to 24 hours after the last dose of the short-acting injectable haloperidol. The short-acting injectable dosage for the preceding 24 hours may be used to approximate the required total daily oral dosage. Monitor individual patient response carefully because this dosage is only an estimate. No bioequivalence data are available for injectable and oral formulations of haloperidol. Adjust the dosage according to individual patient response.

MODERATE SYMPTOMATOLOGY   1 to 6 mg daily orally in two or three divided doses.

SEVERE SYMPTOMATOLOGY   6 to 15 mg daily orally in two or three divided doses.

MAINTENANCE: Upon satisfactory achievement of therapeutic response, reduce the dosage gradually to the lowest effective maintenance dosage.

MAXIMUM: There is no established maximum dosage.

Adults who are resistant to antipsychotic pharmacotherapy or who require long-term haloperidol pharmacotherapy: 6 to 15 mg daily orally in two or three divided doses. Patients who remain severely disturbed, or whose signs and symptoms of psychoses remain inadequately managed, may require an increase in the daily dosage. Daily dosages of up to 100 mg may be needed to achieve optimal therapeutic benefit for some severely resistant patients. However, safety and efficacy of long-term high-dosage haloperidol pharmacotherapy have not been established.

Women who are, or who may become, pregnant: FDA Pregnancy Category C. Safety and efficacy of haloperidol pharmacotherapy for women who are pregnant have not been established. Avoid prescribing haloperidol pharmacotherapy to women who are pregnant. If haloperidol pharmacotherapy is required, advise patients (or their legal guardians in regard to the patient) of potential benefits and possible risks to themselves and the embryo, fetus, or neonate. Collaboration with the patient's obstetrician is required.

Women who are breast-feeding: Safety and efficacy of haloperidol pharmacotherapy for women who are breast-feeding and their neonates and infants have not been established. Haloperidol is excreted in low concentrations in breast milk. Avoid prescribing haloperidol to women who are breast-feeding. If haloperidol pharmacotherapy is required, breast-feeding probably should be discontinued. Collaboration with the patient's pediatrician is indicated.

Elderly, frail, and debilitated patients: Initially, 0.5 to 2 mg daily orally in two or three divided doses. Increase the dosage gradually, if needed, according to individual patient response. Generally prescribe lower dosages for elderly, frail, or debilitated patients. These patients may be more sensitive to the pharmacologic actions of haloperidol than are younger or healthier adult patients.

Children younger than 3 years of age: Safety and efficacy of haloperidol pharmacotherapy for children younger than 3 years of age have not been established. Haloperidol pharmacotherapy is *not* recommended for this age group.

Children 3 to 12 years of age (body weight 15 to 40 kg):   Initially, 0.5 mg daily orally in two or three divided doses. Increase the daily dosage by 0.5 mg at five- to seven-day intervals, as needed, until therapeutic benefit is achieved.

NON-PSYCHOTIC DISORDERS (SEVERE BEHAVIORAL PROBLEMS AND TIC DISORDERS):   0.05 to 0.075 mg/kg/day orally in two or three divided doses

PSYCHOTIC DISORDERS: 0.05 to 0.15 mg/kg/day orally in two or three divided doses. Children who have severe symptomatology may require higher dosages.

MAXIMUM: 6 mg daily orally. There is little evidence of further improvement of signs and symptoms with dosages exceeding 6 mg daily orally.

Notes, Schizophrenia and Other Psychotic Disorders

Initiating and Maintaining Haloperidol Pharmacotherapy

ORAL HALOPERIDOL PHARMACOTHERAPY   Initially, individualize the dosage according to the patient's age and general health, the severity of signs and symptoms, and previous response to antipsychotic pharmacotherapy. Adjust the dosage (i.e., increase or decrease) as rapidly as practical to achieve optimal therapeutic benefit with a minimum of ADRs. Children; elderly, frail, or debilitated patients; and patients who have histories of ADRs associated with previous antipsychotic pharmacotherapy may require lower dosages and more gradual dosage adjustments.

Although not directly associated with oral haloperidol pharmacotherapy, esophageal dysmotility has been reported with other oral antipsychotic pharmacotherapy, particularly olanzapine pharmacotherapy. Attention must be given to the possible occurrence of esophageal dysmotility when oral haloperidol pharmacotherapy is prescribed because of its chemical and pharmacological similarity to olanzapine. Olanzapine-induced esophageal dysmotility has resulted in aspiration pneumonia and death. Elderly patients, particularly those who have Alzheimer's dementia, are at increased risk for this reaction. Whenever possible, prescribe injectable haloperidol pharmacotherapy for these patients rather than the oral pharmacotherapy. If oral haloperidol pharmacotherapy cannot be avoided, monitor these patients carefully for esophageal dysmotility.

INJECTABLE HALOPERIDOL PHARMACOTHERAPY   Safety and efficacy of injectable haloperidol pharmacotherapy for children have not been established. Thus, injectable haloperidol pharmacotherapy is *not* recommended for this age group. Adult patients may benefit from short-acting haloperidol lactate or long-acting haloperidol decanoate injectable pharmacotherapy.

For adults, the deltoid site is recommended for intramuscular injection of the *short-acting* lactate salt. The use of other intramuscular injection sites may result in erratic absorption of the short-acting injectable formulation. The dorsogluteal site is recommended for intramuscular injection of the *long-acting* decanoate salt. A 3.75-cm (1.5-inch), 21-gauge needle is generally recommended, depending on the size and health of the muscle to be injected. Obese patients may require a 6.5-cm (2.5-inch) needle in order to help to ensure that the haloperidol is injected intramuscularly and *not* subcutaneously. Do *not* inject more than 3 ml per any intramuscular injection site. Also avoid getting the injectable solution on the skin or clothing because of associated contact dermatitis.

Initiating Long-Acting Haloperidol Decanoate Pharmacotherapy   Adult patients who have been stabilized with short-acting antipsychotic pharmacotherapy and require long-term antipsychotic pharmacotherapy may benefit from long-acting haloperidol decanoate pharmacotherapy. When replacing short-acting pharmacotherapy with long-acting pharmacotherapy, monitor patients closely during the initial period of dosage adjustment to readily identify the reappearance of psychotic signs and symptoms and to minimize the risk for overdosage. The signs and symptoms of psychosis may reappear before the next injection is due. These signs and symptoms indicate a need for dosage adjustment. During dosage adjustment, or episodes of exacerbation of psychotic signs and symptoms, supplement long-acting haloperidol decanoate pharmacotherapy with short-acting dosage formulations of haloperidol, if required.

Prescribe the dosage of long-acting haloperidol decanoate in terms of haloperidol content. Initially prescribe lower dosages, and adjust the dosage (i.e., increase or decrease), as needed, according to individual patient response. For patients previously maintained on low-dosage oral antipsychotic pharmacotherapy (e.g., up to the equivalent of oral haloperidol 10 mg daily), initially prescribe dosages of haloperidol decanoate 10 to 15 times the previous daily dosage in oral haloperidol equivalents. However, *do not exceed the initial maximal dosage of haloperidol decanoate of 100 mg*, regardless of the patient's previous antipsychotic dosage requirements. As with all injectable pharmacotherapy, local tissue reactions have been reported following haloperidol decanoate injection. Monitor blood pressure and respirations after the first dose and once haloperidol decanoate pharmacotherapy has been stabilized.

Maintaining Long-Acting Haloperidol Decanoate Pharmacotherapy　The recommended interval between intramuscular doses of haloperidol decanoate injections is four weeks. This dosing interval has been found to be effective for the symptomatic management of psychotic disorders for most patients. However, individual patient response may require the adjustment of this dosing interval.

Discontinuing Long-Acting Haloperidol Pharmacotherapy　The discontinuation of long-acting haloperidol pharmacotherapy has been associated with WENS (see Adverse Drug Reactions, CNS).

AVAILABLE DOSAGE FORMS, STORAGE, AND COMPATIBILITY

Concentrate, oral: 2 mg/ml (colorless, odorless, tasteless)
Injectable, intramuscular (short-acting lactate salt): 5 mg/ml
Injectable, intramuscular (long-acting decanoate salt): 50, 100 mg/ml (ampules or prefilled disposable syringe)
Tablets, oral: 0.5, 1, 2, 5, 10, 20 mg

Notes

Injectable Formulations　The injectable formulations of haloperidol are for *intramuscular use only. Do not inject intravenously or subcutaneously.* Inspect injectables visually for particulate matter and discoloration prior to use. Return solutions that are darkly discolored to the dispensing pharmacy or the manufacturer for safe and appropriate disposal.

Store injectables safely protected from light at controlled room temperature (15° to 30°C; 59° to 86°F). Do *not* refrigerate or freeze. A precipitate may form if injectables are refrigerated. However, the injectable solution should become clear upon warming to room temperature. Do *not* dilute injectable formulations with normal saline.

Oral Formulations　The 1.5 and 10 mg oral haloperidol tablets contain tartrazine (FD&C Yellow No. 5). Tartrazine has been associated with hypersensitivity reactions, including bronchial asthma, among susceptible patients, particularly those who have a hypersensitivity to aspirin.

General Instructions for Patients　Instruct patients who are receiving haloperidol pharmacotherapy to

- ingest each dose of the haloperidol oral tablets with food or water.
- dilute each dose of the haloperidol oral concentrate in 2 to 4 ounces (60 to 120 ml) of water, or another compatible beverage, immediately before ingestion to increase its palatability. If preferred, the oral concentrate may be gently mixed in a small amount of cold, soft food (e.g., pudding).
- avoid getting the oral concentrate on the skin or clothing. The oral concentrate has been associated with contact dermatitis.
- safely store haloperidol oral concentrate and oral tablets in tightly closed child- and light-resistant containers out of the reach of children at controlled room temperature (15° to 30°C; 59° to 86°F).
- obtain an available patient information sheet regarding haloperidol pharmacotherapy from their pharmacist at the time that their prescription is dispensed. Encourage patients to clarify any questions that they may have concerning haloperidol pharmacotherapy with their pharmacist or, if needed, to consult their prescribing psychologist.

PROPOSED MECHANISM OF ACTION

The exact mechanism of action of haloperidol is complex and has not yet been fully determined. Its antipsychotic activity appears to be primarily related to its interaction with dopamine-containing neurons, specifically the blockade (antagonism) of dopamine receptors (D2 and D3) both pre- and post-synaptically.

PHARMACOKINETICS/PHARMACODYNAMICS

Haloperidol is rapidly absorbed after oral ingestion and has a mean bioavailability of 60% ($F = 0.6$). Peak blood levels generally are achieved in 2 to 3 hours. Haloperidol is highly plasma protein-bound ($\sim$92%) and has an apparent volume of distribution of approximately 18 L/kg. Its peak effects occur within 30 to 45 minutes after intramuscular injection of the lactate salt. Haloperidol is extensively metabolized in the liver, and less than 1% is excreted in unchanged form in the urine. The mean half-life of elimination is $\sim$20 hours. The mean total body clearance is $\sim$800 ml/minute.

RELATIVE CONTRAINDICATIONS

Coma
CNS depression, severe
Hypersensitivity to haloperidol or other butyrophenones
Parkinsonism

CAUTIONS AND COMMENTS

Prescribe haloperidol pharmacotherapy cautiously to patients who have

- bipolar disorders. When haloperidol is prescribed for these patients, there may be a rapid mood swing to depression.
- cardiovascular disorders (severe). Haloperidol pharmacotherapy has been associated with transient hypotension and anginal pain. In the event of hypotension, collaboration with the patient's family physician or a specialist (e.g., cardiologist) is required, particularly if

a vasopressor is needed. In this regard, epinephrine should *not* be used because haloperidol may block its vasopressor action and result in a paradoxical further lowering of blood pressure. Metaraminol (Aramine®), phenylephrine (Neo-Synephrine®), or norepinephrine (Levophed®) are generally recommended in this situation.

- have histories of breast cancer. Antipsychotic drugs, including haloperidol, elevate prolactin levels. Elevations in prolactin levels persist during long-term pharmacotherapy. Approximately one-third of human breast cancers are associated with elevated prolactin levels. Collaboration with the patient's oncologist is indicated.
- have histories of hypersensitivity to other antipsychotic drugs
- have histories of seizure disorders. Haloperidol may lower the seizure threshold. Adequate anticonvulsant pharmacotherapy should be maintained for patients who have seizure disorders. Collaboration with the prescriber of the anticonvulsant is indicated.
- require or are receiving anticonvulsant pharmacotherapy or have EEG abnormalities. These patients may be at increased risk for seizures.
- require or are receiving anti-parkinsonian pharmacotherapy. The difference in excretion rates between haloperidol and some anti-parkinsonians may prove problematic in regard to optimal dosing. Anti-parkinsonian pharmacotherapy may need to be withheld until haloperidol pharmacotherapy is no longer needed. If both drugs are discontinued simultaneously, EPRs may occur.
- have thyrotoxicosis. The possibility of severe neurotoxicity with signs and symptoms of rigidity, or an inability to walk or talk, may be increased among these patients.

Caution patients who are receiving haloperidol pharmacotherapy against performing activities that require attention, judgment, and physical coordination (e.g., driving an automobile, operating dangerous equipment, supervising children). Haloperidol may impair these mental and physical functions.

In addition to this general precaution, caution patients to inform their prescribing psychologist if they begin or discontinue any other pharmacotherapy while receiving haloperidol pharmacotherapy.

CLINICALLY SIGNIFICANT DRUG INTERACTIONS

Concurrent haloperidol pharmacotherapy and the following may result in clinically significant drug interactions:

Alcohol Use

Concurrent alcohol use may increase the CNS depressant action of haloperidol. Advise patients to avoid, or limit, their use of alcohol while receiving haloperidol pharmacotherapy.

Lithium Pharmacotherapy

Concurrent haloperidol and lithium (Duralith®, Lithane®) pharmacotherapy rarely has been associated with an encephalopathic syndrome with signs and symptoms of confusion, EPRs, fever, lethargy, leukocytosis, tremulousness, and weakness. These signs and symptoms may be followed by irreversible brain damage. Although the existence of this interaction remains inconclusive, patients who are prescribed concurrent haloperidol and lithium pharmacotherapy require close monitoring for early signs and symptoms of this syndrome. If signs and symptoms of this syndrome are identified, discontinue haloperidol and lithium pharmacotherapy immediately.

Pharmacotherapy With Central Nervous System Depressants and Other Drugs That Produce Central Nervous System Depression

Concurrent haloperidol pharmacotherapy with opiate analgesics, sedative-hypnotics, or other drugs that produce CNS depression (e.g., antihistamines, TCAs) may result in additive CNS depression and hypotension. Avoid concurrent pharmacotherapy. If concurrent pharmacotherapy is required, monitor individual patient response carefully.

ADVERSE DRUG REACTIONS

Haloperidol pharmacotherapy has been associated with the following ADRs, listed according to body system. These ADRs include those associated with injectable haloperidol decanoate pharmacotherapy:

Cardiovascular

Various ECG changes, including tachycardia, prolongation of the Q-T interval, and other changes compatible with the polymorphous configuration of torsade de pointes. Hypertension or hypotension also have been associated with haloperidol pharmacotherapy. However, haloperidol pharmacotherapy has been associated with less sedation and hypotension than has phenothiazine pharmacotherapy. Thus, haloperidol may be a better choice than the phenothiazine, chlorpromazine, for rapid tranquillization because of its less pronounced hypotensive action.

Central Nervous System

Agitation, anxiety, confusion, depression, drowsiness, euphoria, and insomnia. Haloperidol pharmacotherapy also has been associated with the exacerbation of signs and symptoms of psychosis, including catatonic-like behavior and hallucinations among susceptible patients. These ADRs may be responsive to the discontinuation of haloperidol pharmacotherapy or to the prescription of concurrent anticholinergic pharmacotherapy. Other potentially serious ADRs involving the CNS include EPRs with TD and tardive dystonia, NMS, and WENS.

Extrapyramidal Reactions   Haloperidol pharmacotherapy commonly has been associated with EPRs, often during the first few days of pharmacotherapy. The margin between optimal therapeutic response and EPRs is narrow. The EPRs occur frequently, particularly among children.

Monitor for parkinsonian-like signs and symptoms including akathisia, dystonia, opisthotonos, and oculogyric crisis. The EPRs can occur at relatively low dosages. However, they occur more commonly, and with greater severity, at higher dosages. Dose reductions, or concurrent anti-parkinsonian pharmacotherapy (e.g., benztropine [Cogentin®], trihexyphenidyl [Artane®]), may be required for the symptomatic management of EPRs. Persistent EPRs may require discontinuation of haloperidol pharmacotherapy. The most serious EPR is TD.

Tardive Dyskinesia   As with other antipsychotic pharmacotherapy, haloperidol pharmacotherapy has been associated with persistent TD (see Phenothiazines General Monograph). Tardive dystonia, not associated with TD, also has been reported. Tardive dystonia is characterized by a delayed onset of choreic or dystonic movements. It is often persistent and, similar to TD, may be irreversible.

Neuroleptic (Antipsychotic) Malignant Syndrome Haloperidol pharmacotherapy has been associated with NMS (see Phenothiazines General Monograph).

Withdrawal Emergent Neurological Signs The abrupt discontinuation of short-term haloperidol pharmacotherapy usually is associated with few ADRs. However, some patients may experience dyskinesia with abrupt discontinuation of long-term haloperidol pharmacotherapy. For some patients, the dyskinesia is indistinguishable from the dyskinetic movements associated with TD, except for the duration of signs and symptoms. The long-acting formulation of haloperidol decanoate provides a gradual discontinuation of pharmacotherapy after the last dose. However, it is not known whether gradual discontinuation of haloperidol pharmacotherapy will reduce the occurrence of WENS.

Cutaneous

Rarely, acneiform and maculopapular skin reactions; photosensitivity; loss of hair (alopecia); and sweating (excessive). Other cutaneous reactions have been associated with similar antipsychotic pharmacotherapy.

Genitourinary

Impotence, increased sex drive, priapism, and urinary retention (see also Metabolic/Endocrine)

Gastrointestinal

Constipation, diarrhea, dry mouth, dyspepsia, salivation (excessive), and vomiting

Hematologic

Anemia, leukocytosis, leukopenia (mild and usually transient), slight lowering of red blood cell counts, and tendency toward lymphomonocytosis

Hepatic

Jaundice and liver dysfunction

Metabolic/Endocrine

Abnormal breast enlargement among males (gynecomastia), abnormal lactation and breast pain (mastalgia), hyperglycemia or hypoglycemia, hyponatremia, and menstrual irregularities. Hyperammoniemia (i.e., excess of ammonia in the blood) involving a 5-year-old child who had citrullinemia, an inherited disorder of ammonia excretion, has been associated with haloperidol pharmacotherapy.

Ocular

Blurred vision, cataracts, retinopathy, and visual disturbances. Other ADRs involving the ocular system have been reported with similar antipsychotic drugs.

Respiratory

Bronchospasm, increased depth of respiration, and laryngospasm. A number of cases of bronchopneumonia, some fatal, have been associated with haloperidol and other antipsychotic pharmacotherapy. It is thought that the lethargy and decreased sensation of thirst associated with haloperidol's central inhibitory action may lead to dehydration, hemoconcentration, and reduced pulmonary ventilation. If common signs and symptoms of possible respiratory infection appear, especially among elderly patients, refer patients immediately for medical evaluation and treatment. Collaboration with the patient's family physician or a specialist (e.g., gerontologist) is indicated.

Miscellaneous

Sudden unexpected death has been associated with haloperidol pharmacotherapy.

OVERDOSAGE

Haloperidol overdosage is more likely to occur with oral pharmacotherapy than with injectable pharmacotherapy. Signs and symptoms of haloperidol overdosage generally are an exaggeration of desired therapeutic actions and associated ADRs, of which the most prominent are severe EPRs, hypotension, and sedation. The EPRs include muscular weakness or rigidity and a generalized or localized tremor of the akinetic or agitans types, respectively. Signs and symptoms of severe haloperidol overdosage include coma, respiratory depression, and hypotension, which may be severe enough to produce a shock-like state. The risk for ECG changes associated with torsade de pointes also should be considered. Haloperidol overdosage requires emergency symptomatic medical support of body systems with attention to increasing haloperidol elimination. There is no known antidote. Associated EPRs may require anti-parkinsonian pharmacotherapy. Anti-parkinsonian pharmacotherapy may need to be continued for several weeks following the overdosage episode before being discontinued gradually.

HEROIN [Diacetylmorphine] [Diamorphine]

(her'o in)

TRADE NAMES

Generally available in Canada under the generic name of diamorphine

CLASSIFICATION

Opiate analgesic (C-I)

See also Opiate Analgesics General Monograph

APPROVED INDICATIONS FOR PSYCHOLOGICAL DISORDERS

Adjunctive pharmacotherapy for the symptomatic management of:

Pain Disorders: Severe Pain, particularly that associated with cancer

USUAL DOSAGE AND ADMINISTRATION

Pain Disorders: Severe Pain, particularly that associated with cancer

Adults: 0.05 to 0.1 mg/kg intramuscularly, intravenously, or subcutaneously every 4 hours

Women who are, or who may become, pregnant: FDA Pregnancy Category "not established." Safety and efficacy of heroin pharmacotherapy for women who are pregnant have not been established. Heroin crosses the placenta. However, it does not appear to be associated with the development of congenital malformations (i.e., birth defects). Neonates born to women who have received heroin pharmacotherapy, or have regularly used heroin, during their pregnancies, especially near term, will display the opiate withdrawal syndrome. Avoid prescribing heroin pharmacotherapy to women who are pregnant. If heroin pharmacotherapy is required, advise patients of potential benefits and possible risks to themselves and the embryo, fetus, or neonate. Collaboration with the patient's obstetrician, oncologist, or pediatrician is indicated.

Women who are breast-feeding: Safety and efficacy of heroin pharmacotherapy for women who are breast-feeding and their neonates and infants have not been established. Heroin is excreted in breast milk. Neonates and infants may display expected pharmacological actions (e.g., drowsiness, lethargy). They also may become addicted. In addition, neonatal addiction developed in utero may be prolonged among breast-fed neonates. Do not prescribe heroin pharmacotherapy to women who are breast-feeding. If heroin pharmacotherapy is required, breast-feeding should be discontinued. Collaboration with the patient's pediatrician is indicated.

Elderly, frail, or debilitated patients: Generally prescribe lower dosages for elderly, frail, or debilitated patients. Increase the dosage gradually, if needed, according to individual patient response. These patients may be more sensitive to the pharmacologic actions of heroin than are younger or healthier adult patients.

Children and adolescents: Safety and efficacy of heroin pharmacotherapy for children and adolescents have not been established. Heroin pharmacotherapy is *not* recommended for this age group.

Notes, Severe Pain, particularly that associated with cancer

Dosage must be individualized according to patient response. Heroin pharmacotherapy for the symptomatic management of cancer pain has had limited use in Canada and the United Kingdom. Studies have not shown heroin pharmacotherapy to be superior to other opiate analgesic pharmacotherapy for this indication. Heroin officially is referred to as *diamorphine* in Canada.

AVAILABLE DOSAGE FORMS, STORAGE, AND COMPATIBILITY

Injectables, intramuscular, intravenous, or subcutaneous: 30, 100 mg/ampule

Notes

Reconstitute heroin injectables with 1 ml of sterile water for injection. The injectable formulation is incompatible with normal saline.

PROPOSED MECHANISM OF ACTION

Heroin elicits its analgesic and CNS and respiratory depressant actions primarily by binding to the endorphin (opiate) receptors in the CNS. The exact mechanism of action has not yet been fully determined.

See also Opiate Analgesics General Monograph

PHARMACOKINETICS/PHARMACODYNAMICS

Heroin is converted in the GI tract to morphine (see Morphine Monograph) following oral ingestion. Following injection, it is first converted to monoacetylmorphine and then rapidly (within minutes) converted to morphine. The duration of analgesic action is 3 to 5 hours. The intramuscular injection of 5 mg of heroin provides approximately the same pain relief as the intramuscular injection of 10 mg of morphine (see Opiate Analgesics General Monograph for other opiate analgesic dosage equivalents). Additional data are unavailable.

RELATIVE CONTRAINDICATIONS

Chronic obstructive lung disease
Hypersensitivity to heroin or other opiate analgesics
Intracranial hypertension
MAOI pharmacotherapy, concurrent or within 14 days
Respiratory depression, acute

CAUTIONS AND COMMENTS

Prescribe heroin pharmacotherapy cautiously to patients who have histories of problematic patterns of opiate analgesic or other abusable psychotropic use. Heroin is addicting and habituating.

Caution patients who are receiving heroin pharmacotherapy to inform their prescribing psychologist if they begin or discontinue any other pharmacotherapy while receiving heroin pharmacotherapy.

See also Opiate Analgesics General Monograph

CLINICALLY SIGNIFICANT DRUG INTERACTIONS

Concurrent heroin pharmacotherapy and the following may result in clinically significant drug interactions:

Pharmacotherapy With Central Nervous System Depressants and Other Drugs That Produce Central Nervous System Depression

Concurrent heroin pharmacotherapy with other opiate analgesics, sedative-hypnotics, or other drugs that produce CNS depression (e.g., antihistamines, phenothiazines, TCAs) may result in additive CNS depression.

See also Opiate Analgesics General Monograph

ADVERSE DRUG REACTIONS

Heroin pharmacotherapy commonly has been associated with constipation and other GI complaints, including nausea and vomiting. It also has been commonly associated with respiratory depression, sedation, and sweating (excessive).

See also Opiate Analgesics General Monograph

OVERDOSAGE

Signs and symptoms of heroin overdosage include an exacerbation of its CNS depressant and other actions. Heroin overdosage requires emergency symptomatic medical support of body systems with attention to increasing heroin elimination. The opiate antagonist naloxone (Narcan®) is generally effective in reversing associated respiratory depression. The duration of action of heroin may exceed that of naloxone. Therefore, repeated doses of naloxone may be required during the course of emergency medical management of heroin overdosage.

HYDROCODONE [Dihydrocodeinone]

(hye droe koe′done)

TRADE NAMES

Lortab® (see Available Dosage Forms, Notes)
Vicodin® (see Available Dosage Forms, Notes)

CLASSIFICATION

Opiate analgesic (C-II)

See also Opiate Analgesics General Monograph

APPROVED INDICATIONS FOR PSYCHOLOGICAL DISORDERS

Adjunctive pharmacotherapy for the symptomatic management of:

Pain Disorders: Acute Pain, Moderate to Moderately Severe

USUAL DOSAGE AND ADMINISTRATION

Acute Pain, Moderate to Moderately Severe

Adults: 20 to 60 mg daily orally in four to six divided doses

MAXIMUM: 60 mg daily orally

Women who are, or who may become, pregnant: FDA Pregnancy Category C. Safety and efficacy of hydrocodone pharmacotherapy for women who are pregnant have not been established. Hydrocodone crosses the placenta. Hydrocodone pharmacotherapy during pregnancy will result in addiction of the neonate, who will display the opiate withdrawal syndrome. Avoid prescribing hydrocodone pharmacotherapy to women who are pregnant. If hydrocodone pharmacotherapy is required, advise patients of potential benefits and possible risks to themselves and the embryo, fetus, or neonate. Collaboration with the patient's obstetrician is indicated.

Women who are breast-feeding: Safety and efficacy of hydrocodone pharmacotherapy for women who are breast-feeding and their neonates and infants have not been established. Avoid prescribing hydrocodone pharmacotherapy for women who are breast-feeding. If hydrocodone pharmacotherapy is required, breast-feeding probably should be discontinued. If desired, lactation may be maintained and breast-feeding resumed following the discontinuation of short-term hydrocodone pharmacotherapy. Collaboration with the patient's pediatrician is indicated.
See also Opiate Analgesics General Monograph

Elderly, frail, or debilitated patients: Generally prescribe lower dosages of hydrocodone for elderly, frail, or debilitated patients. Increase the dosage gradually if needed, according to individual patient response. These patients may be more sensitive to the pharmacologic actions of hydrocodone than are younger or healthier adult patients.

Children: Safety and efficacy of hydrocodone pharmacotherapy for the symptomatic management of acute pain among children have not been established. Hydrocodone pharmacotherapy for this indication is *not* recommended for this age group.

Notes, Acute Pain, Moderate to Moderately Severe

Hydrocodone is for oral pharmacotherapy only. In addition to its use for the symptomatic management of pain disorders, it also is medically prescribed for its antitussive activity (i.e., for the relief of excessive non-productive coughing).

AVAILABLE DOSAGE FORMS, STORAGE, AND COMPATIBILITY

Syrups, oral: 2.5, 5 mg/ml (contains 7% alcohol)
Tablets, oral: 5, 7.5, 10 mg

Notes

The most commonly available dosage formulations (e.g., Lortab®, Vicodin®) contain acetaminophen (generally 500 to 750 mg per dosage unit) in addition to hydrocodone. The acetaminophen provides additional analgesia. It also changes the USDEA schedule from II to III and, thus, reduces the amount of regulation and control over the prescription and dispensing of hydrocodone (i.e., in many jurisdictions, prescriptions for schedule II drugs must be written on special "triplicate" prescription pads, while schedule III drugs carry no such regulatory restriction).

General Instructions for Patients Instruct patients who are receiving hydrocodone pharmacotherapy to

- safely store hydrocodone oral syrups and tablets out of the reach of children in tightly closed child- and light-resistant containers at controlled room temperature (15° to 30°C; 59° to 86°F).
- obtain an available patient information sheet regarding hydrocodone pharmacotherapy from their pharmacist at the time that their prescription is dispensed. Encourage patients to clarify any questions that they may have concerning hydrocodone pharmacotherapy with their pharmacist or, if needed, to consult their prescribing psychologist.

PROPOSED MECHANISM OF ACTION

Hydrocodone elicits its analgesic, CNS depressant, and respiratory depressant actions primarily by binding to the endorphin (opiate) receptors in the CNS. However, its exact mechanism of action has not yet been determined.

See also Opiate Analgesics General Monograph

PHARMACOKINETICS/PHARMACODYNAMICS

Hydrocodone is adequately absorbed following oral ingestion. Peak concentrations generally are achieved within 1.5 hours. Duration of action is 4 to 8 hours. Hydrocodone is extensively metabolized in the liver. The mean half-life of elimination is approximately 4 hours. Additional data are unavailable.

RELATIVE CONTRAINDICATIONS

Hypersensitivity to hydrocodone or other opiate analgesics
Respiratory depression

CAUTIONS AND COMMENTS

Hydrocodone is addicting and habituating and has significant abuse potential. Short-term hydrocodone pharmacotherapy for the management of acute pain rarely results in addiction and habituation. Long-term hydrocodone pharmacotherapy, or regular personal use, will result in addiction and habituation.

Prescribe hydrocodone pharmacotherapy cautiously to patients who

- are post-operative. Hydrocodone, which also is medically prescribed as an antitussive, suppresses the cough reflex. Thus, hydrocodone pharmacotherapy during the post-operative period may impede the removal of bronchial secretions and increase the risk for respiratory complications (e.g., post-operative pneumonia).
- have histories of problematic patterns of opiate or other abusable psychotropic use. These patients may be at risk for the development of problematic patterns of hydrocodone use.

Caution patients who are receiving hydrocodone pharmacotherapy against performing activities that require alertness, judgment, and physical coordination (e.g., driving an automobile, operating dangerous equipment, supervising children) until their response to hydrocodone is known. Hydrocodone's CNS depressant action may adversely affect these mental and physical functions.

In addition to this general precaution, caution patients to inform their prescribing psychologist if they begin or discontinue any other pharmacotherapy while receiving hydrocodone pharmacotherapy.

See also Opiate Analgesics General Monograph

CLINICALLY SIGNIFICANT DRUG INTERACTIONS

Concurrent hydrocodone pharmacotherapy and the following may result in clinically significant drug interactions:

Alcohol Use

Concurrent alcohol use may increase the CNS depressant action of hydrocodone. Advise patients to avoid, or limit, their use of alcohol while receiving hydrocodone pharmacotherapy.

Pharmacotherapy With Central Nervous System Depressants and Other Drugs That Produce Central Nervous System Depression

Concurrent hydrocodone pharmacotherapy with other opiate analgesics, sedative-hypnotics, or other drugs that produce CNS depression (e.g., antihistamines, phenothiazines, TCAs) may result in additive CNS depression.

See also Opiate Analgesics General Monograph

ADVERSE DRUG REACTIONS

Hydrocodone pharmacotherapy has been commonly associated with constipation, dizziness, and drowsiness. It also has been associated with the following ADRs, listed according to body system:

Cardiovascular: hypertension, palpitations, and postural hypotension
CNS: lethargy and sedation
Genitourinary: ureteral spasm and urinary retention
GI: nausea and vomiting
Ocular: blurred vision

See also Opiate Analgesics General Monograph

OVERDOSAGE

Signs and symptoms of hydrocodone overdosage are an exacerbation of its CNS depressant and other actions and include bradycardia; cold, clammy skin; extreme somnolence progressing to stupor or coma; respiratory depression; and skeletal muscle flaccidity. Hydrocodone overdosage requires emergency symptomatic medical support of body systems with attention to increasing hydrocodone elimination. The opiate antagonist naloxone (Narcan®) generally is effective for the medical management of associated respiratory depression. The duration of action of hydrocodone may exceed that of naloxone. Therefore, repeated doses of naloxone may be required during the course of the emergency medical management of hydrocodone overdosage.

HYDROMORPHONE
[Dihydromorphinone]

(hye droe mor'fone)

TRADE NAMES

Dilaudid®
Dilaudid-HP®
Hydromorph Contin®
HydroStat®

CLASSIFICATION

Opiate analgesic (C-II)

See also Opiate Analgesics General Monograph

APPROVED INDICATIONS FOR PSYCHOLOGICAL DISORDERS

Adjunctive pharmacotherapy for the symptomatic management of:

- Pain Disorders: Acute Pain, Moderate to Severe
- Pain Disorders: Chronic Pain, Moderate to Severe, including that associated with cancer

USUAL DOSAGE AND ADMINISTRATION

Moderate to Severe Pain

Adults: Initially, 2 mg orally every four to six hours; *or* 1 mg intramuscularly, intravenously, or subcutaneously every four to six hours; *or* 3 mg rectally every six to eight hours. Adjust dosage according to individual patient response. Patients who have *severe pain* may require 4 mg orally every four to six hours; 2 mg intramuscularly, intravenously, or subcutaneously every four to six hours; or 6 mg rectally every six to eight hours. Patients who have terminal cancer may be tolerant to opiate analgesics. Therefore, these patients may require higher dosages for adequate pain relief. A gradual increase in dosage may be required if analgesia is inadequate or if pain severity increases. For severe pain, or when prompt response is required, initially prescribe the injectable formulation in adequate dosages to control the pain.

Women who are, or who may become, pregnant: FDA Pregnancy Category C. Safety and efficacy of hydromorphone pharmacotherapy for women who are pregnant have not been established. Avoid prescribing hydromorphone pharmacotherapy to women who are pregnant. If hydromorphone pharmacotherapy is required, advise patients of potential benefits and possible risks to themselves and the embryo, fetus, or neonate. Collaboration with the patient's obstetrician or a specialist (e.g., oncologist) is indicated.
See also the Opiate Analgesics General Monograph

Women who are breast-feeding: Safety and efficacy of hydromorphone pharmacotherapy for women who are breast-feeding and their neonates and infants have not been established. It is not known whether hydromorphone is excreted in breast milk. Avoid prescribing hydromorphone pharmacotherapy to women who are breast-feeding. If hydromorphone pharmacotherapy is required, breast-feeding probably should be discontinued. If desired, lactation may be maintained, and breast-feeding resumed, following the discontinuation of short-term pharmacotherapy for the management of acute pain. Collaboration with the patient's pediatrician is indicated.
See also the Opiate Analgesics General Monograph

Elderly, frail, or debilitated patients: Generally prescribe lower dosages for elderly, frail, or debilitated patients. Increase the dosage gradually, if needed, according to individual patient response. Dosage should be guided by the goal of optimal pain management with minimal ADRs. These patients may be more sensitive to the pharmacologic actions of hydromorphone than are younger or healthier adult patients.

Children: Safety and efficacy of hydromorphone pharmacotherapy for the symptomatic management of pain disorders for children have not been established. Hydromorphone pharmacotherapy for this indication is *not* recommended for this age group.

Notes, Moderate to Severe Pain

Hydromorphone pharmacotherapy generally provides adequate pharmacotherapy for the symptomatic management of acute severe pain of short duration. Selected patients may benefit from oral, rectal, or injectable hydromorphone pharmacotherapy.

Oral and Rectal Hydromorphone Pharmacotherapy The advantage of oral hydromorphone pharmacotherapy over other oral opiate analgesic pharmacotherapy, such as morphine or meperidine (Demerol®) pharmacotherapy, is its better oral absorption. In addition, rectal hydromorphone pharmacotherapy may be of benefit to patients for whom the oral route is not feasible or those who require opiate analgesics during the night. Hydromorphone rectal suppositories may provide a longer duration of pain relief for the latter and, thus, obviate the need for dosing during sleeping hours.

Injectable Hydromorphone Pharmacotherapy Subcutaneous and intravenous injections are generally well tolerated. For intravenous pharmacotherapy, inject intravenously *slowly* over 2 to 3 minutes, depending on the dose injected. Rapid injection may increase the incidence of associated ADRs, including hypotension and respiratory depression. Circulatory depression, peripheral circulatory collapse, and cardiac arrest have occurred following rapid intravenous injection.

Patients should lie down for subcutaneous or intravenous hydromorphone pharmacotherapy. They should remain lying down for at least 30 to 60 minutes following the injection. Postural hypotension and fainting may occur if patients suddenly stand after receiving an injection of hydromorphone.

AVAILABLE DOSAGE FORMS, STORAGE, AND COMPATIBILITY

Injectables, *concentrated* intramuscular, intravenous, and subcutaneous: 10, 20, 50 mg/ml (ampules, 10 mg/ml; multidose vials, 10, 20, 50 mg/ml)

Injectables, intramuscular, intravenous, subcutaneous: 1, 2, 4, 10 mg/ml (ampules, 1, 2, 4 mg/ml)

Suppository, rectal: 3 mg (cocoa butter base)

Syrup, oral: 1 mg/ml (unflavored)

Tablets, oral: 1, 2, 3, 4, 8 mg

Notes

The concentrated injectable dosage formulations (i.e., 10, 20, and 50 mg/ml) are *only* intended for hydromorphone pharmacotherapy for patients who are tolerant to opiate analgesics and, thus, require higher dosages. *Do not confuse these concentrated injectable dosage formulations with the less concentrated injectable dosage formulations (i.e., 1, 2, 4 mg/ml). Inadvertent use of the concentrated injectable dosage formulations may result in hydromorphone overdosage and death.*

Inspect injectables visually for particulate matter and discoloration prior to use. A slight yellowish discoloration may develop in hydromorphone ampules and multiple-dose vials. This discoloration does *not* indicate chemical degradation nor a resultant loss of potency. However, do *not* use darkly discolored injectable solutions, and do *not* use products beyond the expiration date indicated on the label.

Store injectables safely protected from light at controlled room temperature (15° to 30°C; 59° to 86°F).

General Instructions for Patients Instruct patients who are receiving hydromorphone pharmacotherapy to

- store hydromorphone suppositories safely out of the reach of children in a refrigerator between 2° and 8°C (36° and 46°F).
- store hydromorphone oral dosage forms safely out of the reach of children in child- and light-resistant containers at controlled room temperature (15° to 30°C; 59° to 86°F).
- obtain an available patient information sheet regarding hydromorphone pharmacotherapy from their pharmacist at the time that their prescription is dispensed. Encourage patients to clarify any questions that they may have concerning hydromorphone pharmacotherapy with their pharmacist or, if needed, to consult their prescribing psychologist.

PROPOSED MECHANISM OF ACTION

Although the exact mechanism of action has not been clearly established, hydromorphone appears to elicit its analgesic, CNS depressant (e.g., drowsiness, changes in mood, and mental clouding), and respiratory depressant actions primarily by binding to the endorphin (opiate) receptors in the CNS.

See also Opiate Analgesics General Monograph

PHARMACOKINETICS/PHARMACODYNAMICS

Hydromorphone's analgesic action is apparent within 15 minutes after injection and may last five or more hours. Hydromorphone is rapidly absorbed after oral ingestion and produces analgesia within 30 minutes. Oral bioavailability is approximately 30%. Hydromorphone is extensively metabolized in the liver. The mean half-life of elimination is approximately 3 hours. Additional data are unavailable.

Although there is no intrinsic limit to hydromorphone's analgesic actions, and adequate doses will relieve even the most severe pain, hydromorphone analgesic pharmacotherapy is limited by its associated ADRs, primarily respiratory depression, nausea, and vomiting.

RELATIVE CONTRAINDICATIONS

Hypersensitivity to hydromorphone or other opiate analgesics
Increased intracranial pressure
Respiratory dysfunction (i.e., including that associated with chronic obstructive lung disease, cor pulmonale, emphysema, kyphoscoliosis, pulmonary edema, and status asthmaticus)

CAUTIONS AND COMMENTS

Hydromorphone is addicting and habituating and has significant abuse potential. Short-term hydromorphone pharmacotherapy for the symptomatic management of acute pain rarely results in addiction and habituation. However, several weeks of continuous pharmacotherapy may result in addiction and habituation among selected patients. Tolerance initially is noted by a shortened duration of analgesia and, subsequently, by decreases in analgesia.

Prescribe hydromorphone pharmacotherapy cautiously to patients who

- are elderly.
- are postoperative. Hydromorphone, which also is medically prescribed as an antitussive, suppresses the cough reflex. Thus, hydromorphone pharmacotherapy may impede the removal of bronchial secretions and increase the risk for respiratory complications (e.g., post-operative pneumonia).
- have head injuries. Hydromorphone, like other opiate analgesics, can increase intracranial pressure. It also can obscure the clinical monitoring of these patients because of its CNS and respiratory depressant actions.
- have histories of problematic patterns of opiate or other abusable psychotropic use.
- have hypothyroidism, Addison's disease, prostatic hypertrophy, or urethral stricture.
- have kidney dysfunction.
- have liver dysfunction.
- have respiratory dysfunction, or are prone to respiratory dysfunction. As with other opiate analgesics, hydromorphone can suppress the cough reflex and depress the rate and depth of respirations. Hydromorphone also produces a dose-related respiratory depression by acting directly on the respiratory center in the brainstem and other centers that affect the control of respiratory rhythm. Thus, hydromorphone may produce irregular and periodic breathing (i.e., apnea) and adversely affect respiratory function among these patients.

Caution patients who are receiving hydromorphone pharmacotherapy against performing activities that require alertness, judgment, or physical coordination (e.g., driving an automobile, operating dangerous equipment, supervising children). Hydromorphone may adversely affect these mental and physical functions.

In addition to this general precaution, caution patients to inform their prescribing psychologist if they begin or discontinue any other pharmacotherapy while receiving hydromorphone pharmacotherapy.

CLINICALLY SIGNIFICANT DRUG INTERACTIONS

Concurrent hydromorphone pharmacotherapy and the following may result in clinically significant drug interactions:

Alcohol Use

Concurrent alcohol use may increase the CNS depressant action of hydromorphone. Advise patients to avoid, or limit, their use of alcohol while receiving hydromorphone pharmacotherapy.

Pharmacotherapy With Central Nervous System Depressants and Other Drugs That Produce Central Nervous System Depression

Concurrent hydromorphone pharmacotherapy with other opiate analgesics, sedative-hypnotics, or other drugs that produce CNS depression (e.g., antihistamines, phenothiazines, TCAs) may result in additive CNS depression.

See also Opiate Analgesics General Monograph

ADVERSE DRUG REACTIONS

Hydromorphone pharmacotherapy commonly has been associated with nausea, respiratory depression, and vomiting. It also has been associated with the following ADRs, listed according to body system:

Cardiovascular: postural hypotension, peripheral circulatory collapse, and cardiac arrest (following rapid intravenous injection)
CNS: dizziness, drowsiness, lethargy, loss of appetite (anorexia), and sedation
Genitourinary: ureteral spasm and urinary retention
GI: constipation, nausea, and vomiting
Respiratory: respiratory depression

See also Opiate Analgesics General Monograph

OVERDOSAGE

Signs and symptoms of hydromorphone overdosage include respiratory depression (decreased rate and tidal volume, Cheyne-Stokes respiration, cyanosis), extreme somnolence progressing to stupor or coma, skeletal muscle flaccidity, cold and clammy skin, and, sometimes, bradycardia and hypotension. Severe overdosage, particularly that associated with intravenous injection, may result in apnea, circulatory collapse, cardiac arrest, and death.

Hydromorphone overdosage requires emergency symptomatic medical support of body systems with attention to increasing hydromorphone elimination, particularly when the overdosage has involved oral dosage forms. The opiate antagonist naloxone (Narcan®) is the specific antidote against respiratory depression. The duration of action of hydromorphone may exceed that of naloxone. Therefore, repeated doses of naloxone may be required during the course of emergency medical management of hydromorphone overdosage.

IMIPRAMINE

(im ip′ra meen)

TRADE NAMES

Novo-Pramine®
Tofranil®

CLASSIFICATION

Antidepressant (tricyclic)

See also Tricyclic Antidepressants General Monograph

APPROVED INDICATIONS FOR PSYCHOLOGICAL DISORDERS

Adjunctive pharmacotherapy for the symptomatic management of:

- Childhood Nocturnal Enuresis. Imipramine pharmacotherapy is indicated for the symptomatic management of nocturnal enuresis among children who are 5 years of age and older for whom possible organic causes have been excluded.
- Mood Disorders, Depressive Disorders: Endogenous Depression

USUAL DOSAGE AND ADMINISTRATION

Childhood Nocturnal Enuresis

Children younger than 5 years of age: Safety and efficacy of imipramine pharmacotherapy for the short-term symptomatic management of nocturnal enuresis for children younger than 5 years of age have not been established. Imipramine pharmacotherapy for this indication is *not* recommended for this age group.

Children 5 years of age or older: 10 to 25 mg daily orally 30 to 60 minutes before bedtime. Increase the dosage gradually by 10 mg daily, if required, according to individual patient response. For children who have enuresis early during the night, a portion of the bedtime dose may be ingested between 1500 and 1700 hours (3 and 5 pm). If satisfactory response is not achieved in one week, increase the dosage to 75 mg daily for children 12 years of age and older. Do *not* exceed 75 mg daily. Daily dosages exceeding 75 mg do not increase therapeutic benefit and may increase the frequency or severity of associated ADRs.

MAXIMUM: 75 mg daily orally. Various ECG changes of unknown significance have been reported among children when higher than recommended dosages have been prescribed. In order to avoid possible cardiovascular ADRs, do *not* exceed a daily dosage of 2.5 mg/kg or 75 mg, whichever is the lower daily dosage.

Notes, Childhood Nocturnal Enuresis

A therapeutic trial period of two to four weeks is usually required to determine the efficacy of imipramine pharmacotherapy for the symptomatic management of childhood nocturnal enuresis. After this therapeutic trial period, institute a drug-free period in order to determine continued need for imipramine pharmacotherapy. However, do not abruptly discontinue imipramine pharmacotherapy. Gradually reduce the dosage over a period of one to two weeks in order to prevent a relapse. Children who relapse following the discontinuation of imipramine pharmacotherapy do not always respond to the reinstitution of imipramine pharmacotherapy.

See also Tricyclic Antidepressants General Monograph

Endogenous Depression

Adults:　Initially, 75 mg daily orally or intramuscularly in three divided doses. Increase the dosage gradually up to 150 mg daily, according to individual patient response. Severely depressed patients may require dosages as high as 300 mg daily. These patients should be hospitalized for high-dosage pharmacotherapy, so that their clinical response can be adequately monitored. Suicide precautions also are indicated. Dosages exceeding 200 mg daily are *not* recommended for patients who are not hospitalized.

MAINTENANCE:　75 to 150 mg daily orally in divided doses. For maintenance imipramine pharmacotherapy, prescribe the lowest effective dosage. Continue imipramine pharmacotherapy for the expected duration of the depressive episode to minimize possible relapse following clinical improvement. Once patients have been stabilized on a maintenance dosage, imipramine pharmacotherapy may be prescribed as a single daily dose 30 minutes before retiring for bed in the evening.

MAXIMUM:　300 mg daily orally

Women who are, or who may become, pregnant:　FDA Pregnancy Category D. Safety and efficacy of imipramine pharmacotherapy for women who are pregnant have not been established. A neonatal distress syndrome may be observed during the first few hours or days following birth among neonates whose mothers received imipramine pharmacotherapy up to delivery. The signs and symptoms of this syndrome include colic, dyspnea, hypertension or hypotension, irritability, lethargy, respiratory distress, spasms, tremor, and urinary retention. Avoid prescribing imipramine pharmacotherapy to women who are pregnant, particularly during the first trimester and the last seven weeks of pregnancy. If imipramine pharmacotherapy is required, advise patients of the potential benefits and possible risks to themselves and the embryo, fetus, or neonate. Collaboration with the patient's obstetrician is indicated.

Women who are breast-feeding:　Safety and efficacy of imipramine pharmacotherapy for women who are breast-feeding and their neonates and infants have not been established. Imipramine is excreted in breast milk in concentrations similar to maternal blood concentrations. If imipramine pharmacotherapy is required, breast-feeding probably should be discontinued. Collaboration with the patient's pediatrician is indicated.

Elderly:　Initially, 25 to 50 mg daily orally in divided doses. Increase the dosage gradually by 10 mg daily, if necessary, according to individual patient response. Imipramine pharmacotherapy has been associated with pharmacogenic (delirious) psychoses among predisposed elderly patients. These psychoses occur particularly during the night. They usually resolve within a few days of discontinuing imipramine pharmacotherapy.

MAXIMUM: 100 mg daily orally

Children younger than 12 years of age: Safety and efficacy of imipramine pharmacotherapy for the symptomatic management of depression among children younger than 12 years of age have not been established. Imipramine pharmacotherapy for this indication is *not* recommended for this age group.

Notes, Endogenous Depression

Initiating, Maintaining, and Discontinuing Short-Term Imipramine Pharmacotherapy
Individualize dosage according to the patient's signs and symptoms of depression and response to imipramine pharmacotherapy. Initiate imipramine pharmacotherapy at the lowest recommended dosage. Increase the dosage gradually according to individual patient response. Monitor patients, particularly adolescent and elderly patients, for intolerance. A delay in therapeutic response usually occurs initially and may last for several days to weeks. Increasing the dosage does not usually shorten this latency period and may increase the incidence or severity of ADRs.

The risk for suicide is high among seriously depressed patients. This risk may persist until a significant remission of the depression occurs. Monitor patients for suicide risk during all phases of imipramine pharmacotherapy. Hospitalization is recommended for severely depressed patients and those who require high-dosage imipramine pharmacotherapy. For patients who are not hospitalized, prescribe the smallest quantity of imipramine feasible for dispensing to help to prevent suicide by intentional imipramine overdosage. Other suicide precautions may be indicated.

Initiating, Maintaining, and Discontinuing Long-Term Imipramine Pharmacotherapy
Obtain the patient's baseline blood pressure before initiating long-term imipramine pharmacotherapy. Patients who have hypotension or labile cardiovascular disorders may react to imipramine pharmacotherapy with a lowering of blood pressure. Monitor blood pressure regularly for patients who are susceptible to postural hypotension. Some patients may require a reduction of their imipramine dosage. Also monitor cardiac function, including ECGs among patients who have heart disease, particularly elderly patients and those who have histories of cardiac conduction disorders. Periodic blood cell counts and liver function tests also are recommended for patients who require long-term imipramine pharmacotherapy. Collaboration with the patient's advanced practice nurse, family physician, cardiologist, or other specialist (e.g., hematologist) is indicated.

Avoid abruptly discontinuing long-term imipramine pharmacotherapy. Abrupt discontinuation of long-term pharmacotherapy has been associated with several ADRs, including anxiety, GI complaints, headache, insomnia, muscle twitching, and nervousness. Discontinue imipramine pharmacotherapy gradually.

AVAILABLE DOSAGE FORMS, STORAGE, AND COMPATIBILITY

Capsules, oral: 75, 100, 125, 150 mg
Injectable, intramuscular: 12.5 mg/ml (ampule)
Tablets, oral: 10, 25, 50, 75, 150 mg

Notes

The injectable formulation of imipramine contains sodium sulfite and sodium bisulfites. These sulfites may cause hypersensitive reactions, including anaphylactic reactions, among susceptible patients. Although relatively uncommon, these reactions appear to occur with a higher incidence among patients who have asthma.

The injectable is for intramuscular use only. Do not inject intravenously. Prior to use, inspect ampules visually for the formation of crystals. If crystals are noted, they can be dissolved by immersing the sealed ampule in hot water for 1 to 2 minutes. Store injectables safely protected from light at controlled room temperature (15° to 30°C; 59° to 86°F).

General Instructions for Patients Instruct patients who are receiving imipramine pharmacotherapy to

- ingest each dose of their imipramine oral tablets with food or milk to decrease associated gastrointestinal upset.
- safely store imipramine oral capsules and tablets out of the reach of children in tightly closed child-resistant containers below 30°C (86°F).
- obtain an available patient information sheet regarding imipramine pharmacotherapy from their pharmacist at the time that their prescription is dispensed. Encourage patients to clarify any questions that they may have concerning imipramine pharmacotherapy with their pharmacist or, if needed, to consult their prescribing psychologist.

PROPOSED MECHANISM OF ACTION

The exact mechanism of action of imipramine has not yet been fully determined. However, it appears to produce its antidepressant action primarily by potentiating the CNS biogenic amines, specifically norepinephrine and serotonin, by blocking their re-uptake at the presynaptic nerve terminals. This inhibition of re-uptake increases the amount of norepinephrine and serotonin in the synapses and, consequently, results in increased activity at the post-synaptic neuron receptor sites. The anticholinergic activity of imipramine appears to be primarily centrally mediated and may be responsible for its efficacy for the symptomatic management of nocturnal childhood enuresis.

See also Tricyclic Antidepressants General Monograph

PHARMACOKINETICS/PHARMACODYNAMICS

Imipramine is moderately and variably absorbed from the GI tract following oral ingestion (mean bioavailability of 40%). Peak blood levels are achieved within 2 to 5 hours. Approximately 90% of imipramine is bound to plasma proteins. The mean apparent volume of distribution is 23 L/kg. Imipramine is metabolized in the liver to several metabolites, including the active metabolite desmethylimipramine. Imipramine is primarily excreted in the urine (~80%) and feces (~20%) as inactive metabolites. Less than 2% is excreted in unchanged form in the urine. The mean half-life of elimination is 12 hours (range 6 to 28 hours), and the mean total body clearance is ~1 L/minute.

Therapeutic Drug Monitoring

Dosage must be determined by individual patient response and *not* imipramine blood concentrations because it is difficult to correlate blood concentrations with therapeutic response and ADRs. Absorption and distribution in body fluids vary. However, blood levels may be useful for monitoring the patient's ability to manage his or her pharmacotherapy or possible overdosage. It is generally recommended that imipramine blood levels be sampled from trough concentrations approximately 12 hours after the last dose. However, in cases of suspected overdosage, sampling can be done at anytime. The usual therapeutic blood concentration ranges from 550 to 1015 nmol/L. Note that these values include the sum total of both imipramine and its active metabolite desmethylimipramine.

RELATIVE CONTRAINDICATIONS

Blood disorders, history of
Convulsive disorders
Glaucoma
Hypersensitivity to imipramine or other TCAs belonging to the dibenzazepine group
Kidney dysfunction, severe
Liver dysfunction, severe
MAOI pharmacotherapy, concurrent or within 14 days. Hypertensive crises with hyperactivity, hyperpyrexia, spasticity, severe convulsions, coma, and death have been associated with imipramine and MAOI pharmacotherapy, concurrent or within 14 days.
Myocardial infarction, acute recovery
Pregnancy, first trimester

CAUTIONS AND COMMENTS

Prescribe imipramine pharmacotherapy cautiously to patients who

- have cardiovascular disorders, including a history of atrioventricular block (grade I to III), dysrhythmias, ischemic heart disease, or myocardial infarction. When prescribed for these patients, cautious monitoring is required, including ECG monitoring, at all dosage levels. Collaboration with the patient's cardiologist is indicated.
- have hyperthyroidism and are receiving thyroid pharmacotherapy. Imipramine pharmacotherapy has been associated with cardiovascular toxicity, including the exacerbation of dysrhythmias and hypotensive episodes among these patients.
- have low seizure thresholds associated with brain injury or concurrent ECT. Monitor these patients carefully. Seizure precautions are indicated.
- have tumors of the adrenal medulla (e.g., neuroblastoma, pheochromocytoma). Imipramine pharmacotherapy may induce a hypertensive crisis among these patients.
- have schizophrenia, family histories of schizophrenia, or other mental disorders, including agitation, bipolar disorders, or hyperactivity. The activation of latent schizophrenia or the aggravation of the signs and symptoms of psychosis may occur among these patients. Agitated or hyperactive patients may become over-stimulated. Patients who have bipolar disorders may experience hypomanic or manic shifts. Discontinue imipramine pharmacotherapy if these signs and symptoms occur among these patients.

Caution patients who are receiving imipramine pharmacotherapy (or their parents or legal guardians in regard to the patient) to inform their prescribing psychologist if they begin or discontinue any other pharmacotherapy while receiving imipramine pharmacotherapy.

CLINICALLY SIGNIFICANT DRUG INTERACTIONS

Concurrent imipramine pharmacotherapy and the following may result in clinically significant drug interactions:

Ketoconazole Pharmacotherapy

Concurrent ketoconazole (Nizoral®) pharmacotherapy may increase the blood concentration of imipramine by approximately 20%. This interaction is postulated to be the result of the inhibition of cytochrome P450 isoenzyme 3A4 (CYP3A4). When concurrent pharmacotherapy cannot be avoided, an adjustment of the imipramine dosage may be required.

See also Tricyclic Antidepressants General Monograph

ADVERSE DRUG REACTIONS

Imipramine pharmacotherapy has been commonly associated with dry mouth; hypotension, particularly postural hypotension; tremors; and weight gain. Imipramine pharmacotherapy also has been associated with the following ADRs, listed according to body system:

Cardiovascular: cardiac dysrhythmias, including tachycardia
CNS: anxiety, confusion, disorientation, dizziness, drowsiness, fatigue, headache, and insomnia
Genitourinary: decreased sex drive, impotence, and urinary retention
GI: dry mouth, gastrointestinal complaints (i.e., nausea, vomiting), and loss of appetite (anorexia)
Hepatic: hepatitis (rarely)
Metabolic/Endocrine: abnormal breast enlargement among men (gynecomastia)
Ocular: blurred vision
Otic: ringing in the ears (tinnitus), which may remit with a decrease in dosage

See also Tricyclic Antidepressants General Monograph

OVERDOSAGE

Children are reportedly more sensitive than adults to acute imipramine overdosage, which may be fatal. Signs and symptoms of imipramine overdosage include abnormally dilated pupils (mydriasis), agitation, athetoid movements, bowel and bladder paralysis, convulsions, cyanosis, delirium, hyperactive reflexes, hyperpyrexia, hypothermia, incoordination (ataxia), muscle rigidity, restlessness, stupor, sweating (severe), and vomiting. The severity of imipramine overdosage depends on the amount of drug absorbed, the patient's age, and the interval between ingestion and the initiation of emergency care.

Serious cardiovascular effects commonly occur, including cardiac dysrhythmias (e.g., atriofibrillation and flutter, premature ventricular beats, ventricular tachycardia), impaired myocardial conduction, atrioventricular and intraventricular block, ECG abnormalities (widened QRS complexes and marked S-T shifts), congestive heart failure, and cardiac arrest. Hypertension may occur initially. However, the usual finding is increasing hypotension, which may lead to shock and coma. Imipramine overdosage requires emergency symptomatic medical support of body systems with attention to increasing imipramine elimination. There is no known antidote.

LEVORPHANOL *

(lee vor'fa nole)

TRADE NAME

Levo-Dromoran®

CLASSIFICATION

Opiate analgesic (C-II)

See also Opiate Analgesics General Monograph

APPROVED INDICATIONS FOR PSYCHOLOGICAL DISORDERS

Adjunctive pharmacotherapy for the symptomatic management of:

Pain Disorders: Acute or Chronic Pain, Moderate to Severe

USUAL DOSAGE AND ADMINISTRATION

Acute or Chronic Pain, Moderate to Severe

Adults: 4 to 12 mg daily orally or subcutaneously in three or four divided doses

Women who are, or who may become, pregnant: FDA Pregnancy Category C. Safety and efficacy of levorphanol pharmacotherapy for women who are pregnant have not been established. Avoid prescribing levorphanol pharmacotherapy to women who are pregnant. If levorphanol pharmacotherapy is required, advise patients of potential benefits and possible risks to themselves and the embryo, fetus, or neonate (see Opiate Analgesics General Monograph). Collaboration with the patient's obstetrician is indicated.

Women who are breast-feeding: Safety and efficacy of levorphanol pharmacotherapy for women who are breast-feeding and their neonates and infants have not been established. Avoid prescribing levorphanol pharmacotherapy to women who are breast-feeding. If levorphanol pharmacotherapy is required, breast-feeding probably should be discontinued. If desired, lactation may be maintained and breast-feeding resumed following the discontinuation of short-term levorphanol pharmacotherapy.

Elderly, frail, or debilitated patients or those who have respiratory dysfunction: 2 to 6 mg daily orally or subcutaneously in three or four divided doses. *Note: Dosage is 50% of the recommended adult dosage.*

Generally prescribe lower dosages for elderly, frail, or debilitated patients and those who have respiratory dysfunction. Increase the dosage gradually, if needed, according to individual patient response. These patients may be more sensitive to the pharmacologic actions of levorphanol than are younger or healthier adult patients.

Children and adolescents younger than 18 years of age: Safety and efficacy of levorphanol pharmacotherapy for children and adolescents have not been established. Levorphanol pharmacotherapy is *not* recommended for this age group.

Notes, Acute or Chronic Pain, Moderate to Severe

Adjust dosage according to the patient's severity of pain, age and weight, concurrent pharmacotherapy, and clinical condition, including kidney and liver function. Higher dosages may be required for patients who are tolerant to opiate analgesics.

Intravenous Levorphanol Pharmacotherapy   Intravenous levorphanol pharmacotherapy is generally reserved for use as a supplement to general anesthesia.

AVAILABLE DOSAGE FORMS, STORAGE, AND COMPATIBILITY

Injectable, intravenous or subcutaneous: 2 mg/ml
Tablets, oral: 2 mg

Notes

Store the levorphanol injectable formulation safely at room temperature below 40°C (104°F). The injectable levorphanol formulation is chemically or physically incompatible with aminophylline, ammonium chloride, amobarbital (Amytal®), chlorothiazide (Diuril®), heparin, methicillin (Staphcillin®), nitrofurantoin (Macrodantin®), pentobarbital (Nembutal®), phenobarbital (Luminal®), phenytoin (Dilantin®), secobarbital (Seconal®), sodium bicarbonate, sodium iodide, and thiopental (Pentothal®).

General Instructions for Patients   Instruct patients who are receiving levorphanol pharmacotherapy to

- safely store levorphanol tablets out of the reach of children in tightly closed child- and light-resistant containers at controlled room temperature (15° to 30°C; 59° to 86°F).
- obtain an available patient information sheet regarding levorphanol pharmacotherapy from their pharmacist at the time that their prescription is dispensed. Encourage patients to clarify any questions that they may have concerning levorphanol pharmacotherapy with their pharmacist or, if needed, to consult their prescribing psychologist.

PROPOSED MECHANISM OF ACTION

Levorphanol primarily elicits its analgesic, CNS depressant, and respiratory depressant actions by binding to the endorphin receptors in the CNS. However, its exact mechanism of action has not yet been fully determined.

See also Opiate Analgesics General Monograph

PHARMACOKINETICS/PHARMACODYNAMICS

Levorphanol appears to be well absorbed following intramuscular injection or oral ingestion. Peak blood concentrations are achieved within 1 hour after oral ingestion. Levorphanol is ~40% plasma protein-bound. The mean half-life of elimination is 12 hours (range 11 to 16 hours), and the mean total body clearance is 1 L/minute (range 0.8 to 1.3 L/minute). Additional data are unavailable.

RELATIVE CONTRAINDICATIONS

Alcoholism, acute
Anoxia
Bronchial asthma
Hypersensitivity to levorphanol
Intracranial pressure, increased
Respiratory depression

CAUTIONS AND COMMENTS

Levorphanol is addicting and habituating. Long-term levorphanol pharmacotherapy, or regular personal use, may result in addiction and habituation. Abrupt discontinuation after long-term pharmacotherapy, or regular personal use, may result in a reportedly mild form of the opiate analgesic withdrawal syndrome.

Prescribe levorphanol pharmacotherapy cautiously for patients who

- have acute cholecystitis or pancreatitis or will be undergoing surgery of the biliary tract. Opiate analgesics generally increase biliary tract pressure. Levorphanol may cause a moderate to marked elevation of biliary pressure. Caution is advised.
- have head injuries, intracranial lesions, or other conditions associated with increased intracranial pressure. The respiratory depressant action associated with levorphanol and its potential for elevating cerebrospinal fluid pressure may markedly exaggerate intracranial pressure among these patients. Levorphanol's analgesic and sedative actions also may obscure the clinical course of these patients.
- have histories of problematic patterns of abusable psychotropic use, including the use of levorphanol or other opiate analgesics. Prescribe the least quantity of drug for dispensing to help to avoid problematic patterns of use, including unadvised patient increases in dosage.
- have liver dysfunction. Serious liver dysfunction appears to predispose patients to a higher incidence of ADRs (e.g., anxiety, marked apprehension, dizziness, drowsiness) even when usual recommended dosages are prescribed. These ADRs may be the result of decreased levorphanol metabolism by the liver and resultant accumulation.

- have respiratory depression, limited respiratory function (e.g., severely limited respiratory reserve, severe bronchial asthma, other obstructive respiratory conditions), or cyanosis. The respiratory depressant action of levorphanol may further compromise the respiratory function of these patients.

Caution patients who are receiving levorphanol pharmacotherapy against performing activities that require alertness, judgment, and physical coordination (e.g., driving an automobile, operating dangerous equipment, supervising children). The CNS depressant action of levorphanol may adversely affect these mental and physical functions.

In addition to this general precaution, caution patients to inform their prescribing psychologist if they begin or discontinue any other pharmacotherapy while receiving levorphanol pharmacotherapy.

CLINICALLY SIGNIFICANT DRUG INTERACTIONS

Concurrent levorphanol pharmacotherapy and the following may result in clinically significant drug interactions:

Alcohol Use

Concurrent alcohol use may increase the CNS depressant action of levorphanol. Advise patients to avoid, or limit, their use of alcohol while receiving levorphanol pharmacotherapy.

Pharmacotherapy With Central Nervous System Depressants and Other Drugs That Produce Central Nervous System Depression

Concurrent levorphanol pharmacotherapy with other opiate analgesics, sedative-hypnotics, or other drugs that produce CNS depression (e.g., antihistamines, phenothiazines, TCAs) may result in additive CNS depression.

See also Opiate Analgesics General Monograph

ADVERSE DRUG REACTIONS

Levorphanol pharmacotherapy commonly has been associated with dizziness, nausea, and vomiting. It also has been associated with the following ADRs, listed according to body system:

Cardiovascular: dysrhythmias (e.g., bradycardia, cardiac arrest, tachycardia)
CNS: abnormal dreams, amnesia, confusion, depression, and lethargy
Cutaneous: flushing, hives, itching, local irritation at the injection site, rash, and sweating (excessive)
Genitourinary: difficulty urinating and urinary retention
GI: constipation, dry mouth, and dyspepsia
Ocular: blurred vision and double vision
Respiratory: apnea and hypoventilation

See also Opiate Analgesics General Monograph

OVERDOSAGE

Signs and symptoms of levorphanol overdosage are similar to the signs and symptoms associated with other opiate analgesic overdosage. Levorphanol overdosage requires emergency symptomatic medical support of body systems with attention to increasing levorphanol elimination. Naloxone (Narcan®) is a specific and effective antidote.

See also Opiate Analgesics General Monograph

LITHIUM

(lith'ee um)

TRADE NAMES

Carbolith®
Eskalith CR®
Lithane®
Lithobid®
Lithonate®

CLASSIFICATION

Antimanic (inorganic element of the alkali-metal group)

APPROVED INDICATIONS FOR PSYCHOLOGICAL DISORDERS

Adjunctive pharmacotherapy for the symptomatic management of:

Bipolar Disorders: Acute Mania. Lithium pharmacotherapy also is indicated for maintenance pharmacotherapy for preventing or decreasing the frequency of subsequent manic episodes among patients who have histories of bipolar disorder with mania.

USUAL DOSAGE AND ADMINISTRATION

Acute Mania

Adults: Individualize dosage according to severity of signs and symptoms, lithium blood concentrations, and clinical response. Initially, prescribe lithium pharmacotherapy according to the following schedule:

Day 1: 600 to 900 mg orally in three divided doses
Day 2: 1200 to 1800 mg orally in three divided doses. Adjust the dosage according to lithium blood concentrations.

ACUTE MANIA   Adjust the dosage to obtain lithium blood concentrations between 0.8 and 1.2 mmol/L (0.8 and 1.2 mEq/L). Obtain blood samples before the patient has ingested the first lithium dose of the day.

FOLLOWING THE ACUTE MANIC EPISODE   After the acute manic episode subsides (usually within a week of initiating lithium pharmacotherapy), reduce the dosage to 450 to 1200 mg daily orally in three divided doses to achieve lithium blood concentrations between 0.6 and 1 mmol/L (0.6 and 1 mEq/L). Maintain the lithium blood concentration below 1.5 mmol/L (1.5 mEq/L)) because there is evidence that patients may have a decreased tolerance to lithium during this time.

Most patients benefit from 900 to 1200 mg daily orally in three divided doses. If satisfactory therapeutic response is not achieved within 14 days, discontinue lithium pharmacotherapy. Patients who are stabilized on lithium may benefit from once daily dosing. For these patients, replace the divided daily dosage of lithium with once daily dosing. The total daily dosage for once daily dosing is approximately 5% to 30% *lower* than the daily dosage when divided over the day. Monitor patient response and lithium blood concentrations when divided doses are replaced with a single daily dose. If therapeutic lithium blood concentrations cannot be maintained with once daily dosing, switch patients to twice daily dosing (i.e., every 12 hours) with the extended-release tablets.

LONG-TERM MAINTENANCE, UNCOMPLICATED CASES   During remission, monitor lithium blood concentrations at least every 2 months. Obtain blood samples immediately prior to the next dose. However, do not rely completely on blood concentrations alone. Monitor also individual patient response.

Women who are, or who may become, pregnant: FDA Pregnancy Category D. Lithium is a known human teratogen. Do *not* prescribe lithium pharmacotherapy to women who are pregnant. Lithium readily crosses the placenta and has been associated with an increased incidence of cardiac and other anomalies, particularly Epstein's anomaly, among neonates. Nephrogenic diabetes insipidus, euthyroid goiter, and hypoglycemia also have been reported among women who have received lithium pharmacotherapy during pregnancy.

Women who are breast-feeding: Safety and efficacy of lithium pharmacotherapy for women who are breast-feeding and their neonates and infants have not been established. Lithium is excreted in breast milk. Avoid prescribing lithium pharmacotherapy to women who are breast-feeding. If lithium pharmacotherapy is required, breast-feeding should be discontinued. Collaboration with the patient's pediatrician is indicated.

Elderly, frail, or debilitated patients and those who have cardiovascular or kidney dysfunction: Initially, do not exceed 300 mg daily, and monitor lithium blood concentrations closely. Maintain lithium blood concentrations in the therapeutic range of 0.4 to 0.8 mmol/L (0.4 and 0.8 mEq/L), or lower. Do not exceed blood concentrations of 1 mmol/L (1 mEq/L). Elderly, frail, or debilitated patients appear to be more sensitive to the pharmacologic actions of lithium than are younger or healthier adult patients. These patients also may be more susceptible for ADRs, even when lithium blood concentrations are within the therapeutic range for younger adults. These patients may experience a higher incidence of neurotoxicity, particularly those who are older than 80 years of age or have cardiovascular or kidney dysfunction. Prescribe lithium pharmacotherapy cautiously to elderly, frail, or debilitated patients and those who have significant cardiovascular or kidney dysfunction.

Children younger than 12 years of age: Safety and efficacy of lithium pharmacotherapy for children younger than 12 years of age have not been established. Lithium pharmacotherapy is *not* recommended for this age group.

Notes, Acute Mania

The ability of patients to tolerate lithium pharmacotherapy is greater during the acute manic phase of the bipolar disorder and decreases when manic signs and symptoms subside. Patients who have bipolar disorders reportedly retain larger amounts of lithium during the active manic phase. Regular monitoring of lithium blood concentrations and individual patient response are required for optimal lithium pharmacotherapy.

Initiating Lithium Pharmacotherapy   Prior to initiating lithium pharmacotherapy, refer patients for medical evaluation with attention to cardiovascular, endocrine, GI and kidney function. Initially, adjust dosage to obtain a lithium blood concentration between 0.8 and 1.2 mmol/L (0.8 and 1.2 mEq/L). Do *not* exceed 1.5 mmol/L (1.5 mEq/L). Upon initiation of pharmacotherapy, monitor 12-hour lithium blood concentrations and the patient's individual response, with attention to mental status and ability to manage his or her lithium pharmacotherapy. Monitor also for ADRs. Adjust the dosage, as needed, to minimize ADRs. A change in dosage form or frequency of dosing, either toward multiple doses or toward a single daily dose, may be required to manage absorption-related ADRs or possible renal toxicity. Maintain lithium blood concentrations between 0.6 and 1 mmol/L (0.6 and 1 mEq/L).

Maintaining Long-Term Lithium Pharmacotherapy   Lithium pharmacotherapy is prescribed and monitored according to the nature and course of the bipolar disorder, rather than by only signs and symptoms of the disorder. The selection of patients for long-term lithium pharmacotherapy requires a firm diagnosis of bipolar disorder. Patients who have had fewer than two episodes annually are likely to benefit from lithium pharmacotherapy. During acute episodes, these patients generally have signs and symptoms that meet DSM-IV criteria for bipolar disorder. They also generally have remissions that do not include significant symptomatology.

Before prescribing long-term lithium pharmacotherapy, establish patient response to lithium pharmacotherapy and assure that the risk for potential ADRs is acceptable. Reevaluate the diagnosis of bipolar disorder and the patient's overall response to pharmacotherapy, including any associated ADRs. Collaboration with the patient's family physician or a specialist (e.g., cardiologist, nephrologist) is indicated in regard to obtaining a medical evaluation of the patient's physical health status. Collaboration with the family physician or a specialist also is indicated for the continued monitoring of the patient's general physical health, weight, fluid and electrolyte balance, kidney function (serum creatinine every 2 months), and thyroid function (plasma thyroid hormone and TSH levels every 6 to 12 months, particularly for women).

Potentially serious ADRs associated with long-term lithium pharmacotherapy include a decrease in the ability of the kidneys to concentrate urine. Signs and symptoms of this ADR include thirst, excessive urination (polyuria), weight gain, and alterations in kidney function tests. Long-term lithium pharmacotherapy also has been associated with nephrogenic diabetes insipidus. In addition, glomerular sclerosis, interstitial fibrosis, and tubular lesions have been associated with long-term lithium pharmacotherapy. Long-term lithium pharmacotherapy for patients who are unresponsive to lithium pharmacotherapy poses unacceptable risk because of these potentially serious ADRs associated with long-term lithium pharmacotherapy.

Monitor kidney function closely among patients who require long-term lithium pharmacotherapy. Progressive or sudden changes in kidney function, even at recommended dosages, indicate the need for reevaluation of lithium pharmacotherapy, including dosage, frequency of dosing, and risk-benefit ratio for long-term pharmacotherapy. Advise patients to avoid dehydration, which can result in lithium retention and toxicity. Kidney dysfunction associated with long-term lithium pharmacotherapy may be only partially reversible upon discontinuation of pharmacotherapy.

AVAILABLE DOSAGE FORMS, STORAGE, AND COMPATIBILITY

Capsules, oral: 150, 300, 600 mg
Liquid, oral: 8 mEq/5 ml (8 mEq of lithium is equivalent to 300 mg of lithium carbonate)
Syrup, oral: 300 mg/5 ml (contains 0.3% alcohol)
Tablets, oral: 300 mg
Tablets, oral extended-release (Eskalith CR®, Lithobid®): 300, 450 mg

Notes

General Instructions for Patients　Instruct patients who are receiving lithium pharmacotherapy to

- ingest each dose of the lithium oral capsules, liquid, syrup, or tablets with meals to decrease associated GI upset.
- swallow each dose of the lithium extended-release tablets whole or broken in half. Advise patients not to chew or crush these tablets.
- safely store lithium oral dosage forms out of the reach of children in tightly closed child-resistant containers at controlled room temperature (15° to 30°C; 59° to 86°F).
- obtain an available patient information sheet regarding lithium pharmacotherapy from their pharmacist at the time that their prescription is dispensed. Encourage patients to clarify any questions that they may have concerning lithium pharmacotherapy with their pharmacist or, if needed, to consult their prescribing psychologist.

PROPOSED MECHANISM OF ACTION

Lithium, a monovalent cation, competes in the body with other monovalent (e.g., potassium, sodium) and divalent (e.g., calcium, magnesium) cations involved in the synthesis, storage, release, and re-uptake of neurotransmitters. Its major actions in the body include alteration of sodium transport in nerves and muscles and alteration in the production and metabolism of central monoamine neurotransmitters, including dopamine and norepinephrine. Bipolar disorders appear to be affected by neurotransmitters, such as dopamine and norepinephrine. However, the exact mechanism of action of lithium for the management of mania associated with bipolar disorder has not yet been fully determined. Lithium does not have sedative action.

PHARMACOKINETICS/PHARMACODYNAMICS

Lithium is completely absorbed (~100%) following oral ingestion. Peak blood levels are obtained with regular oral dosage forms within 3 hours. Extended-release tablets achieve peak blood levels by 12 hours and may be incompletely absorbed. Steady-state concentrations are obtained in 4 days, with the onset of antimanic action usually occurring within 5 to 7 days. Full therapeutic benefit may not be observed for 10 to 21 days following the initiation of lithium pharmacotherapy. Lithium does not bind to plasma proteins but is widely distributed in most body tissues. Its mean apparent volume of distribution is 700 ml/kg. Lithium is not metabolized in the liver. Approximately 100% is eliminated in unchanged form in the urine. Sodium concentrations (i.e., high or low) significantly affect the rate of renal elimination of lithium. Total body clearance ranges from 20 to 40 ml/minute, and the mean half-life of elimination is approximately 22 hours (range 15 to 30 hours). Elimination is directly related to kidney function.

Therapeutic Drug Monitoring

Therapeutic blood levels are generally between 0.5 and 1.5 mmol/L (0.5 to 1.5 mEq/L). These blood levels are generally lower for elderly patients. Recommended maintenance levels generally range from 0.4 to 0.9 mmol/L (0.4 to 0.9 mEq/L). Toxic blood levels generally exceed 1.5 to 2 mmol/L (1.5 to 2 mEq/L). It is generally recommended that blood samples be obtained from trough concentrations approximately 12 hours following the last dose. However, in cases of suspected overdosage, sampling can be done at any time.

RELATIVE CONTRAINDICATIONS

Brain damage
Breast-feeding
Cardiovascular dysfunction
Debilitation, severe
Dehydration
Diuretic pharmacotherapy, concurrent
Kidney dysfunction
Pregnancy
Sodium depletion, including that associated with severe debilitation, dehydration, diuretic pharmacotherapy, and medical disorders that require low sodium ingestion (e.g., congestive heart failure, hypertension). Low salt or "crash diets" also may result in sodium depletion. Sodium depletion increases the risk for lithium toxicity. If lithium pharmacotherapy is required for these patients who are at risk for sodium depletion, initiate lithium pharmacotherapy cautiously under hospitalization at lower dosages than generally recommended. Adjust dosage according to daily lithium blood concentrations and individual patient response.

CAUTIONS AND COMMENTS

Lithium toxicity is closely related to lithium blood concentrations and can occur at levels close to the therapeutic range. Facilities for the prompt and accurate monitoring of lithium blood levels should be available before lithium pharmacotherapy is initiated. Monitor lithium blood levels regularly, and maintain levels below 1.5 mmol/L (1.5 mEq/L) to avoid toxicity.

Caution patients who are receiving lithium pharmacotherapy against performing activities that require alertness, judgment, and physical coordination (e.g., driving an automobile, operating dangerous equipment, supervising children) until their response to lithium pharmacotherapy is known. Lithium may adversely affect these mental and physical functions.

In addition to this general precaution, caution patients to inform their prescribing psychologist if they begin or discontinue any other pharmacotherapy while receiving lithium pharmacotherapy.

CLINICALLY SIGNIFICANT DRUG INTERACTIONS

Concurrent lithium pharmacotherapy and the following may cause clinically significant drug interactions:

Lorsartan Pharmacotherapy

Lorsartan (Cozaar®), an angiotensin II receptor antagonist, reduces blood pressure, in part, by increasing sodium excretion. Concurrent pharmacotherapy may result in decreased lithium renal clearance. This interaction may result in increased lithium blood levels and resultant lithium toxicity. Monitor lithium blood concentrations and patients for signs and symptoms of lithium toxicity (e.g., confusion, incoordination [ataxia], lethargy, loss of appetite [anorexia]). Collaboration with the prescriber of the lorsartan is indicated.

Pharmacotherapy With Angiotensin Converting Enzyme Inhibitors

ACE inhibitors (e.g., Captopril [Capoten®], Enalapril [Vasotec®], Lisinopril [Prinzide®]) induce sodium depletion and may, therefore, decrease the renal clearance of lithium, resulting in lithium toxicity. This interaction may become clinically significant after three to four weeks of concurrent pharmacotherapy, particularly among elderly patients. Monitor lithium blood concentrations and patients for signs and symptoms of lithium toxicity (e.g., confusion, incoordination [ataxia], lethargy, loss of appetite [anorexia]). Collaboration with the prescriber of the ACE inhibitor is indicated.

Pharmacotherapy With Nonsteroidal Anti-Inflammatory Drugs

The NSAIDs (e.g., Ibuprofen [Motrin®], Indomethacin [Indocin®], Naproxen [Naprosyn®]) reduce the renal excretion of lithium. Concurrent pharmacotherapy may result in increased lithium blood concentrations and lithium toxicity. Monitor lithium blood concentrations and patients for signs and symptoms of lithium toxicity (e.g., confusion, incoordination [ataxia], lethargy, loss of appetite [anorexia]). Collaboration with the prescriber of the NSAID is indicated. Note that several NSAIDs (e.g., ibuprofen, naproxen) are available without a prescription. Advise patients who are prescribed lithium pharmacotherapy of this potentially significant drug interaction.

Thiazide Diuretic Pharmacotherapy

Concurrent thiazide diuretic pharmacotherapy (e.g., hydrochlorothiazide [hydroDIURIL®]) may increase lithium blood concentrations and result in lithium toxicity. There is often a 20% to 40% reduction of renal lithium clearance. Patients who are stabilized on lithium pharmacotherapy may require a dosage reduction if concurrent thiazide diuretic pharmacotherapy is prescribed. A reduction in the dosage of the thiazide diuretic will help to avoid lithium toxicity.

When concerned about this drug interaction, monitor lithium blood concentrations and maintain the general therapeutic range of 0.5 to 1.5 mmol/L (0.5 to 1.5 mEq/L). Collaboration with the prescriber of the thiazide diuretic is indicated.

ADVERSE DRUG REACTIONS

Initially, lithium pharmacotherapy is frequently associated with GI complaints, muscle weakness, nausea, and vertigo. These ADRs are thought to be related to a rapid increase in lithium blood levels. However, they also may occur even when lithium blood levels are below 1 mmol/L. These ADRs usually resolve when lithium pharmacotherapy has been stabilized. Lithium pharmacotherapy also has been commonly and persistently associated with fine hand tremor. Long-term pharmacotherapy has been associated with fatigue, nephrogenic diabetes insipidus, and signs and symptoms of kidney dysfunction, such as excessive urination (polyuria) and thirst (polydipsia). Mild to moderate ADRs may occur at lithium blood concentrations of 1.5 to 2 mmol/L (1.5 to 2 mEq/L), and moderate to severe ADRs may occur at concentrations above 2 mmol/L (2 mEq/L). Other ADRs associated with lithium pharmacotherapy are listed according to body system. In order to prevent renal toxicity and other ADRs associated with long-term lithium pharmacotherapy: assure an accurate diagnosis of bipolar disorder; refer patients for medical evaluation of preexisting kidney dysfunction; establish standardized 12-hour lithium blood concentrations that are as low as possible for the achievement of optimal therapeutic benefit; monitor lithium blood concentrations and individual patient response; observe patients carefully for signs and symptoms of ADRs, including lithium toxicity; and adjust pharmacotherapy, including dosage and dosage form, to obtain temporarily periods of low lithium concentration in the kidneys.

Cardiovascular: allergic vasculitis, dysrhythmias, ECG changes (flattening or inversion of T-waves), peripheral circulatory failure, and cardiac collapse

CNS: blackouts, coma, confusion, cranial nerve effects, dizziness (vertigo), dystonia (acute), EEG changes (diffuse slowing, widening of the frequency spectrum, potentiation and disorganization of background rhythm, sensitivity to hyperventilation and paroxysmal bilateral synchronous delta activity), headache, restlessness, somnolence, and stupor. Unlike other antimanics (e.g., carbamazepine), lithium does *not* have a general sedative action.

Cutaneous: dryness and thinning of the hair, leg ulcers, psoriasis (exacerbation), severe itching (pruritus), skin anesthesia, and skin rash

Genitourinary: kidney dysfunction and nephrogenic diabetes insipidus (mild), which presents as excessive urination (polyuria). Sodium and potassium excretion is increased, and the kidney's ability to concentrate urine and reabsorb water is decreased. Excessive urination (polyuria) may persist among some patients even when lithium pharmacotherapy is discontinued.

GI: dry mouth and nausea

Hematologic: abnormal decrease in white blood cells (leukopenia), anemia, and increased number of leukocytes (leukocytosis)

Metabolic/Endocrine: goiter formation, hyperglycemia (transient, and that associated with lithium-induced hyperparathyroidism), and slight elevation of blood magnesium concentration. Lithium suppresses thyroid function and may cause hypothyroidism. Thyroid abnormalities include euthyroid goiter and hypothyroidism with myxedema accompanied by lower T_3 and T_4 levels and elevated TSH. Iodine[131] uptake may be increased. On average, 5% to 15% of patients receiving long-term lithium pharmacotherapy have signs and symptoms of altered serum hormone levels. Paradoxically, rare cases of hyperthyroidism occur.

Musculoskeletal: muscle weakness

Ocular: blurred vision and transient, island-like blind spots in the visual field (scotomata)
Miscellaneous: dehydration, general fatigue, lethargy, metallic taste, peripheral edema, tendency to sleep, and weight loss

OVERDOSAGE

Lithium overdosage is usually associated with blood concentrations exceeding 2 mmol/L (2 mEq/L). Early signs of lithium overdosage occur at lower blood concentrations and may be managed with a reduction in dosage or by withholding lithium pharmacotherapy for 24 to 48 hours. Severe lithium overdosage, which may be fatal, is generally preceded by diarrhea, drowsiness, hand tremor (coarse), lethargy, loss of appetite (anorexia), muscle twitching, sluggishness, and vomiting. These signs and symptoms require immediate discontinuation of lithium pharmacotherapy and emergency symptomatic medical support of body systems with attention to increasing lithium elimination. There is no known antidote.

LORAZEPAM

(lor a′ze pam)

TRADE NAMES

Ativan®
Novo-Lorazem®
Nu-Loraz®

CLASSIFICATION

Sedative-hypnotic (benzodiazepine) (C-IV)

See also Benzodiazepines General Monograph

APPROVED INDICATIONS FOR PSYCHOLOGICAL DISORDERS

Adjunctive pharmacotherapy for the short-term symptomatic management of:

Anxiety Disorders. Lorazepam pharmacotherapy is *not* indicated for the management of everyday anxiety or tension that can be managed with appropriate psychotherapy alone. Lorazepam pharmacotherapy also is *not* recommended for the management of anxiety associated with depression because it has the potential to exacerbate the depression while alleviating the anxiety. The depression associated with anxiety generally resolves with appropriate adjunctive pharmacotherapy (i.e., antidepressant pharmacotherapy) and psychotherapy.

USUAL DOSAGE AND ADMINISTRATION

Anxiety Disorders

Adults: 1 to 6 mg daily intramuscularly, orally, or sublingually in two or three divided doses, with the largest dose administered 30 minutes before retiring for bed in the evening. Most patients require an initial dosage of 2 to 3 mg daily in two or three divided doses. For insomnia associated with anxiety or transient situational stress, 2 to 4 mg orally or sublingually as a single daily dose 30 minutes before retiring for bed in the evening.

Women who are, or who may become, pregnant: FDA Pregnancy Category D. Safety and efficacy of lorazepam pharmacotherapy for women who are pregnant have not been established (see Benzodiazepines General Monograph). Avoid prescribing lorazepam pharmacotherapy to women who are pregnant. If lorazepam pharmacotherapy is required, advise patients of potential benefits and possible risks to themselves and the embryo, fetus, or neonate. Collaboration with the patient's obstetrician may be indicated.

Women who are breast-feeding: Safety and efficacy of lorazepam pharmacotherapy for women who are breast-feeding and their neonates and infants have not been established (see Benzodiazepines General Monograph). Avoid prescribing lorazepam pharmacotherapy for women who are breast-feeding. If lorazepam pharmacotherapy is required, breast-feeding probably should be discontinued. If desired, lactation may be maintained and breast-feeding resumed following the discontinuation of short-term lorazepam pharmacotherapy.

Elderly, frail, or debilitated patients and those who have organic brain syndrome: Initially, 0.5 to 1 mg daily intramuscularly, orally, or sublingually in divided doses. To avoid associated over-sedation, do not initially exceed 2 mg daily. Increase the dosage gradually according to individual patient response. Generally prescribe lower dosages for elderly, frail, or debilitated patients and those who have organic brain syndrome. These patients are reportedly more sensitive to lorazepam's CNS depressant action than are younger or healthier adult patients even when lower dosages are prescribed.

Children and adolescents younger than 18 years of age: Safety and efficacy of lorazepam pharmacotherapy for children and adolescents have not been established. Lorazepam pharmacotherapy is *not* recommended for this age group.

Notes, Anxiety Disorders

The daily dosage, frequency of dosing, and duration of lorazepam pharmacotherapy are determined by the severity of the signs and symptoms of the anxiety disorder and individual patient response. Various oral tablets (e.g., 0.5, 1, 2 mg tablets) and other dosage forms (e.g., oral concentrated solution, sublingual tablets) are available to facilitate individualized pharmacotherapy. To avoid ADRs, increase the dosage of lorazepam gradually, when needed, by increments of 0.5 mg. When higher daily dosages are required, increase the evening dose before increasing the daytime dose. The daily dosage may vary among patients from 1 to 10 mg. The usual dosage range is 2 to 6 mg daily in divided doses, with the largest dose 30 minutes before retiring for bed in the evening. Most adults respond optimally to a total daily dosage of 1 to 4 mg. Elderly, frail, or debilitated patients generally require lower daily dosages. The safety and efficacy of lorazepam pharmacotherapy for longer than 4 months have not been established.

Avoid abruptly discontinuing lorazepam pharmacotherapy. Abrupt discontinuation, particularly after long-term high-dosage pharmacotherapy, or regular personal use, may result in the signs and symptoms of the benzodiazepine withdrawal syndrome, including grand mal seizures. Discontinue lorazepam pharmacotherapy by gradually reducing the dosage according to individual patient response.

AVAILABLE DOSAGE FORMS, STORAGE, AND COMPATIBILITY

Injectables, intravenous: 1, 2, 4 mg/ml
Solution, oral concentrate (Lorazepam Intensol®): 2 mg/ml
Tablets, oral: 0.5, 1, 2 mg
Tablets, sublingual: 1, 2 mg

Notes

Injectable Pharmacotherapy   *The injectable is for intravenous pharmacotherapy only.* Intravenous pharmacotherapy is usually indicated for the initial control of seizures among patients who have status epilepticus. It also is indicated pre-operatively for the management of anxiety and to decrease the recall of events related to the day of surgery. Intravenous lorazepam pharmacotherapy is *not* recommended for the adjunctive symptomatic management of anxiety disorders. Availability of appropriate equipment and properly trained personnel *must* be assured prior to the intravenous injection of lorazepam because of the possibility of heavy sedation and associated partial airway obstruction. The injectable is refrigerated between 2° and 8°C (36° and 46°F) and requires protection from light.

General Instructions for Patients   Instruct patients who are receiving lorazepam pharmacotherapy to

- place each dose of the lorazepam sublingual tablets under the tongue and avoid swallowing for at least 2 minutes for maximal absorption.
- immediately dilute prior to ingestion each dose of the lorazepam oral concentrated solution with 30 ml of carbonated soft drink, juice, or water or mix in 30 ml of cold applesauce or pudding.
- safely store lorazepam tablets out of the reach of children in tightly closed child-resistant containers at controlled room temperature (15° to 30°C; 59° to 86°F).
- obtain an available patient information sheet regarding lorazepam pharmacotherapy from their pharmacist at the time that their prescription is dispensed. Encourage patients to clarify any questions that they may have concerning lorazepam pharmacotherapy with their pharmacist or, if needed, to consult their prescribing psychologist.

PROPOSED MECHANISM OF ACTION

Lorazepam has anticonvulsant, anxiolytic, and sedative actions. The exact mechanism of these actions has not yet been fully determined. However, its anxiolytic action appears to be mediated by or work in concert with the inhibitory neurotransmitter, GABA. This action appears to be accomplished by binding to benzodiazepine receptors within the GABA complex.

See also Benzodiazepines General Monograph

PHARMACOKINETICS/PHARMACODYNAMICS

Lorazepam is well absorbed after oral ingestion, with a mean bioavailability of 93%. Peak blood concentrations of lorazepam are achieved within 2 hours after oral ingestion and 60 minutes after sublingual placement. Lorazepam is 85% bound to plasma proteins. Its mean apparent volume of distribution is 1.3 L/kg. It is rapidly conjugated to an inactive glucuronide. Less than 1% of lorazepam is excreted in unchanged form in the urine. The mean half-life of elimination is approximately 16 hours, and the mean total body clearance is ~80 ml/minute.

RELATIVE CONTRAINDICATIONS

Glaucoma, acute narrow-angle
Hypersensitivity to lorazepam or other benzodiazepines
Myasthenia gravis

CAUTIONS AND COMMENTS

Lorazepam is addicting and habituating. Long-term high-dosage lorazepam pharmacotherapy, or regular personal use, may result in addiction and habituation. Abrupt discontinuation also may result in the benzodiazepine withdrawal syndrome.

See Benzodiazepines General Monograph

Prescribe lorazepam pharmacotherapy cautiously to patients who

- have histories of problematic patterns of alcohol or other abusable psychotropic use. Monitor these patients carefully for the development of problematic patterns of use. These patients may be at increased risk for addiction and habitation.
- have kidney dysfunction. Lorazepam is primarily excreted by the kidneys.

Caution patients who are receiving lorazepam pharmacotherapy against

- increasing the dosage or using lorazepam more often than prescribed. Lorazepam is addicting and habituating. Advise patients not to increase their dosage or use lorazepam more frequently than prescribed without first consulting with their prescribing psychologist.
- performing activities that require alertness, judgment, or physical coordination (e.g., driving an automobile, operating dangerous equipment, supervising children) until their response to lorazepam is known. Lorazepam may adversely affect these mental and physical functions.

In addition to these general precautions, caution patients to inform their prescribing psychologist if they begin or discontinue any other pharmacotherapy while receiving lorazepam pharmacotherapy.

CLINICALLY SIGNIFICANT DRUG INTERACTIONS

Concurrent lorazepam pharmacotherapy and the following may result in clinically significant drug interactions:

Alcohol Use

Concurrent alcohol use may significantly increase the CNS depressant action of lorazepam. Advise patients to avoid, or limit, their use of alcohol while receiving lorazepam pharmacotherapy.

Pharmacotherapy With Central Nervous System Depressants and Other Drugs That Produce Central Nervous System Depression

Concurrent lorazepam pharmacotherapy with opiate analgesics, other sedative-hypnotics, or other drugs that produce CNS depression (e.g., antihistamines, phenothiazines, TCAs) may result in significant additive CNS depression.

See also Benzodiazepines General Monograph

ADVERSE DRUG REACTIONS

Lorazepam pharmacotherapy has been commonly associated with dizziness, drowsiness, sedation, unsteadiness, and weakness. These ADRs occur generally when lorazepam pharmacotherapy is initiated and remit with continued pharmacotherapy or with a reduction in dosage. The incidence of sedation and unsteadiness increases with age. An apparently dose-related anterograde amnesia, decreased or lack of ability to recall events during the period of drug action, also has been associated with lorazepam pharmacotherapy. Other ADRs, listed according to body system, include:

CNS: agitation, confusion, depression, disorientation, fatigue, lethargy, and sleep disturbances
Cutaneous: skin rash
Genitourinary: sexual disturbances
GI: change in appetite, gastrointestinal distress, and nausea
Hematologic: rarely, a reduction in the circulating white blood cell count (leukopenia)

See also Benzodiazepines General Monograph

OVERDOSAGE

Signs and symptoms of lorazepam overdosage include somnolence, confusion, and coma. Lorazepam overdosage requires emergency symptomatic medical support of body systems with attention to increasing lorazepam elimination. The benzodiazepine antagonist flumazenil (Anexate®, Romazicon®) may be required.

LOXAPINE [Oxilapine]

(lox′a peen)

TRADE NAMES

Loxitane®
Loxapac®

CLASSIFICATION

Antipsychotic (dibenzoxazepine)

APPROVED INDICATIONS FOR PSYCHOLOGICAL DISORDERS

Adjunctive pharmacotherapy for the symptomatic management of:

Psychotic Disorders: Schizophrenia and Other Psychotic Disorders

USUAL DOSAGE AND ADMINISTRATION

Schizophrenia and Other Psychotic Disorders

Adults: Initially, 20 mg daily orally in two divided doses. Dosage is based on the severity of the patient's signs and symptoms and previous history of response to antipsychotic pharmacotherapy. Adjust dosage according to individual patient response. See Notes, Schizophrenia and Other Psychotic Disorders.

MAINTENANCE: 60 to 100 mg daily orally in two divided dosages. Prescribe the lowest effective dosage. Most patients benefit from dosages ranging from 20 to 60 mg daily. Dosages exceeding 250 mg daily are *not* recommended.

MAXIMUM: 250 mg daily intramuscularly or orally

Women who are, or who may become, pregnant: FDA Pregnancy Category "not established." Safety and efficacy of loxapine pharmacotherapy for women who are pregnant have not been established. Avoid prescribing loxapine pharmacotherapy to women who are pregnant. If loxapine pharmacotherapy is required, advise patients (or their legal guardian in regard to the patient) of potential benefits and possible risks to themselves and the embryo, fetus, or neonate. Collaboration with the patient's obstetrician is indicated.

Women who are breast-feeding: The safety and efficacy of loxapine pharmacotherapy for women who are breast-feeding and their neonates and infants have not been established. The extent of loxapine excretion in breast milk is unknown. Avoid prescribing loxapine pharmacotherapy to women who are breast-feeding. If loxapine pharmacotherapy is required, breast-feeding probably should be discontinued. Collaboration with the patient's pediatrician is indicated.

Children and adolescents younger than 16 years of age: Safety and efficacy of loxapine pharmacotherapy for children and adolescents younger than 16 years of age have not been established. Loxapine pharmacotherapy is *not* recommended for this age group.

Notes, Schizophrenia and Other Psychotic Disorders

Before initiating loxapine pharmacotherapy, assure that patients (or their legal guardians) are appropriately informed about the associated benefits and potential risks (e.g., TD) associated with loxapine pharmacotherapy. This information is essential, so that they may provide informed consent for loxapine pharmacotherapy.

Intramuscular Loxapine Pharmacotherapy   Intramuscular pharmacotherapy is indicated for the prompt management of acutely agitated patients and patients for whom oral pharmacotherapy is contraindicated or impractical. Inject intramuscularly 12.5 to 50 mg according to the patient's signs and symptoms of psychosis and individual patient response. Twice daily dosing is usually satisfactory. Once an adequate therapeutic response is achieved (usually within five days) and the patient is able to ingest oral dosage forms, replace the injectable formulation of loxapine with the oral capsule or oral concentrate formulation.

There is reportedly a higher incidence of EPRs associated with intramuscular loxapine pharmacotherapy when compared to oral pharmacotherapy. This higher incidence of EPRs may be related to the higher blood concentrations achieved with intramuscular pharmacotherapy.

Oral Loxapine Pharmacotherapy   Initially, 20 mg daily orally in two divided doses. Severely disturbed patients may require up to 50 mg daily. Increase the dosage fairly rapidly over the first 7 to 10 days until the signs and symptoms of psychosis are managed effectively.

AVAILABLE DOSAGE FORMS, STORAGE, AND COMPATIBILITY

Capsules, oral: 5, 10, 25, 50 mg
Concentrate, oral (with calibrated dropper): 25 mg/ml
Injectable, intramuscular: 50 mg/ml

Notes

Loxapine is formulated in oral capsules as the succinate salt and in the oral concentrate and injectable as the hydrochloride salt. *The injectable formulation is for intramuscular injection only. Do not inject intravenously or subcutaneously.* A slight color change of the injectable solution from straw to light amber will not affect potency or therapeutic efficacy.

General Instructions for Patients   Instruct patients who are receiving loxapine pharmacotherapy to

- dilute each dose of loxapine oral concentrate with 60 ml of orange or grapefruit juice just prior to ingestion to increase palatability. *Only* use the calibrated dropper dispensed with the oral concentrate to measure each dose of the oral concentrate.
- obtain an available patient information sheet regarding loxapine pharmacotherapy from their pharmacist at the time that their prescription is dispensed. Encourage patients to clarify any questions that they may have concerning loxapine pharmacotherapy with their pharmacist or, if needed, to consult their prescribing psychologist.

PROPOSED MECHANISM OF ACTION

Loxapine is a tricyclic antipsychotic chemically distinct from thioxanthenes, butyrophenones, and phenothiazines. The exact mechanism of action of loxapine is complex and has not yet been fully determined. However, its antipsychotic activity appears to be primarily related to its interaction with dopamine-containing neurons, specifically the blockade of dopamine receptors both pre- and post-synaptically.

PHARMACOKINETICS/PHARMACODYNAMICS

The absorption of loxapine is rapid and complete following oral ingestion. However, oral ingestion is associated with approximately one-third lower bioavailability than intramuscular injection, probably because of first-pass liver metabolism. Peak blood concentrations are achieved within 1 to 2 hours following oral ingestion and within 4 to 5 hours following intramuscular injection. Loxapine is metabolized extensively in the liver to several metabolites, including the active metabolite 8-hydroxyloxapine. Loxapine is excreted as metabolites in the urine, with little or no loxapine excreted in unchanged form. Additional data are unavailable.

RELATIVE CONTRAINDICATIONS

Blood disorders
Circulatory collapse
CNS depression, severe and including that associated with alcohol, opiate analgesic, and
    sedative-hypnotic overdosage
Coma
Hypersensitivity to loxapine or dibenzoxazepines
Liver dysfunction, severe

CAUTIONS AND COMMENTS

Prescribe loxapine pharmacotherapy cautiously to patients who

- have cardiovascular disorders. Increased pulse rates have been reported among a majority of patients. Transient hypotension also has been reported. Severe hypotension may require medical management with vasopressor pharmacotherapy (i.e., angiotensin or norepinephrine pharmacotherapy). Usual dosages of epinephrine may be ineffective because of loxapine's inhibitory action on epinephrine's vasopressor action.

- have glaucoma (narrow-angle), urinary retention, or are receiving concurrent pharmacotherapy with anticholinergics (e.g., atropine) or other drugs that have anticholinergic actions (e.g., phenothiazines, TCAs). These patients may experience additive anticholinergic reactions.
- have histories of seizure disorders. Loxapine can lower the seizure threshold. Seizures have been reported among patients receiving recommended dosages of loxapine for the symptomatic management of psychotic disorders. Seizures also have been reported among patients who have epilepsy and are concurrently receiving anticonvulsant pharmacotherapy. Collaboration with the patient's family physician or a specialist (e.g., neurologist) is indicated.

Caution patients who are receiving loxapine pharmacotherapy against

- drinking alcohol or using other drugs that can depress the CNS. Concurrent use of alcohol or other drugs that depress the CNS may result in excessive CNS depression.
- performing activities that require alertness, judgment, or psychomotor coordination (e.g., driving an automobile, operating dangerous equipment, supervising children). Loxapine may adversely affect these mental or physical functions, particularly during the first few days of pharmacotherapy.

In addition to these general precautions, caution patients to inform their prescribing psychologist if they begin or discontinue any other pharmacotherapy while receiving loxapine pharmacotherapy.

CLINICALLY SIGNIFICANT DRUG INTERACTIONS

Concurrent loxapine pharmacotherapy and the following may result in clinically significant drug interactions:

Alcohol Use

Concurrent alcohol use may increase the CNS depressant action of loxapine. Advise patients to avoid, or limit, their use of alcohol while receiving loxapine pharmacotherapy.

Epinephrine Pharmacotherapy

Loxapine inhibits the vasopressor action of epinephrine (i.e., the ability of epinephrine to contract the muscles of the arteries and capillaries that results in increased blood pressure). If patients require a vasopressor medically while receiving loxapine pharmacotherapy, norepinephrine (Levophed®) and phenylephrine (Neo-Synephrine®) generally are recommended.

Pharmacotherapy With Drugs That Produce Central Nervous System Depression

Concurrent loxapine pharmacotherapy with opiate analgesics, sedative-hypnotics, or other drugs that produce CNS depression (e.g., antihistamines, phenothiazines, TCAs) may result in additive CNS depression.

ADVERSE DRUG REACTIONS

Loxapine pharmacotherapy commonly has been associated with EPRs, including parkinsonian-like signs and symptoms occurring during the first few days of loxapine pharmacotherapy. Signs and symptoms of TD include excessive salivation, masked facies, rigidity, tremor, and akathisia (motor restlessness). Other signs and symptoms occur less frequently and include dystonia (i.e., spasms of muscles of the neck and face, tongue protrusion, and oculogyric movement) and dyskinetic reactions (i.e., choreoathetoid movements), which may be severe. These reactions may require a reduction of dosage or temporary discontinuation of loxapine pharmacotherapy. Some patients may require concurrent anti-parkinsonian pharmacotherapy. Loxapine pharmacotherapy also has been associated with NMS and TD. Other ADRs associated with loxapine pharmacotherapy, listed according to body system, include:

Cardiovascular: fainting (syncope), hypertension, postural hypotension, and tachycardia

CNS: agitation, akinesia, confusion, dizziness, headache, insomnia, light-headedness, seizures, and tension. Drowsiness, usually mild, is associated with the initiation of loxapine pharmacotherapy or with increases in the dosage. This ADR usually remits with continued pharmacotherapy.

Cutaneous: dermatitis, facial puffiness, flushed face, hair loss (alopecia), rash, seborrhea, and severe itching (pruritus)

GI: constipation, dry mouth, nausea, paralytic ileus, and vomiting

Genitourinary: urinary retention

Hematologic: rarely, abnormal reduction in the blood neutrophil count (neutropenia [agranulocytosis, granulocytopenia]), which often results in an increased susceptibility to bacterial and fungal infections; abnormal reduction in the circulating white blood cell count (leukopenia); and abnormal reduction in the number of blood platelets (thrombocytopenia)

Hepatic: hepatocellular injury

Musculoskeletal: muscle twitching, numbness (paresthesias), shuffling or staggering gait, slurred speech, and weakness

Ocular: blurred vision

Respiratory: difficult or labored breathing (dyspnea) and nasal congestion

Miscellaneous: body temperature exceeding 41°C (106°F) (hyperpyrexia), excessive thirst (polydipsia), and weight gain or loss.

OVERDOSAGE

Signs and symptoms of loxapine overdosage range from mild cardiovascular and CNS depression to profound hypotension, respiratory depression, and unconsciousness. Extrapyramidal reactions, kidney failure, and seizures also have been reported. Loxapine overdosage requires emergency symptomatic medical support of body systems with attention to increasing loxapine elimination. There is no known antidote.

MAPROTILINE

(ma proe'ti leen)

TRADE NAME

Ludiomil®

CLASSIFICATION

Antidepressant (tetracyclic)

APPROVED INDICATIONS FOR PSYCHOLOGICAL DISORDERS

Adjunctive pharmacotherapy for the symptomatic management of:

Mood Disorders, Depressive Disorders: Moderate to Severe Depression. Maprotiline is prescribed according to the severity of the signs and symptoms of depression.

USUAL DOSAGE AND ADMINISTRATION

Moderate Depression

Adults (non-hospitalized):   Initially, 75 mg daily orally in two or three divided doses. Maintain this dosage for two weeks in order to monitor appropriately individual patient response because maprotiline has a long half-life of elimination. Increase the dosage gradually by 25 mg increments, as needed, according to individual patient response. Prescribe dosage increases for the late afternoon or evening dose in order to avoid associated daytime sedation.

MAXIMUM: 150 mg daily orally

Women who are, or who may become, pregnant: FDA Pregnancy Category B. Safety and efficacy of maprotiline pharmacotherapy for women who are pregnant have not been established. A possible association between maprotiline pharmacotherapy and adverse fetal effects has been suggested. Withdrawal-like effects (e.g., irritability and tremors) have been noted among neonates. Avoid prescribing maprotiline pharmacotherapy to women who are pregnant. If maprotiline pharmacotherapy is required, advise patients of potential benefits and possible risks to themselves and the embryo, fetus, or neonate. Collaboration with the patient's obstetrician is indicated.

Women who are breast-feeding: Safety and efficacy of maprotiline pharmacotherapy for women who are breast-feeding and their neonates and infants have not been established. Maprotiline is readily excreted into breast milk. The concentration of maprotiline in breast milk may generally exceed the concentration in maternal blood by approximately 50%. Do *not* prescribe maprotiline pharmacotherapy to women who are breast-feeding. If maprotiline pharmacotherapy is required, breast-feeding should be discontinued. Collaboration with the patient's pediatrician is indicated.

Elderly, frail, or debilitated patients: Initially, 30 mg daily orally in three divided doses. Increase the dosage gradually, if needed, according to individual patient response. Generally prescribe lower dosages for elderly, frail, or debilitated patients. These patients may be more sensitive to the pharmacologic actions of maprotiline than are younger or healthier adult patients.

MAXIMUM: 75 mg daily orally

Children and adolescents younger than 18 years of age: Safety and efficacy of maprotiline pharmacotherapy for children and adolescents have not been established. Maprotiline pharmacotherapy for the symptomatic management of moderate depressive disorders is *not* recommended for this age group.

Severe Depression

Adults (hospitalized):   Initially, 100 mg daily orally in two or three divided doses. The usual optimal dosage is 150 mg daily. Some patients may require up to 225 mg daily in divided doses. Before initiating high-dosage pharmacotherapy, exclude a history of seizure disorders among these patients.

MAXIMUM: 225 mg daily orally

Women who are, or who may become, pregnant: FDA Pregnancy Category B. Safety and efficacy of maprotiline pharmacotherapy for women who are pregnant have not been established. A possible association between maprotiline pharmacotherapy and adverse fetal effects has been suggested. Withdrawal-like effects (e.g., irritability and tremors) have been noted among neonates. Avoid prescribing maprotiline pharmacotherapy to women who are pregnant. If maprotiline pharmacotherapy is required, advise patients of potential benefits and possible risks to themselves and the embryo, fetus, or neonate. Collaboration with the patient's obstetrician is indicated.

Women who are breast-feeding: Safety and efficacy of maprotiline pharmacotherapy for women who are breast-feeding and their neonates and infants have not been established. Maprotiline is readily excreted into breast milk. The concentration of maprotiline in breast milk may generally exceed the concentration in maternal blood by approximately 50%. Do not prescribe maprotiline pharmacotherapy to women who are breast-feeding. If maprotiline pharmacotherapy is required, breast-feeding should be discontinued. Collaboration with the patient's pediatrician is indicated.

Elderly, frail, and debilitated patients (hospitalized):   Initially, 50 mg daily orally in two divided doses. Increase the dosage gradually, if needed, according to individual patient response. Generally prescribe lower dosages for elderly, frail, or debilitated patients. These patients may be more sensitive to the pharmacologic actions of maprotiline than are younger or healthier adult patients.

Children and adolescents younger than 18 years of age: Safety and efficacy of maprotiline pharmacotherapy for children and adolescents have not been established. Maprotiline pharmacotherapy for the symptomatic management of severe depressive disorders is *not* recommended for this age group.

Notes, Moderate to Severe Depression

An increased risk for suicide among severely depressed patients may persist until significant remission of the depressive disorder occurs. Therefore, monitor patients carefully during all phases of maprotiline pharmacotherapy and prescribe for dispensing the smallest quantity of drug feasible (i.e., a two-week supply). Other suicide precautions may be indicated.

Initiating Maprotiline Pharmacotherapy Initially prescribe the lowest recommended dosage. Increase the dosage gradually according to individual patient response. Initial therapeutic benefit may be delayed for several days or weeks. Increasing the dosage does not appear to shorten this latency period and may increase the incidence or severity of ADRs. Obtain white blood cell counts periodically, during the first few months of maprotiline pharmacotherapy, and monitor patients for signs and symptoms associated with low white blood cell counts (e.g., fever, sore throat).

Seizures also have been associated with maprotiline pharmacotherapy. Seizures have been reported among patients who have no previous known history of seizures and who are receiving maprotiline pharmacotherapy at recommended dosages. The risk for seizures may be increased when the recommended dosage of maprotiline is rapidly exceeded. Risk also may be increased when maprotiline pharmacotherapy is prescribed with phenothiazine pharmacotherapy or when the dosage of concurrent benzodiazepine pharmacotherapy is rapidly reduced. The risk for seizures among patients who require maprotiline pharmacotherapy may be minimized by initiating pharmacotherapy at lower dosages, maintaining the initial dosage for two weeks before gradually increasing the dosage, prescribing the lowest effective maintenance dosage (dosages below 200 mg daily), avoiding the concurrent prescription of drugs that lower the seizure threshold (e.g., phenothiazines), and, if necessary, gradually reducing concurrent benzodiazepine pharmacotherapy.

Maintaining Long-Term High-Dosage Maprotiline Pharmacotherapy Patients who require long-term high-dosage maprotiline pharmacotherapy, especially those who have heart disease or are elderly, require periodic monitoring of heart function, including ECG. Patients who are susceptible to postural hypotension require regular monitoring of blood pressure. Periodic blood cell counts and liver function tests are recommended for all patients who require long-term maprotiline pharmacotherapy. Collaboration with the patient's family physician or a specialist (e.g., cardiologist, hematologist) is indicated.

AVAILABLE DOSAGE FORMS, STORAGE, AND COMPATIBILITY

Tablets, oral: 10, 25, 50, 75 mg

Notes

General Instructions for Patients Instruct patients who are receiving maprotiline pharmacotherapy to

- safely store maprotiline tablets out of the reach of children in tightly closed child-resistant containers below 30°C (86°F).

- obtain an available patient information sheet regarding maprotiline pharmacotherapy from their pharmacist at the time that their prescription is dispensed. Encourage patients to clarify any questions that they may have concerning maprotiline pharmacotherapy with their pharmacist or, if needed, to consult their prescribing psychologist.

PROPOSED MECHANISM OF ACTION

The exact mechanism of action of maprotiline has not yet been established. Maprotiline appears to produce its antidepressant action primarily by potentiating the CNS biogenic amines, particularly norepinephrine, by blocking their re-uptake at the pre-synaptic nerve terminals. This inhibition of re-uptake increases their concentration at the synapses and, consequently, results in increased activity at the post-synaptic neuron receptor sites. The anticholinergic activity of maprotiline appears to be primarily centrally mediated. The pharmacology of maprotiline is similar to that of the TCAs.

PHARMACOKINETICS/PHARMACODYNAMICS

Maprotiline is slowly but well absorbed after oral ingestion. Average time to peak blood concentration is 12 hours (range 8 to 24 hours). It is moderately plasma protein-bound (88%). Maprotiline is metabolized by N-demethylation, deamination, aliphatic and aromatic hydroxylations, and formation of aromatic methoxy derivatives. It is primarily excreted in the urine (two-thirds) and bile (one-third) as metabolites. The mean half-life of elimination is 51 hours (range 27 to 60 hours). The half-life of elimination and renal excretion are not significantly affected by the presence of kidney dysfunction when liver function is normal. Although the urinary excretion of metabolites may be reduced for these patients, it generally is offset by increased fecal elimination of metabolites through biliary excretion. Additional data are unavailable.

RELATIVE CONTRAINDICATIONS

Blood disorders, history of severe
Breast-feeding
Cardiac conduction defects
Glaucoma, narrow-angle
Hypersensitivity to maprotiline
Kidney dysfunction, severe
Liver dysfunction, severe
MAOI pharmacotherapy, concurrent or within 14 days
Myocardial infarction, acute recovery phase
Overdosage, acute alcohol or other psychotropic
Pregnancy
Seizure disorders, known or suspected. Maprotiline can lower the seizure threshold.
Urinary retention (e.g., that associated with prostatic hypertrophy). Maprotiline's anticholinergic action may exacerbate this condition.

CAUTIONS AND COMMENTS

Prescribe maprotiline pharmacotherapy cautiously to patients who

- are concurrently receiving anticholinergic (e.g., atropine) or sympathomimetic (e.g., amphetamine, phenylpropanolamine) pharmacotherapy. Concurrent anticholinergic or sympathomimetic pharmacotherapy may result in additive anticholinergic actions. Monitor patients closely for excessive anticholinergic actions (e.g., blurred vision, delayed urination), hot flushes, paralytic ileus, and sublingual adenitis (inflammation of the lymph nodes). Adjust the maprotiline dosage carefully, if needed.
- are concurrently receiving guanethidine (Ismelin®) pharmacotherapy or similar sympatholytic antihypertensive pharmacotherapy (e.g., bethanidine, clonidine, reserpine). Maprotiline may block the action of these drugs with subsequent loss of blood pressure control. Collaboration with the prescriber of the guanethidine is indicated.
- are elderly or bedridden. Although not directly associated with maprotiline pharmacotherapy, paralytic ileus has been associated with TCA pharmacotherapy, particularly among elderly and bedridden patients. Monitor these patients for the signs and symptoms of constipation because maprotiline has anticholinergic actions similar to the TCAs. Plan to prevent constipation and implement appropriate measures should constipation occur. Collaboration with the patient's advanced practice nurse, family physician, or specialist (e.g., gerontologist) is indicated.
- have bipolar disorder. Hypomanic or manic episodes have been reported among patients who have bipolar disorder and are receiving TCA pharmacotherapy during the depressed phase. The possibility of the occurrence of this reaction must be considered when maprotiline pharmacotherapy is prescribed because of its chemical and pharmacological similarity to the TCAs. These ADRs, should they occur, may require a reduction in the dosage or the discontinuation of maprotiline pharmacotherapy.
- have cardiovascular disorders. Tricyclic antidepressant pharmacotherapy, particularly when high dosages are required, has been associated with cardiac dysrhythmias, sinus tachycardia, and prolongation of conduction time. Myocardial infarction, stroke, and unexpected death rarely have been reported among patients who had histories of cardiovascular disorders. The pharmacology of maprotiline is similar to that of the TCAs. Thus, extreme caution is advised when maprotiline pharmacotherapy is prescribed to patients who have known cardiovascular disorders, including elderly patients and those who have histories of myocardial infarction, dysrhythmias, and ischemic heart disease. Maprotiline pharmacotherapy, when required, should be initiated at low dosages and increased gradually, only as needed, with close monitoring of patient response at all dosage levels. Collaboration with the patient's family physician or a specialist (e.g., cardiologist) is indicated, so that cardiac function, including ECG, can be monitored appropriately.
- have histories of increased intraocular pressure or urinary retention. Maprotiline can exacerbate these conditions because of its anticholinergic actions.
- have hyperthyroidism or are concurrently receiving thyroid pharmacotherapy. Maprotiline pharmacotherapy has been associated with cardiotoxic effects among these patients, including the potentiation of the cardiovascular actions of epinephrine and norepinephrine.
- require elective surgery. Maprotiline pharmacotherapy has been associated with cardiotoxic effects among these patients, including the potentiation of the cardiovascular actions of epinephrine and norepinephrine. Discontinue maprotiline pharmacotherapy as early as possible before elective surgery.
- require ECT. Concurrent maprotiline pharmacotherapy and ECT may be hazardous because of the increased risk for seizures.
- have schizophrenia. Although not directly associated with maprotiline pharmacotherapy, an activation of psychosis among patients who have schizophrenia has occasionally occurred with TCA pharmacotherapy. The possibility of the occurrence of this reaction must be considered when maprotiline pharmacotherapy is prescribed because of its chemical and pharmacological similarity to the TCAs. This ADR, should it occur, may require a reduction in the dosage or the discontinuation of maprotiline pharmacotherapy. Antipsychotic pharmacotherapy may be required.

Caution patients who are receiving maprotiline pharmacotherapy against performing activities that require alertness, judgment, and physical coordination (e.g., driving an automobile, operating dangerous equipment, supervising children) until their individual response to maprotiline pharmacotherapy is known. Maprotiline may produce sedation and, thus, adversely affect these mental and physical functions.

In addition to this general precaution, caution patients to inform their prescribing psychologist if they begin or discontinue any other pharmacotherapy while receiving maprotiline pharmacotherapy.

CLINICALLY SIGNIFICANT DRUG INTERACTIONS

Concurrent maprotiline pharmacotherapy and the following may result in clinically significant drug interactions:

Alcohol Use

Concurrent alcohol use may increase the CNS depressant action of maprotiline. Advise patients to avoid, or limit, their use of alcohol while receiving maprotiline pharmacotherapy.

Pharmacotherapy With Central Nervous System Depressants and Other Drugs That Produce Central Nervous System Depression

Concurrent maprotiline pharmacotherapy with opiate analgesics, sedative-hypnotics, or other drugs that produce CNS depression (e.g., antihistamines, phenothiazines, TCAs) may result in additive CNS depression.

See also Tricyclic Antidepressants General Monograph

ADVERSE DRUG REACTIONS

It is often difficult to differentiate the ADRs associated with maprotiline pharmacotherapy from the signs and symptoms of depression (e.g., agitation, anxiety, constipation, depressed mood, dry mouth, fatigue, sleep disorders), particularly because they do not always correlate with dosage or blood concentration levels. The most common ADRs associated with maprotiline pharmacotherapy are related to its anticholinergic actions. These ADRs include blurred vision, constipation, dry mouth, headache, nervousness, sedation (daytime), and vertigo. Maprotiline pharmacotherapy also has been associated with confusion, GI complaints, hypotension, and seizures. Most of these ADRs reportedly are mild and transient and usually resolve with continued pharmacotherapy or a reduction in dosage.

Severe ADRs, particularly those involving the central and peripheral nervous systems, require immediate discontinuation of maprotiline pharmacotherapy. Elderly, frail, or debilitated patients may be particularly sensitive to these reactions. Other ADRs that have been less commonly associated with maprotiline pharmacotherapy are listed according to body system. The ADRs generally associated with TCA pharmacotherapy also have been included because of the chemical and pharmacological similarities between maprotiline and the TCAs. It is recommended that prescribing psychologists also monitor for these ADRs:

Cardiovascular: atrial flutter, atypical ventricular tachycardia, dysrhythmias, fainting (syncope), heart block, hypertension, postural hypotension (particularly among elderly patients who have histories of cardiovascular disorders), Q-T prolongation, reversible T-wave changes, and tachycardia

CNS: agitation, anxiety, confusion with hallucinations (especially among elderly patients), delusions, disorientation, dizziness, drowsiness, EEG pattern alterations, exacerbation of psychosis, extrapyramidal reactions (e.g., akathisia, tremors), fatigue, feelings of unreality, hypomania, lightheadedness, mania, memory impairment, nightmares, and restlessness

Cutaneous: cutaneous vasculitis, flushing, hair loss (alopecia), hives (urticaria), petechiae, photosensitivity (advise patients to avoid excessive exposure to sunlight), skin rash, and sweating (excessive)

Genitourinary: changes in sex drive (increase or decrease), delayed urination, dilation of the urinary tract, impotence, and urinary frequency or retention

GI: abdominal cramps, bitter taste, black tongue, difficulty swallowing (dysphagia), epigastric distress, excessive salivation, loss of appetite (anorexia), paralytic ileus, stomatitis, sublingual adenitis (inflammation of the lymph nodes), taste disturbances, and vomiting

Hematologic: rarely, abnormal reduction in blood platelets (thrombocytopenia); bone marrow depression, including a reduction in blood neutrophil count that can result in an increased susceptibility to bacterial or fungal infections (i.e., neutropenia [agranulocytosis, granulocytopenia]), eosinophilia, and purpura. White blood cell and differential counts should be obtained for patients who develop a fever or sore throat during maprotiline pharmacotherapy. Collaboration with the patient's family physician or a specialist (e.g., hematologist) is required for the confirmation of blood disorders and related medical treatment, if needed. Maprotiline pharmacotherapy should be discontinued in the event of neutrophil depression.

Hepatic: rarely, liver dysfunction, hepatitis with or without jaundice, and increased serum transaminases

Metabolic/Endocrine: abnormal breast enlargement among males (gynecomastia) and abnormal breast enlargement and lactation (galactorrhea) among females, changes in blood sugar levels (increase or decrease), testicular swelling, and weight gain or loss

Musculoskeletal: rarely, joint pain (dysarthria), incoordination (ataxia), numbness or tingling of the extremities (paresthesias), twitching or clonic spasm of a muscle or group of muscles (myoclonus), and weakness

Ocular: disturbances of accommodation and abnormal dilation of the pupils (mydriasis)

Otic: ringing in the ears (tinnitus)

Respiratory: rarely, allergic alveolitis, with or without eosinophilia, and nasal congestion

Miscellaneous: rarely, drug fever and edema (general edema or edema involving the face and tongue).

See also Tricyclic Antidepressants General Monograph

OVERDOSAGE

Signs and symptoms of maprotiline overdosage may vary according to the severity of the overdosage. Generally, signs and symptoms reflect maprotiline's CNS, anticholinergic, and cardiotoxic actions. Accidental childhood ingestion of any amount of maprotiline is serious and potentially fatal. Initial signs and symptoms of overdosage may be observed 1 to 2 hours after ingestion and include abnormal dilation of the pupils (mydriasis), convulsions, cyanosis, disturbances of consciousness to coma, dysrhythmias, hyperreflexia followed by hyporeflexia, hyperpyrexia, hypotension, impaired cardiac conduction, incoordination (ataxia), motor restlessness, muscle twitching and rigidity, respiratory depression, shock, tachycardia, tremor, vertigo, and vomiting. Actual or suspected maprotiline overdosage requires emergency symptomatic medical support of body systems with attention to increasing maprotiline elimination. There is no known antidote. Accidental and intentional overdosages involving the antidepressants have been fatal.

MAZINDOL

(may′zin dole)

TRADE NAME

Sanorex®

CLASSIFICATION

CNS Stimulant (anorexiant, amphetamine-congener) (C-IV)

See also Amphetamines General Monograph

APPROVED INDICATIONS FOR PSYCHOLOGICAL DISORDERS

Adjunctive pharmacotherapy for the short-term (no longer than six weeks) symptomatic management of:

Eating Disorders: Exogenous Obesity. Prescribe mazindol pharmacotherapy as an adjunct to appropriate psychotherapy and a medically supervised weight reduction program based on dietary caloric restrictions and exercise.

USUAL DOSAGE AND ADMINISTRATION

Exogenous Obesity

Adults: 3 mg daily orally in three divided doses one hour before meals. If preferred, 1 to 2 mg orally as a single daily dose one hour before the first main meal of the day (usually 2 mg before lunch). Prescribe the lowest effective dosage for no longer than six weeks. Monitor patients for the development of tolerance to the anorexiant action of mazindol, which may occur within a few weeks of pharmacotherapy. When tolerance occurs, *discontinue* mazindol pharmacotherapy. Do *not* increase the dosage in an attempt to prolong mazindol's anorexiant action.

Women who are, or who may become, pregnant: FDA Pregnancy Category "not established." Safety and efficacy of mazindol pharmacotherapy for women who are pregnant have not been established. Avoid prescribing mazindol pharmacotherapy to women who are pregnant. If mazindol pharmacotherapy is required, advise patients of potential benefits and possible risks to themselves and the embryo, fetus, or neonate. Collaboration with the patient's obstetrician is indicated.

Women who are breast-feeding: Safety and efficacy of mazindol pharmacotherapy for women who are breast-feeding and their neonates and infants have not been established. Avoid prescribing mazindol pharmacotherapy to women who are breast-feeding. If mazindol pharmacotherapy is required, breast-feeding probably should be discontinued. If desired, lactation may be maintained and breast-feeding resumed following the discontinuation of short-term mazindol pharmacotherapy. Collaboration with the patient's pediatrician is indicated.

Children younger than 12 years of age: Safety and efficacy of mazindol pharmacotherapy for children who are younger than 12 years of age have not been established. Mazindol pharmacotherapy is *not* recommended for this age group.

Notes, Exogenous Obesity

Mazindol pharmacotherapy, like other anorexiant pharmacotherapy, is of limited benefit for the symptomatic management of exogenous obesity. Generally patients lose only a fraction of a kilogram or pound per week more than patients who do not receive anorexiant pharmacotherapy as part of their weight reduction programs. As with other similar anorexiants, rebound weight gain may occur following the discontinuation of mazindol pharmacotherapy.

AVAILABLE DOSAGE FORMS, STORAGE, AND COMPATIBILITY

Tablets, oral: 1, 2 mg

Notes

The Sanorex® tablets contain tartrazine (FD&C Yellow No. 5). Tartrazine has been associated with hypersensitivity reactions, including bronchial asthma, among susceptible patients, particularly those who have a hypersensitivity to aspirin.

General Instructions for Patients   Instruct patients who are receiving mazindol pharmacotherapy to

- ingest each dose of mazindol oral tablets with a small amount of food or milk. Mazindol tablets may be irritating to the stomach and may cause stomach upset.
- safely store mazindol oral tablets out of the reach of children in tightly closed child-resistant containers below 25°C (77°F).
- obtain an available patient information sheet regarding mazindol pharmacotherapy from their pharmacist at the time that their prescription is dispensed. Encourage patients to clarify any questions that they may have concerning mazindol pharmacotherapy with their pharmacist or, if needed, to consult their prescribing psychologist.

PROPOSED MECHANISM OF ACTION

Mazindol is an imidazo-isoindole anorexiant that shares many pharmacological actions with the amphetamines and their congeners. Mazindol has CNS stimulant and anorexiant (anorectant; anorectic) actions. Tolerance to the anorexiant action reportedly occurs with all drugs in this class, including mazindol. The exact mechanism of mazindol's anorexiant action for the management of exogenous obesity has not been fully determined. It appears to involve appetite suppression and other, as yet unspecified, CNS actions.

PHARMACOKINETICS/PHARMACODYNAMICS

Mazindol is well absorbed after oral ingestion. Its onset of action is within 30 to 60 minutes. Peak blood levels are generally achieved within 1 to 2 hours. Mazindol has a high tissue affinity, so that the blood contains the lowest relative concentration 2 hours after oral ingestion. It has a duration of action of 8 to 15 hours and is slowly excreted in the urine and feces. The excretion rate can be increased with continued use. Additional data are unavailable.

Therapeutic Drug Monitoring

Therapeutic blood levels of mazindol reportedly range from 3 to 12 ng/ml.

RELATIVE CONTRAINDICATIONS

Addiction or habituation to mazindol or other CNS stimulants (e.g., amphetamines), history of
Agitation
Cardiac decompensation
Cerebral ischemia
Glaucoma
Hypersensitivity to mazindol
Hypertension, severe
MAOI pharmacotherapy, concurrent or within 14 days
Myocardial infarction, recent
Schizophrenia
Uremia

CAUTIONS AND COMMENTS

Long-term mazindol pharmacotherapy, or regular personal use, has been associated with severe habituation. Mazindol is chemically and pharmacologically related to the amphetamines, which have high abuse potential. Patients may increase their dosages to many times those recommended. Monitor patients for signs and symptoms of problematic patterns of use. Avoid abrupt discontinuation of mazindol use among these patients. Abrupt discontinuation of long-term pharmacotherapy, or regular personal use, may be associated with an amphetamine-like withdrawal syndrome. The signs and symptoms of this syndrome include extreme fatigue and mental depression. Prescribe for dispensing the smallest quantity of mazindol feasible to minimize the possible development of problematic patterns of use, and do not prescribe mazindol pharmacotherapy for longer than six weeks.

Prescribe mazindol pharmacotherapy cautiously to patients who

- have hypertension. Mazindol pharmacotherapy may exacerbate this condition. Monitor blood pressure regularly during mazindol pharmacotherapy. Collaboration with the patient's advanced practice nurse or family physician is indicated.
- have symptomatic cardiovascular disorders, including dysrhythmias. Mazindol's stimulant actions may adversely affect heart function among these patients. Collaboration with the patient's cardiologist is indicated.

Caution patients who are receiving mazindol pharmacotherapy against performing activities that require alertness, judgment, and physical coordination (e.g., driving an automobile, operating hazardous equipment, supervising children) until their response to mazindol pharmacotherapy is known. Mazindol's CNS actions may adversely affect these mental and physical functions.

In addition to this general precaution, caution patients to inform their dentist, family physician, or other prescribers that they are receiving mazindol pharmacotherapy. Advise them to carry an emergency identification card stating that they are receiving mazindol pharmacotherapy. Pressor drugs, which may be required in an emergency, should be prescribed with caution to patients who are receiving mazindol pharmacotherapy.

CLINICALLY SIGNIFICANT DRUG INTERACTIONS

Concurrent mazindol pharmacotherapy and the following may result in clinically significant drug interactions:

Guanethidine Pharmacotherapy

Mazindol may decrease the neuronal uptake of guanethidine (Ismelin®) and, thus, decrease its antihypertensive action. An adjustment in the guanethidine dosage may be required. Collaboration with the prescriber of the guanethidine is indicated.

Monoamine Oxidase Inhibitor Pharmacotherapy

Mazindol may interact with MAOIs (e.g., phenelzine [Nardil®], tranylcypromine [Parnate®]) and cause the release of large amounts of catecholamines and associated effects, including hypertensive crisis. Hypertensive crisis is characterized by a severe headache and hypertension. Concurrent mazindol and MAOI pharmacotherapy is *contraindicated*.

See also Amphetamines General Monograph

ADVERSE DRUG REACTIONS

Mazindol pharmacotherapy is commonly associated with constipation, dry mouth, insomnia, nausea, and nervousness. Other ADRs associated with mazindol pharmacotherapy, listed according to body system, include:

Cardiovascular: hypertension or hypotension, palpitations, and tachycardia
CNS: anxiety, depression, dizziness, drowsiness, dysphoria, headache, and overstimulation
Cutaneous: clamminess of the skin, flushing, pallor, rash, and sweating (excessive)
Genitourinary: changes in sex drive, impotence, and painful urination (dysuria)
GI: abdominal discomfort, diarrhea, unpleasant taste, and vomiting
Musculoskeletal: numbness and tingling of the hands, motor restlessness, tremor, and weakness
Ocular: abnormal dilation of the pupils (mydriasis) and blurred vision

See also Amphetamines General Monograph

OVERDOSAGE

Mazindol overdosage rarely has been reported. Signs and symptoms of mazindol overdosage include agitation, hyperactivity, irritability, and tachycardia. Mazindol overdosage requires emergency symptomatic medical support of body systems with attention to increasing mazindol elimination. There is no known antidote.

MEPERIDINE [Pethidine]

(me per'i deen)

TRADE NAME

Demerol®

CLASSIFICATION

Opiate analgesic (C-II)

See also Opiate Analgesics General Monograph

APPROVED INDICATIONS FOR PSYCHOLOGICAL DISORDERS

Adjunctive pharmacotherapy for the symptomatic management of:

Pain Disorders: Acute Pain, Moderate to Severe, and Cancer Pain, Moderate to Severe

USUAL DOSAGE AND ADMINISTRATION

Acute Pain, Moderate to Severe, and Cancer Pain, Moderate to Severe

Adults: 1 to 3 mg/kg orally every three or four hours, as needed; or 0.5 to 1.5 mg/kg intramuscularly, intravenously, or subcutaneously every three or four hours, as needed.

MAXIMUM: 4 mg/kg/dose intramuscularly, intravenously, or subcutaneously to a maximum of 150 mg/dose

Women who are, or who may become, pregnant: FDA Pregnancy Category B. Safety and efficacy of meperidine pharmacotherapy for women who are pregnant have not been established. Neonatal addiction and withdrawal are associated with maternal meperidine pharmacotherapy, or regular personal use, near term. Avoid prescribing meperidine pharmacotherapy to women who are pregnant. If meperidine pharmacotherapy is required, advise patients of potential benefits and possible risks to themselves and the embryo, fetus, or neonate. Collaboration with the patient's obstetrician is indicated.

Women who are breast-feeding: Safety and efficacy of meperidine pharmacotherapy for women who are breast-feeding and their neonates and infants have not been established. Meperidine is excreted into breast milk. Repeated doses can result in significant concentrations in breast milk of both meperidine and its active metabolite, normeperidine. These concentrations may place breast-fed neonates and infants at risk for expected pharmacologic actions (e.g., drowsiness) and addiction. Avoid prescribing meperidine pharmacotherapy to women who are breast-feeding. If meperidine pharmacotherapy is required, breast-feeding probably should be discontinued. If desired, lactation may be maintained and breast-feeding resumed following the discontinuation of short-term meperidine pharmacotherapy. Collaboration with the patient's pediatrician is indicated.

Elderly, frail, or debilitated patients: Generally prescribe lower dosages for elderly, frail, or debilitated patients. Increase the dosage gradually, if needed, according to individual patient response. These patients may be more sensitive to the pharmacologic actions of meperidine than are younger or healthier adult patients.

Children: 1 to 3 mg/kg orally every three or four hours, as needed; or 0.5 to 1.5 mg/kg intramuscularly, intravenously, or subcutaneously every three or four hours, as needed

MAXIMUM: 2 mg/kg/dose intramuscularly, intravenously, or subcutaneously to a maximum of 100 mg/dose

Adolescents: 1 to 1.5 mg/kg intramuscularly, intravenously, or subcutaneously every three or four hours, as needed

MAXIMUM: 4 mg/kg/dose intramuscularly, intravenously, or subcutaneously to a maximum of 150 mg/dose

Notes, Acute Pain, Moderate to Severe, and Cancer Pain, Moderate to Severe

Adjust the dosage according to severity of pain and individual patient response. Note difference between recommended oral and injectable dosages. Meperidine is less effective when ingested orally than when injected intramuscularly, intravenously, or subcutaneously. Poor drug absorption following oral ingestion requires generally higher oral dosages. Following intravenous injection, meperidine is excreted into the stomach and reabsorbed. Thus, it may have a late increased action. As tolerance to meperidine's analgesic action develops, do *not* exceed recommended dosages. Higher dosages have been associated with seizures, even among patients who have no previous history of seizure disorders.

Injectable Meperidine Pharmacotherapy

INTRAMUSCULAR PHARMACOTHERAPY   Absorption from intramuscular injection sites may vary. Inject meperidine into healthy muscle sites. The dorsogluteal and ventrogluteal sites are recommended. Identify recommended sites carefully before injection. Inadvertent injection at a nerve trunk may result in sensory-motor paralysis (usually transitory). Intramuscular injections of meperidine also have been associated with pain at the injection site. Rotate injection sites carefully when repeated injections are required.

INTRAVENOUS PHARMACOTHERAPY   Dilute injectable prior to intravenous injection. Inject slowly over 3 to 5 minutes with the patient lying down. Rapid intravenous injection increases the incidence of associated ADRs, including apnea, hypotension, peripheral circulatory collapse, severe respiratory depression, and cardiac arrest. Do *not* inject meperidine intravenously unless an opiate antagonist (i.e., naloxone [Narcan®]) and the facilities and equipment needed for emergency symptomatic medical support of body systems, including equipment for assisted respiration, are immediately available.

SUBCUTANEOUS PHARMACOTHERAPY   Avoid subcutaneous injections because they are generally painful and have been associated with local tissue irritation and induration, particularly when repeated injections are required. Although subcutaneous injections may be used occasionally, intramuscular injections are preferred, particularly when repeated injections are required.

AVAILABLE DOSAGE FORMS, STORAGE, AND COMPATIBILITY

Injectables, intramuscular, intravenous, subcutaneous: 10, 25, 50, 75, 100 mg/ml
Syrup, oral: 50 mg/5 ml (banana flavored)
Tablets, oral: 50, 100 mg

Notes

Injectable Formulations   Do not combine the injectable meperidine solution with an injectable barbiturate solution because of physical incompatibility. Store injectables safely at controlled room temperature (15° to 25°C; 59° to 77°F).

General Instructions for Patients   Instruct patients who are receiving meperidine pharmacotherapy to

- ingest each dose of the meperidine oral syrup with water (30 to 60 ml [1 to 2 ounces]) to minimize associated topical anesthesia of the mouth and throat.
- safely store the meperidine oral syrup and tablets out of the reach of children in tightly closed child- and light-resistant containers at controlled room temperature (15° to 30°C; 59° to 86°F).
- obtain an available patient information sheet regarding meperidine pharmacotherapy from their pharmacist at the time that their prescription is dispensed. Encourage patients to clarify any questions that they may have concerning meperidine pharmacotherapy with their pharmacist or, if needed, to consult their prescribing psychologist.

PROPOSED MECHANISM OF ACTION

Meperidine appears to elicit its analgesic and CNS and respiratory depressant actions primarily by binding to the endorphin receptors in the CNS. However, the exact mechanism of action has not yet been fully determined.

See also Opiate Analgesics General Monograph

PHARMACOKINETICS/PHARMACODYNAMICS

Meperidine has several therapeutic actions qualitatively similar to those of morphine, one of which is analgesia. When injected in doses of 80 to 100 mg, meperidine is approximately equivalent in analgesic action to 10 mg of morphine. The onset of action is slightly more rapid than that for morphine, although the duration of action is slightly shorter. Meperidine is significantly less effective following oral ingestion than when injected. However, the exact ratio of oral to injectable analgesia has not been determined.

Meperidine is moderately absorbed (approximately 52%) following oral ingestion. Peak analgesia occurs generally within 1 hour after oral ingestion or intramuscular, intravenous, or subcutaneous injection. Analgesia may last for up to 2 to 4 hours. Meperidine is extensively metabolized, primarily in the liver, with only approximately 5% eliminated in unchanged form in the urine. Total body clearance is approximately 850 ml/minute. The mean half-life of elimination is approximately 3 hours. Normeperidine, an active metabolite of meperidine, is associated with CNS excitation and may accumulate among patients who have kidney dysfunction.

Meperidine is a weak acid. Therefore, alkalinization of the urine will decrease its excretion, and acidification of the urine will increase its excretion. These changes in urinary pH may significantly affect the amount of meperidine, or its metabolite, that is excreted in the urine, the total body clearance, and the half-life of elimination. Additional data are unavailable.

RELATIVE CONTRAINDICATIONS

Coma

Hypersensitivity to meperidine

MAOI pharmacotherapy, concurrent or within 14 days. Concurrent pharmacotherapy may result in the occurrence of serious ADRs. The mechanism of these reactions is unknown. However, they may be related to a pre-existing hyperphenylalaninemia. Some reactions resemble acute opiate analgesic overdosage and are characterized by coma, cyanosis, hypotension, and respiratory depression. Other reactions have been predominantly associated with convulsions, hyperexcitability, hyperpyrexia (body temperature of 41°C [106°F]), hypertension, and tachycardia. If opiate analgesic pharmacotherapy is required for patients who are receiving MAOI pharmacotherapy, or have received such pharmacotherapy within 14 days, a morphine sensitivity test should be performed prior to initiating meperidine or other opiate analgesic pharmacotherapy. Small, repeated incremental doses of morphine are injected over the course of several hours with direct medical monitoring of body systems. Collaboration with the patient's family physician or a specialist in morphine sensitivity testing is required.

Porphyria. Meperidine pharmacotherapy can precipitate an acute attack of porphyria among these patients.

Ritonavir pharmacotherapy. See Clinically Significant Drug Interactions.

CAUTIONS AND COMMENTS

Meperidine is referred to in Canada and the United Kingdom as "pethidine."

Meperidine is addicting and habituating. Meperidine pharmacotherapy can produce addiction and habituation similar to that associated with morphine and other opiate analgesics. Thus, it has high abuse potential.

Using a reduced dosage, prescribe meperidine pharmacotherapy cautiously to patients who

- have acute abdominal disorders (e.g., appendicitis). Meperidine may obscure the medical diagnosis or clinical course of these disorders.
- have atrial flutter and other supraventricular tachycardias. Meperidine pharmacotherapy may cause a possible vagolytic action that may produce a significant increase in the ventricular response rate among these patients.
- have head injuries, other medical disorders associated with increased intracranial pressure, or pre-existing increased intracranial pressure. The respiratory depressant action of meperidine and its ability to increase cerebrospinal fluid pressure may be markedly exaggerated among these patients. Opiate analgesics also produce ADRs that may obscure the clinical course of these patients. Meperidine pharmacotherapy must be prescribed with extreme caution for these patients.
- have histories of problematic patterns of meperidine or other abusable psychotropic use. Meperidine has high abuse potential. Prescribe meperidine pharmacotherapy cautiously to these patients, and monitor them closely for problematic patterns of use.
- regularly drink alcohol or are receiving concurrent pharmacotherapy with other opiate analgesics, sedative-hypnotics, or other drugs that depress the CNS (e.g., phenothiazines, TCAs). Hypotension, profound sedation, respiratory depression, and coma may occur among these patients.
- have seizure disorders. Meperidine pharmacotherapy may aggravate seizure disorders.
- have severe kidney or liver dysfunction because of the potential accumulation of meperidine's metabolite, normeperidine. Observe for associated signs and symptoms of CNS stimulation (e.g., agitation, irritability, nervousness, seizures) among these patients.
- have status asthmaticus (acute asthmatic attack), chronic obstructive pulmonary disease, cor pulmonale, substantially decreased respiratory reserve, or pre-existing respiratory depression, hypoxia, or hypercapnia. Even usual recommended dosages of meperidine for these patients may decrease their respiratory drive while simultaneously increasing airway resistance to the point of apnea.

Caution patients who are receiving meperidine pharmacotherapy against performing activities that require alertness, judgment, and physical coordination (e.g., driving an automobile, operating dangerous equipment, supervising children) until their response to meperidine is known. Meperidine may adversely affect these mental and physical functions.

In addition to this general precaution, caution patients to inform their prescribing psychologist if they begin or discontinue any other pharmacotherapy while receiving meperidine pharmacotherapy.

CLINICALLY SIGNIFICANT DRUG INTERACTIONS

Concurrent meperidine pharmacotherapy and the following may result in clinically significant drug interactions:

Alcohol Use

Concurrent alcohol use may increase the CNS depressant action of meperidine. Advise patients to avoid, or limit, their use of alcohol while receiving meperidine pharmacotherapy.

Pharmacotherapy With Central Nervous System Depressants and Other Drugs That Produce Central Nervous System Depression

Concurrent meperidine pharmacotherapy with other opiate analgesics, sedative-hypnotics, or other drugs that produce CNS depression (e.g., antihistamines, phenothiazines, TCAs) may result in additive CNS depression.

Ritonavir Pharmacotherapy

Ritonavir (Norvir®), an antiretroviral drug indicated for the pharmacologic management of HIV infection, can significantly inhibit the hepatic microsomal enzyme metabolism of meperidine. This interaction may result in severe toxicity, including cardiac dysrhythmias and seizures. Concurrent meperidine and ritonavir pharmacotherapy is *contraindicated*.

See also Opiate Analgesics General Monograph

ADVERSE DRUG REACTIONS

The most serious ADRs associated with meperidine pharmacotherapy include respiratory depression, circulatory depression, respiratory arrest, shock, and cardiac arrest. Other ADRs are listed according to body system. Some of these ADRs reportedly are more common among non-hospitalized or ambulatory patients and those who are not experiencing severe pain. Prescribing lower dosages, or advising these patients to lie down following the administration of meperidine, may be of benefit.

Cardiovascular: bradycardia, cardiovascular depression, fainting (syncope), hypotension, palpitations, phlebitis (following intravenous injection), and tachycardia
CNS: agitation, CNS depression, disorientation, dizziness, dysphoria, euphoria, hallucinations (transient), headache, lightheadedness, sedation, and seizures (severe)
Cutaneous: hives (urticaria), severe itching (pruritus), and other skin rashes; sweating (excessive); and wheal and flare at intravenous injection sites
Genitourinary: diminished amount of urine formation (oliguria) and urinary retention
GI: biliary tract spasm, constipation, dry mouth, nausea, and vomiting
Musculoskeletal: incoordinated muscle movements, tremor, and weakness
Ocular: visual disturbances
Respiratory: respiratory depression

See also Opiate Analgesics General Monograph

OVERDOSAGE

Signs and symptoms of meperidine overdosage include respiratory depression with a decrease in rate and tidal volume, Cheyne-Stokes respiration, cyanosis, extreme somnolence progressing to stupor or coma, skeletal muscle flaccidity, cold and clammy skin, and, sometimes, bradycardia and hypotension. In severe overdosage, particularly that involving intravenous injection, apnea, circulatory collapse, cardiac arrest, and death may occur. Meperidine overdosage requires emergency symptomatic medical support of respiratory and other body systems with attention to increasing meperidine elimination. The opiate antagonist naloxone (Narcan®) is a specific antidote for treating the respiratory depression associated with meperidine and other opiate analgesic overdosage. If patients are addicted to opiates, the use of the opiate antagonist will precipitate an acute opiate withdrawal syndrome. The severity of the withdrawal syndrome depends on the patient's degree of opiate analgesic addiction, the amount of opiate involved in the overdosage, the time elapsed before seeking emergency treatment, and the dose of the antagonist injected. Lower dosages of the opiate analgesic antagonist (10% to 20% of the usual recommended initial dosage) are generally recommended for these patients.

MEPHOBARBITAL *

(me foe bar'bi tal)

TRADE NAME

Mebaral®

CLASSIFICATION

Sedative-hypnotic (barbiturate) (C-IV)

See also Barbiturates General Monograph

APPROVED INDICATIONS FOR PSYCHOLOGICAL DISORDERS

Adjunctive pharmacotherapy for the symptomatic management of:

Anxiety Disorders. Mephobarbital pharmacotherapy is *not* indicated for the management of everyday anxiety or tension or of anxiety that can be managed with psychotherapy alone. Mephobarbital also is *not* recommended for the management of anxiety associated with depression because it has the potential to exacerbate the depression while alleviating the anxiety. The depression associated with anxiety generally resolves with appropriate adjunctive pharmacotherapy (i.e., antidepressant pharmacotherapy) and psychotherapy.

USUAL DOSAGE AND ADMINISTRATION

Anxiety Disorders

Adults: 96 to 400 mg daily orally in three or four divided doses

Women who are, or who may become, pregnant: FDA Pregnancy Category D. Safety and efficacy of mephobarbital pharmacotherapy for women who are pregnant have not been established. Mephobarbital readily crosses the placenta after injection, resulting in fetal blood levels that approach maternal blood levels. Its use during pregnancy has been associated with a wide variety of congenital malformations (i.e., birth defects) including atrial septal defect, cleft lip and palate, congenital hip dislocation, inguinal hernia, talipes equinus, and ventricular septal defect. Do *not* prescribe mephobarbital pharmacotherapy to women who are pregnant.

Women who are breast-feeding: Safety and efficacy of mephobarbital pharmacotherapy for women who are breast-feeding and their neonates and infants have not been established. Small amounts of barbiturate are excreted in breast milk. Avoid prescribing mephobarbital pharmacotherapy to women who are breast-feeding. If mephobarbital pharmacotherapy is required, breast-feeding probably should be discontinued. If desired, lactation may be maintained and breast-feeding resumed following the discontinuation of short-term mephobarbital pharmacotherapy. Collaboration with the patient's pediatrician is indicated.

Elderly, frail, or debilitated patients and those who have kidney or liver dysfunction: Generally prescribe lower dosages for elderly, frail, or debilitated patients. Increase the dosage gradually, if needed, according to individual patient response. These patients may be more sensitive to the pharmacologic actions of mephobarbital than are younger or healthier adult patients.

Children: 48 to 128 mg daily orally in three or four divided doses

Notes, Anxiety Disorders

Although mephobarbital and other barbiturates may be prescribed for the symptomatic management of anxiety disorders, they are *not* the sedative-hypnotics of first choice. The benzodiazepines are the sedative-hypnotics of first choice when adjunctive pharmacotherapy is required for the symptomatic management of anxiety disorders. The benzodiazepines have greater clinical efficacy, safety, and lower incidence and severity of ADRs when compared to the barbiturates and other sedative-hypnotics. Mephobarbital pharmacotherapy for the symptomatic management of anxiety disorders should be reserved for patients who are hypersensitive to the benzodiazepines or, for any other reason (e.g., contraindication), cannot be prescribed benzodiazepine pharmacotherapy.

AVAILABLE DOSAGE FORMS, STORAGE, AND COMPATIBILITY

Tablets, oral: 32, 50, 100 mg

Notes

General Instructions for Patients   Instruct patients who are receiving mephobarbital pharmacotherapy to

- safely store mephobarbital oral tablets out of the reach of children in tightly closed child- and light-resistant containers.

• obtain an available patient information sheet regarding mephobarbital pharmacotherapy from their pharmacist at the time that their prescription is dispensed. Encourage patients to clarify any questions that they may have concerning mephobarbital pharmacotherapy with their pharmacist or, if needed, to consult their prescribing psychologist.

PROPOSED MECHANISM OF ACTION

The exact mechanism of mephobarbital's sedative or anxiolytic action has not yet been fully determined. However, mephobarbital appears to act primarily at the level of the thalamus, where it interferes with impulse transmission to the cortex.

See also Barbiturates General Monograph

PHARMACOKINETICS/PHARMACODYNAMICS

Mephobarbital has strong sedative action but relatively weak hypnotic action. Thus, mephobarbital pharmacotherapy is usually associated with little or no drowsiness or lassitude. When prescribed as a sedative for the symptomatic management of anxiety, patients usually become more calm, cheerful, and better adjusted to their surroundings without significant mental impairment. After oral ingestion, approximately half of the mephobarbital dose is absorbed from the GI tract. It has an onset of action of 30 to 60 minutes and its duration of action is 10 to 16 hours.

The lipid solubility of barbiturates, such as mephobarbital, results in their rapid and widespread distribution throughout the body. Particularly high concentrations are achieved in the brain, kidneys, and liver. Therapeutic blood levels have not been established nor has the half-life of elimination. Mephobarbital is metabolized primarily (i.e., approximately 75% of a single dose in 24 hours) by the microsomal enzymes of the liver to phenobarbital. The phenobarbital is excreted in the urine in unchanged form or as glucuronide or sulfate conjugates. Thus, long-term mephobarbital pharmacotherapy, such as that required for the symptomatic management of seizure disorders, may result in the accumulation of phenobarbital in the blood. It is unclear whether mephobarbital or phenobarbital is the active drug during long-term mephobarbital pharmacotherapy.

See also Phenobarbital and Barbiturates General Monographs

RELATIVE CONTRAINDICATIONS

Hypersensitivity to mephobarbital or other barbiturates
Liver dysfunction, severe
Porphyria, active or latent

CAUTIONS AND COMMENTS

Addiction and habituation have been associated with long-term mephobarbital pharmacotherapy and regular personal use. Abrupt discontinuation of long-term mephobarbital pharmacotherapy, or regular personal use, may result in the signs and symptoms of the barbiturate withdrawal syndrome. These signs and symptoms include status epilepticus. Prescribe the smallest quantity of mephobarbital feasible for dispensing at one time to minimize the possible development of problematic patterns of use or overdosage.

Prescribe mephobarbital pharmacotherapy cautiously for patients who

- are receiving oral anticoagulant pharmacotherapy because of the associated difficulty in stabilizing prothrombin times. Avoid prescribing mephobarbital pharmacotherapy to patients who are receiving oral anticoagulant pharmacotherapy. If mephobarbital pharmacotherapy is required, collaboration with the prescriber of the anticoagulant is indicated.
- have CNS depression. Mephobarbital pharmacotherapy may increase CNS depression among these patients.
- have kidney dysfunction. Adjust the dosage carefully for these patients.
- have liver dysfunction. Adjust the dosage carefully for these patients.
- have respiratory dysfunction, including respiratory depression

Caution patients who are receiving mephobarbital pharmacotherapy against

- drinking alcohol or using other drugs that can produce CNS depression. Concurrent use of alcohol or other drugs that produce CNS depression can result in excessive CNS depression.
- performing activities that require alertness, judgment, and physical coordination (e.g., driving an automobile, operating dangerous equipment, supervising children) until their response to mephobarbital pharmacotherapy is known. Mephobarbital may adversely affect these mental and physical functions.

In addition to these general precautions, caution patients to inform their prescribing psychologist if they begin or discontinue any other pharmacotherapy while receiving mephobarbital pharmacotherapy.

CLINICALLY SIGNIFICANT DRUG INTERACTIONS

Concurrent mephobarbital pharmacotherapy and the following may result in clinically significant drug interactions:

Alcohol Use

Concurrent alcohol use may increase the CNS depressant action of mephobarbital. Advise patients to avoid, or limit, their use of alcohol while receiving mephobarbital pharmacotherapy.

Pharmacotherapy With Central Nervous System Depressants and Other Drugs That Produce Central Nervous System Depression

Concurrent mephobarbital pharmacotherapy with opiate analgesics, other sedative-hypnotics, or other drugs that produce CNS depression (e.g., antihistamines, phenothiazines, TCAs) may result in additive CNS depression.
See also Barbiturates General Monograph

Pharmacotherapy With Drugs That are Primarily Metabolized in the Liver

Mephobarbital may stimulate the production of the hepatic microsomal enzymes that are responsible for the metabolism of many different drugs. Whenever mephobarbital is added to or removed from a patient's pharmacotherapy, attention must be given to the effect on concurrent pharmacotherapy (e.g., corticosteroid, oral anticoagulant, oral contraceptive, or quinidine [Biquin®] pharmacotherapy). Dosage adjustments (i.e., an increase or decrease in dosage) may be required. Collaboration with the patient's family physician or other prescribers (e.g., dentist, advanced practice nurse) is indicated.

ADVERSE DRUG REACTIONS

Mephobarbital pharmacotherapy has been associated with drowsiness and, rarely, vertigo. It also may cause ADRs that are associated with other barbiturates because of its chemical and pharmacological similarity to the other drugs in this class.

See Phenobarbital and Barbiturates General Monographs

OVERDOSAGE

The signs and symptoms of mephobarbital overdosage are similar to those associated with other barbiturate overdosage.

See Phenobarbital and Barbiturates General Monographs

MEPROBAMATE

(me proe ba′mate)

TRADE NAMES

Equanil®
Meprospan®
Miltown®
Novo-Mepro®

CLASSIFICATION

Sedative-hypnotic (carbamate derivative) (C-IV)

APPROVED INDICATIONS FOR PSYCHOLOGICAL DISORDERS

Adjunctive pharmacotherapy for the short-term symptomatic management of:

Anxiety Disorders. Meprobamate pharmacotherapy is *not* indicated for the management of everyday anxiety or tension or of anxiety that can be managed with psychotherapy alone.

Meprobamate also is *not* recommended for the management of anxiety associated with depression because it has the potential to exacerbate the depression while alleviating the anxiety. The depression associated with anxiety generally resolves with appropriate adjunctive pharmacotherapy (i.e., antidepressant pharmacotherapy) and psychotherapy.

USUAL DOSAGE AND ADMINISTRATION

Anxiety Disorders

Adults: 1,200 to 1,600 mg daily orally in three or four divided doses, *or* 800 to 1,600 mg extended-release capsules daily orally in two divided doses (i.e., upon awakening in the morning and before retiring for bed in the evening)

MAXIMUM: 2,400 mg daily orally

Women who are, or who may become, pregnant: FDA Pregnancy Category D. Safety and efficacy of meprobamate pharmacotherapy for women who are pregnant have not been established. Meprobamate crosses the placenta. Pharmacotherapy during the first trimester of pregnancy has been associated with an increased risk for congenital malformations (i.e., birth defects). Do *not* prescribe meprobamate pharmacotherapy to women who are pregnant.

Women who are breast-feeding: Safety and efficacy of meprobamate pharmacotherapy for women who are breast-feeding and their neonates and infants have not been established. Meprobamate is excreted in breast milk at concentrations two to four times that of maternal blood. This higher concentration in breast milk as compared to maternal blood may result in expected pharmacologic actions among breast-fed neonates and infants (e.g., drowsiness, lethargy), who also may become addicted. Do *not* prescribe meprobamate pharmacotherapy to women who are breast-feeding. If meprobamate pharmacotherapy is required, breast-feeding should be discontinued. If desired, lactation may be maintained and breast-feeding resumed following the discontinuation of short-term meprobamate pharmacotherapy. (See Relative Contraindications)

Elderly, frail, or debilitated patients: Generally prescribe lower dosages for elderly, frail, or debilitated patients. Increase the dosage gradually, if needed, according to individual patient response. These patients may be more sensitive to the pharmacologic actions of meprobamate than are younger or healthier adult patients. Prescribe the lowest effective dosage to avoid over-sedation among these patients.

Children younger than 6 years of age: Safety and efficacy of meprobamate pharmacotherapy for children who are younger than 6 years of age have not been established. Meprobamate pharmacotherapy is *not* recommended for this age group.

Children 6 to 12 years of age: 200 to 600 mg daily orally in two or three divided doses, *or* 400 mg extended-release capsules daily orally in two divided doses, morning and evening 30 minutes before bedtime

MAXIMUM: 1,000 mg daily orally

Notes, Anxiety Disorders

The safety and efficacy of meprobamate pharmacotherapy for longer than four months have not been established. Reevaluate therapeutic benefit periodically for patients who appear to require longer pharmacotherapy. Avoid abrupt discontinuation of long-term, high-dosage pharmacotherapy, or regular personal use. Abrupt discontinuation may precipitate a recurrence of the initial signs and symptoms of the anxiety disorder, including anorexia, anxiety, and insomnia. Abrupt discontinuation of pharmacotherapy can also precipitate the meprobamate withdrawal syndrome.

Signs and symptoms of the meprobamate withdrawal syndrome include confusion, hallucinations, incoordination (ataxia), muscle twitching, vomiting, and, rarely, seizures. Seizures are more likely to occur among patients who have histories of CNS injury or dysfunction or pre-existing or latent seizure disorders. The signs and symptoms of meprobamate withdrawal occur within 12 to 48 hours after its discontinuation. In order to avoid precipitating the meprobamate withdrawal syndrome, reduce the dosage gradually over one to two weeks. A short-acting barbiturate may be required during this period for the symptomatic management of the signs and symptoms of withdrawal.

AVAILABLE DOSAGE FORMS, STORAGE, AND COMPATIBILITY

Capsules, oral extended-release (Meprospan®): 200, 400 mg
Tablets, oral: 200, 400, 600 mg

Notes

General Instructions for Patients   Instruct patients who are receiving meprobamate pharmacotherapy to

- safely store meprobamate oral tablets out of the reach of children in tightly closed child-resistant containers at controlled room temperature (15° to 30°C; 59° to 86°F).
- obtain an available patient information sheet regarding meprobamate pharmacotherapy from their pharmacist at the time that their prescription is dispensed. Encourage patients to clarify any questions that they may have concerning meprobamate pharmacotherapy with their pharmacist or, if needed, to consult their prescribing psychologist.

PROPOSED MECHANISM OF ACTION

Although the exact mechanism of action for meprobamate has not yet been determined, it appears to act at multiple sites in the CNS, including the thalamus and the limbic system.

PHARMACOKINETICS/PHARMACODYNAMICS

Meprobamate is well absorbed following oral ingestion. Its onset of action is within 1 hour. Peak blood levels are achieved within 1 to 3 hours. It is only slightly bound to plasma proteins (~20%) but appears to be uniformly distributed throughout the body tissues. Meprobamate is metabolized extensively in the liver to several inactive metabolites. Approximately 10% is excreted in unchanged form in the urine. The mean half-life of elimination is 10 hours (range 6 to 16 hours). Additional data are unavailable.

Therapeutic Drug Monitoring

Optimal therapeutic meprobamate blood concentrations have not been determined. However, meprobamate blood concentrations may be useful for the management of overdosage and related toxicity. In this regard, blood concentrations of 30 to 100 μg/ml are generally associated with stupor or light coma, 100 to 200 μg/ml are generally associated with deep coma and are potentially fatal, and >200 μg/ml increasingly result in death.

RELATIVE CONTRAINDICATIONS

Breast-feeding. The concentration of meprobamate in breast milk is 2 to 4 times that of the
  maternal blood concentration.
Hypersensitivity to meprobamate or related drugs (e.g., carisoprodol [Soma®])
Porphyria, acute intermittent
Pregnancy

CAUTIONS AND COMMENTS

Meprobamate pharmacotherapy is associated with addiction and habituation, particularly long-term pharmacotherapy with higher than recommended dosages, or regular personal use. Signs and symptoms of problematic patterns of use may include incoordination (ataxia), slurred speech, and vertigo.
Prescribe meprobamate pharmacotherapy cautiously to patients who

* have histories of problematic patterns of alcohol or other abusable psychotropic use. These patients may be more likely to develop problematic patterns of meprobamate use.
* have kidney or liver dysfunction. Meprobamate is metabolized in the liver and is excreted by the kidneys. Meprobamate accumulation and toxicity may occur among these patients.
* have seizure disorders, including epilepsy. Meprobamate may occasionally induce seizures among these patients.

Caution patients who are receiving meprobamate pharmacotherapy against performing activities that require alertness, judgment, and physical coordination (e.g., driving an automobile, operating dangerous equipment, supervising children) until their response to meprobamate pharmacotherapy is known. Meprobamate may adversely affect these mental and physical functions.
In addition to this general precaution, caution women to inform their prescribing psychologist if they become, or intend to become, pregnant while receiving meprobamate pharmacotherapy, so that their pharmacotherapy can be safely discontinued.

CLINICALLY SIGNIFICANT DRUG INTERACTIONS

Concurrent meprobamate pharmacotherapy and the following may result in clinically significant drug interactions:

Alcohol Use

Concurrent alcohol use may increase the CNS depressant action of meprobamate. Advise patients to avoid, or limit, their use of alcohol while receiving meprobamate pharmacotherapy.

Pharmacotherapy With Central Nervous System Depressants and Other Drugs That Produce Central Nervous System Depression

Concurrent meprobamate pharmacotherapy with opiate analgesics, other sedative-hypnotics, or other drugs that produce CNS depression (e.g., antihistamines, phenothiazines, TCAs) may result in additive CNS depression.

ADVERSE DRUG REACTIONS

Meprobamate pharmacotherapy has been associated with hypersensitivity or idiosyncratic reactions. These hypersensitivity reactions have been observed among susceptible patients who have reported no previous meprobamate pharmacotherapy. These reactions generally have occurred between the first and fourth doses of meprobamate pharmacotherapy. Reactions can be mild or severe. A milder reaction may be generalized or confined to the groin and involve an itchy, urticarial, or erythematous maculopapular rash. Other reactions may include adenopathy, ecchymoses, eosinophilia, fever, fixed drug eruptions (with cross-reaction to carisoprodol, as well as cross-sensitivity between meprobamate and mebutamate and meprobamate and carbromal), leukopenia, nonthrombocytopenic purpura, peripheral edema, and petechiae. More severe reactions rarely may include anaphylaxis, angioneurotic edema, anuria, bullous dermatitis, bronchospasm, chills, erythema multiforme, exfoliative dermatitis, hyperpyrexia, oliguria, proctitis, Stevens-Johnson syndrome, and stomatitis. In the event of hypersensitivity, or idiosyncratic reactions, discontinue meprobamate pharmacotherapy *immediately*. Refer patients for medical evaluation and treatment of presenting symptomatology. Emergency symptomatic medical support of body systems may be required.

Meprobamate pharmacotherapy also has been associated with the following ADRs, listed according to body system:

Cardiovascular: dysrhythmias (various), ECG changes, fainting (syncope), hypotensive crisis, palpitations, and tachycardia

CNS: dizziness, drowsiness, euphoria, headache, incoordination (ataxia), overstimulation, paradoxical excitement, paresthesias, rapid EEG activity, slurred speech, vertigo, and weakness

Cutaneous: rarely thrombocytopenic purpura

GI: diarrhea, nausea, and vomiting

Hematologic: rarely, aplastic anemia and fatal reduction in the blood neutrophil count (neutropenia [agranulocytosis, granulocytopenia]), which may result in an increased susceptibility to infections. Meprobamate pharmacotherapy may exacerbate the signs and symptoms of porphyria.

OVERDOSAGE

Signs and symptoms of meprobamate overdosage include coma, drowsiness, incoordination (ataxia), lethargy, stupor, and vasomotor and respiratory collapse. Meprobamate overdosage has been associated with the concurrent use of alcohol or other psychotropic drugs. It also has been associated with suicide attempts, some of which have been successful. Meprobamate overdosage, alone, or in combination with other psychotropic drugs, requires emergency symptomatic medical support of body systems with attention to increasing meprobamate (and other drug) elimination. There is no known antidote.

MESORIDAZINE

(mez oh rid′a zeen)

TRADE NAME

Serentil®

CLASSIFICATION

Antipsychotic (phenothiazine)

See also Phenothiazines General Monograph

APPROVED INDICATIONS FOR PSYCHOLOGICAL DISORDERS

Adjunctive pharmacotherapy for the symptomatic management of:

- Behavioral Problems (e.g., combativeness, uncooperativeness) Among Patients Who Have Mental Retardation or Organic Brain Syndrome
- Neuroses: Anxiety and Tension. The prescription of mesoridazine for the symptomatic management of anxiety neuroses, although officially approved, is considered to be outdated and inappropriate. The anxiety appears to be ameliorated by mesoridazine's anticholinergic actions (i.e., drowsiness, sedation). A more rational therapeutic approach would be to prescribe specific sedative-hypnotic anxiolytic pharmacotherapy, such as benzodiazepine pharmacotherapy. Benzodiazepine pharmacotherapy is associated with greater safety and efficacy and significantly fewer ADRs. See Benzodiazepines General Monograph
- Psychotic Disorders: Schizophrenia and Other Psychotic Disorders
- Substance-Related Disorders: Acute Alcohol Withdrawal. Mesoridazine pharmacotherapy ameliorates anxiety, delirium tremens (DTs), tension, nausea, and vomiting without further compromising liver function. Acute alcohol withdrawal that is not accompanied by DTs or related symptoms generally should be managed with appropriate benzodiazepine pharmacotherapy rather than mesoridazine pharmacotherapy.

See Benzodiazepines General Monograph

USUAL DOSAGE AND ADMINISTRATION

Behavioral Problems Among Patients Who Have Mental Retardation or Chronic Brain Syndrome

Adults: Initially, 75 mg daily orally in three divided doses. Adjust the dosage gradually according to individual patient response.

MAINTENANCE: 75 to 300 mg daily orally in three divided doses

Women who are, or who may become, pregnant: FDA Pregnancy Category "not established." Safety and efficacy of mesoridazine pharmacotherapy for women who are pregnant, particularly during the first trimester, have not been established. Avoid prescribing mesoridazine to women who are pregnant. If mesoridazine pharmacotherapy is required, advise patients (or their legal guardians in regard to the patient) of potential benefits and possible risks to themselves and the embryo, fetus, or neonate. Collaboration with the patient's obstetrician is required.

Women who are breast-feeding: Safety and efficacy of mesoridazine pharmacotherapy for women who are breast-feeding and their neonates and infants have not been established. Mesoridazine is excreted into breast milk. Avoid prescribing mesoridazine pharmacotherapy to women who are breast-feeding. If mesoridazine pharmacotherapy is required, breast-feeding probably should be discontinued. Collaboration with the patient's pediatrician is indicated.

Elderly, frail, or debilitated patients: Generally prescribe lower dosages for elderly, frail, or debilitated patients. Increase the dosage gradually, if needed, according to individual patient response. These patients may be more sensitive to the pharmacologic actions of mesoridazine than are younger or healthier adult patients.

Children younger than 12 years of age: Safety and efficacy of mesoridazine pharmacotherapy for children younger than 12 years of age have not been established. Mesoridazine pharmacotherapy is *not* recommended for this age group.

Notes, Behavioral Problems Among Patients Who Have Mental Retardation or Chronic Brain Syndrome

Initially, prescribe lower dosages and adjust the dosage according to individual patient response. When maximal therapeutic benefit is achieved, reduce the dosage gradually to the lowest effective maintenance dosage.

Schizophrenia and Other Psychotic Disorders

Adults: Initially, 150 mg daily orally in three divided doses. Adjust the dosage gradually according to individual patient response.

MAINTENANCE: 75 to 400 mg daily orally in three divided doses, *or* 25 to 200 mg daily intramuscularly. Optimal therapeutic benefit generally may be achieved without exceeding 200 mg daily.

MAXIMUM: 400 mg daily

Women who are, or who may become, pregnant: FDA Pregnancy Category "not established." Safety and efficacy of mesoridazine pharmacotherapy for women who are pregnant, particularly during the first trimester, have not been established. Avoid prescribing mesoridazine to women who are pregnant. If mesoridazine pharmacotherapy is required, advise patients (or their legal guardians in regard to the patient) of potential benefits and possible risks to themselves and the embryo, fetus, or neonate. Collaboration with the patient's obstetrician is required.

Women who are breast-feeding: Safety and efficacy of mesoridazine pharmacotherapy for women who are breast-feeding and their neonates and infants have not been established. Mesoridazine is excreted into breast milk. Avoid prescribing mesoridazine pharmacotherapy to women who are breast-feeding. If mesoridazine pharmacotherapy is required, breast-feeding probably should be discontinued. Collaboration with the patient's pediatrician is indicated.

Elderly, frail, or debilitated patients and those who have kidney dysfunction: Initiate mesoridazine pharmacotherapy with one-fourth to one-half of the usual adult dosage. Increase the dosage gradually, if needed, according to individual patient response. Generally prescribe lower dosages for elderly, frail, or debilitated patients. Patients who have kidney dysfunction may also require lower dosages. These patients may be more sensitive to the pharmacologic action of mesoridazine than are younger or healthier adult patients.

Children younger than 12 years of age: Safety and efficacy of mesoridazine pharmacotherapy for children younger than 12 years of age have not been established. Mesoridazine pharmacotherapy is *not* recommended for this age group.

Children and adolescents 12 years of age and older: 75 to 400 mg daily orally in three or four divided doses, *or* 25 to 200 mg daily intramuscularly. *Note: dosage is the same as the adult maintenance dosage.*

MAXIMUM: 400 mg daily

Notes, Schizophrenia and Other Psychotic Disorders

Initially, prescribe lower dosages, and adjust the dosage according to individual patient response. When maximal therapeutic benefit is achieved, reduce the dosage gradually to the lowest effective maintenance dosage.

Intramuscular Mesoridazine Pharmacotherapy   Patients should be lying down for intramuscular mesoridazine pharmacotherapy and should remain lying down for 30 to 60 minutes after their injections. Intramuscular pharmacotherapy has been associated with postural (orthostatic) hypotension and falls. Monitor patients for postural hypotension, and also instruct patients to report any changes in vision following intramuscular pharmacotherapy.

Substance-Related Disorders: Acute Alcohol Withdrawal

Adults: Initially, 50 mg daily orally in two divided doses. Adjust dosage according to individual patient response.

MAXIMUM: 200 mg daily orally

Women who are, or who may become, pregnant: FDA Pregnancy Category "not established." Safety and efficacy of mesoridazine pharmacotherapy for women who are pregnant, particularly during the first trimester, have not been established. Avoid prescribing mesoridazine pharmacotherapy to women who are pregnant. If mesoridazine pharmacotherapy is required, advise patients of potential benefits and possible risks to themselves and the embryo, fetus, or neonate. Collaboration with the patient's obstetrician is required.

Women who are breast-feeding: Safety and efficacy of mesoridazine pharmacotherapy for women who are breast-feeding and their neonates and infants have not been established. Mesoridazine is excreted into breast milk. Avoid prescribing mesoridazine pharmacotherapy to women who are breast-feeding. If mesoridazine pharmacotherapy is required, breast-feeding probably should be discontinued. Collaboration with the patient's pediatrician is indicated.

Elderly, frail, or debilitated patients: Generally prescribe lower dosages for elderly, frail, or debilitated patients. Increase the dosage gradually, if needed, according to individual patient response. These patients may be more sensitive to the pharmacologic actions of mesoridazine than are younger or healthier adult patients.

Children younger than 12 years of age: Safety and efficacy of mesoridazine pharmacotherapy for children younger than 12 years of age have not been established. Mesoridazine pharmacotherapy is *not* recommended for this age group.

Notes, Substance-Related Disorders: Acute Alcohol Withdrawal

Initially, prescribe lower dosages, and adjust the dosage according to individual patient response. When maximal therapeutic benefit is achieved, reduce the dosage gradually to the lowest effective maintenance dosage.

AVAILABLE DOSAGE FORMS, STORAGE, AND COMPATIBILITY

Injectable, intramuscular: 25 mg/ml (ampule)
Concentrate, oral: 25 mg/ml (contains 0.61% alcohol)
Tablets, oral: 10, 25, 50, 100 mg

Notes

The injectable formulation is for intramuscular use only. Do *not* inject intravenously.

General Instructions for Patients Instruct patients who are receiving mesoridazine pharmacotherapy (or those responsible for their pharmacotherapy) to

- dilute each dose of the mesoridazine oral concentrate with acidified tap water, distilled water, grape juice, or orange juice immediately prior to ingestion. Advise patients *against* preparing and storing bulk dilutions for later use.

- measure each dose of the mesoridazine oral concentrate with the accompanying calibrated dropper to help to assure that an accurate dose is measured.
- safely store the mesoridazine oral concentrate and tablets out of the reach of children in tightly closed child- and light-resistant containers below 30°C (86°F).
- obtain an available patient information sheet regarding mesoridazine pharmacotherapy from their pharmacist at the time that their prescription is dispensed. Encourage patients to clarify any questions that they may have concerning mesoridazine pharmacotherapy with their pharmacist or, if needed, to consult their prescribing psychologist.

PROPOSED MECHANISM OF ACTION

The exact mechanism of action of mesoridazine is complex and has not yet been fully determined. However, its antipsychotic activity appears to be related primarily to its interaction with dopamine-containing neurons, specifically the blockade of dopamine receptors both pre-synaptically and post-synaptically.

See also Phenothiazines General Monograph

PHARMACOKINETICS/PHARMACODYNAMICS

Mesoridazine is well absorbed after oral ingestion and attains peak blood levels within 4 hours. Approximately 40% of an oral or intramuscular dose is excreted in the urine, and approximately 30% is excreted in the feces. Additional data are unavailable.

RELATIVE CONTRAINDICATIONS

Blood disorders
Bone marrow depression
Cardiovascular disorders, severe
CNS depression, severe
Coma
Hypersensitivity to mesoridazine or other phenothiazines
Hypertension, severe
Hypotension, severe
Liver dysfunction, severe

CAUTIONS AND COMMENTS

Prescribe mesoridazine pharmacotherapy cautiously to patients who have histories of heart disease. Prolongation of the Q-T interval, flattening and inversion of the T-wave, and the appearance of a wave tentatively identified as a bifid T or U wave, all of which are generally reversible, have been associated with mesoridazine and other phenothiazine pharmacotherapy. Collaboration with the patient's cardiologist is indicated. Additional precautions have been advised for patients who require mesoridazine and other phenothiazine pharmacotherapy.

Caution patients who are receiving mesoridazine pharmacotherapy against performing activities that require alertness, judgment, and physical coordination (e.g., driving an automobile, operating dangerous equipment, supervising children) until their response to mesoridazine is known. Mesoridazine may adversely affect these mental and physical functions.

CLINICALLY SIGNIFICANT DRUG INTERACTIONS

Concurrent mesoridazine pharmacotherapy and the following may result in clinically significant drug interactions:

Guanethidine Pharmacotherapy

Mesoridazine may decrease the neuronal uptake of guanethidine (Ismelin®) and, thus, decrease its antihypertensive action. The dosage of the guanethidine may require adjustment. Collaboration with the prescriber of the guanethidine is indicated.

Pharmacotherapy With Anticholinergics or Other Drugs That Produce Anticholinergic Actions

Concurrent mesoridazine pharmacotherapy with anticholinergics (e.g., atropine) and other drugs that produce anticholinergic actions (e.g., TCAs) may result in additive anticholinergic actions.

See also Phenothiazines General Monograph

ADVERSE DRUG REACTIONS

Mesoridazine pharmacotherapy commonly has been associated with drowsiness, sedation, and other ADRs related to its anticholinergic actions (e.g., blurred vision, dry mouth, decreased GI motility, tachycardia, urinary retention). These ADRs generally occur when mesoridazine pharmacotherapy is initiated or when high dosages are prescribed. These ADRs generally can be managed by reducing the dosage. Hypotension also has been reported. Although hypotension is usually mild, collaboration with the patient's advanced practice nurse, family physician, or a specialist (e.g., cardiologist) is required for its appropriate management.

Ocular pigmentary changes and other potentially serious ADRs, including TD, other EPRs, over-sedation, and unexpected, sudden death, have been associated with phenothiazines of the piperidine class, to which mesoridazine belongs. Although not directly associated with mesoridazine pharmacotherapy, the possible occurrence of these ADRs cannot be excluded for patients who are receiving mesoridazine pharmacotherapy. Monitor patients, particularly those who are receiving long-term high-dosage pharmacotherapy, for these ADRs. Collaboration with the patient's ophthalmologist is indicated for the regular periodic monitoring, including complete eye examinations, for possible ocular reactions.

See also Phenothiazines General Monograph

OVERDOSAGE

Signs and symptoms of mesoridazine overdosage include agitation, confusion, delirium, and drowsiness. Areflexia and coma may occur with severe overdosage. Unlike other phenothiazine overdosages, respiratory depression, a late sign of severe phenothiazine overdosage, and acute EPRs (e.g., dystonia, oculogyric crisis), convulsions, and restlessness have not been directly associated with mesoridazine overdosage. However, these signs and symptoms may occur with mesoridazine overdosage because of its chemical and pharmacological similarity to other phenothiazines. Mesoridazine overdosage requires emergency symptomatic medical support of body systems with attention to increasing mesoridazine elimination. There is no known antidote.

METHADONE

(meth'a done)

TRADE NAMES

Dolophine®
Methadose®

CLASSIFICATION

Opiate analgesic (C-II)

See also Opiate Analgesics General Monograph

APPROVED INDICATIONS FOR PSYCHOLOGICAL DISORDERS

Adjunctive pharmacotherapy for the symptomatic management of:

- Pain Disorders: Acute Pain, Moderate to Severe
- Substance Use Disorders: Opiate Addiction Detoxification
- Substance Use Disorders: Opiate Addiction Maintenance

USUAL DOSAGE AND ADMINISTRATION

Acute Pain, Moderate to Severe

Adults: 0.1 mg/kg (generally 2.5 to 10 mg) intramuscularly, orally, or subcutaneously every three or four hours, as needed

MAXIMUM: 10 mg/dose

Women who are, or who may become, pregnant: FDA Pregnancy Category C. Safety and efficacy of methadone pharmacotherapy for women who are pregnant have not been established. Methadone crosses the placenta. Long-term pharmacotherapy, or regular personal use, during pregnancy will result in the neonatal addiction syndrome. Avoid prescribing methadone pharmacotherapy to women who are pregnant. If methadone pharmacotherapy is required, advise patients of potential benefits and possible risks to themselves and the embryo, fetus, or neonate. Collaboration with the patient's obstetrician is indicated.

Women who are breast-feeding: Safety and efficacy of methadone pharmacotherapy for women who are breast-feeding and their neonates and infants have not been established. Methadone is excreted in breast milk in concentrations up to 85% of those in the maternal blood. Expected pharmacologic actions (e.g., drowsiness, lethargy, respiratory depression) may be observed among breast-fed neonates and infants, who also may become addicted. Avoid prescribing methadone pharmacotherapy to women who are breast-feeding. If methadone pharmacotherapy is required, breast-feeding probably should be discontinued. If desired, lactation may be maintained and breast-feeding resumed following the discontinuation of short-term methadone pharmacotherapy. Collaboration with the patient's pediatrician is indicated.

Elderly, frail, or debilitated patients and those who have kidney dysfunction: Generally prescribe lower dosages for elderly, frail, or debilitated patients. Increase the dosage gradually, if needed, according to individual patient response. These patients may be more sensitive to the pharmacologic actions of methadone than are younger or healthier adult patients. Patients who have kidney dysfunction also may require lower dosages.

Children: Safety and efficacy of methadone pharmacotherapy for the symptomatic management of acute pain for children have not been established. Methadone pharmacotherapy for this indication is *not* recommended for this age group.

Notes, Acute Pain, Moderate to Severe

Adjust the dosage according to the severity of the patient's pain and individual response to methadone pharmacotherapy. Patients who have severe pain, or those who have developed a tolerance to the analgesic action of methadone or other opiate analgesics, may require dosages that exceed the usual recommended dosages. Also note the differences in duration of action for injectable and oral dosage formulations.

Oral Methadone Pharmacotherapy Too frequent oral dosing over a few days may result in the signs and symptoms of drug accumulation and toxicity (e.g., somnolence, respiratory depression).

Injectable Methadone Pharmacotherapy An injectable dose of 10 mg of methadone is approximately equivalent in analgesic action to 10 mg of morphine. Intramuscular injection is preferred when repeated doses are required for patients who are unable to swallow, are vomiting, or for any other reason are unable to ingest the oral dosage formulations. Subcutaneous injection is suitable for occasional use.

Opiate Addiction Detoxification

Adults: Initially, 15 to 20 mg daily orally or intramuscularly in a single dose. Intramuscular pharmacotherapy is usually reserved for patients who are unable to ingest the oral dosage forms. Additional doses may be required to prevent the opiate withdrawal syndrome. Some patients may require 40 mg daily in single or divided doses. Stabilize patients for two to three days, and then gradually reduce the dosage at one or two day intervals, according to individual patient response. Maintain an adequate dosage to prevent the occurrence of the signs and symptoms of the opiate withdrawal syndrome. A daily reduction of 20% of the total daily dosage is usually tolerated by patients who are hospitalized, or otherwise closely monitored. Non-hospitalized patients may require a more gradual reduction in dosage (e.g., 10% daily).

If methadone pharmacotherapy for the symptomatic management of opiate detoxification is required for longer than three weeks (21 consecutive days), methadone pharmacotherapy is considered by U.S. federal regulation (Title 21, Section 291.505) to have changed from opiate addiction detoxification to opiate addiction maintenance.

Women who are, or who may become, pregnant: FDA Pregnancy Category C. Safety and efficacy of methadone pharmacotherapy for women who are pregnant have not been established. Methadone crosses the placenta. During pregnancy, long-term pharmacotherapy, or regular personal use, will result in the neonatal addiction syndrome. Avoid prescribing methadone pharmacotherapy to women who are pregnant. If methadone pharmacotherapy is required, advise patients of potential benefits and possible risks to themselves and the embryo, fetus, or neonate. Collaboration with the patient's obstetrician is indicated.

Women who are breast-feeding: Safety and efficacy of methadone pharmacotherapy for women who are breast-feeding, and their neonates and infants, have not been established. Methadone is excreted in breast milk in concentrations up to 85% of those of the maternal blood. Expected pharmacologic actions (e.g., drowsiness, lethargy, respiratory depression) may be observed among breast-fed neonates and infants, who also may become addicted. Avoid prescribing methadone pharmacotherapy to women who are breast-feeding. If methadone pharmacotherapy is required, breast-feeding should be discontinued. If desired, lactation may be maintained and breast-feeding resumed following the discontinuation of short-term methadone pharmacotherapy.

Elderly, frail, or debilitated patients and those who have kidney dysfunction: Generally prescribe lower dosages for elderly, frail, or debilitated patients. Patients who have kidney dysfunction also may require lower dosages. These patients may be more sensitive to the pharmacologic actions of methadone than are younger or healthier adult patients. Generally follow the recommended adult dosage guidelines while monitoring individual patient response.

Children younger than 12 years of age: Safety and efficacy of methadone pharmacotherapy for opiate addiction detoxification for children younger than 12 years of age have not been established. Methadone pharmacotherapy for this indication is *not* recommended for this age group.

Children and adolescents 12 years of age and older: Initially, 10 to 15 mg daily orally in a single dose. Generally follow the recommended adult dosage guidelines while monitoring individual patient response.

Notes, Opiate Addiction Detoxification

Methadone pharmacotherapy is ingested daily under close supervision.

Opiate Addiction Maintenance

Adults: 10 to 120 mg daily orally in a single dose

Women who are, or who may become, pregnant: FDA Pregnancy Category C. Safety and efficacy of methadone pharmacotherapy for women who are pregnant have not been established. Methadone crosses the placenta. During pregnancy, long-term pharmacotherapy, or regular personal use, will result in the neonatal addiction syndrome. Avoid prescribing methadone pharmacotherapy to women who are pregnant. If methadone pharmacotherapy is required, advise patients of potential benefits and possible risks to themselves and the embryo, fetus, or neonate. Collaboration with the patient's obstetrician is indicated.

Women who are breast-feeding: Safety and efficacy of methadone pharmacotherapy for women who are breast-feeding, and their neonates and infants, have not been established. Methadone is excreted in breast milk in concentrations up to 85% of those of the maternal blood. Expected pharmacologic actions (e.g., drowsiness, lethargy, respiratory depression) may be observed among breast-fed neonates and infants, who also may become addicted. Avoid prescribing methadone pharmacotherapy to women who are breast-feeding. If methadone pharmacotherapy is required, breast-feeding should be discontinued. Collaboration with the patient's pediatrician is indicated.

Elderly, frail, or debilitated patients: Generally prescribe lower dosages for elderly, frail, or debilitated patients. Increase the dosage gradually, if needed, according to individual patient response. These patients may be more sensitive to the pharmacologic actions of methadone than are younger or healthier adult patients. However, the dosage should be sufficient to prevent the occurrence of the signs and symptoms of the opiate withdrawal syndrome.

Children and adolescents younger than 16 years of age: Safety and efficacy of methadone pharmacotherapy for opiate addiction maintenance for children and adolescents younger than 16 years of age have not been established. Methadone pharmacotherapy for this indication is *not* recommended for this age group. In addition, U.S. federal regulations specifically prohibit children and adolescents younger than 16 years of age from being admitted to opiate addiction (methadone) maintenance programs.

Adolescents 16 to 18 years of age: 10 to 120 mg daily orally in a single dose. *Note: dosage is the same as the usual adult dosage.* In order to qualify for admittance to an opiate addiction (methadone) maintenance program, these adolescents must meet the following two minimum criteria: (1) a documented history of two or more unsuccessful attempts at opiate analgesic detoxification and (2) a documented history of addiction to heroin or related opiate analgesics beginning two years or more prior to application for admittance to the program.

Notes, Opiate Addiction Maintenance

Methadone pharmacotherapy for the maintenance of opiate addiction requires patients to be enrolled in an opiate addiction maintenance program. Methadone pharmacotherapy is individualized according to each patient's degree of opiate addiction and other factors. The individualized dosage of methadone is ingested once daily under close supervision. Additional doses may be required to prevent the opiate withdrawal syndrome. Intramuscular injection may be required by patients who are unable to ingest the oral dosage form. Some patients may require 40 mg or more daily in a single or divided doses, depending on their opiate addiction. The dosage always should be sufficient to prevent the opiate withdrawal syndrome.

The methadone withdrawal syndrome, although qualitatively similar to that of morphine and other opiates, differs in several ways from these opiate withdrawal syndromes. The onset of the methadone withdrawal syndrome is slower, its course is more prolonged, and the signs and symptoms are more intense or severe. Patients who want to decrease their dosage, or completely discontinue their methadone use, require opiate addiction detoxification.

Patients who require methadone pharmacotherapy for the management of their opiate addiction react to problems and stresses of everyday life with similar anxiety as other people. Avoid confusing the signs and symptoms of anxiety with the signs and symptoms of the opiate withdrawal syndrome. Also avoid prescribing increased dosages of methadone for the symptomatic management of anxiety for which it is not indicated. The goal of methadone pharmacotherapy for the maintenance of opiate addiction is to prevent the occurrence of the signs and symptoms of the opiate withdrawal syndrome. Methadone pharmacotherapy is *not* indicated for, nor is it effective for, the symptomatic management of anxiety.

AVAILABLE DOSAGE FORMS, STORAGE, AND COMPATIBILITY

Injectable, intramuscular, subcutaneous: 10 mg/ml
Solution, oral: 1, 2 mg/ml (contains 8% alcohol) (citrus flavored)
Solution, oral concentrate (Methadone Intensol®, Methadose Concentrate®): 10 mg/ml (for opiate addiction maintenance program use *only*)
Syrup, oral: 5 mg/15 ml
Tablets, oral: 5, 10 mg
Tablets, oral dispersible (Methadone Diskets®): 40 mg

Notes

Safely store methadone oral and injectable formulations at controlled room temperature (15° to 30°C; 59° to 86°F). All methadone dosage formulations should be stored and used in accordance with federal regulations for controlled substances.

General Instructions for Patients   Instruct patients who are receiving methadone pharmacotherapy, as appropriate (i.e., in some jurisdictions [e.g., Canada] outpatient take-home dosages of methadone are permitted under certain circumstances), to

- safely store methadone syrup and tablets out of the reach of children in tightly closed child- and light-resistant containers.
- obtain an available patient information sheet regarding methadone pharmacotherapy from their pharmacist at the time that their prescription is dispensed. Encourage patients to clarify any questions that they may have concerning methadone pharmacotherapy with their pharmacist or, if needed, to consult their prescribing psychologist.

PROPOSED MECHANISM OF ACTION

Methadone is a synthetic opiate analgesic with multiple actions quantitatively similar to those of morphine. The most prominent actions involve the CNS and body organs composed of smooth muscle (e.g., intestines, lungs). However, the major actions of concern to psychologists are its analgesic and CNS depressant actions and its use as adjunctive pharmacotherapy for the symptomatic management of pain disorders, opiate addiction detoxification, and opiate addiction maintenance.

Methadone elicits its analgesic and CNS depressant actions primarily by binding to the endorphin receptors in the CNS. However, the exact mechanism of action has not yet been fully determined.

See Opiate Analgesics General Monograph

PHARMACOKINETICS/PHARMACODYNAMICS

Methadone is well absorbed (~90%) following oral ingestion. However, when orally ingested, methadone is approximately one-half as potent as when injected, presumably because of its significant first-pass hepatic metabolism. Oral ingestion is associated with a delay in the onset of action, a lowering of the peak blood level, and an increase in the duration of analgesic action. Methadone's duration of action is 3 to 5 hours following intramuscular or subcutaneous injection. Following oral ingestion, it is 6 to 8 hours. A prolonged duration of action makes methadone an effective drug for the symptomatic management of cancer pain and for opiate addiction maintenance. Methadone is approximately 90% bound to plasma proteins and has a mean apparent volume of distribution of approximately 4 L/kg. The total body clearance is approximately 90 ml/minute, and the mean half-life of elimination is 36 hours.

RELATIVE CONTRAINDICATIONS

Hypersensitivity to methadone or other opiate analgesics

See also Opiate Analgesics General Monograph

CAUTIONS AND COMMENTS

Methadone is addicting and habituating. Thus, it has the potential to be abused. Prescribe methadone pharmacotherapy cautiously to patients who

- have acute abdominal conditions (e.g., appendicitis) for which the use of methadone may obscure the monitoring of the clinical course of the condition.
- are receiving pharmacotherapy with other drugs that produce CNS depression (e.g., antihistamines, phenothiazines, sedative-hypnotics). Additive actions may result in hypotension, respiratory depression, and profound sedation or coma. For these reasons, avoid prescribing methadone pharmacotherapy to patients who are receiving pharmacotherapy with other drugs that produce CNS depression.
- have difficulty maintaining normal blood pressure (e.g., have a depleted blood volume, are concurrently receiving phenothiazines or other pharmacotherapy that can lower blood pressure). Methadone pharmacotherapy for these patients may result in severe hypotension.
- have head injuries or other medical disorders associated with increased intracranial pressure. Methadone's associated respiratory depressant actions and its ability to elevate cerebrospinal spinal fluid pressure may be exaggerated among these patients. In addition, methadone pharmacotherapy may obscure the monitoring of the clinical course of these patients. Methadone also has been associated with postural (orthostatic) hypotension among these patients. Prescribe methadone pharmacotherapy cautiously for these patients.

- have status asthmaticus, chronic obstructive lung disease, cor pulmonale, substantially reduced respiratory reserve, pre-existing respiratory depression, hypoxia, or hypercapnia. Even usual therapeutic dosages of methadone for these patients may decrease respiratory drive while simultaneously increasing airway resistance to the point of apnea.

Caution patients who are receiving methadone pharmacotherapy against performing activities that require alertness, judgment, and physical coordination (e.g., driving an automobile, operating dangerous equipment, supervising children). Methadone may adversely affect these mental and physical functions.

In addition to this general precaution, caution patients who are enrolled in opiate addiction maintenance programs to carry a card in order to alert medical personnel in the event of an emergency identifying that they are receiving methadone for opiate addiction maintenance. These patients may experience the opiate withdrawal syndrome if they receive opiate agonist-antagonist (e.g., pentazocine [Talwin®]) or antagonist (e.g., naloxone [Narcan®]) pharmacotherapy.

CLINICALLY SIGNIFICANT DRUG INTERACTIONS

Concurrent methadone pharmacotherapy and the following may result in clinically significant drug interactions:

Alcohol Use

Concurrent alcohol use may increase the CNS depressant action of methadone. Advise patients to avoid, or limit, their use of alcohol while receiving methadone pharmacotherapy.

Pharmacotherapy With Drugs That Produce Central Nervous System Depression

Concurrent methadone pharmacotherapy with other opiate analgesics, sedative-hypnotics, and other drugs that produce CNS depression (e.g., antihistamines, phenothiazines, TCAs) may result in additive CNS depression.

Phenytoin Pharmacotherapy

Phenytoin (Dilantin®), an anticonvulsant, may increase the hepatic metabolism of methadone, resulting in decreased methadone blood levels and diminished pharmacologic action.

Rifampin Pharmacotherapy

Rifampin (Rimactane®), an antibacterial, may increase the hepatic metabolism of methadone, resulting in decreased methadone blood levels and diminished pharmacologic action.
See also Opiate Analgesics General Monograph

ADVERSE DRUG REACTIONS

Methadone has a low incidence of ADRs when compared to morphine and produces less euphoria than heroin. Methadone pharmacotherapy is commonly associated with dizziness, drowsiness, excessive sweating, GI complaints, light-headedness, nausea, sedation, and vomiting. Methadone also may produce the ADRs commonly associated with other opiate analgesics because of its chemical and pharmacological similarity.

See Opiate Analgesics General Monograph

OVERDOSAGE

Signs and symptoms of methadone overdosage are similar to those observed with morphine overdosage. These signs and symptoms, which begin within seconds after intravenous injection or within minutes after oral ingestion, nasal insufflation, or rectal insertion, include abnormal contraction of the pupils (miosis), coma, cool and clammy skin, respiratory depression, skeletal muscle flaccidity, and somnolence. In severe overdosages, these signs and symptoms can progress to apnea, bradycardia, hypotension, and death.

Methadone overdosage requires emergency symptomatic medical support of body systems with attention to increasing methadone elimination. The opiate antagonist naloxone (Narcan®) is an essential component of the emergency medical management of methadone and other opiate analgesic overdosage. *Repeated doses* of naloxone are usually required because methadone's duration of action is prolonged (36 to 48 hours) and that of naloxone is short (1 to 3 hours).

Naloxone will precipitate the opiate withdrawal syndrome among patients who are addicted to methadone, including those who are enrolled in opiate addiction maintenance programs. The signs and symptoms of the opiate withdrawal syndrome include abdominal cramps, diarrhea, dilated pupils, piloerection (goose flesh), restlessness, salivation, sweating, tearing, vomiting, and yawning. These signs and symptoms generally remit as the action of naloxone abates.

See also Naloxone and Opiate Analgesics General Monographs

METHAMPHETAMINE *
[Desoxyephedrine]

(meth am fet′a meen)

TRADE NAME

Desoxyn®

CLASSIFICATION

CNS stimulant (amphetamine) (C-II)

See also Amphetamines General Monograph

APPROVED INDICATIONS FOR PSYCHOLOGICAL DISORDERS

Adjunctive pharmacotherapy for the symptomatic management of:

- Attention-Deficit/Hyperactivity Disorder
- Eating Disorders: Exogenous Obesity
- Sleep Disorders: Narcolepsy. *Note:* Methamphetamine is *not* indicated to combat fatigue or replace normal rest requirements. Indication is *not* FDA approved.

USUAL DOSAGE AND ADMINISTRATION

Attention-Deficit/Hyperactivity Disorder

Adults: Safety and efficacy of methamphetamine pharmacotherapy for the symptomatic management of A-D/HD among adults have not been established. Methamphetamine pharmacotherapy for this indication is *not* recommended for this age group.

Children younger than 6 years of age: Safety and efficacy of methamphetamine pharmacotherapy for children younger than 6 years of age have not been established. Methamphetamine pharmacotherapy is *not* recommended for this age group.

Children 6 years of age or older: Initially, 5 to 10 mg daily orally in two divided doses. Increase the daily dosage weekly by increments of 5 mg until optimal therapeutic benefit is achieved. The usual effective dosage is 20 to 25 mg daily. Avoid prescribing late afternoon or evening doses because of associated insomnia. Once the optimal daily dosage has been established, it may be prescribed as a single daily dose with the extended-release tablet formulation. The extended-release tablet formulation is not indicated for the initiation of methamphetamine pharmacotherapy and should not be prescribed until the optimal daily dosage is equal to, or greater than, the dosage provided by the extended-release formulation.

Notes, Attention-Deficit/Hyperactivity Disorder

Adjunctive pharmacotherapy is not indicated for all children who are diagnosed with A-D/HD. Adjunctive pharmacotherapy should be considered only after the child has had a complete psychological assessment with attention to the severity of the child's signs and symptoms and their appropriateness for his or her age. Collaboration with the parents, pediatrician, and teachers is indicated. A comprehensive multidisciplinary (e.g., psychological, educational, and social) therapeutic program generally is required. This program should be guided by the goal of achieving optimal symptomatic management of A-D/HD among children 6 years of age and older with a minimum of ADRs.

Decrements in predicted growth (i.e., height and weight) have been associated with long-term methamphetamine pharmacotherapy among children. Monitor height and weight closely among children who require long-term methamphetamine pharmacotherapy. Collaboration with the child's pediatrician may be indicated. Whenever possible, interrupt methamphetamine pharmacotherapy occasionally to reevaluate the need for continued pharmacotherapy.

See also Amphetamines General Monograph

Exogenous Obesity

Adults: Initially, 5 to 15 mg daily orally in two or three divided doses 30 minutes before meals *or* 10 to 15 mg extended-release tablets daily orally in a single dose in the morning. Adjunctive methamphetamine pharmacotherapy for the symptomatic management of exogenous obesity is only indicated for short-term pharmacotherapy. Do *not* prescribe methamphetamine pharmacotherapy for this indication for longer than 12 weeks.

Women who are, or who may become, pregnant: FDA Pregnancy Category C. Safety and efficacy of methamphetamine pharmacotherapy for women who are pregnant have not been established. Women who are addicted or habituated to methamphetamine have an increased risk for premature delivery and low birth weight among their neonates. Neonates also may display signs and symptoms of the methamphetamine withdrawal syndrome, including agitation and lassitude. Avoid prescribing methamphetamine pharmacotherapy to women who are pregnant. If methamphetamine pharmacotherapy is required, advise patients of potential benefits and possible risks to themselves and the embryo, fetus, or neonate. Collaboration with the patient's obstetrician is indicated.

Women who are breast-feeding: Safety and efficacy of methamphetamine pharmacotherapy for women who are breast-feeding and their neonates and infants have not been established. Methamphetamine is excreted into breast milk (see Amphetamines General Monograph). Avoid prescribing methamphetamine pharmacotherapy to women who are breast-feeding. If methamphetamine pharmacotherapy is required, breast-feeding probably should be discontinued. Collaboration with the patient's pediatrician may be indicated.

Elderly: Generally prescribe lower dosages of methamphetamine for elderly patients. Increase the dosage gradually, if needed, according to individual patient response. These patients may be more sensitive to the pharmacologic actions of methamphetamine than are younger adult patients.

Children younger than 12 years of age: Safety and efficacy of methamphetamine pharmacotherapy for the symptomatic management of obesity for children who are younger than 12 years of age have not been established. Methamphetamine pharmacotherapy for this indication is *not* recommended for this age group.

Notes, Exogenous Obesity

Short-term (i.e., a maximum of 12 weeks) adjunctive methamphetamine pharmacotherapy may be of limited benefit as a component in a medically monitored weight reduction program based on caloric restriction and exercise for patients whose obesity is refractory to alternative therapies (e.g., group programs, hypnosis, repeated diets, other pharmacotherapy). The limited benefit associated with methamphetamine pharmacotherapy must be weighed against possible risks, including the risk for addiction and habituation.

Prescribe the lowest effective dosage adjusted according to individual patient response. Avoid prescribing late evening doses because of associated insomnia. Monitor patients for the development of tolerance. Tolerance to methamphetamine's anorexiant action usually develops within a few weeks. Discontinue methamphetamine pharmacotherapy when tolerance occurs. *Do not exceed the recommended dosage in an attempt to extend methamphetamine's anorexiant action.* Increasing the dosage or prolonging pharmacotherapy will not extend therapeutic benefit and may increase the incidence or severity of ADRs. It also will increase the risk for addiction and habituation.

Sleep Disorders: Narcolepsy (Indication is *not* FDA approved)

Adults: 15 to 60 mg daily orally in a single or divided doses

Women who are, or who may become, pregnant: FDA Pregnancy Category C. Safety and efficacy of methamphetamine pharmacotherapy for women who are pregnant have not been established. Women who are addicted or habituated to methamphetamine have an increased risk for premature delivery and low birth weight among their neonates. Neonates also may display signs and symptoms of the methamphetamine withdrawal syndrome, including agitation and lassitude (see Amphetamines General Monograph). Avoid prescribing methamphetamine pharmacotherapy to women who are pregnant. If methamphetamine pharmacotherapy is required, advise patients of potential benefits and possible risks to themselves and the embryo, fetus, or neonate. Collaboration with the patient's obstetrician is indicated.

Women who are breast-feeding: Safety and efficacy of methamphetamine pharmacotherapy for women who are breast-feeding and their neonates and infants have not been established. Methamphetamine is excreted into breast milk. Avoid prescribing methamphetamine pharmacotherapy to women who are breast-feeding. If methamphetamine pharmacotherapy is required, breast-feeding probably should be discontinued.

Elderly, frail, or debilitated patients: Generally prescribe lower dosages for elderly, frail, or debilitated patients. Increase the dosage gradually, if needed, according to individual patient response. These patients may be more sensitive to the pharmacologic actions of methamphetamine than are younger or healthier adult patients.

Children and adolescents younger than 18 years of age: Safety and efficacy of methamphetamine pharmacotherapy for the symptomatic management of narcolepsy among children and adolescents have not been established. Methamphetamine pharmacotherapy for this indication is *not* recommended for this age group.

AVAILABLE DOSAGE FORMS, STORAGE, AND COMPATIBILITY

Tablets, oral: 5 mg
Tablets, oral extended-release (Desoxyn Gradumet®): 5, 10, 15 mg
　　The Gradumet® is an inert, porous plastic matrix that is filled with the drug. The drug is slowly released from the matrix as it passes through the GI tract. The expended matrix is not absorbed and is excreted in the feces. The 15 mg Gradumet® tablets contain tartrazine. Tartrazine is a coloring agent (FD&C Yellow No. 5) that has been associated with hypersensitivity reactions, including bronchial asthma, among susceptible patients. Patients who have a hypersensitivity to aspirin appear to be at particular risk.

General Instructions for Patients   Instruct patients who are receiving methamphetamine pharmacotherapy, as appropriate, to

- swallow whole each dose of the methamphetamine oral extended-release tablets without breaking, crushing, or chewing.
- safely store regular and extended-release methamphetamine oral tablets out of the reach of children in child-resistant containers at temperatures below 30°C (86°F).
- obtain an available patient information sheet regarding methamphetamine pharmacotherapy from their pharmacist at the time that their prescription is dispensed. Encourage patients to clarify any questions that they may have concerning methamphetamine pharmacotherapy with their pharmacist or, if needed, to consult their prescribing psychologist.

PROPOSED MECHANISM OF ACTION

Methamphetamine is a potent CNS stimulant. It appears to elicit its stimulant actions by increasing the release of norepinephrine from central adrenergic neurons. A direct effect on α- and β-adrenergic receptors, inhibition of the enzyme amine oxidase, and the release of dopamine also may be involved. However, the exact mechanism of action has not yet been fully determined.

The mechanism of action of methamphetamine in relation to producing beneficial behavioral changes among children who have A-D/HD is unknown. When prescribed as adjunctive pharmacotherapy for the symptomatic management of obesity, amphetamines are commonly referred to as "anorexiants," "anorectics," or "anorexigenics." However, it is unknown whether their action for this indication is primarily associated with appetite suppression, other centrally mediated actions, or metabolic actions. The exact mechanism of action for the symptomatic management of narcolepsy is related to methamphetamine's action as a CNS stimulant.

PHARMACOKINETICS/PHARMACODYNAMICS

Methamphetamine is rapidly absorbed following oral ingestion. The primary site of metabolism is the liver. Excretion of both metabolites and unchanged drug occurs primarily in the urine and is pH dependent. Thus, in alkaline urine, excretion will be significantly decreased and the half-life of elimination will be increased. In acidic urine, excretion will be significantly increased, and the half-life of elimination will be decreased. The usual mean half-life of elimination is approximately 4 hours. Additional data are unavailable.

RELATIVE CONTRAINDICATIONS

Addiction and habituation to methamphetamine or other amphetamines, history of
Agitation
Arteriosclerosis, advanced
Cardiac disease, symptomatic
Glaucoma
Hypersensitivity to amphetamine, methamphetamine, or sympathomimetic amines (e.g., phenylpropanolamine [Acutrim®, Dexatrim®])
Hypertension, moderate to severe
Hyperthyroidism
MAOI pharmacotherapy, concurrent of within 14 days (see Clinically Significant Drug Interactions)
Phenothiazine pharmacotherapy (see Clinically Significant Drug Interactions)

CAUTIONS AND COMMENTS

Methamphetamine has a high potential for addiction and habituation. Thus, it should be cautiously prescribed as adjunctive pharmacotherapy for the symptomatic management of A-D/HD, exogenous obesity, and narcolepsy. Long-term methamphetamine pharmacotherapy, or regular personal use, may lead to addiction and habituation. Thus, attention must be given to the possibility that some patients may become addicted or habituated to methamphetamine as a result of their pharmacotherapy. Attention also must be given to the possibility that some patients may seek methamphetamine prescriptions to support their addiction or habituation (i.e., regular personal use).

Methamphetamine has been associated with problematic patterns of use since its synthesis. Reportedly, patients have increased their dosages to many times the usual recommended dosage. Intoxication with methamphetamine is characterized by the following signs and symptoms: hyperactivity, irritability, marked insomnia, personality changes, and severe dermatoses. Psychosis also has been associated with methamphetamine intoxication. Psychosis, often clinically indistinguishable from paranoid schizophrenia, is probably one of the most severe signs and symptoms of intoxication.

Abrupt discontinuation of methamphetamine following high-dosage, long-term pharmacotherapy, or regular personal use, may result in the amphetamine withdrawal syndrome. Signs and symptoms of this syndrome include EEG changes during sleep, fatigue, and mental depression. Limit prescriptions to the smallest quantity that is feasible for dispensing at one time in order to minimize the possible development of problematic patterns of use.

Prescribe methamphetamine pharmacotherapy cautiously to patients who

- have cardiovascular disorders, including mild hypertension. Methamphetamine pharmacotherapy has been associated with cardiac dysrhythmias and hypertension among these patients.
- have histories of schizophrenia or other psychotic disorders. Methamphetamine pharmacotherapy for children and adults who have psychotic disorders may exacerbate the signs and symptoms of the behavior disturbance and thought disorder. Amphetamines reportedly exacerbate motor and phonic tics and Tourette's disorder (i.e., Gilles de la Tourette's syndrome). Clinical assessment of children and adults for tics and Gilles de la Tourette's syndrome should precede the prescription of methamphetamine pharmacotherapy.
- have insulin-dependent diabetes mellitus. Methamphetamine pharmacotherapy may alter insulin requirements among these patients.

CLINICALLY SIGNIFICANT DRUG INTERACTIONS

Concurrent methamphetamine pharmacotherapy and the following may result in clinically significant drug interactions:

Guanethidine Pharmacotherapy

Methamphetamine pharmacotherapy may decrease the neuronal uptake of guanethidine (Ismelin®) and, thus, decrease its antihypertensive action. An adjustment of the guanethidine dosage may be required. Collaboration with the prescriber of the guanethidine is indicated.

Insulin Pharmacotherapy

Methamphetamine pharmacotherapy may alter insulin requirements among patients who have insulin-dependent diabetes mellitus, particularly those who also have a restricted caloric diet.

Monoamine Oxidase Inhibitor Pharmacotherapy

Methamphetamine may interact with MAOIs (e.g., phenelzine [Nardil®]). This interaction may cause the release of large amounts of catecholamines and associated pharmacologic actions, including the hypertensive crisis. The hypertensive crisis is characterized by severe headaches and hypertension. Thus, this combination of pharmacotherapy, concurrent or within 14 days, is *contraindicated*. See Relative Contraindications

Pharmacotherapy With Urinary Acidifiers

Drugs that acidify the urine (e.g., ammonium chloride) increase the urinary excretion of methamphetamine and, hence, decrease its half-life of elimination. This interaction may result in a decrease in the pharmacologic action of methamphetamine.

Pharmacotherapy With Urinary Alkalinizers

Drugs that alkalinize the urine (e.g., acetazolamide, sodium bicarbonate) decrease the urinary excretion of methamphetamine and, hence, increase its half-life of elimination. This interaction may result in methamphetamine toxicity.

Phenothiazine Pharmacotherapy

Phenothiazines (i.e., chlorpromazine) reportedly antagonize the CNS stimulatory actions of methamphetamine and other amphetamines. Concurrent methamphetamine and phenothiazine pharmacotherapy is *contraindicated* except in situations of methamphetamine overdosage.

Tricyclic Antidepressant Pharmacotherapy

Concurrent methamphetamine and TCA pharmacotherapy (as with amphetamine and other sympathomimetic pharmacotherapy) may result in additive CNS stimulation. When concurrent pharmacotherapy is required, monitor patients closely and adjust the dosage of both drugs carefully according to individual patient response.

See also Amphetamines General Monograph

ADVERSE DRUG REACTIONS

Methamphetamine pharmacotherapy has been associated with the following ADRs, listed according to body system:

Cardiovascular: increased systolic and diastolic blood pressures, palpitations, and tachycardia. Methamphetamine pharmacotherapy also has been associated with weak bronchodilator and respiratory stimulant actions.

CNS: dizziness, dysphoria, euphoria, headache, insomnia, and overstimulation. Psychotic episodes rarely have been reported at recommended dosages.

Cutaneous: hives (urticaria)

Genitourinary: changes in sex drive and impotence

GI: constipation, diarrhea, dry mouth, gastrointestinal complaints, and unpleasant taste

Musculoskeletal: restlessness and tremor. Suppression of growth also has been reported among children who have received long-term methamphetamine or other amphetamine pharmacotherapy.

See also Amphetamines General Monograph

OVERDOSAGE

Signs and symptoms of acute methamphetamine overdosage include assaultiveness, cardiovascular reactions (e.g., dysrhythmias, hypertension or hypotension, and circulatory collapse), confusion, destruction of skeletal muscle (rhabdomyolysis), GI complaints (e.g., abdominal cramps, diarrhea, nausea, and vomiting), hallucinations, hyperpyrexia, hyperreflexia, panic, rapid respirations, restlessness, and tremor. Depression and fatigue usually follow the central stimulation. Fatal overdosage usually terminates in convulsions and coma.

Methamphetamine overdosage requires emergency symptomatic medical support of body systems with attention to increasing methamphetamine elimination. Increasing methamphetamine elimination is particularly important when the extended-release tablet formulation has been involved in the overdosage. The extended-release formulation gradually releases methamphetamine over a prolonged period. Although there is no known antidote, chlorpromazine blocks dopamine and norepinephrine re-uptake. This action inhibits the central stimulant actions of the amphetamines.

METHOTRIMEPRAZINE
[Levomepromazine]

(meth oh trye mep′ra zeen)

TRADE NAMES

Levoprome®
Novo-Meprazine®
Nozinan®

CLASSIFICATION

Antipsychotic (phenothiazine)

See also Phenothiazines General Monograph

APPROVED INDICATIONS FOR PSYCHOLOGICAL DISORDERS

Adjunctive pharmacotherapy for the symptomatic management of:

- Pain Disorders: Moderate to Severe Intractable Pain Among Hospitalized Patients
- Psychotic Disorders: Schizophrenia and Other Psychotic Disorders. Indication is *not* FDA approved.

USUAL DOSAGE AND ADMINISTRATION

Pain Disorders: Moderate to Severe Intractable Pain Among Hospitalized Patients

Adults (hospitalized):   Moderate to severe intractable pain, 10 to 20 mg intramuscularly every four to six hours, as needed. Injections should be made into large healthy muscle sites. Initially prescribe lower dosages. Increase the dosage gradually until therapeutic benefit is achieved.

Women who are, or who may become, pregnant: FDA Pregnancy Category C. Safety and efficacy of methotrimeprazine pharmacotherapy for women who are pregnant have not been established. Methotrimeprazine crosses the placenta. Reports indicate a higher incidence of cardiac defects among neonates born to women who received methotrimeprazine and related phenothiazine pharmacotherapy during pregnancy (see Phenothiazines General Monograph). Avoid prescribing methotrimeprazine pharmacotherapy to women who are pregnant, particularly during the first trimester of pregnancy. If methotrimeprazine pharmacotherapy is required, advise patients of potential benefits and possible risks to themselves and the embryo, fetus, or neonate. Collaboration with the patient's obstetrician is indicated.

Women who are breast-feeding: Safety and efficacy of methotrimeprazine pharmacotherapy for women who are breast-feeding and their neonates and infants have not been established. Methotrimeprazine is excreted into breast milk (see Phenothiazines General Monograph). Avoid prescribing methotrimeprazine pharmacotherapy to women who are breast-feeding. If methotrimeprazine pharmacotherapy is required, breast-feeding probably should be discontinued. Collaboration with the patient's pediatrician is indicated.

Elderly, frail, or debilitated patients: Generally prescribe lower dosages for elderly, frail, or debilitated patients. Increase the dosage gradually, if needed, according to individual patient response. These patients may be more sensitive to the pharmacologic actions of methotrimeprazine than are younger or healthier adult patients.

Children younger than 12 years of age: Safety and efficacy of methotrimeprazine pharmacotherapy for the symptomatic management of acute moderate to severe intractable pain for children younger than 12 years of age have not been established. Methotrimeprazine pharmacotherapy for this indication is *not* recommended for this age group.

Notes, Pain Disorders: Moderate to Severe Intractable Pain Among Hospitalized Patients

Initiating Methotrimeprazine Pharmacotherapy   Prescribe the initial dosage according to the severity of the patient's pain, with the goal of achieving adequate pain relief with a minimum of ADRs. Adjust the dosage according to individual patient response. Postural hypotension has been initially associated with high-dosage (100 to 200 mg daily) oral or injectable pharmacotherapy. Prescribe the total daily dosage in divided doses, and maintain patients on bed rest for the first few days of pharmacotherapy. Psychomotor functions also may be adversely affected during initial pharmacotherapy. Advise hospitalized patients to avoid activities that require alertness, judgment, or physical coordination (e.g., ambulating without assistance or going up and down stairs, signing legal papers) until their response to methotrimeprazine pharmacotherapy is known.

INJECTABLE PHARMACOTHERAPY   Injectable pharmacotherapy is generally reserved for the symptomatic management of moderate to severe intractable pain. It also may be prescribed for the initial symptomatic management of psychosis or for patients who are unable to ingest methotrimeprazine oral dosage formulations (e.g., have nausea and vomiting).

Intramuscular pharmacotherapy.   Inject methotrimeprazine deeply into large healthy muscle sites. Do *not* inject subcutaneously because the injectable formulation is irritating to subcutaneous tissues and may cause local irritation.

Intravenous pharmacotherapy.   The safety and efficacy of intravenous methotrimeprazine pharmacotherapy for the symptomatic management of moderate to severe intractable pain have not been established. Intravenous pharmacotherapy is *not* recommended for this indication.

Maintaining Methotrimeprazine Pharmacotherapy   Monitor blood counts regularly, particularly during the first two to three months of methotrimeprazine pharmacotherapy. Observe patients for any signs and symptoms of blood disorders (i.e., neutropenia), such as those suggesting an increased susceptibility to infection (e.g., sore throat). Monitor liver function periodically among patients who require long-term methotrimeprazine pharmacotherapy. Collaboration with the patient's family physician or a specialist (hematologist, oncologist) may be required.

Methotrimeprazine pharmacotherapy for the symptomatic management of pain disorders generally should be limited to periods of less than 30 days unless either opiate analgesics are contraindicated (e.g., the patient has a hypersensitivity to opiates) or pharmacotherapy is required for the symptomatic management of terminal cancer pain.

Schizophrenia and Other Psychotic Disorders (Indication HPB, but *not* FDA approved)

Adults: Mild to moderate symptoms, 6 to 25 mg daily orally in three divided doses with meals. Severe symptoms, 50 to 100 mg daily orally in three divided doses with meals, *or* 75 to 100 mg daily intramuscularly in three or four divided doses. Injections should be made into large healthy muscle sites. Increase the dosage gradually until desired therapeutic response is achieved.

MAXIMUM: 1,000 mg daily

Women who are, or who may become, pregnant: FDA Pregnancy Category C. Safety and efficacy of methotrimeprazine pharmacotherapy for women who are pregnant have not been established. Methotrimeprazine crosses the placenta (see Phenothiazines General Monograph). Reports indicate a higher incidence of cardiac defects among neonates born to women who received methotrimeprazine and related phenothiazine pharmacotherapy during pregnancy. Avoid prescribing methotrimeprazine pharmacotherapy to women who are pregnant, particularly during the first trimester of pregnancy. If methotrimeprazine pharmacotherapy is required, advise patients (or their legal guardians in regard to the patient) of potential benefits and possible risks to themselves and the embryo, fetus, or neonate. Collaboration with the patient's obstetrician is indicated.

Women who are breast-feeding: Safety and efficacy of methotrimeprazine pharmacotherapy for women who are breast-feeding and their neonates and infants have not been established. Methotrimeprazine is excreted into breast milk (see Phenothiazines General Monograph). Avoid prescribing methotrimeprazine pharmacotherapy to women who are breast-feeding. If methotrimeprazine pharmacotherapy is required, breast-feeding probably should be discontinued. Collaboration with the patient's pediatrician is indicated.

Elderly, frail, or debilitated patients: Initially, 6 mg daily orally in divided doses. Generally prescribe lower dosages for elderly, frail, or debilitated patients. Increase the dosage gradually, if needed, according to individual patient response. These patients may be more sensitive to the pharmacologic actions of methotrimeprazine than are younger or healthier adult patients.

Children: Initially, 0.25 mg/kg daily orally in two or three divided doses with meals, *or* 0.065 mg/kg/daily intramuscularly in a single or divided dose. Increase the dosage gradually until desired therapeutic response is achieved. Inject only into large healthy muscle sites. Replace injectable pharmacotherapy with oral pharmacotherapy as soon as feasible. Do *not* prescribe dosages exceeding 40 mg daily for children who are younger than 12 years of age.

MAXIMUM: 40 mg daily

Notes, Schizophrenia and Other Psychotic Disorders

Initiating Methotrimeprazine Pharmacotherapy Prescribe the daily dosage according to the severity of the patient's signs and symptoms. Adjust the dosage according to individual patient response. If daytime sedation becomes troublesome, divide the total daily dosage so that lower doses are prescribed during the day and a higher dose is prescribed for the evening.

Postural hypotension has been associated with high dosage (100 to 200 mg daily) oral or injectable methotrimeprazine pharmacotherapy. Prescribe the total daily dosage in divided doses and maintain patients on bed rest for the first few days of pharmacotherapy. Psychomotor function also may be adversely affected during initial pharmacotherapy.

INJECTABLE PHARMACOTHERAPY Injectable pharmacotherapy is generally reserved for the initial symptomatic management of psychosis and for patients who are unable to ingest methotrimeprazine oral dosage forms (e.g., have nausea and vomiting). It also may be prescribed for the symptomatic management of acute moderate to severe intractable pain.

Intramuscular pharmacotherapy. Inject methotrimeprazine deeply into large healthy muscle sites. Do *not* inject subcutaneously because the injectable formulation is irritating to subcutaneous tissues and may cause local irritation.

Intravenous pharmacotherapy. The safety and efficacy of intravenous methotrimeprazine pharmacotherapy for the symptomatic management of psychotic disorders have not been established. Intravenous pharmacotherapy is *not* recommended for this indication.

Maintaining Methotrimeprazine Pharmacotherapy   Monitor blood counts regularly, particularly during the first two to three months of methotrimeprazine pharmacotherapy. Observe patients for any signs and symptoms of blood disorders (i.e., neutropenia) suggestive of increased susceptibility to infection (e.g., sore throat). Monitor liver function periodically for patients who require long-term methotrimeprazine pharmacotherapy. Collaboration with the patient's family physician or a specialist (e.g., hematologist) may be required.

AVAILABLE DOSAGE FORMS, STORAGE, AND COMPATIBILITY

Drops, oral: 40 mg/ml (contains 16.5% alcohol)
Injectable, intramuscular: 20, 25 mg/ml (ampule, vial)
Liquid, oral: 25 mg/5 ml (contains 2% alcohol)
Tablets, oral: 2, 5, 25, 50 mg

Notes

The injectable formulations contain sodium metabisulfite or sodium sulfite. Sulfites have been associated with hypersensitivity reactions, including anaphylactic reactions, among susceptible patients. Although relatively uncommon, these reactions appear to occur with a higher incidence among patients who have asthma.

Store injectables protected from light at controlled room temperature (15° to 30°C; 59° to 86°F).

General Instructions for Patients   Instruct patients who are receiving methotrimeprazine pharmacotherapy (or their legal guardian in regard to the patient) to

- safely store oral dosage forms of methotrimeprazine out of the reach of children in child-resistant containers.
- obtain an available patient information sheet regarding methotrimeprazine pharmacotherapy from their pharmacist at the time that their prescription is dispensed. Encourage patients to clarify any questions that they may have concerning methotrimeprazine pharmacotherapy with their pharmacist or, if needed, to consult their prescribing psychologist.

PROPOSED MECHANISM OF ACTION

Methotrimeprazine's analgesic action appears to be related to its ability to raise the pain threshold. The exact mechanism of its antipsychotic and sedative actions for the symptomatic management of schizophrenia and other psychotic disorders is complex and has not yet been fully determined. These actions appear to be related primarily to its interaction with dopamine-containing neurons, specifically the blockade of dopamine receptors both pre-synaptically and post-synaptically.

See also Phenothiazines General Monograph

PHARMACOKINETICS/PHARMACODYNAMICS

Methotrimeprazine has analgesic and strong antiapomorphine, antispasmodic, and antihistaminic actions. It also potentiates anesthetics strongly and has a hypothermic action three times more potent than chlorpromazine. Following intramuscular injection, maximum analgesic effect occurs within ~30 minutes. Its duration of action is 4 to 6 hours. Methotrimeprazine is significantly metabolized in the liver, with less than 1% excreted in unchanged form in the urine. Additional data are unavailable.

RELATIVE CONTRAINDICATIONS

Antihypertensive pharmacotherapy, concurrent
Blood disorders
CNS depression, including that associated with alcohol, opiate analgesics, and other CNS
    depressants
Coma
Heart disease, severe
Hypersensitivity to methotrimeprazine or other phenothiazines
Hypotension, clinically significant
Kidney dysfunction, severe
Liver dysfunction, severe
MAOI pharmacotherapy, concurrent or within 14 days

CAUTIONS AND COMMENTS

Prescribe methotrimeprazine pharmacotherapy cautiously to patients who

- have glaucoma or prostatic hypertrophy. Methotrimeprazine has anticholinergic actions that may exacerbate these conditions.
- have histories of epilepsy or other seizure disorders. Methotrimeprazine is a phenothiazine. Phenothiazines can generally lower the threshold for cortical excitation. Concurrent anticonvulsive pharmacotherapy may be needed. Collaboration with the patient's family physician or a specialist (e.g., neurologist) is indicated.

Caution patients who are receiving methotrimeprazine pharmacotherapy against performing activities that require alertness, judgment, and physical coordination (e.g., driving an automobile, operating dangerous equipment, supervising children) until their response to methotrimeprazine is known. Methotrimeprazine pharmacotherapy may adversely affect these mental and physical functions.

In addition to this general precaution, caution patients to inform their prescribing psychologist if they begin or discontinue any other pharmacotherapy while receiving methotrimeprazine pharmacotherapy.

CLINICALLY SIGNIFICANT DRUG INTERACTIONS

Concurrent methotrimeprazine pharmacotherapy and the following may result in clinically significant drug interactions:

Alcohol Use

Concurrent alcohol use with methotrimeprazine pharmacotherapy can produce additive CNS depression. Advise patients to avoid, or limit, their use of alcohol while receiving methotrimeprazine pharmacotherapy.

Anticholinergic Pharmacotherapy

Concurrent methotrimeprazine pharmacotherapy with anticholinergics (e.g., atropine) or other drugs that produce anticholinergic actions (e.g., TCAs) may cause additive anticholinergic actions.

Pharmacotherapy With Central Nervous System Depressants and Other Drugs That Produce Central Nervous System Depression

Methotrimeprazine pharmacotherapy and concurrent pharmacotherapy with opiate analgesics, sedative-hypnotics, or other drugs that produce CNS depression (e.g., antihistamines, TCAs) may result in additive CNS depression. Concurrent methotrimeprazine pharmacotherapy with these drugs may require that the usual dosages of these drugs be reduced by half until the dosage of methotrimeprazine has been stabilized.

See also Phenothiazines General Monograph

ADVERSE DRUG REACTIONS

Methotrimeprazine pharmacotherapy has been associated with the following ADRs, listed according to body system. Other potentially serious ADRs associated with phenothiazine pharmacotherapy include TD, other EPRs, over-sedation, and unexpected, sudden death. Methotrimeprazine is a phenothiazine; thus, the possible occurrence of these ADRs cannot be excluded for patients who are receiving methotrimeprazine pharmacotherapy. Caution is recommended, particularly when long-term high-dosage pharmacotherapy is prescribed.

> **Cardiovascular:** postural hypotension may occur during initial pharmacotherapy, particularly with high-dosage oral pharmacotherapy or with injectable pharmacotherapy. Tachycardia may occur as a result of methotrimeprazine's anticholinergic actions. Elderly patients may be more sensitive to the ADRs affecting the cardiovascular system.
>
> **CNS:** drowsiness. Generally this ADR occurs initially and gradually diminishes during the first weeks of pharmacotherapy or with dosage adjustment.
>
> **Cutaneous:** hypersensitivity and photosensitivity reactions (rare)
>
> **GI:** constipation and dry mouth
>
> **Hematologic:** agranulocytosis (rare)
>
> **Liver:** cholestatic jaundice without liver damage (rare)
>
> **Metabolic/Endocrine:** weight gain. This ADR usually is associated with long-term high-dosage methotrimeprazine pharmacotherapy.

See Phenothiazines General Monograph

OVERDOSAGE

Signs and symptoms of acute methotrimeprazine overdosage include convulsions, CNS depression, spasms, tonic or clonic convulsions, tremor, and coma with hypotension and respiratory depression. Methotrimeprazine overdosage requires emergency symptomatic medical support of body systems with attention to increasing methotrimeprazine elimination. There is no known antidote.

METHYLPHENIDATE
[Methylphenidylacetate]

(meth il fen'i date)

TRADE NAMES

Riphenidate®
Ritalin®
Ritalin-SR®

CLASSIFICATION

CNS stimulant (C-II)

APPROVED INDICATIONS FOR PSYCHOLOGICAL DISORDERS

Adjunctive pharmacotherapy for the symptomatic management of:

- Attention-Deficit/Hyperactivity Disorder
- Sleep Disorders: Narcolepsy

USUAL DOSAGE AND ADMINISTRATION

Attention-Deficit/Hyperactivity Disorder

Adults: Safety and efficacy of methylphenidate pharmacotherapy for the symptomatic management of A-D/HD for adults have not been established. Data from controlled clinical trials and clinical experience in this area are limited. See dosage and administration recommendations for "Children 6 years of age and older" for established guidelines.

Women who are, or who may become, pregnant: FDA Pregnancy Category C. Safety and efficacy of methylphenidate pharmacotherapy for women who are pregnant have not been established. Avoid prescribing methylphenidate pharmacotherapy to women who are pregnant. If methylphenidate pharmacotherapy is required, advise patients of potential benefits and possible risks to themselves and the embryo, fetus, or neonate. Collaboration with the patient's obstetrician is indicated.

Women who are breast-feeding:　Safety and efficacy of methylphenidate pharmacotherapy for women who are breast-feeding and their neonates and infants have not been established. Avoid prescribing methylphenidate pharmacotherapy to women who are breast-feeding. If methylphenidate pharmacotherapy is required, breast-feeding probably should be discontinued. Collaboration with the patient's pediatrician is indicated.

Children younger than 6 years of age:　Safety and efficacy of methylphenidate pharmacotherapy for children younger than 6 years of age have not been established. Methylphenidate pharmacotherapy is *not* recommended for this age group.

Children 6 years of age and older:　Initially, 5 to 10 mg daily orally in two divided doses. Increase the daily dosage weekly by 5 to 10 mg, as needed, to 60 mg daily orally in two divided doses (usually in the morning before breakfast and at noon). If preferred, initially prescribe 0.25 mg/kg daily orally in two divided doses. If significant ADRs are *not* noted, double the daily dosage each week to achieve an optimum dosage of 2 mg/kg daily orally. Dosages exceeding 60 mg daily are *not* recommended. Dosing should coincide with periods of greatest academic and other difficulties. However, late afternoon dosing may result in insomnia. If therapeutic benefit is not achieved over a one-month period with appropriate dosage adjustments, discontinue methylphenidate pharmacotherapy.

MAXIMUM:　2 mg/kg daily orally or 60 mg daily orally, whichever is less

Notes, Attention-Deficit/Hyperactivity Disorder

Initiating Childhood Methylphenidate Pharmacotherapy　Adjunctive methylphenidate pharmacotherapy provides one component of a comprehensive multidisciplinary (e.g., educational, family, medical, psychological, social) therapeutic program guided by the goal of optimal symptomatic management of A-D/HD among children 6 years of age and older. Adjunctive pharmacotherapy is not indicated for all children diagnosed with A-D/HD. Adjunctive pharmacotherapy should be considered only after children have received a complete psychological assessment, with attention to the severity of their signs and symptoms. Collaboration with their parents, pediatricians, social workers, and teachers is required. Children who are agitated may adversely react to methylphenidate pharmacotherapy. These children require discontinuation of pharmacotherapy.

Maintaining Childhood Methylphenidate Pharmacotherapy　The safety and efficacy of long-term methylphenidate pharmacotherapy for children have not been clearly established. Prescribe dosages according to individual patient response. Whenever possible, occasionally interrupt methylphenidate pharmacotherapy to provide "drug holidays" (i.e., withhold methylphenidate pharmacotherapy on weekends and during school holidays) in order to reevaluate the need for continued pharmacotherapy.

For optimal therapeutic benefit and a minimum of ADRs, monitor the following at regular intervals:

- blood pressure, particularly for patients who have histories of hypertension
- complete blood counts, differential, and platelet counts
- growth (i.e., height and weight). Long-term methylphenidate pharmacotherapy has been associated with growth suppression when prescribed during childhood. Collaboration with the patient's pediatrician is indicated.

- the child's ability to manage his or her pharmacotherapy. Monitor also for signs and symptoms of problematic patterns of use (e.g., increasing the dosage or using methylphenidate more often than prescribed without first checking with the prescribing psychologist). Long-term methylphenidate pharmacotherapy, or regular personal use, may result in addiction and habituation. Long-term methylphenidate pharmacotherapy during childhood and adolescence also may be associated with an increased predisposition for later development of problematic patterns of abusable psychotropic use (e.g., addiction to amphetamines, cocaine, or other abusable psychotropics).
- psychosis. Varying degrees of psychosis and other abnormal behavior have been associated with long-term methylphenidate pharmacotherapy during childhood, particularly injectable pharmacotherapy.

Discontinuing Long-Term Methylphenidate Pharmacotherapy Discontinue long-term methylphenidate pharmacotherapy cautiously. Severe depression and chronic over-activity have been associated with the discontinuation of long-term pharmacotherapy. The potential for the occurrence of basic personality disturbances also may require continued monitoring at regular intervals after the discontinuation of pharmacotherapy.

Narcolepsy

Adults: 20 to 60 mg daily orally in two or three divided doses one-half hour before meals. Some patients may ingest their last daily dose before 6 pm (1800 hours) to prevent associated insomnia.

Women who are, or who may become, pregnant: FDA Pregnancy Category C. Safety and efficacy of methylphenidate pharmacotherapy for women who are pregnant have not been established. Avoid prescribing methylphenidate pharmacotherapy to women who are pregnant. If methylphenidate pharmacotherapy is required, advise patients of potential benefits and possible risks to themselves and the embryo, fetus, or neonate. Collaboration with the patient's obstetrician may be indicated.

Women who are breast-feeding: Safety and efficacy of methylphenidate pharmacotherapy for women who are breast-feeding and their neonates and infants have not been established. Avoid prescribing methylphenidate pharmacotherapy to women who are breast-feeding. If methylphenidate pharmacotherapy is required, breast-feeding probably should be discontinued. Collaboration with the patient's pediatrician may be indicated.

Elderly, frail, or debilitated patients: Generally prescribe lower dosages for elderly, frail, or debilitated patients. Increase the dosage gradually according to individual patient response. These patients may be more sensitive to the pharmacologic actions of methylphenidate than are younger or healthier adult patients.

Children younger than 12 years of age: Safety and efficacy of methylphenidate pharmacotherapy for the symptomatic management of narcolepsy have not been established for children younger than 12 years of age. Methylphenidate pharmacotherapy for this indication is *not* recommended for this age group.

Notes, Narcolepsy

If paradoxical aggravation of the signs and symptoms of narcolepsy occur, reduce the dosage. If necessary, discontinue methylphenidate pharmacotherapy.

AVAILABLE DOSAGE FORMS, STORAGE, AND COMPATIBILITY

Tablets, oral: 5, 10, 20 mg
Tablets, oral extended-release (i.e., Ritalin-SR®): 20 mg

Notes

Methylphenidate oral extended-release tablets (Ritalin-SR®) have a duration of action of approximately 8 hours. These tablets are indicated for patients whose signs and symptoms have been managed with regular oral tablets (Ritalin®) and who prefer 8 hour dosing.

General Instructions for Patients   Instruct patients who are receiving methylphenidate pharmacotherapy to

- swallow whole each dose of the methylphenidate extended-release tablets without breaking, chewing, or crushing. Also instruct them to ingest each dose with adequate liquid chaser (e.g., 60 to 120 ml of water or compatible beverage).
- safely store methylphenidate oral regular and extended-release tablets out of the reach of children and at temperatures below 30°C (86°F) in tightly closed child- and light-resistant containers protected from moisture.
- obtain an available patient information sheet regarding methylphenidate pharmacotherapy from their pharmacist at the time that their prescription is dispensed. Encourage patients to clarify any questions that they may have concerning methylphenidate pharmacotherapy with their pharmacist or, if needed, to consult their prescribing psychologist.

PROPOSED MECHANISM OF ACTION

The exact mechanism of methylphenidate's CNS stimulant action for the symptomatic management of A-D/HD has not yet been fully determined. However, it appears to primarily involve stimulation of the CNS by activation of the brain stem arousal system and cortex. This action also is probably involved in the symptomatic management of narcolepsy.

PHARMACOKINETICS/PHARMACODYNAMICS

Methylphenidate is rapidly and well absorbed after oral ingestion. However, bioavailability is low (i.e., F = 0.3), and peak blood concentrations vary among patients because of extensive hepatic first-pass metabolism. When compared to regular oral tablets (i.e., Ritalin®), methylphenidate extended-release oral tablets (i.e., Ritalin-SR®) are absorbed more slowly but to the same extent. The apparent volume of distribution among children, although varying, is approximately 20 L/kg. Methylphenidate is excreted into the urine mainly as metabolites, with less than 5% excreted in unchanged form. Methylphenidate has a mean half-life of elimination of approximately

2 hours among children and adults. Thus, the pharmacokinetic parameters appear to be similar for children who have A-D/HD and normal adults. Additional data are unavailable.

RELATIVE CONTRAINDICATIONS

Agitation
Angina pectoris, severe
Anxiety
Glaucoma
Heart disease, severe
Hypersensitivity to methylphenidate
MAOI pharmacotherapy, concurrent or within 14 days
Tachycardia
Thyrotoxicosis
Tourette's disorder (Gilles de la Tourette's syndrome), or family history of

CAUTIONS AND COMMENTS

Long-term methylphenidate pharmacotherapy, or regular personal use, may result in addiction and habituation.

Prescribe methylphenidate pharmacotherapy cautiously to patients who

- have histories of seizure disorders or EEG abnormalities in the absence of seizures. The safety and efficacy of concurrent methylphenidate and anticonvulsant pharmacotherapy have not been established. If seizures occur, methylphenidate pharmacotherapy should be discontinued.
- have hypertension. Methylphenidate pharmacotherapy may exacerbate this medical disorder. Avoid prescribing methylphenidate pharmacotherapy to these patients. If methylphenidate pharmacotherapy is required, monitor blood pressure regularly. Collaboration with the patient's advanced practice nurse or family physician may be indicated.

Caution patients who are receiving methylphenidate pharmacotherapy against performing activities that require alertness, judgment, and physical coordination (e.g., driving an automobile, operating dangerous equipment, supervising children) until their response to methylphenidate pharmacotherapy is known. Methylphenidate may adversely affect these mental and physical functions.

In addition to this general precaution, caution patients to inform their prescribing psychologist if they begin or discontinue any other pharmacotherapy while receiving methylphenidate pharmacotherapy.

CLINICALLY SIGNIFICANT DRUG INTERACTIONS

Concurrent methylphenidate pharmacotherapy and the following may result in clinically significant drug interactions:

Anticoagulant (Oral) Pharmacotherapy

Concurrent methylphenidate and oral anticoagulant (i.e., coumadin [Warfarin®]) pharmacotherapy may result in the inhibition of the metabolism of the oral anticoagulant. Lower dosages of the anticoagulant may be required. Collaboration with the prescriber of the anticoagulant pharmacotherapy is indicated.

Anticonvulsant Pharmacotherapy

Concurrent methylphenidate and anticonvulsant (e.g., diphenylhydantoin [Dilantin®], phenobarbital [Luminal®], primidone [Mysoline®]) pharmacotherapy may result in the inhibition of the metabolism of the anticonvulsant. Lower dosages of the anticonvulsant may be required. Collaboration with the prescriber of the anticonvulsant pharmacotherapy is indicated.

Guanethidine Pharmacotherapy

Concurrent methylphenidate and guanethidine (Ismelin®) pharmacotherapy may result in a decrease in the antihypertensive action of guanethidine. Higher dosages of the antihypertensive may be required. Collaboration with the prescriber of the guanethidine pharmacotherapy is indicated.

Monoamine Oxidase Inhibitor Pharmacotherapy

Methylphenidate may interact with MAOIs (e.g., phenelzine [Nardil®]), resulting in the release of large amounts of catecholamines and the hypertensive crisis. The hypertensive crisis is characterized by severe headache and hypertension. Thus, methylphenidate pharmacotherapy, concurrent or within 14 days of MAOI pharmacotherapy, is *contraindicated*.

Phenylbutazone Pharmacotherapy

Concurrent methylphenidate and phenylbutazone (Nova-Butazone®) pharmacotherapy may result in the inhibition of the metabolism of the phenylbutazone. Lower dosages of the phenylbutazone may be required. Collaboration with the prescriber of the phenylbutazone is indicated.

Tricyclic Antidepressant Pharmacotherapy

Concurrent methylphenidate and TCA (e.g., desipramine [Norpramin®], imipramine [Tofranil®]) pharmacotherapy may result in the inhibition of the metabolism of the TCA. Lower dosages of the TCA may be required.

ADVERSE DRUG REACTIONS

Methylphenidate pharmacotherapy is commonly associated with insomnia, particularly if the last dose of the day is ingested late in the afternoon or early evening. This ADR may be managed by reducing the dosage of the methylphenidate or by omitting the afternoon or evening dose. Anorexia, which is usually transient, and nervousness also commonly occur. The latter may be managed with a reduction in dosage. Other ADRs associated with methylphenidate pharmacotherapy, listed according to body system, include:

Cardiovascular: angina, blood pressure changes (increase or decrease), cardiac dysrhythmias (e.g., tachycardia), and changes in pulse rate (increase or decrease)

CNS: addiction and habituation with long-term pharmacotherapy, convulsions, depressed mood (transient), dizziness, drowsiness, dyskinesia, headache, insomnia, psychotic episodes, including hallucinations, tics, or their exacerbation, and Tourette's disorder (i.e., Gilles de la Tourette's syndrome). Psychotic episodes and Tourette's disorder usually subside with discontinuation of methylphenidate pharmacotherapy.

Cutaneous: hair loss (alopecia), itchy hives or wheals (urticaria), rash, and severe itching (pruritus). Rarely, abnormal decrease in the number of blood platelets (thrombocytopenia purpura); reddened areas of the skin, usually involving the extremities (erythema multiforme), with inflammation and necrosis of blood or lymph vessels (necrotizing vasculitis); and redness of the skin followed by scaling and loss of skin with associated enlargement of the liver, fever, and edema (exfoliative dermatitis).

GI: initially, abdominal pain, loss of appetite (anorexia), and nausea. These ADRs may be relieved by ingesting each dose with food.

Hematologic: rarely, abnormal decrease in red blood cells (anemia), abnormal decrease in white blood cells (leukopenia), and abnormal decrease in the number of blood platelets (thrombocytopenia)

Metabolic/Endocrine: weight loss

Musculoskeletal: defect in voluntary movement (dyskinesia); growth retardation among children (minor, usually associated with long-term pharmacotherapy), and joint pain (arthralgia); rarely, choreoathetoid movements (e.g., extreme range of motion; jerky, involuntary movement more proximal than distal; fluctuating muscle tone from hypo- to hypertonia)

Ocular: blurring of the vision and difficulties with accommodation (adjustment of the eye for seeing various distances)

Miscellaneous: fever

OVERDOSAGE

Signs and symptoms of acute methylphenidate overdosage are associated with its CNS stimulant and sympathomimetic actions. These signs and symptoms may include abnormal dilation of the pupils (mydriasis), agitation, cardiac dysrhythmias, confusion, convulsions, delirium, dryness of the mouth and other mucous membranes, euphoria, flushing, hallucinations, headache, increase in body temperature above 41°C (106°F) (hyperpyrexia), increased action of the reflexes (hyperreflexia), hypertension, muscle twitching, palpitations, sweating, tremors, tachycardia, and vomiting. Acute methylphenidate overdosage requires emergency symptomatic medical support of body systems with attention to increasing methylphenidate elimination, particularly when overdosage involves extended-release tablets. There is no known antidote.

MIRTAZAPINE *

(mir taz′a peen)

TRADE NAME

Remeron®

CLASSIFICATION

Antidepressant (tetracyclic, piperazinoazepine)

APPROVED INDICATIONS FOR PSYCHOLOGICAL DISORDERS

Adjunctive pharmacotherapy for the symptomatic management of:

Mood Disorders, Depressive Disorders: Major Depressive Disorder

USUAL DOSAGE AND ADMINISTRATION

Major Depressive Disorder

Adults: Initially, 15 mg daily orally in a single dose 30 minutes before retiring for bed in the evening. After 7 days, if needed, according to individual patient response, increase the oral dosage to 30 mg daily in a single dose 30 minutes before retiring for bed in the evening.

MAXIMUM: 45 mg daily orally

Women who are, or who may become, pregnant: FDA Pregnancy Category C. Safety and efficacy of mirtazapine pharmacotherapy for women who are pregnant have not been established. Avoid prescribing mirtazapine pharmacotherapy to women who are pregnant. If mirtazapine pharmacotherapy is required, advise patients of potential benefits and possible risks to themselves and the embryo, fetus, or neonate. Collaboration with the patient's obstetrician is indicated.

Women who are breast-feeding: Safety and efficacy of mirtazapine pharmacotherapy for women who are breast-feeding and their neonates and infants have not been established. Avoid prescribing mirtazapine pharmacotherapy to women who are breast-feeding. If mirtazapine pharmacotherapy is required, breast-feeding probably should be discontinued. Collaboration with the patient's pediatrician may be indicated.

Elderly, frail, or debilitated patients and those who have kidney or liver dysfunction: Generally prescribe lower dosages for elderly, frail, or debilitated patients and those who have kidney or liver dysfunction. Increase the dosage gradually, if needed, according to individual patient response. Total body clearance may be reduced by up to one-third among these patients. These patients also may be more sensitive to the pharmacologic actions of mirtazapine than are younger or healthier adult patients.

Children: Safety and efficacy of mirtazapine pharmacotherapy for children have not been established. Mirtazapine pharmacotherapy is *not* recommended for this age group.

Notes, Major Depressive Disorder

Safety and efficacy of mirtazapine pharmacotherapy exceeding 6 weeks have not been established.

AVAILABLE DOSAGE FORMS, STORAGE, AND COMPATIBILITY

Tablets, oral: 15, 30 mg

Notes

General Instructions for Patients Instruct patients who are receiving mirtazapine pharmacotherapy to

- safely store mirtazapine tablets out of the reach of children in tightly closed light- and child-resistant containers at controlled room temperature (20° to 25°C; 68° to 77°F).
- obtain an available patient information sheet regarding mirtazapine pharmacotherapy from their pharmacist at the time that their prescription is dispensed. Encourage patients to clarify any questions that they may have concerning mirtazapine pharmacotherapy with their pharmacist or, if needed, to consult their prescribing psychologist.

PROPOSED MECHANISM OF ACTION

The exact mechanism of action of mirtazapine has not yet been fully determined. Mirtazapine is a potent antagonist of central serotonin receptors (i.e., 5-HT$_2$ and 5-HT$_3$ receptors) and of central pre-synaptic adrenergic receptors (i.e., α-2 receptors). Its antidepressant activity is believed to be due to its ability to increase norepinephrine and serotonin levels in the CNS. Mirtazapine also is a central histamine (H$_1$) receptor and peripheral adrenergic (α-1) receptor antagonist. These actions may help to explain its sedative and postural hypotensive actions, respectively.

PHARMACOKINETICS/PHARMACODYNAMICS

Mirtazapine is rapidly and completely absorbed following oral ingestion. However, bioavailability is significantly reduced (F = 0.5) because of extensive first-pass hepatic metabolism. The ingestion of food has no significant effect on the bioavailability of mirtazapine. Peak blood levels are obtained within 2 hours. Mirtazapine is moderately ($\sim$85%) bound to plasma proteins and is extensively metabolized in the liver. The mean half-life of elimination across age and gender groups ranges from 20 to 40 hours. Significant gender effects in the half-life of elimination have been noted (i.e., mean = 26 hours for males versus mean = 37 hours for females). Variability also is significant between the chemical structural mirror images (i.e., enantiomers) of mirtazapine. Formulated as a racemic mixture that has equal proportions of (+) and (−) enantiomers, the (−) enantiomer has a half-life of elimination and achieves blood levels approximately twice that of the (+) enantiomer. Additional data are unavailable.

RELATIVE CONTRAINDICATIONS

Hypersensitivity to mirtazapine

MAOI pharmacotherapy, concurrent or within 14 days. Although not yet directly associated with mirtazapine, concurrent MAOI and other antidepressant pharmacotherapy have been associated with the potentially fatal serotonin syndrome.

CAUTIONS AND COMMENTS

Mirtazapine pharmacotherapy has been associated with the development of severe neutropenia (i.e., agranulocytosis, granulocytopenia), a potentially fatal reduction in the blood neutrophil (granulocyte) count, often resulting in an increased susceptibility to bacterial and fungal infections. This reaction may or may not be associated with signs and symptoms of fever and infection in approximately one out of one thousand patients. Although potentially fatal, recovery is generally complete and uneventful upon discontinuation of mirtazapine pharmacotherapy. Instruct patients to report any signs and symptoms suggesting neutropenia (i.e., chills, fever, mucous membrane ulceration, sore throat, stomatitis [inflammation of the mouth]). Obtain for these patients laboratory white blood cell counts immediately, and, if low, discontinue mirtazapine pharmacotherapy. Collaboration with and referral to the patient's family physician or a specialist (e.g., hematologist) are indicated for the confirmation of neutropenia and its medical management.

Prescribe mirtazapine pharmacotherapy cautiously to patients who

have cardiovascular disorders, such as arteriosclerosis or hypercholesterolemia. Mirtazapine pharmacotherapy has been associated with significant increases in both non-fasting cholesterol and triglyceride serum concentrations. Collaboration with the patient's family physician or a specialist (e.g., cardiologist) is indicated.

Caution patients who are receiving mirtazapine pharmacotherapy against performing activities that require alertness, judgment, and physical coordination (e.g., driving an automobile, operating dangerous equipment, supervising children) until their response to mirtazapine pharmacotherapy is known. The drowsiness and somnolence associated with mirtazapine pharmacotherapy may adversely affect these mental and physical functions.

CLINICALLY SIGNIFICANT DRUG INTERACTIONS

Concurrent mirtazapine pharmacotherapy and the following may result in clinically significant drug interactions:

Alcohol Use

Concurrent mirtazapine pharmacotherapy may increase the CNS depression associated with alcohol use. Advise patients to avoid, or limit, their use of alcohol while receiving mirtazapine pharmacotherapy.

ADVERSE DRUG REACTIONS

Mirtazapine pharmacotherapy commonly has been associated with constipation, dry mouth, increased appetite, increased serum cholesterol, somnolence, and weight gain. Other ADRs, listed according to body system, include

Cardiovascular: edema, hypertension, postural hypotension, and vasodilation
CNS: abnormal dreams, agitation, amnesia, anxiety, confusion, and dizziness
Cutaneous: dry skin, itching (severe), and rash
Genitourinary: urinary frequency
GI: abdominal pain, anorexia, nausea, and vomiting

Musculoskeletal: arthritis; joint pain (arthralgia); muscle pain (myalgia); muscular weakness and abnormal fatigue (asthenia; myasthenia); numbness, prickling, or tingling sensations (paresthesias); and tremor

Ocular: abnormal accommodation, conjunctivitis, eye pain, and glaucoma

Otic: deafness and ear pain

Respiratory: cough (increased), difficult or labored breathing (dyspnea), and sinusitis

Miscellaneous: chills, malaise, and thirst

OVERDOSAGE

Signs and symptoms of mirtazapine overdosage include disorientation, drowsiness, memory impairment, and tachycardia. Mirtazapine overdosage requires emergency symptomatic medical support of body systems with attention to increasing mirtazapine elimination. There is no known antidote.

MOCLOBEMIDE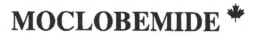

(moe kloe′be mide)

TRADE NAME

Manerix®

CLASSIFICATION

Antidepressant (reversible inhibitor of monoamine oxidase, type A [RIMA])

APPROVED INDICATIONS FOR PSYCHOLOGICAL DISORDERS

Adjunctive pharmacotherapy for the symptomatic management of:

Mood Disorders, Depressive Disorders: Major Depressive Disorder

USUAL DOSAGE AND ADMINISTRATION

Major Depressive Disorder

Adults: Initially, 300 mg daily orally in two or three divided doses immediately after meals. Increase the dosage gradually according to individual patient response. Note that therapeutic response may be delayed for two or three weeks.

MAXIMUM: 600 mg daily orally

Women who are, or who may become, pregnant: FDA Pregnancy Category "not established." Safety and efficacy of moclobemide pharmacotherapy for women who are pregnant have not been established. Avoid prescribing moclobemide pharmacotherapy to women who are pregnant. If moclobemide pharmacotherapy is required, advise patients of potential benefits and possible risks to themselves and the embryo, fetus, or neonate. Collaboration with the patient's obstetrician is indicated.

Women who are breast-feeding: Safety and efficacy of moclobemide pharmacotherapy for women who are breast-feeding and their neonates and infants have not been established. Small quantities (~1%) of moclobemide are excreted into breast milk. Avoid prescribing moclobemide pharmacotherapy to women who are breast-feeding. If moclobemide pharmacotherapy is required, breast-feeding probably should be discontinued. Collaboration with the patient's pediatrician is indicated.

Elderly, frail, or debilitated patients and those who have liver dysfunction: Initially, 300 mg daily orally in two or three divided doses. Do not exceed the recommended adult maximum dosage of 600 mg daily orally. Generally, no dosage adjustments are required for elderly patients. However, prescribe lower dosages for frail or debilitated patients and those who have liver dysfunction. Increase the dosage gradually, if needed, according to individual patient response. These patients may be more sensitive to the pharmacologic actions of moclobemide than are younger or healthier adult patients.

MAXIMUM: 600 mg daily orally

Children and adolescents younger than 18 years of age: Safety and efficacy of moclobemide pharmacotherapy for children and adolescents have not been established. Moclobemide pharmacotherapy is *not* recommended for this age group.

Notes, Major Depressive Disorder

Prescribe doses for ingestion after meals. Moclobemide may interact with tyramine-containing foods. This interaction may be minimized by ingesting moclobemide after, rather than prior to, meals. Other special dietary restrictions in regard to tyramine generally are not required. See Clinically Significant Drug Interactions.

AVAILABLE DOSAGE FORMS, STORAGE, AND COMPATIBILITY

Tablets, oral: 100, 150, 300 mg

Notes

General Instructions for Patients Instruct patients who are receiving moclobemide pharmacotherapy to

- always ingest each dose of moclobemide oral tablets immediately after a meal in order to minimize possible interactions with tyramine-containing foods (see Clinically Significant Drug Interactions).

- safely store moclobemide oral tablets out of the reach of children in child-resistant containers at controlled room temperature (15° to 30°C; 59° to 86°F).
- obtain an available patient information sheet regarding moclobemide pharmacotherapy from their pharmacist at the time that their prescription is dispensed. Encourage patients to clarify any questions that they may have concerning moclobemide pharmacotherapy with their pharmacist or, if needed, to consult their prescribing psychologist.

PROPOSED MECHANISM OF ACTION

The exact mechanism of action of moclobemide has not been fully determined. However, its antidepressant action appears to be directly related to the inhibition of monoamine oxidase, particularly type A (i.e., ~80% inhibition of type A and ~20% inhibition of type B). The inhibition of monoamine oxidase type A is brief (i.e., less than 24 hours) and reversible.

PHARMACOKINETICS/PHARMACODYNAMICS

Moclobemide is well and completely absorbed (~98%) following oral ingestion. However, bioavailability is significantly reduced (i.e., $F = 0.55$ after single dosing; $F = 0.9$ after multiple dosing) because of significant first-pass hepatic metabolism. Food reduces the rate, but not the extent, of absorption. Peak blood levels generally are achieved within 1 hour. Moclobemide is moderately (i.e., ~50%) bound to plasma proteins and is widely distributed throughout the body with a mean apparent volume of distribution of 1.2 L/kg. Moclobemide is metabolized extensively in the liver to several inactive metabolites. Its mean half-life of elimination is 1.5 hours. Mean total body clearance is ~32 L/hour. Note that ~2% of the Caucasian population and 15% of the Asian population are genetically phenotyped as slow metabolizers in relation to oxidative hepatic metabolism. The total area under the blood concentration time curve (AUC) for these patients (i.e., the total amount of moclobemide absorbed and available to the systemic or general circulation) may be increased up to 50% when compared to extensive metabolizers (i.e., the majority of the population) when given an equal oral dose. Additional data are unavailable.

RELATIVE CONTRAINDICATIONS

Clomipramine pharmacotherapy, concurrent. Concurrent moclobemide and clomipramine pharmacotherapy may result in severe ADRs. Although clomipramine is a TCA, its associated SSRI activity is most likely responsible for these severe ADRs. Concurrent moclobemide and clomipramine pharmacotherapy is *contraindicated*.

Confusional states, acute

Hypersensitivity to moclobemide

Meperidine pharmacotherapy, concurrent. Although not yet directly associated with moclobemide pharmacotherapy, concurrent meperidine and MAOI (i.e., phenelzine, tranylcypromine) pharmacotherapy has resulted in death. Thus, concurrent moclobemide and meperidine pharmacotherapy is *contraindicated*.

SSRI pharmacotherapy, concurrent. Although not yet directly associated with moclobemide pharmacotherapy, concurrent SSRI and MAOI pharmacotherapy has been associated with an exacerbation of serotonergic ADRs, including the potentially fatal serotonin syndrome (see Clinically Significant Drug Interactions). Concurrent moclobemide and SSRI pharmacotherapy is generally *contraindicated*.

CAUTIONS AND COMMENTS

Prescribe moclobemide pharmacotherapy cautiously to patients who

have pheochromocytoma or thyrotoxicosis. Although not yet reported with moclobemide, MAOI pharmacotherapy has precipitated serious hypertensive reactions among these patients.

Caution patients who are receiving moclobemide pharmacotherapy against performing activities that require alertness, judgment, and physical coordination (e.g., driving an automobile, operating dangerous equipment, supervising children) until their response to moclobemide pharmacotherapy is known. Moclobemide may adversely affect these physical and mental functions.

In addition to this general precaution, caution patients to inform their prescribing psychologist if they begin or discontinue any other pharmacotherapy while receiving moclobemide pharmacotherapy.

CLINICALLY SIGNIFICANT DRUG INTERACTIONS

Concurrent moclobemide pharmacotherapy and the following may result in clinically significant drug interactions:

Antihypertensive Pharmacotherapy

Concurrent moclobemide pharmacotherapy and antihypertensive pharmacotherapy may result in varying changes in blood pressure, both increases and decreases. Monitor patients carefully when concurrent pharmacotherapy is necessary. Some patients may require an adjustment in the dosage of the antihypertensive. Collaboration with the prescriber of the antihypertensive is indicated.

Tyramine-containing Beverages and Foods

Moclobemide may interact with beverages and foods that contain high concentrations of tyramine. Ingesting each dose of moclobemide after meals appears to be the only precaution required to prevent this interaction. However, the excessive consumption of beverages or foods that have high tyramine content should probably be avoided (see Phenelzine and Tranylcypromine Monographs). Advise patients to ingest each dose of their moclobemide after meals and to avoid beverages and foods that have high tyramine concentrations. Also advise them to report immediately the sudden occurrence of bradycardia, neck stiffness, palpitations, tachycardia, or other unusual signs and symptoms suggestive of a moclobemide and tyramine interaction.

Cimetidine Pharmacotherapy

Cimetidine (Tagamet®) inhibits the hepatic microsomal metabolism of moclobemide. This interaction may result in a doubling of the area under the curve (AUC) and moclobemide's steady-state concentrations. When concurrent pharmacotherapy is required, decrease by 50% the initial moclobemide dosage.

Clomipramine Pharmacotherapy

Concurrent moclobemide and clomipramine (Anafranil®) pharmacotherapy is *contraindicated*. See Relative Contraindications.

Monoamine Oxidase Inhibitor Pharmacotherapy

Concurrent moclobemide and MAOI pharmacotherapy increases the risk for the potentially fatal serotonin syndrome. This combination of pharmacotherapy is *contraindicated*. See Relative Contraindications.

Nefazodone Pharmacotherapy

Concurrent moclobemide and nefazodone (Serzone®) pharmacotherapy may result in increased serotonin effects. This interaction may increase the risk for the potentially fatal serotonin syndrome.

Pharmacotherapy With Sympathomimetics

Concurrent moclobemide and sympathomimetic pharmacotherapy (e.g., amphetamines, ephedrine, methylphenidate [Ritalin®], phenylephrine [Neo-Synephrine®]) may potentiate the actions of the sympathomimetic (e.g., increase blood pressure excessively), particularly long-term high-dosage moclobemide pharmacotherapy.

Selegiline Pharmacotherapy

Selegiline (Eldepryl®) is a selective MAO-type B inhibitor. Concurrent moclobemide (a MAO-type A inhibitor) and selegiline pharmacotherapy may result in combined activity resembling that of a classic MAOI. Thus, concurrent pharmacotherapy requires associated cautions and dietary restrictions (e.g., avoidance of beverages and foods high in tyramine content).

See Phenelzine and Tranylcypromine Monographs

ADVERSE DRUG REACTIONS

Moclobemide pharmacotherapy commonly has been associated with a dry mouth, headache, and insomnia. Other ADRs, listed according to body system, include

Cardiovascular: hypotension, palpitations, and tachycardia
CNS: agitation, anxiety, dizziness, nervousness, nightmares, and restlessness
Cutaneous: dry skin, itching, rash, and sweating (excessive)
Genitourinary: abnormal bleeding from the uterus at any time other than during the menstrual period (metrorrhagia), difficult or painful urination (dysuria), and frequent or excessive urination (polyuria)
GI: constipation, diarrhea, indigestion, and vomiting
Metabolic/Endocrine: see Genitourinary
Musculoskeletal: muscular pain and tremor
Ocular: blurred vision and conjunctivitis

OVERDOSAGE

Signs and symptoms of moclobemide overdosage include amnesia, drowsiness, mild disorientation, nausea, reduced reflexes, slurred speech, and stupor. Moclobemide overdosage requires emergency symptomatic medical support of body systems with attention to increasing moclobemide elimination. There is no known antidote.

MOLINDONE *

(moe lin'done)

TRADE NAME

Moban®

CLASSIFICATION

Antipsychotic (dihydroindolone)

APPROVED INDICATIONS FOR PSYCHOLOGICAL DISORDERS

Adjunctive pharmacotherapy for the symptomatic management of:

Psychotic Disorders: Schizophrenia and Other Psychotic Disorders

USUAL DOSAGE AND ADMINISTRATION

Schizophrenia and Other Psychotic Disorders

Adults: Initially, 50 to 75 mg daily orally in three or four divided doses. In three or four days, increase the dosage to 100 mg daily, according to the severity of signs and symptoms and individual patient response. Some patients may require up to 225 mg daily, depending on the severity of their symptomatology and clinical response.

MAINTENANCE: 10 to 225 mg daily orally in three or four divided doses. Adjust the dosage according to the severity of signs and symptoms and individual patient response.
Mild symptomatology: 10 to 60 mg daily orally in three or four divided doses
Moderate symptomatology: 30 to 100 mg daily orally in three or four divided doses
Severe symptomatology: 225 mg daily orally in three or four divided doses

MAXIMUM: 300 mg daily

Women who are, or who may become, pregnant: FDA Pregnancy Category "not established." Safety and efficacy of molindone pharmacotherapy for women who are pregnant have not been established. Avoid prescribing molindone pharmacotherapy to women who are pregnant. If molindone pharmacotherapy is required, advise patients of potential benefits and possible risks to themselves and the embryo, fetus, or neonate. Collaboration with the patient's obstetrician may be indicated.

Women who are breast-feeding: Safety and efficacy of molindone pharmacotherapy for women who are breast-feeding and their neonates and infants have not been established. Molindone is excreted into breast milk. Avoid prescribing molindone pharmacotherapy for women who are breast-feeding. If molindone pharmacotherapy is required, breast-feeding probably should be discontinued. Collaboration with the patient's pediatrician is indicated.

Elderly, frail, or debilitated patients and those who have kidney dysfunction: Initiate molindone pharmacotherapy with lower dosages. Increase the dosage gradually according to the severity of signs and symptoms and individual patient response. Generally prescribe lower dosages for elderly, frail, or debilitated patients. These patients may be more sensitive to the pharmacologic actions of molindone than are younger or healthier adult patients. Patients who have kidney dysfunction also may require lower dosages.

Children younger than 12 years of age: Safety and efficacy of molindone pharmacotherapy for children younger than 12 years of age have not been established. Molindone pharmacotherapy is *not* recommended for this age group.

Notes, Schizophrenia and Other Psychotic Disorders

Prescribe initial and maintenance dosages according to the severity of signs and symptoms and individual patient response.

AVAILABLE DOSAGE FORMS, STORAGE, AND COMPATIBILITY

Capsules, oral: 5, 10, 25 mg
Concentrate, oral: 20 mg/ml (cherry flavored, contains alcohol)
Tablets, oral: 5, 10, 25, 50, 100 mg

Notes

Molindone Oral Concentrate The oral concentrate (i.e., Moban Concentrate®) contains sodium metabisulfite. Sulfites have been associated with hypersensitivity reactions, including life-threatening anaphylactic reactions, among susceptible patients. Sulfite hypersensitivity may occur more frequently among people who have histories of asthma.

General Instructions for Patients Instruct patients who are receiving molindone pharmacotherapy to

- safely store oral dosage forms of molindone out of the reach of children in child- and light-resistant containers at controlled room temperature (15° to 30°C; 59° to 86°F).
- obtain an available patient information sheet regarding molindone pharmacotherapy from their pharmacist at the time that their prescription is dispensed. Encourage patients to clarify any questions that they may have concerning molindone pharmacotherapy with their pharmacist or, if needed, to consult their prescribing psychologist.

PROPOSED MECHANISM OF ACTION

The exact mechanism of action of molindone is complex and has not yet been fully determined. Its antipsychotic activity appears to be related primarily to its interaction with dopamine-containing neurons, specifically the blockade of dopamine receptors both pre-synaptically and post-synaptically. EEG evidence provides some support for action on the ascending reticular activating system (RAS) (i.e., alerting system of the brain), including the hypothalamus, sub-thalamus, and medial thalamus. The RAS extends from the central core of the brain stem to all parts of the cerebral cortex. It is essential for initiating and maintaining wakefulness and introspection and for directing attention. Some of the antipsychotics may act to depress this system.

PHARMACOKINETICS/PHARMACODYNAMICS

Molindone is absorbed rapidly and metabolized extensively after oral ingestion, with peak blood levels occurring within 1 hour. It is distributed widely in the body. Molindone is metabolized extensively in the liver to over 30 different inactive metabolites. Less than 3% of molindone is excreted in unchanged form in the urine. The mean half-life of elimination is 1.5 hours. Additional data are unavailable.

RELATIVE CONTRAINDICATIONS

CNS depression, severe, including that associated with the use of alcohol, opiate analgesics, and sedative-hypnotics (e.g., barbiturates)
Coma
Hypersensitivity to molindone

CAUTIONS AND COMMENTS

Caution patients who are receiving molindone pharmacotherapy against performing activities that require alertness, judgment, and physical coordination (e.g., driving an automobile, operating dangerous equipment, supervising children) until their response to molindone pharmacotherapy is known. Molindone may adversely affect these mental and physical functions.

CLINICALLY SIGNIFICANT DRUG INTERACTIONS

None commonly identified at present

ADVERSE DRUG REACTIONS

Drowsiness commonly has been associated with the initiation of molindone pharmacotherapy. This ADR generally can be managed with continued pharmacotherapy or by lowering the dosage. Molindone pharmacotherapy also has been associated with depression, euphoria, and hyperactivity. In addition to these ADRs, attention to the ADRs associated with other antipsychotic pharmacotherapy is required because of molindone's chemical and pharmacological similarities to these other antipsychotics (see Phenothiazines General Monograph). These ADRs, listed according to body system, include

Cardiovascular

Hypotension, tachycardia (associated with molindone's anticholinergic action), and, rarely, transient nonspecific T-wave changes on ECG.

Central Nervous System

EPRs. These ADRs generally are reversible with appropriate management, including the reduction of dosage, concurrent sedative-hypnotic pharmacotherapy, or concurrent antiparkinsonian (other than levodopa [Dopar®]) pharmacotherapy. EPRs include the following:

Akathisia (Motor Restlessness)   Akathisia is usually associated with initial pharmacotherapy and is characterized by an inability to sit still. The thought of sitting down causes severe anxiety and restlessness. Patients generally have an urgent need for movement and feelings of muscular "quivering."

Dystonic Syndrome   The dystonic syndrome involves prolonged abnormal contractions of muscle groups.

Parkinsonian Syndrome   Immobility, rigidity, and reduction of voluntary movements and tremor characterize the Parkinsonian syndrome. This syndrome occurs less frequently than akathisia.

Tardive Dyskinesia   TD, or involuntary movement, characterized by slow, rhythmical, automatic stereotyped movements, can be generalized or involve a single group of muscles (see also Phenothiazines General Monograph).

Cutaneous

Rash (nonspecific, probably a hypersensitivity reaction)

Genitourinary

Increase in sex drive (conscious or unconscious) and urinary retention

Gastrointestinal

Constipation, dry mouth, excessive salivation, and nausea

Hematologic

Rarely, an abnormal decrease in white blood cells (leukopenia), including mainly the lymphocytes, but also basophils, eosinophils, and monocytes. An increase in the number of leukocytes (leukocytosis), which generally is associated with the presence of infection, also may rarely occur.

Hepatic

Rarely, clinically significant alterations in liver function

Metabolic/Endocrine

Abnormal absence of menses (amenorrhea), abnormal breast enlargement (gynecomastia), abnormal lactation (galactorrhea), resumption of menses among previously amenorrheic women, heavy menses (usually associated with initial pharmacotherapy), and weight gain or loss in the direction of normal or ideal weight.

Musculoskeletal

See CNS

Ocular

Blurred vision

OVERDOSAGE

Molindone overdosage requires emergency symptomatic medical support of body systems with attention to increasing molindone elimination. There is no known antidote.

MORPHINE

(mor'feen)

TRADE NAMES

Duramorph®
Morphitec®

M.O.S.®
MS Contin®
Oramorph SR®

CLASSIFICATION

Opiate analgesic (C-II)

See also Opiate Analgesics General Monograph

APPROVED INDICATIONS FOR PSYCHOLOGICAL DISORDERS

Adjunctive pharmacotherapy for the symptomatic management of:

- Pain Disorders: Acute Pain, Moderate to Severe. Morphine is indicated for the symptomatic management of acute pain of six months' or shorter duration. Dosage generally is prescribed according to type and severity of pain and method of administration.
- Pain Disorders: Chronic Cancer Pain, Moderate to Severe. Morphine is indicated for the symptomatic management of chronic pain of six months' or longer duration. Dosage generally is prescribed according to type and severity of pain and method of administration.

USUAL DOSAGE AND ADMINISTRATION

Acute Pain, Moderate to Severe

Adults: Initially, 5 to 20 mg intramuscularly, *or* 2.5 to 15 mg intravenously slowly over four to five minutes, *or* 10 to 30 mg orally, *or* 10 to 20 mg rectally. Repeat the initial dose every four hours, as needed, according to individual patient response (see Notes). Some patients may benefit from patient controlled analgesia (PCA).

PCA MULTIPLE, SLOW INTRAVENOUS INJECTION OF MORPHINE   Dosage is adjusted according to the severity of pain and individual patient response. Assure that patients understand the safe and correct use of the PCA infusion device. Care must be used to determine and set the maximum parameters of the PCA infusion pump to avoid overdosage and resultant respiratory depression. Abrupt cessation of prolonged opiate analgesic pharmacotherapy may result in not only a loss of analgesia, but also the opiate withdrawal syndrome.

Women who are, or who may become, pregnant: FDA Pregnancy Category C. Safety and efficacy of morphine pharmacotherapy for women who are pregnant have not been established. Although morphine pharmacotherapy during pregnancy has not been associated with congenital malformations (i.e., birth defects), high-dosage pharmacotherapy, or regular personal use, near term may result in the neonatal opiate withdrawal syndrome (see Opiate Analgesics General Monograph). Avoid prescribing morphine pharmacotherapy to women who are pregnant. If morphine pharmacotherapy is required, advise patients of potential benefits and possible risks to themselves and the embryo, fetus, or neonate. Collaboration with the patient's advanced practice nurse or obstetrician is indicated. Morphine pharmacotherapy is not recommended for women prior to labor unless potential benefits outweigh possible risks to the embryo, fetus, or neonate. Opiate pharmacotherapy during labor may result in drowsiness and other expected pharmacologic actions (e.g., respiratory depression) among neonates.

Women who are breast-feeding: Safety and efficacy of morphine pharmacotherapy for women who are breast-feeding and their neonates and infants have not been established. Morphine is excreted into breast milk. The concentration of morphine in breast milk generally is higher than that in the maternal blood. Expected pharmacologic actions (e.g., CNS or respiratory depression, constipation) may be observed among breast-fed neonates and infants, who also may become addicted (see Opiate Analgesics General Monograph). Avoid prescribing morphine pharmacotherapy to women who are breast-feeding. If morphine pharmacotherapy is required, breast-feeding should be discontinued. If desired, lactation may be maintained and breast-feeding resumed following the discontinuation of short-term morphine pharmacotherapy. Collaboration with the patient's advanced practice nurse or pediatrician is indicated.

Elderly, frail, or debilitated patients: Generally prescribe lower dosages for elderly, frail, or debilitated patients. Increase the dosage gradually, if needed, according to individual patient response. These patients may be more sensitive to the pharmacologic actions of morphine than are younger or healthier adult patients.

Children: Initially, 0.1 to 0.2 mg/kg intramuscularly or subcutaneously, *or* 0.05 to 0.1 mg/kg intravenously slowly over four to five minutes, *or* 0.15 to 0.3 mg/kg orally, *or* 0.15 to 0.3 mg/kg rectally. Repeat the initial dose every four hours, as needed, according to individual patient response (see Notes, Pain Disorders).

MAXIMUM: 15 mg/dose

Chronic Cancer Pain, Moderate to Severe

Adults: Initially, 0.2 to 0.4 mg/kg orally or rectally every four to six hours, as needed; *or* 2.5 to 15 mg intravenously or subcutaneously every four to six hours, as needed. For intravenous injection, dilute in 4 to 5 ml of sterile water for injection and inject slowly over 3 to 5 minutes with the patient lying down. Patients whose chronic moderate to severe pain has been managed with short-acting morphine formulations may benefit from long-acting oral extended-release formulations of morphine (to replace short-acting morphine pharmacotherapy with long-acting morphine pharmacotherapy see Notes, Chronic Cancer Pain, Moderate to Severe). Other patients may require continuous intravenous or subcutaneous pharmacotherapy.

CONTINUOUS INTRAVENOUS OR SUBCUTANEOUS INFUSION FOR RELIEF OF SEVERE CHRONIC PAIN ASSOCIATED WITH CANCER   Initially, 0.8 to 10 mg/hour. Adjust to lowest effective dosage. An intravenous loading dose of 15 mg or more may be injected for initial relief of pain prior to initiating continuous intravenous infusion.

Loading dose for patients whose pain is poorly controlled: 1 to 2 mg/minute until pain is relieved. Dilute in 4 to 5 ml of intravenous solution and infuse slowly over 1 minute while monitoring heart rate, respiratory rate, and blood pressure. Withhold morphine pharmacotherapy if respiratory rate slows to less than 10 respirations per minute or if the diastolic pressure decreases more than 10%. Resume morphine pharmacotherapy when respiratory rate and blood pressure have stabilized.

Loading dose, for patients whose pain is presently controlled: Using the previous day's 24-hour opiate requirement, calculate hourly dose with attention to method of administration and analgesic equivalents.

Maintenance: 0.8 to 80 mg/hour. Dosages of 150 mg/hour have occasionally been required. Relatively high dosages (275 to 440 mg/hour) have occasionally been infused for several hours or days to provide relief of exacerbations of chronic pain among adults previously stabilized on lower dosages or whose dosage had been gradually titrated to relatively high levels. Subsequent dosage reductions, according to patient response, generally were possible.

MULTIPLE SLOW INTRAVENOUS INJECTION FOR PATIENT CONTROLLED ANALGESIA Dosage is adjusted according to the severity of pain and individual patient response. Assure that the patient understands the safe and correct use of the PCA infusion device. Care must be used to determine and set the maximum parameters of the PCA infusion pump to avoid overdosage and resultant respiratory depression. Also avoid inadvertent abrupt cessation of pharmacotherapy. Abrupt cessation of pharmacotherapy may result in a loss of analgesia and the opiate withdrawal syndrome.

Women who are, or who may become, pregnant: FDA Pregnancy Category C. Safety and efficacy of morphine pharmacotherapy for women who are pregnant have not been established. Although morphine pharmacotherapy during pregnancy has not been associated with congenital malformations (i.e., birth defects), high-dosage pharmacotherapy, or regular personal use, near term may result in the neonatal opiate withdrawal syndrome (see Opiate Analgesics General Monograph). Avoid prescribing morphine pharmacotherapy to women who are pregnant. If morphine pharmacotherapy is required, advise patients of potential benefits and possible risks to themselves and the embryo, fetus, or neonate. Collaboration with the patient's advanced practice nurse or obstetrician is indicated.

Women who are breast-feeding: Safety and efficacy of morphine pharmacotherapy for women who are breast-feeding and their neonates and infants have not been established. Morphine is excreted into breast milk. The concentration of morphine in breast milk generally is higher than that in maternal blood. Expected pharmacological actions (e.g., CNS or respiratory depression, constipation) may be observed among breast-fed infants, who also may become addicted (see also Opiate Analgesics General Monograph). Avoid prescribing morphine pharmacotherapy to women who are breast-feeding. If morphine pharmacotherapy is required, breast-feeding should be discontinued. Collaboration with the patient's advanced practice nurse or pediatrician may be indicated.

Elderly, frail, or debilitated patients: Generally prescribe lower dosages for elderly, frail, or debilitated patients. Increase the dosage gradually, if needed, according to individual patient response. These patients may be more sensitive to the pharmacologic actions of morphine than are younger or healthier adult patients.

Children: Initially, 0.2 to 0.4 mg/kg orally or rectally every four to six hours, as needed, *or* 0.1 to 0.2 mg/kg subcutaneously every four hours, as needed, *or* 0.05 to 0.1 mg/kg intravenously. Inject intravenously slowly over three to five minutes. Adjust dosage according to patient response.

MAXIMUM: For palliative care, the maximum dosage is guided by patient response.

Notes, Acute Pain and Chronic Cancer Pain, Moderate to Severe

Prescribe morphine pharmacotherapy at regular intervals throughout the 24-hour day for the symptomatic management of pain. Do not prescribe morphine on an "as needed" basis. This recommendation is particularly important for patients who have chronic pain associated with malignant disease. These patients usually need to be awakened during the night to maintain pain management so that they will not awaken with morning pain. The dosage range for morphine is wide. There is no "usual" recommended dosage because of such varying factors as general health, pharmacokinetic parameters, and individual experience of pain, including its cause, intensity, and duration. A general rule is to prescribe the *lowest effective dosage* as infrequently as possible. This recommendation will help to provide optimal therapeutic benefit while minimizing the development of tolerance to morphine's analgesic action and addiction and habituation.

When adjusting the dosage, do not increase the dosage more frequently than every 24 hours. It generally takes approximately 5 morphine half-lives to attain a new steady-state concentration among patients who have normal kidney and liver function. Monitor patients closely following all increases in dosage for ADRs, particularly constipation, hypotension, sedation, nausea, respiratory depression, and vomiting.

During the first two to three days of effective pain management, patients may sleep for several hours. This somnolence may be incorrectly attributed to excessive CNS depression rather than effective pain management among exhausted patients who previously had ineffective pain management. Maintain the dosage for approximately 3 days before reducing the dosage, given that respiratory function and other physiological parameters are adequate. Following the relief of severe pain, attempt periodically to reduce the morphine dosage. Lower dosages or complete discontinuation of morphine pharmacotherapy may become possible as a result of physiological change or improved psychological health among patients.

Injectable Morphine Pharmacotherapy   Injectable pharmacotherapy may be prescribed by intramuscular or subcutaneous injection or by subcutaneous infusion with a portable infusion pump. It also may be prescribed by slow intravenous injection over three to five minutes or by continuous intravenous infusion.

INTRAMUSCULAR PHARMACOTHERAPY   Usually prescribe intramuscular morphine pharmacotherapy every four hours, around the clock.

INTRAVENOUS PHARMACOTHERAPY   Dilute each dose in intravenous solution (5% dextrose in water or sodium chloride injection) to the desired concentration (usually 0.1 to 0.5 mg/ml) before injection. Inject intravenously slowly over three to five minutes. Rapid intravenous injection may result in an increased severity and frequency of associated ADRs, including apnea, cardiac arrest, chest wall rigidity, hypotension, peripheral circulatory collapse, possible anaphylaxis, and severe respiratory depression. The opiate analgesic antagonist Naloxone (Narcan®), emergency equipment for assisted breathing, and trained medical personnel should be immediately available whenever intravenous morphine pharmacotherapy is administered.

SUBCUTANEOUS PHARMACOTHERAPY WITH AN INFUSION PUMP   Subcutaneous infusion is indicated for patients who have limited muscle mass or have inadequate or unaccessible peripheral veins. When replacing intravenous morphine pharmacotherapy with subcutaneous infusion, use the same dose, and monitor the same parameters. The maximum dosage has not been determined, but dosages as high as 480 mg daily may be required. Erythema, bruising, induration, or tenderness around the subcutaneous injection site may occur. Inspect the injection site daily for these ADRs and for leakage of drug around the site. Irritation at venipuncture sites may be minimized by changing needle sites every 7 to 10 days (some prescribers prefer every 48 hours).

Oral Morphine Pharmacotherapy   Prescribe oral morphine pharmacotherapy rather than injectable pharmacotherapy whenever possible with the end goal of pain relief. As a general rule, when replacing injectable morphine pharmacotherapy with oral pharmacotherapy, double the dose (e.g., 5 mg intravenously = 10 mg orally) because of the decreased oral bioavailability of morphine. Whenever possible, prescribe the extended-release tablets or capsules. The extended-release tablets and capsules will allow some patients to be dosed every eight to twelve hours (e.g., MS Contin® and Oramorph SR® extended-release tablets) or every twenty four hours (e.g., Kadian® extended-release capsules).

EXTENDED-RELEASE FORMULATIONS   Morphine pharmacotherapy with the oral extended-release formulation is indicated for patients who have been stabilized on a set dosage of morphine. To replace this pharmacotherapy with the oral extended-release formulation, approximate the dosage according to the entire daily dosage in either a single dose with the extended-release *capsules* or two or three equally divided doses with the extended-release *tablets* every twelve or eight hours, respectively. Do not generally adjust the dosage more frequently than every 48 hours because of the pharmacokinetic properties of the oral extended-release formulations. A short-acting opiate analgesic may be required during the interim 48 hours in order to provide relief for breakthrough pain. If the oral extended-release formulation is replacing a different opiate analgesic, use the approximate analgesic equivalents to determine the initial daily dosage requirements provided in the Opiate Analgesics General Monograph.

Following the control of chronic, severe pain, periodically attempt to reduce the dosage or discontinue morphine pharmacotherapy. Always prescribe the lowest effective dosage of the extended-release formulation according to individual patient response. Unfortunately, oral formulations may not always achieve therapeutic efficacy among patients who have chronic cancer pain.

AVAILABLE DOSAGE FORMS, STORAGE, AND COMPATIBILITY

Capsules, oral: 15, 30 mg
Capsules, oral extended-release: 20, 50, 100 mg
Concentrate, oral with calibrated dropper (M.O.S.®, M.O.S.-SR®, Roxanol® concentrated oral solution): 20, 50 mg/ml (unflavored)
Injectables, intramuscular, intravenous, subcutaneous: 0.5, 1, 2, 3, 4, 5, 8, 10, 15, 25, 30, 50 mg/ml. Injectable morphine is incompatible with aminophylline, calcium chloride, heparin, or sodium bicarbonate.
Injectables, cartridges: 1, 5 mg/ml
Injectables, cartridges for Patient-Controlled Analgesia Infusor: 1, 2, 3, 5 mg in 30 ml
Injectables, Rapiject® prefilled single-dose syringe: 1, 2, 50 mg in 50 ml (the 50 mg formulation is prepared without a preservative)
Solutions, oral: 5, 10, 20 mg/5 ml
Suppositories, rectal (RMS®): 5, 10, 20, 30 mg
Syrups, oral: 1, 5, 10, 20 mg/ml (orange-flavored, contains 5% alcohol; unflavored, alcohol free)
Tablets, oral: 5, 10, 15, 20, 25, 30, 35, 40, 50, 60 mg
Tablets, oral extended-release (MS Contin®, Oramorph SR®): 15, 30, 60, 100, 200 mg

Notes

Injectable Morphine Formulations   Store injectables safely between 15° and 30°C (59° and 86°F). Do *not* autoclave. Neither loss of potency nor increased toxicity has been associated with a discolored injectable solution of morphine.

Some injectable formulations (e.g., those manufactured by Abbott or Faulding) contain sodium metabisulfite. Sulfites may cause hypersensitivity reactions, including anaphylactic reactions, among susceptible patients. Although relatively uncommon, these reactions appear to occur with a higher incidence among patients who have asthma.

MORPHINE INJECTABLES (1, 2 mg/ml)   When stored at room temperature, morphine injection diluted to concentrations of 0.1 to 0.5 mg/ml in PVC bags containing dextrose 5% injection or sterile water for injection should be used within 24 hours after dilution in order to avoid risk of microbial contamination. Morphine injectables and dilutions in dextrose 5% injection or sodium chloride 0.9% injection may be stored in portable infusion pump cassettes, syringes, or PVC infusion bags. Protected from light, they will remain stable for 24 hours at room temperature, or for 72 hours when refrigerated. Proper aseptic technique for the preparation and handling of solutions is required to minimize contamination of solutions.

As with all injectables, prior to use intravenous admixtures should be inspected visually, whenever packaging permits, for clarity, particulate matter, precipitates, and leakage. Do not use solutions that are hazy or those that contain particulate matter, precipitates, or are leaking. Discard these solutions appropriately. A yellow discoloration does not indicate a loss of potency or toxicity.

HIGHLY CONCENTRATED INJECTABLE SOLUTIONS   Highly concentrated solutions of morphine for injection (e.g., Morphine HP®) may be used with or without dilution. These injectable formulations are indicated exclusively for the relief of severe pain among patients who require intramuscular or subcutaneous opiate analgesia in doses higher than those usually required (i.e., *these injectable formulations are for patients who are tolerant to opiate analgesics*). These formulations allow smaller injection volumes and, thus, less discomfort, usually associated with the injection of larger volumes of drug at subcutaneous or intramuscular injection sites. These formulations also may be diluted in large-volume intravenous solutions (e.g., dextrose 5% in water; sodium chloride injection) for slow, continuous intravenous infusion.

It is strongly recommended that the use of these highly concentrated formulations be avoided for patients who are not opiate tolerant because of the potential for overdosage error. When a less concentrated morphine injection is being replaced with the highly concentrated solution formulation, similar dosages should be prescribed, depending on individual patient need and response. If a highly concentrated morphine solution is replacing a different opiate analgesic, an equivalency table (see Opiate Analgesics General Monograph) should be used as a guide to determine the appropriate initial dose.

Do *not* confuse concentrated solutions of morphine for injection with nonconcentrated injectable formulations, which have lower dosage strengths. *Fatal overdosage may result.*

RAPIJECT® PREFILLED SYRINGES   The Rapiject® prefilled syringe is considered to be sterile as long as it is in a sealed, intact condition with caps in place. This formulation contains no bacteriostatics or antimicrobials and is intended as a single-dose unit. Any unused portion should be discarded appropriately. Store at room temperature below 25°C (77°F). Protect from light. Do not autoclave.

Directions for Rapiject® prefilled syringe:

- remove protective caps from vial and injector
- insert vial into injector
- rotate vial three turns in clockwise direction until some resistance occurs
- rotate vial another turn or two. The needle will then be in contact with the morphine solution
- remove the needle cap and expel any air
- the Rapiject® is ready for use

Oral Morphine Formulations   Do not confuse the regular capsules, tablets, oral solutions, or oral syrups with the extended-release capsules and tablets or more concentrated oral solutions. *Fatal overdosage may result.*

EXTENDED-RELEASE CAPSULES AND TABLETS   The extended-release *capsules* are formulated to be dosed every twelve hours. The extended-release *tablets* are formulated to be dosed every eight or twelve hours, depending on individual patient requirements.

SYRUPS   The Morphitec® syrup contains tartrazine (FD&C No. 5). Tartrazine has been associated with hypersensitivity reactions, including bronchial asthma, among susceptible patients. These reactions appear to occur more commonly among patients who have a hypersensitivity to aspirin.

The M.O.S.® syrup contains sodium metabisulfite. Sulfites have been associated with hypersensitivity reactions, including anaphylactic reactions, among susceptible patients. Although relatively uncommon, these reactions appear to occur with a higher incidence among patients who have asthma. M.O.S. flavored syrup also contains 5% alcohol.

General Instructions for Patients   Instruct patients who are receiving morphine pharmacotherapy to

- safely store morphine oral capsules, tablets, and other oral dosage forms out of the reach of children in tightly closed child- and light-resistant containers at controlled room temperature (15° to 30°C; 59° to 86°F).
- swallow whole each dose of the morphine oral extended-release capsules and tablets without breaking, crushing, or chewing. Crushing or chewing these formulations could result in rapid release and absorption of large doses of morphine and associated toxicity. Also instruct patients to ingest their oral capsules and tablets with adequate liquid chaser (e.g., 60 to 120 ml of water). If patients have difficulty swallowing the oral extended-release capsules, instruct them to take the capsule apart gently and sprinkle the timed beads onto a small amount of applesauce, pudding, jam, yogurt, or other cold soft food, and ingest within 30 minutes. To assure that the entire dose is ingested, advise them to rinse their mouth with water or another beverage immediately following the ingestion of the timed beads and to swallow the rinse. Caution them not to chew or crush the timed beads.
- obtain an available patient information sheet regarding morphine pharmacotherapy from their pharmacist at the time that their prescription is dispensed. Encourage patients to clarify any questions that they may have concerning morphine pharmacotherapy with their pharmacist or, if needed, to consult their prescribing psychologist.

PROPOSED MECHANISM OF ACTION

Morphine acts as an agonist at specific opiate receptor sites in the CNS, producing analgesia. It also produces alterations in endocrine and autonomic nervous system function (e.g., decreased GI motility), drowsiness, mood changes, nausea, respiratory depression, and vomiting.

See also Opiate Analgesics General Monograph

PHARMACOKINETICS/PHARMACODYNAMICS

Morphine is fairly well absorbed following oral ingestion. However, only about 40% reaches the systemic circulation because of significant first-pass hepatic metabolism. Thus, oral pharmacotherapy is less potent than intramuscular or subcutaneous pharmacotherapy. Plasma protein binding is low (~36%). The mean apparent volume of distribution is ~3 L/kg (range 1 to 5 L/kg). Among elderly patients, the volume of distribution is considerably smaller, and initial concentrations of morphine are, thus, correspondingly higher. Peak analgesic action occurs within 20 minutes after intravenous injection and within 1 hour after intramuscular, oral, rectal, or subcutaneous administration. Morphine is metabolized rapidly and extensively primarily in the liver. Less than 10% is eliminated in unchanged form in the urine. Morphine's total body clearance ranges from 900 to 1200 ml/minute. The half-life of elimination is approximately 2 to 4 hours. Morphine's duration of action is 4 to 5 hours when administered by the oral or injectable routes.

RELATIVE CONTRAINDICATIONS

Alcoholism, acute
Biliary tract surgery or biliary or renal colic. Morphine causes smooth muscle spasms.
Cirrhosis, severe
CNS depression, severe
Delirium tremens
Heart failure secondary to chronic lung disease
Hypersensitivity to morphine or any of the components of the morphine formulation (e.g., Rapiject® syringes contain sodium metabisulfite, which may cause hypersensitivity reactions among susceptible patients, particularly those who have a history of asthma).
Hypotension, severe. Opiate analgesics may exacerbate this condition.
MAOI pharmacotherapy, concurrent or within 14 days
Respiratory depression, severe
Respiratory disorders characterized by hypoxia, such as status asthmaticus (acute asthma attack), chronic obstructive pulmonary disease, or cor pulmonale, or patients who for any other reason, have a substantially decreased respiratory reserve (e.g., pre-existing respiratory depression, hypoxia, or hypercapnia). Among these patients, even low therapeutic doses may decrease respiratory drive while simultaneously increasing airway resistance to the point of apnea.
Upper airway obstruction

CAUTIONS AND COMMENTS

Morphine generally is considered the prototype for all opiate analgesics and, thus, is the measure by which they are compared. Morphine has high abuse potential, and long-term morphine pharmacotherapy, or regular personal use, may result in addiction and habituation.

Prescribe morphine pharmacotherapy cautiously to patients who

- have acute abdominal conditions (e.g., acute appendicitis). Morphine pharmacotherapy may obscure the medical diagnosis or clinical course of these conditions.
- are elderly, frail, or debilitated or have severe kidney or liver dysfunction. Morphine may have prolonged duration and cumulative actions among these patients.
- are in shock. Associated impaired perfusion may prevent absorption after intramuscular or subcutaneous injection. Repeated injections may result in overdosage due to an excessive amount of morphine being absorbed when the patient's circulation is restored.
- have atrial flutter and other supraventricular tachycardias. Morphine's vagolytic action may produce a significant increase in the ventricular response rate among these patients.
- have compromised ability to maintain blood pressure due to excessive blood loss (e.g., injury, surgery) or the use of phenothiazines or other drugs that can lower blood pressure. Morphine pharmacotherapy may produce severe hypotension among these patients.
- have head injuries, brain tumors, other intracranial lesions, or pre-existing increased intracranial pressure. The respiratory depressant action of morphine and its ability to increase cerebrospinal fluid pressure may be exaggerated markedly among these patients. Morphine pharmacotherapy also may obscure the clinical course of these conditions.
- have hypothyroidism, Addison's disease, and prostatic hypertrophy or urethral stricture. Morphine pharmacotherapy may exacerbate these conditions.
- regularly drink alcohol or are concurrently receiving pharmacotherapy with other opiate analgesics, phenothiazines, sedative-hypnotics, TCAs, or other drugs that produce CNS depression. Additive CNS depression may occur among these patients.

Caution patients who are receiving morphine pharmacotherapy against performing activities that require alertness, judgment, and physical coordination (e.g., driving an automobile, operating dangerous equipment, supervising children) until their response to morphine is known. The CNS depressant action of morphine may adversely affect these mental and physical functions.

In addition to this general precaution, caution patients to inform their prescribing psychologist if they begin or discontinue any other pharmacotherapy while receiving morphine pharmacotherapy.

CLINICALLY SIGNIFICANT DRUG INTERACTIONS

Concurrent morphine pharmacotherapy and the following may result in clinically significant drug interactions:

Alcohol Use

Concurrent alcohol use may increase the CNS depressant action of morphine. Advise patients to avoid, or limit, their use of alcohol while receiving morphine pharmacotherapy. Caution patients that their usual responses to alcohol may be exaggerated.

Pharmacotherapy With Central Nervous System Depressants and Other Drugs That Produce Central Nervous System Depression

Concurrent morphine pharmacotherapy with other opiate analgesics, sedative-hypnotics, or other drugs that produce CNS depression (e.g., antihistamines, phenothiazines, TCAs) may result in additive CNS depression. When concurrent pharmacotherapy is required, the dosage of one or both drugs should be reduced.

Pharmacotherapy With Drugs that Acidify the Urine

The renal elimination of morphine is decreased by urinary acidifiers (e.g., ammonium chloride). Thus, this interaction may result in morphine accumulation and toxicity.

Pharmacotherapy With Drugs that Alkalinize the Urine

The renal elimination of morphine is enhanced by urinary alkalinizers (e.g., sodium bicarbonate). Thus this interaction may result in increased morphine elimination, a shortened half-life of elimination, and decreased pain relief.

See also Opiate Analgesics General Monograph

ADVERSE DRUG REACTIONS

Morphine pharmacotherapy has been associated with serious ADRs. These ADRs include respiratory depression, cardiac arrest, circulatory depression, respiratory arrest, and shock. Morphine pharmacotherapy also has been commonly associated with constipation, dizziness, lightheadedness, nausea, sedation, sweating, and vomiting.

See also Opiate Analgesics General Monograph

OVERDOSAGE

Signs and symptoms of morphine overdosage include respiratory depression (i.e., decrease in respiratory rate and tidal volume, Cheyne-Stokes respiration, cyanosis), extreme somnolence progressing to stupor or coma, skeletal muscle flaccidity, and cold and clammy skin. Bradycardia and hypotension also may occur. Severe morphine overdosage may result in apnea, cardiac arrest, circulatory collapse, and death.

Morphine overdosage requires emergency symptomatic medical support of body systems with attention to increasing morphine elimination. The opiate antagonist naloxone (Narcan®) is the specific antidote against respiratory depression. Usual dosages of naloxone will precipitate the opiate withdrawal syndrome among patients addicted to morphine. The severity of the syndrome depends on the degree of the patient's addiction and the dose of naloxone administered. For these patients, 10% to 20% of the usual dosage should be administered initially and then adjusted (increased) according to individual patient response.

NALBUPHINE

(nal'byoo feen)

TRADE NAME

Nubain®

CLASSIFICATION

Opiate analgesic (mixed agonist/antagonist)

See also Opiate Analgesics General Monograph

APPROVED INDICATIONS FOR PSYCHOLOGICAL DISORDERS

Adjunctive pharmacotherapy for the symptomatic management of:

- Pain Disorders: Acute Pain, Moderate to Severe
- Pain Disorders: Chronic Cancer Pain, Moderate to Severe

USUAL DOSAGE AND ADMINISTRATION

Acute Pain, Moderate to Severe

Adults: 40 to 80 mg daily intramuscularly, intravenously, or subcutaneously in four to eight divided doses according to individual patient response

MAXIMUM: 20 mg/dose; 160 mg daily

Women who are, or who may become, pregnant: FDA Pregnancy Category "not established." Safety and efficacy of nalbuphine pharmacotherapy for women who are pregnant have not been established. Nalbuphine crosses the placenta rapidly and may achieve fetal blood concentrations approximately equivalent to maternal blood concentrations. Associated fetal and neonatal effects have been reported, including fetal bradycardia and neonatal bradycardia and respiratory depression (see also Opiate Analgesics General Monograph). Avoid prescribing nalbuphine pharmacotherapy to women who are pregnant. If nalbuphine pharmacotherapy is required, advise patients of potential benefits and possible risks to themselves and the embryo, fetus, or neonate. Collaboration with the patient's obstetrician is indicated.

Women who are breast-feeding: Safety and efficacy of nalbuphine pharmacotherapy for women who are breast-feeding and their neonates and infants have not been established (see Opiate Analgesics General Monograph). Avoid prescribing nalbuphine pharmacotherapy to women who are breast-feeding. If nalbuphine pharmacotherapy is required, breast-feeding probably should be discontinued. If desired, lactation may be maintained and breast-feeding resumed following the discontinuation of short-term nalbuphine pharmacotherapy. Collaboration with the patient's pediatrician is indicated.

Elderly, frail, or debilitated patients: Generally prescribe lower dosages for elderly, frail, or debilitated patients. Increase the dosage gradually, if needed, according to individual patient response. These patients may be more sensitive to the pharmacologic actions of nalbuphine than are younger or healthier adult patients.

Children and adolescents younger than 18 years of age: Safety and efficacy of nalbuphine pharmacotherapy for children and adolescents have not been established. Nalbuphine pharmacotherapy is *not* recommended for this age group.

Chronic Cancer Pain, Moderate to Severe

See Acute Pain, Moderate to Severe

AVAILABLE DOSAGE FORMS, STORAGE, AND COMPATIBILITY

Injectables, intramuscular, intravenous, subcutaneous: 10, 20 mg/ml

Notes

The injectable formulations of some manufacturers (e.g., Astra, Du Pont) contain sodium metabisulfite. Sulfites have been associated with hypersensitivity reactions, including anaphylactic reactions, among susceptible patients. Although relatively uncommon, these reactions appear to occur with a higher incidence among patients who have asthma.

Store nalbuphine injectable formulations safely protected from light at controlled room temperature (15° to 30°C; 59° to 86°F).

PROPOSED MECHANISM OF ACTION

Nalbuphine elicits its analgesic, CNS depressant, and respiratory depressant actions primarily by binding to the endorphin receptors in the CNS. However, the exact mechanism of action has not yet been fully determined.

See also Opiate Analgesics General Monograph

PHARMACOKINETICS/PHARMACODYNAMICS

Nalbuphine has limited oral bioavailability (~20%). Thus, injectable pharmacotherapy is required for optimal bioavailability. Onset of action occurs within 3 minutes following intravenous injection and within 15 minutes following intramuscular or subcutaneous injection. The mean apparent volume of distribution is 4 L/kg. Nalbuphine is metabolized in the liver, and less than 5% is excreted in unchanged form in the urine. The mean half-life of elimination is ~5 hours, and the mean total body clearance is 1.5 L/minute.

RELATIVE CONTRAINDICATIONS

Hypersensitivity to nalbuphine

See also Opiate Analgesics General Monograph

CAUTIONS AND COMMENTS

Nalbuphine is addicting and habituating. Long-term nalbuphine pharmacotherapy, or regular personal use, may result in addiction and habituation. Abrupt discontinuation after long-term pharmacotherapy, or regular personal use, may result in a reportedly mild form of the opiate analgesic withdrawal syndrome. Nalbuphine also may cause signs and symptoms of the opiate analgesic withdrawal syndrome among patients who are receiving long-term opiate analgesic pharmacotherapy with pure opiate agonist analgesics (e.g., morphine). Nalbuphine, a mixed opiate agonist/antagonist, has weak opiate antagonist actions.

Prescribe nalbuphine pharmacotherapy cautiously for patients who

- have cholecystitis or pancreatitis (acute) or will be undergoing surgery of the biliary tract. Opiate analgesics generally increase biliary tract pressure. Nalbuphine may cause spasms of the circular muscle constricting the opening of the common bile duct (i.e., sphincter of Oddi).
- have head injuries, intracranial lesions, or other conditions associated with increased intracranial pressure. The respiratory depressant action associated with nalbuphine and its potential for elevating cerebrospinal fluid pressure may markedly increase intracranial pressure among these patients. Nalbuphine's analgesic and sedative actions also may obscure the clinical course of these conditions.
- have histories of problematic patterns of opiate analgesic or other abusable psychotropic use. These patients may be at risk for developing problematic patterns of use. In addition, patients who are addicted to opiates may experience signs and symptoms of the opiate analgesic withdrawal syndrome. Nalbuphine, a mixed agonist/antagonist, has weak opiate antagonist action.
- have liver dysfunction. Serious liver dysfunction appears to predispose patients to a higher incidence of ADRs (e.g., anxiety, dizziness, drowsiness, marked apprehension) even when usual recommended dosages are prescribed. These ADRs may be the result of decreased nalbuphine metabolism by the liver and resultant accumulation.
- have respiratory depression, limited respiratory function (e.g., severely limited respiratory reserve, severe bronchial asthma, other obstructive respiratory conditions), or cyanosis. The respiratory depressant action of nalbuphine may further compromise the respiratory function of these patients.

Caution patients who are receiving nalbuphine pharmacotherapy against performing activities that require alertness, judgment, and physical coordination (e.g., driving an automobile, operating dangerous equipment, supervising children) until their response to nalbuphine is known. The CNS depressant action of nalbuphine may adversely affect these mental and physical functions.

In addition to this general precaution, caution patients to inform their prescribing psychologist if they begin or discontinue any other pharmacotherapy while receiving nalbuphine pharmacotherapy.

CLINICALLY SIGNIFICANT DRUG INTERACTIONS

Concurrent nalbuphine pharmacotherapy and the following may result in clinically significant drug interactions:

Alcohol Use

Concurrent alcohol use may increase the CNS depressant action of nalbuphine. Advise patients to avoid, or limit, their use of alcohol while receiving nalbuphine pharmacotherapy.

Pharmacotherapy With Central Nervous System Depressants and Other Drugs That Produce Central Nervous System Depression

Concurrent nalbuphine pharmacotherapy with other opiate analgesics, sedative-hypnotics, or other drugs that produce CNS depression (e.g., antihistamines, phenothiazines, TCAs) may result in additive CNS depression.

ADVERSE DRUG REACTIONS

Nalbuphine pharmacotherapy commonly has been associated with dizziness, nausea, sedation, a sweaty-clammy feeling, and vomiting. It also has been associated with the following ADRs, listed according to body system:

Cardiovascular: hypertension and tachycardia
CNS: depression and headache
Cutaneous: flushing, hives, and itching (severe)
Genitourinary: urinary urgency
GI: constipation, cramps, and dyspepsia
Ocular: blurred vision
Respiratory: labored or difficult breathing (dyspnea) and respiratory depression

See also Opiate Analgesics General Monograph

OVERDOSAGE

Signs and symptoms of nalbuphine overdosage are similar to the signs and symptoms associated with other opiate analgesic overdosages, although respiratory depression is reportedly less severe. Nalbuphine overdosage requires emergency symptomatic medical support of body systems with attention to increasing nalbuphine elimination. Naloxone (Narcan®) is a specific and effective antidote.

NALOXONE

(nal ox'own)

TRADE NAME

Narcan®

CLASSIFICATION

Opiate Antagonist

APPROVED INDICATIONS FOR PSYCHOLOGICAL DISORDERS

Adjunctive pharmacotherapy for the symptomatic management of:

Substance-Related Disorders: Opiate Analgesic Overdosage, Known or Suspected. *Note:* Naloxone is an opiate antagonist that produces complete or partial reversal of the signs and symptoms of opiate overdosage, particularly respiratory depression. Naloxone also is indicated for the diagnosis of suspected acute opiate overdosage. Although overdosages involving opiate analgesics and other psychotropics require emergency symptomatic medical support of body systems, prescribing psychologists require a knowledge of the use and action of naloxone and other antagonists, such as those indicated for the management of benzodiazepine overdosage (e.g., flumazenil [Anexate®, Romazicon®]).

USUAL DOSAGE AND ADMINISTRATION

Opiate Analgesic Overdosage, Known or Suspected

Adults: 0.4 to 2 mg intravenously. If therapeutic response is not achieved, repeat at two to three minute intervals. If therapeutic response is not noted after 10 mg, reevaluate the diagnosis of opiate analgesic overdosage. Intramuscular or subcutaneous injection may be required if intravenous injection is not feasible.

INTRAVENOUS INFUSION   2 mg per 500 ml of 5% dextrose or normal saline solution to obtain a concentration of 4 μg/ml (0.004 mg/ml). Use admixture within 24 hours. Discard remaining unused admixture after 24 hours. Generally infuse at 100 ml/hour (i.e., 0.4 mg/hour). Infusion is generally initiated for opiate overdosage associated with long-acting opiates (e.g., methadone [Dolophine®], propoxyphene [Darvon®]). Individualize concentration and infusion rate to obtain desired antagonist response without intravenous fluid overload or precipitation of the acute opiate analgesic withdrawal syndrome.

Women who are, or who may become, pregnant: FDA Pregnancy Category B. Safety and efficacy of naloxone pharmacotherapy for women who are pregnant (other than during labor) have not been established. Naloxone has no known direct pharmacologic action other than its opiate antagonist action. When indicated for the management of acute opiate overdosage, potential benefit significantly outweighs minor potential risk to the embryo, fetus, or neonate. Collaboration with the patient's obstetrician is indicated.

Women who are breast-feeding: Safety and efficacy of naloxone pharmacotherapy for women who are breast-feeding and their neonates and infants have not been established. It is unknown whether naloxone is excreted in breast milk. However, risk to breast-fed neonates and infants, other than reversal of opiate analgesic action, appears minimal. Collaboration with the patient's pediatrician is indicated.

Elderly, frail, or debilitated patients: Same dosage and administration as generally recommended for younger adult patients

Children: 0.01 mg/kg intravenously. If therapeutic response is not achieved, a subsequent dose of 0.1 mg/kg may be injected. This dosage can be repeated at two to three minute intervals, if required. Intramuscular or subcutaneous pharmacotherapy may be required, in divided doses, if intravenous pharmacotherapy is not feasible. If necessary, may dilute naloxone with sterile water for injection.

INTRAVENOUS INFUSION   Intravenous infusion is generally initiated for opiate overdosage involving long-acting opiates (e.g., methadone [Dolophine®], propoxyphene [Darvon®]). The infusion rate for children should be adjusted according to individual patient factors (e.g., body weight; heart, kidney, and liver function) and clinical response.

Neonates: 0.01 mg/kg intravenously. If therapeutic response is not achieved, inject a subsequent dose of 0.1 mg/kg intravenously. Intramuscular or subcutaneous pharmacotherapy may be required, in divided doses, if intravenous pharmacotherapy is not feasible. If necessary, may dilute naloxone with sterile water for injection.

INTRAVENOUS INFUSION   Intravenous infusion is generally initiated for opiate overdosage involving long-acting opiates (e.g., methadone [Dolophine®], propoxyphene [Darvon®]). The infusion rate for neonates should be adjusted according to individual patient factors (e.g., body weight; heart, kidney, and liver function) and clinical response.

Notes, Acute Opiate Analgesic Overdosage, Known or Suspected

Naloxone pharmacotherapy generally may be prescribed for intramuscular, intravenous, or subcutaneous pharmacotherapy. The most rapid onset of action is achieved with intravenous injection. Intravenous injection is recommended for the emergency symptomatic medical management of acute opiate analgesic overdosage. In emergency situations where injectable pharmacotherapy is not feasible, naloxone has been successfully administered by endotracheal tube.
Repeated doses of naloxone at periodic intervals for up to 48 hours may be required because of the relatively long duration of action of some opiate analgesics (e.g., methadone

[*Dolophine*®]). Medical monitoring of respiratory rate is necessary to evaluate the need for repeated doses of naloxone (i.e., respiratory rate less than 10 respirations/minute) because of its relatively short half-life of elimination and duration of action.

AVAILABLE DOSAGE FORMS, STORAGE, AND COMPATIBILITY

Injectables, intramuscular, intravenous, subcutaneous: 0.02, 0.4 mg/ml (neonatal formulations); 1 mg/ml (child and adult formulation)

Notes

Inspect injectable formulations visually for particulate matter and discoloration prior to use whenever solution and container permit. Do not mix naloxone injectable with formulations containing bisulfite, metabisulfite, long-chain or high molecular weight anions, or any solution that has an alkaline pH. Do not add any other drug to injectable naloxone unless its chemical and physical compatibility with naloxone is known.

Store the injectable safely at controlled room temperature (15° to 30°C; 59° to 86°F).

PROPOSED MECHANISM OF ACTION

Naloxone essentially exhibits no direct pharmacologic action other than antagonizing the actions of opiate analgesics by competitively blocking the endogenous endorphin receptors in the CNS. This action reverses analgesia and the signs and symptoms of opiate analgesic overdosage, particularly respiratory depression. It also produces the acute opiate analgesic withdrawal syndrome among patients who are addicted to opiate analgesics.

PHARMACOKINETICS/PHARMACODYNAMICS

Naloxone is well absorbed (~90%) following oral ingestion. However, bioavailability is very low (i.e., F = 0.02) because of significant first-pass hepatic metabolism. The onset of action for naloxone is usually within 2 minutes of intravenous injection. Its onset of action is only slightly less rapid when injected intramuscularly or subcutaneously. The duration of naloxone's action is 1 to 4 hours and depends on the dose and method of administration. Intramuscular injection produces a more prolonged action than intravenous injection. The requirement for repeat doses of naloxone depends on the opiate analgesic being antagonized (i.e., short- or long-acting opiate) for the symptomatic management of opiate analgesic overdosage and the severity of the overdosage.

Following intramuscular, intravenous, or subcutaneous injection, naloxone is distributed rapidly in the body. Its mean apparent volume of distribution is approximately 2 L/kg. Naloxone is metabolized in the liver and excreted in the urine. Total body clearance is approximately 1.5 L/minute. The mean half-life of elimination is approximately 1 hour (range 30 to 90 minutes). Due to immature mechanisms of liver metabolism and urinary excretion among neonates, the mean half-life of elimination is prolonged to approximately 3 hours for this age group.

RELATIVE CONTRAINDICATIONS

Hypersensitivity to naloxone

CAUTIONS AND COMMENTS

Prescribe naloxone pharmacotherapy cautiously to patients who

- are known, or suspected, to be addicted to opiate analgesics. Abrupt and complete reversal of opiate analgesic action may produce the opiate analgesic withdrawal syndrome among these patients. The severity of the syndrome depends on the degree of addiction (i.e., opiate analgesic used, dosage, and duration of use), the naloxone dose, the method of administration, and individual patient factors (e.g., personality and concomitant disorders).
- have respiratory depression (severe). These patients require lower dosages than usually recommended and close medical monitoring. Close medical monitoring should be maintained even after satisfactory response has been achieved. Repeated doses may be required because the duration of action of some opiate analgesics (e.g., methadone [Dolophine®]) may exceed that of naloxone.

CLINICALLY SIGNIFICANT DRUG INTERACTIONS

There have been no reports of drug interactions involving naloxone other than its expected antagonism of opiate analgesics.

ADVERSE DRUG REACTIONS

Although naloxone essentially exhibits no pharmacologic action, abrupt reversal of opiate overdosage may result in nausea, vomiting, sweating, tachycardia, increased blood pressure, tremulousness, and cardiac arrest.

OVERDOSAGE

There have been no reports of naloxone overdosage.

NALTREXONE

(nal trex′one)

TRADE NAME

ReVia® (formerly known as Trexan®)

CLASSIFICATION

Opiate Antagonist

APPROVED INDICATIONS FOR PSYCHOLOGICAL DISORDERS

Adjunctive pharmacotherapy for the symptomatic management of:

- Substance-Related Disorders: Maintenance of Abstinence From Alcohol Use. Naltrexone pharmacotherapy is indicated for patients who have completed detoxification for alcohol addiction. If there is any question concerning opiate analgesic addiction among patients for whom naltrexone pharmacotherapy is considered for the maintenance of abstinence from alcohol use, perform a naloxone (Narcan®) challenge test *prior* to initiating naltrexone pharmacotherapy (see Notes, Maintenance of Abstinence From Opiate Analgesic Use, Naloxone [Narcan®] Challenge Test).
- Substance-Related Disorders: Maintenance of Abstinence From Opiate Analgesic Use. Naltrexone pharmacotherapy is indicated for patients who have completed detoxification for opiate analgesic addiction. Prescribe naltrexone pharmacotherapy only for patients who have remained opiate-free for 10 days or more. Patient self-report of abstinence requires *verification* with a urine test and/or a naloxone challenge test (see Notes, Maintenance of Abstinence From Opiate Analgesic Use). Patients should not display any signs and symptoms of the opiate analgesic withdrawal syndrome upon initiation of naltrexone pharmacotherapy.

USUAL DOSAGE AND ADMINISTRATION

Maintenance of Abstinence From Alcohol Use

Adults: 50 mg daily orally in a single dose. The safety and efficacy of naltrexone pharmacotherapy have not been established for the maintenance of abstinence from alcohol use for longer than 12 weeks.

Women who are, or who may become, pregnant: FDA Pregnancy Category "not established." Safety and efficacy of naltrexone pharmacotherapy for women who are pregnant have not been established. Risk to the embryo, fetus, or neonate does not appear to be significant based upon the known pharmacology of naltrexone. However, avoid prescribing naltrexone pharmacotherapy to women who are pregnant. If naltrexone pharmacotherapy is required, advise patients of potential benefits and possible risks to themselves and the embryo, fetus, or neonate. Collaboration with the patient's obstetrician is indicated.

Women who are breast-feeding: Safety and efficacy of naltrexone pharmacotherapy for women who are breast-feeding and their neonates and infants have not been established. It is unknown whether naltrexone is excreted in breast milk. Avoid prescribing naltrexone pharmacotherapy to women who are breast-feeding. If naltrexone pharmacotherapy is required, breast-feeding probably should be discontinued. Collaboration with the patient's pediatrician is indicated.

Elderly, frail, or debilitated patients: Safety and efficacy of naltrexone pharmacotherapy for the maintenance of abstinence from alcohol use have not been established for elderly, frail, or debilitated patients.

Children and adolescents younger than 18 years of age: Safety and efficacy of naltrexone pharmacotherapy for the maintenance of abstinence from alcohol use have not been established for children and adolescents. Naltrexone pharmacotherapy is *not* recommended for this age group.

Notes, Maintenance of Abstinence from Alcohol Use

See Notes, Maintenance of Abstinence from Opiate Analgesic Use

Maintenance of Abstinence From Opiate Analgesic Use

Adults: Initially, 25 mg orally. Observe the patient for one hour. If there are no signs and symptoms of opiate analgesic withdrawal, administer an additional 25 mg orally.

MAINTENANCE: 50 mg daily orally. If preferred, prescribe *one* of the following schedules:

50 mg orally every weekday and 100 mg orally on Saturday; or
100 mg orally every other day; or
150 mg orally every third day; or
100 mg orally on Monday and Wednesday and 150 mg orally on Friday.

The degree of opiate blockade may be somewhat reduced when higher dosages are prescribed at longer dosing intervals. However, some patients may be better able to follow their pharmacotherapy when dosing is every two to three days (48 to 72 hours) rather than daily (every 24 hours).

Women who are, or who may become, pregnant: FDA Pregnancy Category "not established." Safety and efficacy of naltrexone pharmacotherapy for women who are pregnant have not been established. Risk to the embryo, fetus, or neonate does not appear to be significant based upon the known pharmacology of naltrexone. However, avoid prescribing naltrexone pharmacotherapy to women who are pregnant. If naltrexone pharmacotherapy is required, advise patients of potential benefits and possible risks to themselves and the embryo, fetus, or neonate. Collaboration with the patient's obstetrician is indicated.

Women who are breast-feeding: Safety and efficacy of naltrexone pharmacotherapy for women who are breast-feeding and their neonates and infants have not been established. It is unknown whether naltrexone is excreted in breast milk. Avoid prescribing naltrexone pharmacotherapy to women who are breast-feeding. If naltrexone pharmacotherapy is required, breast-feeding probably should be discontinued. Collaboration with the patient's pediatrician is indicated.

Elderly, frail, or debilitated patients: Safety and efficacy of naltrexone pharmacotherapy for the maintenance of abstinence from opiate analgesic use have not been established for elderly, frail, or debilitated patients.

Children and adolescents younger than 18 years of age: Safety and efficacy of naltrexone pharmacotherapy for the maintenance of abstinence from opiate analgesic use have not been established for children and adolescents. Naltrexone pharmacotherapy is *not* recommended for this age group.

Notes, Maintenance of Abstinence From Opiate Analgesic Use

Adjunctive naltrexone pharmacotherapy discourages opiate analgesic use among patients previously addicted to opiate analgesics by blocking their desired action. The oral ingestion of 50 mg of naltrexone blocks the action of 25 mg of heroin (an average heroin dose on the street) for 24 hours. However, the opiate blockade produced by naltrexone is surmountable. Naltrexone also may precipitate acute opiate analgesic withdrawal among patients who are currently using opiates analgesics.

Naloxone (Narcan®) Challenge Test Following appropriate screening (i.e., self-report of abstinence or urine screen for opiate analgesics), a naloxone challenge test is recommended prior to initiating naltrexone pharmacotherapy to confirm that patients are opiate-free. In the event that they are not, the test can be repeated in 24 hours. Prepare a syringe with 0.8 mg naloxone. Inject 0.2 mg intravenously, and monitor the patient for 30 seconds for any signs and symptoms of opiate analgesic withdrawal (e.g., abdominal cramps, feeling of temperature change, joint or bone pain, muscle pain, piloerection [goose flesh], skin crawling, stuffiness or runny nose, sweating, tearing, tremor, vomiting, yawning). If no signs and symptoms of opiate analgesic withdrawal are noted, inject the remaining 0.6 mg intravenously. Continue monitoring the patient for an additional 20 minutes. See Naloxone Monograph for additional information.

Subcutaneous Challenge Inject 0.8 mg naloxone subcutaneously. Monitor the patient for 45 minutes for any signs and symptoms of opiate analgesic withdrawal (e.g., abdominal cramps, feeling of temperature change, joint or bone pain, muscle pain, piloerection [goose flesh], skin crawling, stuffiness or runny nose, sweating, tearing, tremor, vomiting, yawning). The observation of these signs and symptoms indicates opiate analgesic use and potential risk to patients if naltrexone pharmacotherapy is initiated. Withhold naltrexone pharmacotherapy until abstinence from opiate analgesic use can be assured. If no signs and symptoms of withdrawal are noted, initiate naltrexone pharmacotherapy. However, if there is any doubt, readminister naloxone as a confirmatory re-challenge. See Naloxone Monograph for additional information.

Confirmatory Rechallenge (if necessary) Inject 1.6 mg of naloxone intravenously. Monitor the patient for signs and symptoms of opiate analgesic withdrawal (e.g., abdominal cramps, feeling of temperature change, joint or bone pain, muscle pain, piloerection [goose flesh], skin crawling, stuffiness or runny nose, sweating, tearing, tremor, vomiting, yawning). If no signs and symptoms of withdrawal are noted, initiate naltrexone pharmacotherapy. If signs and symptoms of withdrawal are noted, withhold naltrexone pharmacotherapy until repeated naloxone challenge indicates that the patient is opiate-free.

AVAILABLE DOSAGE FORMS, STORAGE, AND COMPATIBILITY

Tablets, oral: 50 mg

Notes

General Instructions for Patients   Instruct patients who are receiving naltrexone pharmacotherapy to

- ingest each dose of naltrexone with food or milk to decrease associated GI irritation
- safely store naltrexone tablets out of the reach of children in tightly closed child- and light-resistant containers at controlled room temperature (15° to 30°C; 59° to 86°F)
- obtain an available patient information sheet regarding naltrexone pharmacotherapy from their pharmacist at the time that their prescription is dispensed. Encourage patients to clarify any questions that they may have concerning naltrexone pharmacotherapy with their pharmacist or, if needed, to consult their prescribing psychologist.

PROPOSED MECHANISM OF ACTION

Naltrexone is a synthetic congener of oxymorphone. However, it has no opiate agonist actions. It also is related to the potent opiate antagonist naloxone (Narcan®). Naltrexone, also an opiate antagonist, markedly blocks completely and reversibly the CNS action of intravenously injected opiate analgesics. When ingested concurrently with opiate analgesics on a long-term basis, naltrexone blocks the CNS actions thought to be associated with addiction and habituation. Naltrexone has few, if any, intrinsic actions other than its opiate analgesic blocking action. However, its use will precipitate the acute opiate analgesic withdrawal syndrome among people addicted to opiate analgesics. While the mechanism of action has not yet been fully determined, naltrexone appears to act primarily by blocking the actions of opiate analgesics by means of competitively binding to the opiate receptors. Although the mechanism has not been fully determined, opiate receptor blockade by opiate antagonists also is associated with decreased alcohol consumption.

PHARMACOKINETICS/PHARMACODYNAMICS

Naltrexone is well absorbed (i.e., ~96%) after oral ingestion. However, it is subject to extensive first-pass hepatic metabolism and, consequently, has a low bioavailability (range $F = 0.05$ to 0.4). Peak plasma levels occur within 1 hour. Naltrexone is only partially bound to plasma proteins (~21%) and has a fairly large volume of distribution (~1350 L). It is metabolized extensively in the liver and, to a lesser extent, at other sites. Total body clearance is approximately 3.5 L/minute. Less than 2% of naltrexone is excreted in unchanged form in the urine. The major metabolite (i.e., 6-β-naltrexol) also is thought to be a pure opiate antagonist and may contribute to the pharmacological blockade of the opiate receptors. The pharmacokinetics of naltrexone suggest that its metabolites undergo enterohepatic recycling. The mean half-life of elimination is 3 hours. Additional data are unavailable.

RELATIVE CONTRAINDICATIONS

Hepatitis, acute
Hypersensitivity to naltrexone
Liver failure
Naloxone (Narcan®) challenge, failure of
Opiate analgesic pharmacotherapy, or regular personal use, concurrent or within 10 days (or 5 half-lives of elimination)
Opiate analgesic withdrawal, acute
Urine screen for opiate analgesics, positive

CAUTIONS AND COMMENTS

Prescribe naltrexone pharmacotherapy cautiously to patients who

have liver dysfunction. Naltrexone pharmacotherapy may produce dose-related hepatotoxicity among patients who have liver dysfunction (e.g., patients who have alcoholic cirrhosis or who have histories of hepatitis associated, for example, with their use of contaminated needles and syringes). Naltrexone pharmacotherapy is contraindicated among patients who have acute hepatitis or liver failure. Its use among patients who have less severe liver dysfunction, or a history of liver disease, must be carefully considered in relation to its potential for hepatotoxicity.

Caution patients who are receiving naltrexone pharmacotherapy against

- attempting to overcome the naltrexone blockade. Naltrexone has a prolonged pharmacologic action ranging from 24 to 72 hours. The blockade produced is surmountable. Although useful for patients who require emergency analgesia (e.g., victims of a car crash), this action poses a potential risk to patients who attempt to overcome the blockade by injecting large amounts of opiate analgesics, such as formerly opiate analgesic addicted patients who choose to resume opiate analgesic use. Any attempt by a patient to overcome naltrexone's antagonistic action is associated with extreme risk and may lead to fatal opiate analgesic overdosage.
  The blood concentration attained immediately following the intravenous injection of opiate analgesics may be sufficient to overcome the naltrexone blockade. Thus, patients may be at extreme risk for life-threatening opiate analgesic overdosage and associated respiratory arrest and circulatory collapse. The use of smaller amounts of opiates also may be associated with extreme risk if they are used by patients prior to the next dose of naltrexone, when naltrexone blood concentrations are low, or in an amount that persists in the body longer than the effective concentrations of naltrexone and its metabolites. Advise patients of the serious consequences associated with attempts to surmount naltrexone's opiate analgesic blockade.
- giving, selling, or trading this drug to any relatives, friends, or others. Naltrexone pharmacotherapy is part of a comprehensive treatment program designed to help previously addicted patients maintain their abstinence from alcohol or opiate analgesic use.
- performing activities that require alertness, judgment, or physical coordination (e.g., driving an automobile, operating dangerous equipment, supervising children) until their response to naltrexone pharmacotherapy is known. Naltrexone may adversely affect these mental and physical functions.

In addition to these general precautions, caution patients to

- carry a card, or wear a medic alert bracelet, to alert medical personnel in the event of an emergency that they are receiving naltrexone pharmacotherapy. Advise patients, if they require surgery or other medical or dental treatment, to inform their surgeon, family physician, or dentist that they are receiving naltrexone pharmacotherapy.
- inform their prescribing psychologist if they begin or discontinue any other pharmacotherapy while receiving naltrexone pharmacotherapy.

CLINICALLY SIGNIFICANT DRUG INTERACTIONS

None commonly identified at present other than the expected antagonism of opiate analgesics.

ADVERSE DRUG REACTIONS

Naltrexone pharmacotherapy is generally reported to be well tolerated. Associated GI irritation may be minimized by instructing patients to ingest each dose with food or milk. Although naltrexone can precipitate, or exacerbate, the signs and symptoms of the opiate analgesic withdrawal syndrome among patients who are not opiate-free, it is essentially a pure opiate antagonist that has little pharmacologic activity at recommended dosages in the absence of an opiate. The ADRs associated directly with naltrexone pharmacotherapy generally are mild. However, naltrexone has the capacity to cause dose-related hepatocellular injury and has been associated with significant hepatotoxicity at dosages of 300 mg daily.

OVERDOSAGE

There have been no reports of naltrexone overdosage.

NEFAZODONE

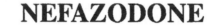

(nef ay′zoe done)

TRADE NAME

Serzone®

CLASSIFICATION

Antidepressant, nonselective (phenylpiperazine)

APPROVED INDICATIONS FOR PSYCHOLOGICAL DISORDERS

Adjunctive pharmacotherapy for the symptomatic management of:

Mood Disorders, Depressive Disorders: Major Depressive Disorder

USUAL DOSAGE AND ADMINISTRATION

Major Depressive Disorder

Adults: Initially, 200 mg daily orally in two divided doses. Increase the daily dosage weekly by 100 to 200 mg, as needed, according to individual patient response.

MAXIMUM: 600 mg daily orally

Women who are, or who may become, pregnant: FDA Pregnancy Category C. Safety and efficacy of nefazodone pharmacotherapy for women who are pregnant have not been established. Avoid prescribing nefazodone pharmacotherapy to women who are pregnant. If nefazodone pharmacotherapy is required, advise patients of potential benefits and possible risks to themselves and the embryo, fetus, or neonate. Collaboration with the patient's obstetrician is indicated.

Women who are breast-feeding: Safety and efficacy of nefazodone pharmacotherapy for women who are breast-feeding and their neonates and infants have not been established. Avoid prescribing nefazodone pharmacotherapy to women who are breast-feeding. If nefazodone pharmacotherapy is required, breast-feeding probably should be discontinued. Collaboration with the patient's pediatrician is indicated.

Elderly, frail, or debilitated patients and those who have significant liver dysfunction: Initially, 100 mg daily orally in two divided doses. Generally prescribe lower dosages for elderly, frail, or debilitated patients and those who have liver dysfunction. Increase the dosage gradually, if needed, according to individual patient response. These patients may be more sensitive to the pharmacologic actions of nefazodone than are younger or healthier adult patients.

MAXIMUM: 400 mg daily orally

Children and adolescents younger than 18 years of age: Safety and efficacy of nefazodone pharmacotherapy for children and adolescents have not been established. Nefazodone pharmacotherapy is *not* recommended for this age group.

Notes, Major Depressive Disorder

Several weeks of pharmacotherapy are generally required before optimal therapeutic benefit is achieved. Suicide precautions may be indicated.

AVAILABLE DOSAGE FORMS, STORAGE, AND COMPATIBILITY

Tablets, oral: 50, 100, 150, 200, 250, 300 mg

Notes

General Instructions for Patients   Instruct patients who are receiving nefazodone pharmacotherapy to

- safely store nefazodone tablets out of the reach of children in tightly closed child-resistant containers at room temperature below 40°C (104°F).
- obtain an available patient information sheet regarding nefazodone pharmacotherapy from their pharmacist at the time that their prescription is dispensed. Encourage patients to clarify any questions that they may have concerning nefazodone pharmacotherapy with their pharmacist or, if needed, to consult their prescribing psychologist.

PROPOSED MECHANISM OF ACTION

The exact mechanism of action of nefazodone has not yet been fully determined. Nefazodone appears to produce its antidepressant action primarily by potentiating the CNS biogenic amines, particularly norepinephrine and serotonin, by blocking their re-uptake at the pre-synaptic nerve receptor sites, particularly the serotonin-2 receptor (5-HT_2). Nefazodone also has demonstrated adrenergic receptor (i.e., α-1) blocking activity.

PHARMACOKINETICS/PHARMACODYNAMICS

Nefazodone is virtually completely absorbed following oral ingestion. However, the absolute bioavailability is low (i.e., F = 0.2) probably because of extensive first-pass hepatic metabolism. Food delays the absorption of nefazodone and increases the amount of drug subject to first-pass metabolism (i.e., the ingestion of nefazodone with food decreases bioavailability by approximately 20%). Peak blood concentrations occur within 1 to 3 hours after ingestion. Nefazodone is highly plasma protein-bound (greater than 99%). It is widely distributed in body tissues and has an apparent volume of distribution ranging from 0.22 to 0.87 L/kg. Nefazodone is metabolized extensively in the liver, with less than 1% excreted in unchanged form in the urine. Several active metabolites are produced. The half-life of elimination is approximately 2 to 4 hours. Nefazodone reportedly is subject to nonlinear kinetics (i.e., $T_{1/2}$ = 1.9 hours following a daily oral dosage of 100 mg; $T_{1/2}$ = 2.9 hours following a daily oral dosage of 200 mg; and $T_{1/2}$ = 3.7 hours following a daily oral dosage of 400 mg).

RELATIVE CONTRAINDICATIONS

Astemizole (Hismanal®), cisapride (Prepulsid®), or terfenadine (Seldane® [removed from the U.S. market in 1998 at the request of the FDA]) pharmacotherapy, concurrent (see Clinically Significant Drug Interactions)
Hypersensitivity to nefazodone
MAOI pharmacotherapy, concurrent or within 14 days

CAUTIONS AND COMMENTS

Prescribe nefazodone pharmacotherapy cautiously to patients who

- are elderly, are receiving antihypertensive pharmacotherapy, or have cardiovascular disorders. These patients may be particularly susceptible to postural (orthostatic) hypotension and its related sequelae (e.g., dizziness, fainting [syncope], tachycardia). The incidence of postural hypotension associated with nefazodone pharmacotherapy is ~5%. This incidence, and the severity of related sequelae (e.g., falls), would be expected to be significantly increased among these patients.

- have histories of bipolar disorder. Nefazodone may increase the frequency of the occurrence of manic episodes among these patients.

Caution patients who are receiving nefazodone pharmacotherapy against

- drinking alcohol or using other drugs that produce CNS depression. These drugs may increase the CNS depression associated with nefazodone pharmacotherapy.
- performing activities that require alertness, judgment, and physical coordination (e.g., driving an automobile, operating dangerous equipment, supervising children) until their individual response to nefazodone is known. Nefazodone may adversely affect these mental and physical functions.

In addition to these general precautions, caution patients to inform their prescribing psychologist if they begin or discontinue any other pharmacotherapy while receiving nefazodone pharmacotherapy.

CLINICALLY SIGNIFICANT DRUG INTERACTIONS

Concurrent nefazodone pharmacotherapy and the following may result in clinically significant drug interactions:

Monoamine Oxidase Inhibitor Pharmacotherapy

Concurrent MAOI and SSRI pharmacotherapy may result in the serotonin syndrome. Signs and symptoms of this potentially fatal syndrome include autonomic nervous system instability with rapid, wide fluctuations in blood pressure, heart rate, and respiratory rate; hyperthermia; mental status changes (e.g., agitation, delirium, coma); myoclonus; and rigidity. Although not yet associated directly with nefazodone pharmacotherapy, concurrent pharmacotherapy is *contraindicated* because of the ability of nefazodone to inhibit both norepinephrine and serotonin re-uptake.

Pharmacotherapy With Drugs That Are Metabolized by Hepatic Microsomal Enzymes, Primarily, Cytochrome P450 Isoenzyme CYP3A3/4

Nefazodone may inhibit hepatic microsomal enzyme metabolism, particularly that which is mediated by isoenzyme CYP3A3/4. This interaction may result in significantly increased blood concentrations and half-lives of elimination for affected drugs. These drugs include alprazolam (Xanax®), astemizole (Hismanal®), calcium channel blockers (nifedipine [Adalat®, Procardia®]), carbamazepine [Tegretol®], cisapride (Prepulsid®), clozapine (Clozaril®), corticosteroids, cyclosporine (Sandimmune®), diazepam (Valium®), diltiazem (Cardizem®), erythromycin (E-Mycin®), imipramine (Tofranil®), felodipine (Plendil®), lidocaine (Xylocaine®), loratadine (Claritin®), lovastatin (Mevacor®), midazolam (Versed®), quinidine (Quinidex®), simvastatin (Zocor®), terfenadine (Seldane®) [removed from the U.S. market in 1998 at the request of the FDA], triazolam (Halcion®), and verapamil (Isoptin®).

For example, concurrent nefazodone and alprazolam or triazolam pharmacotherapy has resulted in blood concentrations of alprazolam or triazolam that are increased severalfold. Thus, concurrent nefazodone pharmacotherapy requires an initial dosage reduction of 50% for these interacting drugs. Concurrent nefazodone and astemizole, cisapride, or terfenadine pharmacotherapy also has been associated with increased blood concentrations with resultant QT-interval prolongation and potentially fatal cardiac dysrhythmias. Thus, concurrent nefazodone pharmacotherapy and pharmacotherapy with any drugs that are subject to hepatic microsomal enzyme metabolism, primarily metabolism by cytochrome P450 isoenzyme CYP3A3/4, is *contraindicated* (see Relative Contraindications).

Pharmacotherapy With Other Drugs That Are Highly Bound to Plasma Protein

Nefazodone may displace other highly plasma protein-bound drugs (e.g., phenytoin [Dilantin®], warfarin [Coumadin®]). It may also be displaced by them, depending upon the concentration and relative binding affinity of each interacting drug.

ADVERSE DRUG REACTIONS

Nefazodone pharmacotherapy commonly has been associated with abnormal vision, blurred vision, confusion, constipation, dizziness, dry mouth, headache, light-headedness, nausea, somnolence, and weakness or lack of strength (asthenia). Other ADRs associated with nefazodone pharmacotherapy, listed according to body system, include

Cardiovascular: angina pectoris; fainting (syncope); hypertension; hypotension, including postural hypotension; and tachycardia

CNS: apathy, hallucinations, and insomnia

Cutaneous: acne, eczema, itching (severe), loss of hair (alopecia), and rash

Genitourinary: abnormal absence of menses (amenorrhea), bladder infection (cystitis), breast enlargement, breast pain, impotence, painful menses (dysmenorrhea), urinary frequency, urinary retention, vaginal hemorrhage, and vaginitis

GI: belching (eructation), diarrhea, inflammation of the stomach (gastritis), inflammation of the stomach and intestinal tract (gastroenteritis), loss of appetite (anorexia), mouth ulceration, and peptic ulcer

Musculoskeletal: arthralgia, arthritis, bursitis, difficult and defective speech due to impairment of the tongue or other muscles essential to speech (dysarthria), inflammation of a tendon sheath (tenosynovitis), muscle stiffness, neck pain, and neck rigidity

Ocular: abnormal dilation of the pupil (mydriasis), double vision (diplopia), dry eyes, eye pain, inflammation of the conjunctiva (mucous membrane that lines eyelids and is reflected onto eyeball, conjunctivitis), and unusual intolerance of light (photophobia)

Otic: ear pain and ringing in the ear (tinnitus)

Respiratory: bronchitis, cough (increased), difficult or labored breathing (dyspnea), hiccups, and inflammation of the pharynx (pharyngitis)

Miscellaneous: chills, fever, thirst, and weight loss

OVERDOSAGE

Signs and symptoms of nefazodone overdosage include drowsiness, nausea, somnolence, and vomiting. Nefazodone overdosage requires emergency symptomatic medical support of body systems with attention to increasing nefazodone elimination. There is no known antidote.

NICOTINE

(nik oh'teen)

TRADE NAMES

Habitrol®
Nicoderm®
Nicorette®
Nicotrol NS®
Prostep®

CLASSIFICATION

CNS stimulant

APPROVED INDICATIONS FOR PSYCHOLOGICAL DISORDERS

Adjunctive pharmacotherapy for the symptomatic management of:

Substance-Related Disorders: Nicotine Withdrawal Syndrome Associated With the Cessation of Tobacco Smoking

USUAL DOSAGE AND ADMINISTRATION

Nicotine Withdrawal Syndrome

Adults: Dosage must be prescribed according to the severity of signs and symptoms of nicotine withdrawal, the dosage form prescribed (i.e., chewing gum, nasal spray, transdermal drug delivery system), and individual patient response.

CHEWING GUM: Instruct patients to chew a 2 or 4 mg gum square for 15 to 30 minutes and to repeat when the urge arises to smoke tobacco. Alternatively, instruct patients to bite the 4 mg gum square once or twice, place it between the cheek and gum for a minute, then repeat the procedure for up to 30 minutes.
Maximum: 2 mg chewing gum squares, 24 pieces daily; 4 mg chewing gum squares, 24 pieces daily

NASAL SPRAY: Initially, one or two sprays in *each* nostril every hour. Increase the dosage as needed (one spray equals 0.5 mg).

Maximum: 40 mg daily (80 sprays daily, divided evenly in each nostril)

TRANSDERMAL NICOTINE DELIVERY SYSTEM (TNDS):   Transdermal nicotine pharmacotherapy requires the selection of an initial dosage and a maintenance phase of up to 8 weeks, followed by a weaning phase of 2 to 4 weeks. Most patients initially should be prescribed the 15 mg/16 hour system. However, the initial dosage strength selected and the duration of pharmacotherapy for each dosage strength should be based on a consideration of the patient's level of addiction to tobacco smoking, body weight, concomitant medical and psychological disorders, and individual response to nicotine pharmacotherapy. Patients who have histories of cardiovascular disease, weigh less than 45 kg (100 lbs), or smoke less than one-half a package of cigarettes daily, may require lower dosages.

Dosage schedule, 16-hour TNDS (Nicotrol®):   Apply a 16-hour system upon awakening, and remove prior to retiring for bed in the evening, according to the following recommended 12-week schedule:

Weeks	Dose
1 to 8	15 mg/16 hours
9 and 10	10 mg/16 hours
11 and 12	5 mg/16 hours

If patients are unable to cease tobacco smoking within 4 weeks of initiating transdermal nicotine pharmacotherapy, discontinue pharmacotherapy.

Dosage schedule, 24-hour TNDS (Nicoderm®, Prostep®):   Initiate 24-hour transdermal nicotine pharmacotherapy with the 14 mg/day Nicoderm® system (or the 11 mg/day Prostep® system) for 6 weeks. Decrease the dosage to 7 mg/day (or remain constant with Prostep®) for the final 2 to 4 weeks of pharmacotherapy. Assess all patients for the need for dosage adjustment during the first 2 weeks of 24-hour transdermal nicotine pharmacotherapy. Depending on the initial dose, the entire course of transdermal nicotine pharmacotherapy requires 8 to 12 weeks, including the gradual discontinuation of pharmacotherapy. Do *not* exceed 12 weeks of 24-hour transdermal nicotine pharmacotherapy.

Weeks	Dose and comments
1 through 6	Initiate nicotine pharmacotherapy with the 21 mg/day system (or 22 mg/day Prostep®). Instruct patients to cease tobacco smoking during this period. If unable to cease smoking within 4 weeks, discontinue nicotine pharmacotherapy. For patients who are able to cease smoking, continue pharmacotherapy with a reduced dosage.
7 and 8	Continue pharmacotherapy with the 14 mg/day system. For patients who are able to maintain smoking cessation, continue pharmacotherapy with a further reduction in dosage.
9 and 10	Continue pharmacotherapy with a 7 mg/day system.

Women who are, or who may become, pregnant: FDA Pregnancy Category D. The safety and efficacy of nicotine pharmacotherapy for women who are pregnant have not been established. Although safer for the fetus than tobacco smoking (i.e., the fetus is not exposed to additional chemicals that are present in tobacco smoke), nicotine pharmacotherapy has been associated, as has tobacco smoking, with spontaneous abortion. Long-term nicotine pharmacotherapy also may result in expected pharmacologic actions among neonates, including addiction and signs and symptoms of the nicotine withdrawal syndrome. Avoid prescribing nicotine pharmacotherapy to women who are pregnant. Nicotine pharmacotherapy should be used during pregnancy *only* if the risk to the mother and embryo, fetus, or neonate is justified by the risk posed by continued maternal tobacco smoking. If nicotine pharmacotherapy is required, advise patients of potential benefits and possible risks to themselves and the embryo, fetus, or neonate. Advise women who may become pregnant to take adequate precautions to avoid pregnancy while receiving nicotine pharmacotherapy. Collaboration with the patient's obstetrician is indicated.

Women who are breast-feeding: Safety and efficacy of nicotine pharmacotherapy for women who are breast-feeding and their neonates and infants have not been established. Nicotine, whether obtained from nicotine pharmacotherapy or tobacco smoking, is excreted in breast milk. The concentrations of nicotine and its metabolite, cotinine, in breast milk may be as much as three times the concentrations in maternal blood. Breast-fed infants may display related signs and symptoms of nicotine ingestion, including diarrhea, increased heart rate, restlessness, and vomiting. Advise women who are breast-feeding of the potential risks to their neonates and infants. If nicotine pharmacotherapy is required, breast-feeding should be discontinued. Collaboration with the patient's pediatrician may be indicated.

Elderly patients: Nicotine pharmacotherapy is generally well-tolerated by elderly patients (see Usual Dosage and Administration, Adults).

Children and adolescents younger than 18 years of age: Safety and efficacy of nicotine pharmacotherapy for children and adolescents who want to cease tobacco smoking have not been established. Nicotine pharmacotherapy (e.g., chewing gum, nasal spray, transdermal delivery system) is *not* recommended for children and adolescents.

Notes, Nicotine Withdrawal Syndrome

For optimal therapeutic response, initiate nicotine pharmacotherapy based on the individual patient's level of nicotine addiction as determined by the Fragerström Nicotine Tolerance Scale[1]:

---

[1] Instructions for using the scale: Assign the appropriate score indicated in each column according to the patient's response to the question (Note: Not all questions have an answer in Column C). The highest possible score is 11.

	A = 0 points	B = 1 point	C = 2 points	Score
How soon after you wake do you smoke your first cigarette?	After 30 minutes	Within 30 minutes		
How many cigarettes a day do you smoke?	1 to 15	16 to 25	More than 26	
Does the brand you smoke have a low, medium, or high nicotine content?	Low, less than 0.4 mg	Medium, between 0.5 and 0.8 mg	High, more than 0.9 mg	
Which of all the cigarettes you smoke a day is the most satisfying one?	Any other than the first one in the morning	The first one in the morning		
Do you smoke more during the morning than during the rest of the day?	No	Yes		
Do you smoke when you are so ill that you are in bed most of the day?	No	Yes		
Do you find it difficult to refrain from smoking in places where it is forbidden, such as the library, theater, doctor's office?	No	Yes		
How often do you inhale smoke from your cigarette?	Never	Sometimes	Always	

Score: _____

Chewing Gum Formulations   Before prescribing nicotine pharmacotherapy using the chewing gum formulation, determine the patient's level of nicotine addiction using the Fragerström Nicotine Tolerance Scale (see above). For scores of 6 or less, prescribe the 2 mg chewing gum formulation. For scores of 7 or more, prescribe the 4 mg chewing gum formulation. Most patients require approximately 10 pieces daily of the 2 mg chewing gum formulation (e.g., Nicorette®) during the first month of pharmacotherapy (i.e., 20 mg daily).

Instruct patients to chew one piece of gum for up to 30 minutes when they have a desire to smoke tobacco. Advise patients not to drink beverages or ingest other liquids (e.g., soup) while chewing nicotine gum formulations. Drinking beverages or other liquids may reduce the pH of the mouth or otherwise interfere with the buccal absorption of nicotine. Decrease the dosage and discontinue use over a 1 to 2 week period. Advise patients not to swallow chewing gum formulations and to discard chewed gum appropriately, to prevent access by children or pets.

Nicotine pharmacotherapy using the chewing gum formulations may require 6 months for optimal benefit. Discontinue pharmacotherapy when patients demonstrate an ability to maintain abstinence from tobacco smoking. Advise abstinent patients to carry gum with them for up to 3 months to use in situations where they have a sudden overpowering urge to smoke.

Nasal Spray   The dose of nicotine nasal spray (e.g., Nicotrol NS®) should be administered into the nostril(s) with the head tilted slightly back. Instruct patients *not* to sniff, swallow, or inhale through the nose as the spray is being administered. One dose is defined as 1 mg of nicotine (i.e., one 0.5 mg spray in *each* nostril).

Discontinue nicotine nasal spray pharmacotherapy gradually (e.g., reduce the dosage of one spray in each nostril to one spray in a single nostril). Some patients may simply discontinue their nicotine spray pharmacotherapy without gradually reducing the dosage.

Transdermal Nicotine Delivery Systems The transdermal nicotine delivery systems (TNDS) are available in 16-hour or 24-hour formulations. Some TNDS are available without a prescription in some states and provinces.

16-HOUR TNDS. The 16-hour transdermal formulation (e.g., Nicotrol®) is a multilayered, laminated thin film containing nicotine as the active ingredient. Proceeding from the visible surface toward the surface attached to the skin are three distinct layers: an outer backing layer composed of a laminated polyester film; a middle layer containing an adhesive, a structural non-woven material, and nicotine (the adhesive controls the rate of delivery of nicotine to the skin); and a disposable liner that protects the system, which is removed prior to use.

The 16-hour TNDS is designed to provide a 16-hour rate-controlled delivery of nicotine following its application to intact skin. For optimal therapeutic benefit, the system should be applied during the day and removed at night prior to retiring for bed in the evening. This procedure reflects generally common smoking patterns and minimizes possible ADRs that may disturb sleep. The 16-hour transdermal formulation reportedly increases the success rate of tobacco smoking cessation among smokers who are motivated to quit.

24-HOUR TNDS. From the visible surface of the TNDS to the surface attached to skin, the 24-hour transdermal formulation (e.g., Habitrol®, Nicoderm®) has an occlusive backing, a drug reservoir containing nicotine, a rate-controlling membrane, a polyisobutylene adhesive, and a protective liner that covers the adhesive layer that must be removed before the system is applied to the skin.

APPLICATION AND CARE OF 16- AND 24-HOUR TNDS. Apply the 16- or 24-hour transdermal system promptly upon its removal from the protective pouch to prevent loss of nicotine from the system. Store the pouch safely to use for the disposal of the used system. Apply one active system once per day to a non-hairy, clean, and dry skin site on the upper arm or the hip. Use a different application site each day. Each day a new active system should be applied upon awakening.

Depending on the TNDS prescribed, the active system should not be worn for longer than 16 or 24 hours daily. If other people are assisting with the application of the system, they should avoid unnecessary contact with the active systems and should only wash their hands with water after applying the system. The use of soap may increase nicotine absorption through the skin. They also should avoid touching the eyes to prevent inadvertently getting nicotine in the eyes. When the used system is removed from the skin, it should be folded over and placed in its original pouch for disposal. The used system should be immediately disposed of to prevent inadvertent access by children or pets. Used TNDS generally contain, on average, over 50% of their initial drug content (i.e., enough nicotine to cause serious, even fatal, poisoning if accidentally ingested by small children or pets).

Before initiating transdermal nicotine pharmacotherapy, advise patients to read the patient instruction leaflet on transdermal nicotine pharmacotherapy, and encourage them to ask any questions that they may have. Instruct patients to cease smoking upon initiation of transdermal nicotine pharmacotherapy. Also caution them not to smoke tobacco while receiving transdermal nicotine pharmacotherapy because they may experience ADRs associated with peak nicotine levels higher than those experienced with smoking only. If ADRs are experienced, particularly those affecting the cardiovascular system, the dose should be reduced or the transdermal nicotine pharmacotherapy discontinued. Discourage the use of transdermal nicotine pharmacotherapy beyond 12 weeks by patients who cease smoking because long-term use of nicotine by any method of use is addicting and habituating and otherwise harmful. Discontinue nicotine pharmacotherapy for patients who continue to smoke.

Transdermal nicotine delivery systems generally are well tolerated by patients who have normal skin. However, they may be irritating for some patients who have sensitive skin or skin disorders (e.g., atopic or eczematous dermatitis). Advise patients to discontinue transdermal nicotine pharmacotherapy promptly if they experience severe or persistent local skin reactions (e.g., generalized rash, hives [urticaria]). Concurrent transdermal nicotine pharmacotherapy with other transdermal pharmacotherapy may result in local skin reactions at both application sites and, thus, limits the number of available sites. Advise use of one system or discontinuation of both systems. Serious hypersensitivity reactions rarely may occur.

AVAILABLE DOSAGE FORMS, STORAGE, AND COMPATIBILITY

Chewing gum, buccal (e.g., Nicorette®): 2, 4 mg. The chewing gum formulation is flavored (Nicorette®, mint flavored) and sugar-free. Instruct patients to store chewing gum formulations safely at room temperature, below 30°C (86°F) protected from light. These formulations generally are available for patients without a prescription.

Nasal spray: 10 mg/ml (e.g., Nicotrol NS®). The nasal spray is supplied in a glass container capped with a metered spray pump and child-resistant cap. Each metered-dose spray contains approximately 0.5 mg of nicotine. The unit delivers approximately 200 sprays. Each unit consists of a glass container, which may break if dropped.

Instruct patients to clean up the nicotine solution immediately and carefully if they should break a container (note that the nicotine solution may be extremely toxic, particularly to children and pets). Advise them to rinse well immediately with water *only* any nicotine solution that comes into direct contact with the skin. Instruct patients to store their nasal spray formulation safely out of the reach of children and pets at room temperature below 30°C (86°F).

Transdermal nicotine delivery systems, 16-hour (e.g., Nicotrol®): 5, 10, 15 mg/16 hours. Some transdermal formulations are available for patients without a prescription. In regard to the 16-hour TNDS, instruct patients to

- safely store transdermal nicotine delivery systems out of the reach of children and pets at room temperature below 30°C (86°F).
- only use transdermal systems that are packaged in intact pouches to assure that they have not been tampered with. Advise patients that skin application sites should not be reused for at least one week.
- immediately apply the system once it has been removed from the protective pouch because nicotine is volatile and the system may lose its potency if not immediately applied.

Caution patients against

- storing the system after the pouch has been opened.
- using a system for longer than 16 hours.

Transdermal nicotine delivery systems, 24-hour (e.g., Habitrol®, Nicoderm®): 7, 14, 21 mg/day (11, 22 mg/day [Prostep®]). In regard to the 24-hour TNDS, instruct patients to

- safely store transdermal nicotine delivery systems out of the reach of children and pets at room temperature below 30°C (86°F).
- only use transdermal systems that are packaged in intact pouches to assure that they have not been tampered with. Advise patients that skin application sites should not be reused for at least one week.
- immediately apply the system once removed from the protective pouch because nicotine is volatile and the system may lose potency if not immediately applied.

Caution patients against

- storing the system after the pouch has been opened.
- using a system for longer than 24 hours.

Notes

General Instructions for Patients   Instruct patients who are receiving nicotine pharmacotherapy to obtain an available patient information sheet regarding nicotine pharmacotherapy from their pharmacist at the time that their prescription is dispensed. Encourage patients to clarify any questions that they may have concerning nicotine pharmacotherapy with their pharmacist or, if needed, to consult their prescribing psychologist (see also Available Dosage Forms, Storage, and Compatibility)

PROPOSED MECHANISM OF ACTION

Nicotine binds to acetylcholine receptors in various body organs and tissues, including the adrenal medulla, autonomic ganglia, CNS, and neuromuscular junctions. The pharmacologic action of nicotine is dose-dependent. Lower doses stimulate autonomic ganglia, whereas higher doses block autonomic ganglia. The action on autonomic ganglia also varies according to the degree of tolerance to nicotine. The major action of nicotine is CNS stimulation, which is modulated primarily in the cortex via the locus ceruleus. The CNS stimulant action produces increased alertness and cognitive performance. A CNS "reward" effect, which is modulated primarily in the limbic system, produces a "pleasurable" sensation. Nicotine also has cardiovascular actions associated with its stimulation of sympathetic ganglia and the adrenal medulla and from the activation of chemoreceptors of the aortic and carotid bodies. These actions result in tachycardia, vasoconstriction, and increased blood pressure. The available nicotine replacement products work simply by providing nicotine to patients in dosage forms that are associated with significantly less morbidity and mortality than are associated with smoking tobacco.

PHARMACOKINETICS/PHARMACODYNAMICS

Nicotine absorption following oral ingestion is low (i.e., $F = 0.3$). The pharmacokinetics of nicotine favor buccal absorption, which is rapid and avoids first-pass metabolism in the liver that would otherwise result in its immediate and rapid inactivation. Buccally absorbed chewing gum formulations (e.g., Nicorette®) provide nicotine blood levels that approximate those obtained by the inhalation of smoke from a tobacco cigarette (i.e., F = 0.9). The nicotine, which is in the form of a natural extract from the tobacco plant, is bound to an ion exchange resin and is released only during chewing. Thus, the rate of nicotine release and resultant blood levels are related to the rate and vigor with which the gum is chewed. It is possible to obtain nicotine blood levels of the same order as those produced by smoking cigarettes.

Nicotine is only slightly bound to plasma proteins (i.e., less than 5%). The volume of distribution is approximately 2 to 3 L/kg. Nicotine is primarily metabolized by the liver. Its hepatic clearance rate is approximately 1.2 L/minute. Over 20 different metabolites of nicotine have been identified, all of which are less pharmacologically active than the parent compound. Both nicotine and its metabolites are rapidly excreted in the urine (approximately 15% in unchanged form). Elimination is affected by urinary pH. An alkaline urine can decrease elimination, whereas an acidic urine can increase elimination (i.e., acidification of the urine to below a pH of 5 can result in up to 30% of the dose being eliminated in unchanged form). The mean half-life of elimination is 2 hours.

RELATIVE CONTRAINDICATIONS

> Angina pectoris, severe or worsening
> Breast-feeding
> Cardiac disease, severe
> Children
> Dysrhythmias, life threatening
> Myocardial infarction, immediately post-myocardial infarction
> Nonsmokers
> Peptic ulcer disease, active
> Pregnancy
> Skin disorders, generalized (transdermal nicotine delivery system)
> Temporomandibular joint disease, active (nicotine chewing gum)

CAUTIONS AND COMMENTS

Nicotine, regardless of its method of use, is addicting and habituating. Patients can become addicted to nicotine chewing gum, nasal spray, or transdermal delivery systems. Addiction has been associated with the chewing gum formulations. Transdermal pharmacotherapy has a lower abuse potential probably because it has a much slower rate of absorption, produces much smaller fluctuations in blood levels, maintains lower blood levels of nicotine, and requires less frequent use (i.e., once daily application). To minimize the risk for addiction, advise patients to follow the instructions for use and gradually discontinue their nicotine pharmacotherapy according to their planned schedules. *Nicotine pharmacotherapy should not exceed 12 weeks.*

Prescribe nicotine pharmacotherapy cautiously to patients who

- have cardiovascular disorders. Patients who have coronary artery disease, including a history of myocardial infarction or angina pectoris, serious cardiac dysrhythmias, or vasospastic diseases (e.g., Buerger's disease, Prinzmetal variant angina) should be carefully screened and evaluated. Collaboration with the patient's family physician or a specialist (e.g., cardiologist) is required. If an increase in cardiovascular signs and symptoms occurs, nicotine pharmacotherapy should be discontinued. Tachydysrhythmias have been occasionally reported among patients who have histories of heart disease.

- have hyperthyroidism, pheochromocytoma, or insulin-dependent diabetes mellitus. Nicotine acts on the adrenal medulla. This action can result in the release of catecholamines, which may exacerbate these medical conditions. Collaboration with the patient's advanced practice nurse or family physician is required.
- have systemic hypertension. Nicotine pharmacotherapy, similar to tobacco smoking, has been associated with exacerbating hypertension. Avoid prescribing nicotine pharmacotherapy to patients who have hypertension. If nicotine pharmacotherapy is required, advise patients to weigh potential benefits and possible risks. Collaboration with the patient's advanced practice nurse, family physician, or a specialist (e.g., cardiologist) is required.

In addition, prescribe *nicotine chewing gum formulations* cautiously to patients who

- are ex-smokers and who, after a course of nicotine pharmacotherapy, desire to continue their pharmacotherapy beyond the recommended schedule. The relative risks for resuming tobacco smoking should be weighed against the long-term use of nicotine chewing gum by these patients.
- have dental problems that may be exacerbated by the use of the chewing gum formulation, including dentures, dental caps, or partial bridges to which the gum formulation may stick. Although generally formulated to be sugar-free with minimal stickiness, the degree to which gum formulations stick to dental work may depend on the materials from which the dental work is made and other factors (e.g., salivation, interaction with dental adhesives; denture cleaning compounds). Dental evaluation may be indicated prior to the use of the chewing gum formulation. In the event of excessive adhesion to dental work, advise patients to discontinue their use of the chewing gum formulation to prevent further damage to their dental work and to consult their dentist.
- have oral pharyngeal inflammation, histories of esophagitis, or histories of peptic ulcer disease (active or inactive) that may be exacerbated by the chewing gum formulation. Collaboration with the patient's family physician is indicated.

In addition to these general precautions for patients, caution women to inform their prescribing psychologist if they become or intend to become pregnant while receiving nicotine pharmacotherapy, so that their pharmacotherapy can be safely discontinued.

CLINICALLY SIGNIFICANT DRUG INTERACTIONS

Although no clinically significant drug interactions have been associated with nicotine pharmacotherapy, the cessation of tobacco smoking, with or without nicotine pharmacotherapy, may alter patient response to concurrent pharmacotherapy with a number of different drugs. Tobacco smoking increases, by enzyme induction, the metabolism of acetaminophen (Tylenol®), caffeine, theophylline (Theo-Dur®) (a bronchodilator), imipramine (Tofranil®), oxazepam (Serax®), and pentazocine (Talwin®). Thus, the cessation of tobacco smoking may result in increased blood concentrations of these drugs. Collaboration with other prescribers is indicated in order to help to assure optimal pharmacotherapy.

ADVERSE DRUG REACTIONS

The ADRs associated with nicotine pharmacotherapy include both local and systemic reactions. The local reactions generally are related to the dosage formulation (e.g., oral irritation with chewing gum or local skin irritation with transdermal delivery systems). The systemic reactions are related to the pharmacologic actions of nicotine.

Local Adverse Drug Reactions

Gum Formulation Jaw muscle ache and traumatic injury to the oral tissues, teeth, and jaw are related to the mechanical chewing of the gum formulations. Eructation (belching) secondary to air swallowing also may occur. These ADRs may be minimized by advising patients to modify their chewing techniques. Small (aphthous) ulcers on the mucous membranes of the mouth and inflammation of the gums (gingivitis), tongue (glossitis), pharynx (pharyngitis), and mouth (stomatitis), as well as changes in taste perception, can occur among smokers who have ceased tobacco smoking with or without the chewing gum formulation.

Transdermal Formulation Nicotine transdermal delivery systems are generally associated with local skin irritation. The most common ADR associated with transdermal nicotine pharmacotherapy is a redness (erythema) and itching of the skin (pruritus) at the application site, which may be severe. These ADRs are usually insignificant and resolve within an hour of removal of the system. Some cases of local redness of the skin (erythema) may resolve within 24 hours.

Systemic Adverse Drug Reactions

Nicotine pharmacotherapy, regardless of the dosage formulation or method of use, has been associated with the following systemic ADRs, listed according to body system:

Cardiovascular: chest pains, fainting (syncope), hypertension, rapid heart rate (tachycardia), rapid heart rate and irregular heartbeat (tachydysrhythmias), and rapid throbbing or fluttering of the heart (palpitations). Nicotine pharmacotherapy also has been associated with fatal cardiac arrest, congestive heart failure, myocardial infarction, and stroke.

CNS: concentration, impaired; confusion; convulsions; depression; dizziness or lightheadedness; euphoria; headache; insomnia; irritability; and signs and symptoms of nicotine intoxication

Cutaneous: edema, flushing, itching, itchy hives or wheals (urticaria), rash, and redness of the skin (erythema). These cutaneous reactions may be generalized or affect skin areas other than the actual sites of transdermal delivery system application

GI: belching (eructation), constipation or diarrhea, dry mouth, excessive intestinal gas (flatulence), hiccups, GI complaints (nonspecific), indigestion, loss of appetite (anorexia), mouth or throat soreness, nausea and vomiting, and salivation (excessive) (see also Miscellaneous)

Musculoskeletal: sensation of numbness, prickling or tingling (paresthesia), and weakness

Otic: ringing in the ears (tinnitus)

Respiratory: congestion, cough, difficulty breathing, hoarseness, sneezing, and wheezing

Miscellaneous: Excessive weight gain has been associated with smoking cessation among smokers. This weight gain is thought to be caused by a combination of the discontinuation of the oral habit of tobacco smoking and its replacement with an increased ingestion of food. It also may be associated with reduced GI motility in the absence of nicotine. Monitor patients for weight gain. A weight maintenance program may be indicated.

OVERDOSAGE

Overdosage associated with nicotine pharmacotherapy has been related to simultaneously chewing, or chewing in rapid succession, more than the recommended number of chewing gum squares. The risk for overdosage associated with swallowing gum is low because absorption without chewing is slow and incomplete. In addition, any absorbed nicotine undergoes extensive first-pass liver metabolism. The toxicity associated with overdosage may be minimized by the associated early nausea and vomiting that occurs with excessive nicotine use. The signs and symptoms of acute nicotine overdosage can be mild to moderate, or moderate to severe.

> **Mild to moderate:** abdominal pain, cold sweat, confusion, diarrhea, dizziness, headache, hearing and vision disturbances, nausea, salivation (excessive), vomiting, and weakness (marked)
>
> **Moderate to severe:** breathing difficulty; circulatory collapse; faintness and prostration; hypotension; rapid, weak, irregular pulse; and terminal convulsions, with death occurring within minutes due to the respiratory failure caused by paralysis of the muscles of respiration

There have been reports of patients simultaneously applying several transdermal nicotine delivery systems or swallowing these systems. Signs and symptoms of overdosage associated with transdermal delivery systems are the same as for those associated with other nicotine overdosage. Hypotension, prostration, and respiratory failure may be observed with severe overdosage. Convulsions and death may follow as a result of peripheral or central respiratory paralysis or, less frequently, cardiac failure. In cases of overdosage, discontinue nicotine pharmacotherapy immediately, including immediate removal of the transdermal delivery system. For the latter patients, the skin surface should be flushed with water. Soap must not be used because it may increase nicotine absorption. Nicotine will continue to be delivered into the bloodstream for several hours after the removal of the system because of the depot of nicotine that is formed in the skin.

The minimal single acute lethal dose for orally ingested nicotine among adults is approximately 50 mg. However, the amounts of nicotine that are tolerated by adult tobacco smokers can be fatal if ingested by children or pets. Suspected or actual nicotine overdosage requires emergency symptomatic medical support of body systems with attention to increasing nicotine elimination. There is no known antidote. Caution patients to keep nicotine formulations safely stored out of the reach of children and pets. Also caution patients against concurrent tobacco smoking while receiving nicotine pharmacotherapy.

NITRAZEPAM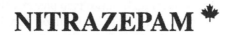

(nye tra′ze pam)

TRADE NAME

Mogadon®

CLASSIFICATION

Sedative-hypnotic (benzodiazepine) (C-IV)

See also Benzodiazepines General Monograph

APPROVED INDICATIONS FOR PSYCHOLOGICAL DISORDERS

Adjunctive pharmacotherapy for the short-term symptomatic management of:

Sleep Disorders: Insomnia (difficulty falling asleep, frequent nocturnal awakenings, and/or early morning awakenings)

USUAL DOSAGE AND ADMINISTRATION

Insomnia

Adults: Initially, 5 mg daily orally 30 minutes before retiring for bed in the evening. Generally limit pharmacotherapy to 7 to 10 consecutive evenings.

MAXIMUM: 10 mg daily orally

Women who are, or who may become, pregnant: FDA Pregnancy Category "not established." Safety and efficacy of nitrazepam pharmacotherapy for women who are pregnant have not been established (see Benzodiazepines General Monograph). Avoid prescribing nitrazepam pharmacotherapy to women who are pregnant. If nitrazepam pharmacotherapy is required, advise patients of potential benefits and possible risks to themselves and the embryo, fetus, or neonate. Collaboration with the patient's obstetrician is indicated.

Women who are breast-feeding: Safety and efficacy of nitrazepam pharmacotherapy for women who are breast-feeding and their neonates and infants have not been established. Nitrazepam is excreted in breast milk in concentrations that are ~25% of those of the maternal blood (see also Benzodiazepines General Monograph). Avoid prescribing nitrazepam pharmacotherapy to women who are breast-feeding. If nitrazepam pharmacotherapy is required, breast-feeding probably should be discontinued. If desired, lactation may be maintained and breast-feeding resumed following the discontinuation of short-term nitrazepam pharmacotherapy.

Elderly, frail, or debilitated patients: Initially, 2.5 mg daily orally 30 minutes before retiring for bed in the evening. Initiate nitrazepam pharmacotherapy with the lowest dosage to avoid associated incoordination (ataxia) or over-sedation, which could result in falls or other injuries. Increase the dosage gradually, if needed, according to individual patient response. Do *not* exceed 5 mg per dose for elderly, frail, or debilitated patients. These patients may be more sensitive to the pharmacologic actions of nitrazepam than are younger or healthier adult patients.

MAXIMUM: 5 mg daily orally

Children and adolescents younger than 18 years of age: Safety and efficacy of nitrazepam pharmacotherapy for children and adolescents have not been established. Nitrazepam pharmacotherapy is *not* recommended for this age group.

Notes, Insomnia

Adjust dosage according to individual patient response for optimal therapeutic benefit. While usual dosages will meet the needs of most patients, some patients may require higher dosages. Increase the dosage gradually for these patients to avoid associated ADRs.

The safety and efficacy of nitrazepam pharmacotherapy for longer than 30 days have not been established. Reevaluate patients who appear to require nitrazepam pharmacotherapy for longer than 30 days. A benzodiazepine withdrawal syndrome similar to the alcohol withdrawal syndrome has been associated with the abrupt discontinuation of long-term nitrazepam pharmacotherapy, or regular personal use. Discontinue nitrazepam pharmacotherapy gradually for these patients.

AVAILABLE DOSAGE FORMS, STORAGE, AND COMPATIBILITY

Tablets, oral: 5, 10 mg

Notes

General Instructions for Patients   Instruct patients who are receiving nitrazepam pharmacotherapy to

- safely store nitrazepam tablets out of the reach of children in child-resistant containers at controlled room temperature (15° to 30°C; 59° to 86°F).
- obtain an available patient information sheet regarding nitrazepam pharmacotherapy from their pharmacist at the time that their prescription is dispensed. Encourage patients to clarify any questions that they may have concerning nitrazepam pharmacotherapy with their pharmacist or, if needed, to consult their prescribing psychologist.

PROPOSED MECHANISM OF ACTION

Nitrazepam is a benzodiazepine with anticonvulsant and hypnotic actions. The exact mechanism of action of nitrazepam has not yet been fully determined. It appears to be mediated by, or work in concert with, the inhibitory neurotransmitter GABA.

See also the Benzodiazepines General Monograph

PHARMACOKINETICS/PHARMACODYNAMICS

Nitrazepam is well and rapidly absorbed (bioavailability ~80%) following oral ingestion. Peak levels generally are achieved within 3 hours. Nitrazepam is ~90% protein-bound. Its mean apparent volume of distribution is ~3 L/kg. It is extensively metabolized in the liver and, with its metabolites, is primarily excreted in the urine. However, less than 1% of nitrazepam is excreted in unchanged form in the urine. The mean half-life of elimination is ~26 hours, and the mean total body clearance is ~73 ml/minute.

RELATIVE CONTRAINDICATIONS

Acute narrow-angle glaucoma. Nitrazepam may be prescribed to patients who have open-angle glaucoma and who are receiving appropriate pharmacotherapy for its management. Collaboration with the patient's ophthalmologist is indicated.
Hypersensitivity to nitrazepam or other benzodiazepines
Myasthenia gravis
Sleep apnea syndrome

CAUTIONS AND COMMENTS

Long-term nitrazepam pharmacotherapy, or regular personal use, may result in addiction and habituation. Abrupt discontinuation has been associated with a benzodiazepine withdrawal syndrome similar to the alcohol withdrawal syndrome. Signs and symptoms of the severe benzodiazepine withdrawal syndrome may include abdominal and muscle cramps, convulsions, tremor, vomiting, and sweating. Severe withdrawal signs and symptoms have been associated with the discontinuation of long-term high-dosage pharmacotherapy, or regular personal use. Milder withdrawal signs and symptoms, such as dysphoria and insomnia, have been observed among patients following the abrupt discontinuation of benzodiazepine pharmacotherapy with recommended dosages. Avoid abrupt discontinuation of nitrazepam pharmacotherapy, particularly when pharmacotherapy has been extended over several months. A gradual reduction of dosage is recommended before nitrazepam pharmacotherapy is completely discontinued.

Prescribe nitrazepam pharmacotherapy cautiously to patients who

- have histories of problematic patterns of alcohol or other abusable psychotropic use. These patients may be at particular risk for the development of problematic patterns of nitrazepam use. Closely monitor these patients for signs and symptoms of problematic patterns of use.
- have kidney or liver dysfunction. Nitrazepam's half-life of elimination may be significantly increased among these patients.
- have latent depression. Benzodiazepine pharmacotherapy may exacerbate depression. Monitor these patients carefully for increased suicide risk. Suicide precautions may be indicated.

Caution patients who are receiving nitrazepam pharmacotherapy against

- drinking alcohol or using other drugs that produce CNS depression. Concurrent use may result in severe CNS depression.
- increasing their prescribed dosage, using nitrazepam more often than prescribed, or abruptly discontinuing their pharmacotherapy without first consulting with their prescribing psychologist. Nitrazepam is addicting and habituating. Abrupt discontinuation of pharmacotherapy, or regular personal use, may result in the benzodiazepine withdrawal syndrome.
- performing activities that require alertness, judgment, and physical coordination (e.g., driving an automobile; operating dangerous equipment; supervising children) until their response to nitrazepam pharmacotherapy is known. The CNS depressant action of nitrazepam may adversely affect these mental and physical functions.

In addition to these general precautions, caution patients to inform their prescribing psychologist if they begin or discontinue any other pharmacotherapy while receiving nitrazepam pharmacotherapy.

CLINICALLY SIGNIFICANT DRUG INTERACTIONS

Concurrent nitrazepam pharmacotherapy and the following may result in clinically significant drug interactions:

Alcohol Use

Concurrent alcohol use may increase the CNS depressant action of nitrazepam. Advise patients to avoid, or limit, their use of alcohol while receiving nitrazepam pharmacotherapy.

Pharmacotherapy With Central Nervous System Depressants and Other Drugs That Produce Central Nervous System Depression

Concurrent nitrazepam pharmacotherapy with opiate analgesics, other sedative-hypnotics, or other drugs that produce CNS depression (e.g., antihistamines, phenothiazines, TCAs), may result in additive CNS depressant actions.

See also the Benzodiazepines General Monograph

Pharmacotherapy With Drugs That Inhibit Cytochrome P450-Mediated Hepatic Metabolism

Concurrent nitrazepam pharmacotherapy with drugs that inhibit cytochrome P450-mediated hepatic metabolism (e.g., cimetidine [Tagamet®]) may result in the delayed or decreased elimination of nitrazepam.

ADVERSE DRUG REACTIONS

Nitrazepam pharmacotherapy commonly has been associated with dizziness, drowsiness, falling, fatigue, incoordination (ataxia), lethargy, lightheadedness, mental confusion, and a staggering gait. Other ADRs, listed according to body system, include:

CNS: depression and nightmares. Paradoxical reactions, including agitation, anxiety (acute), and violent behavior have been reported. If these ADRs are observed, discontinue nitrazepam pharmacotherapy.
GI: constipation, diarrhea, heartburn, and nausea
Hematologic: rarely, granulocytopenia and leukopenia

See also Benzodiazepines General Monograph

OVERDOSAGE

Signs and symptoms of nitrazepam overdosage include confusion, diminished reflexes, drowsiness, increased sedation, and coma. Nitrazepam overdosage requires emergency symptomatic medical support of body systems with attention to increasing nitrazepam elimination. Flumazenil (Anexate®, Romazicon®), the benzodiazepine antagonist, may be required.

See Benzodiazepines General Monograph

NORTRIPTYLINE

(nor trip'ti leen)

TRADE NAMES

Aventyl®
Pamelor®

CLASSIFICATION

Antidepressant (tricyclic)

See also Tricyclic Antidepressants General Monograph

APPROVED INDICATIONS FOR PSYCHOLOGICAL DISORDERS

Adjunctive pharmacotherapy for the symptomatic management of:

Mood Disorders, Depressive Disorders: Endogenous Depression

USUAL DOSAGE AND ADMINISTRATION

Endogenous Depression

Adults: 75 to 100 mg daily orally in three or four divided doses. If preferred, the total daily dosage may be prescribed as a single dose.

MAXIMUM: 150 mg daily orally

Women who are, or who may become, pregnant: FDA Pregnancy Category D. Safety and efficacy of nortriptyline pharmacotherapy for women who are pregnant have not been established. Nortriptyline pharmacotherapy during pregnancy has been associated with a neonatal distress syndrome characterized by hypertonia, respiratory distress, and urinary retention (see also Tricyclic Antidepressants General Monograph). Avoid prescribing nortriptyline pharmacotherapy to women who are pregnant. If nortriptyline pharmacotherapy is required, advise patients of potential benefits and possible risks to themselves and the embryo, fetus, or neonate. Collaboration with the patient's obstetrician is indicated.

Women who are breast-feeding: Safety and efficacy of nortriptyline pharmacotherapy for women who are breast-feeding and their neonates and infants have not been established. Nortriptyline is excreted in low concentrations in breast milk (see also Tricyclic Antidepressants

General Monograph). Avoid prescribing nortriptyline pharmacotherapy to women who are breast-feeding. If nortriptyline pharmacotherapy is required, breast-feeding probably should be discontinued. Collaboration with the patient's pediatrician is indicated.

Elderly, frail, or debilitated patients: Initially, 30 to 50 mg daily orally in three or four divided doses. Generally prescribe lower dosages for elderly, frail, or debilitated patients. Increase the dosage gradually, if needed, according to individual patient response. These patients may be more sensitive to the pharmacologic actions of nortriptyline than are younger or healthier adult patients.

Children: Safety and efficacy of nortriptyline pharmacotherapy for children have not been established. Nortriptyline pharmacotherapy is *not* recommended for this age group.

Adolescents: 30 to 50 mg daily orally in three or four divided doses

Notes, Endogenous Depression

The risk for suicide is increased among depressed patients. Prescribe for dispensing the smallest quantity of nortriptyline feasible (i.e., two-week supply) until the risk for suicide has been judged to be minimal. Following the remission of the depressive episode (approximately three months), long-term maintenance nortriptyline pharmacotherapy may be required. Prescribe for dispensing no more than a one month supply of nortriptyline for these patients.

Initiating Nortriptyline Pharmacotherapy   Initially prescribe lower dosages, and increase the dosage gradually according to individual patient response. Lower dosages are generally recommended for non-hospitalized patients, who may not be as closely monitored as hospitalized patients. Reduce the dosage if patients develop mild ADRs. Discontinue nortriptyline pharmacotherapy promptly if patients develop hypersensitivity reactions or other serious ADRs.

Maintaining Nortriptyline Pharmacotherapy   Prescribe the lowest dosage that will maintain remission. When dosages exceed 100 mg daily, monitor nortriptyline blood concentrations. However, individual patient response should predominate over blood concentrations as the primary determinant of optimal dosage. Maintenance dosages exceeding 150 mg daily are *not* recommended.

AVAILABLE DOSAGE FORMS, STORAGE, AND COMPATIBILITY

Capsules, oral: 10, 25, 50, 75 mg
Solution, oral: 10 mg/5 ml (contains 4% alcohol)

Notes

The 50 mg oral capsules contain sodium bisulfite. Sulfites have been associated with hypersensitivity reactions, including anaphylactic reactions, among susceptible patients. Although relatively uncommon, these reactions appear to occur with a higher incidence among patients who have asthma.

General Instructions for Patients   Instruct patients who are receiving nortriptyline pharmacotherapy to

- safely store nortriptyline oral dosage forms out of the reach of children in tightly closed child- and light-resistant containers at controlled room temperature (15° to 30°C; 59° to 86°F).
- obtain an available patient information sheet regarding nortriptyline pharmacotherapy from their pharmacist at the time that their prescription is dispensed. Encourage patients to clarify any questions that they may have concerning nortriptyline pharmacotherapy with their pharmacist or, if needed, to consult their prescribing psychologist.

PROPOSED MECHANISM OF ACTION

The exact mechanism of action for nortriptyline has not yet been fully determined. It appears to produce its antidepressant action by potentiating the action of the CNS biogenic amines. Specifically, nortriptyline appears to block the re-uptake of norepinephrine and serotonin at the pre-synaptic nerve terminals. This inhibition of re-uptake is thought to increase the amount of norepinephrine and serotonin at the synapses and, consequently, results in increased activity at the post-synaptic neuron receptor sites. The anticholinergic activity of nortriptyline appears to be primarily centrally mediated.

See also Tricyclic Antidepressants General Monograph

PHARMACOKINETICS/PHARMACODYNAMICS

Nortriptyline is moderately absorbed (51%) following oral ingestion. Peak blood levels are generally achieved within 8 hours. Approximately 92% of nortriptyline is bound to plasma proteins. Nortriptyline is extensively metabolized primarily in the liver. Less than 5% of an absorbed dose is eliminated in unchanged form in the urine. Total body clearance ranges from 370 to 630 ml/minute, and the half-life of elimination is approximately 31 hours (range 16 to 90 hours).

Therapeutic Drug Monitoring

The optimal dosage must be determined by individual patient response and not by nortriptyline blood concentrations. It is difficult to correlate blood concentrations with therapeutic response and ADRs. Absorption and distribution in body fluids vary. However, blood concentrations may be useful for monitoring the patient's ability to manage his or her nortriptyline pharmacotherapy or possible overdosage. It generally is recommended that blood samples be obtained from trough blood concentrations approximately 12 hours after the last dose of nortriptyline. However, in cases of suspected overdosage, sampling may be done at anytime. The usual therapeutic blood concentration range is from 170 to 495 nmol/L (50 to 150 ng/ml). Toxic blood concentrations exceed generally 500 ng/ml.

RELATIVE CONTRAINDICATIONS

Hypersensitivity to nortriptyline or other TCAs

MAOI pharmacotherapy, concurrent or within 14 days. Hypertensive crisis, including severe convulsions and death, have been associated with concurrent TCA and MAOI pharmacotherapy.

Myocardial infarction, acute recovery

CAUTIONS AND COMMENTS

Prescribe nortriptyline pharmacotherapy cautiously to patients who

- have acute, narrow-angle glaucoma or histories of urinary retention. Nortriptyline's anticholinergic action may exacerbate these conditions.
- are receiving anticholinergic (e.g., atropine) pharmacotherapy or pharmacotherapy with other drugs that produce anticholinergic actions (e.g., phenothiazines). Nortriptyline's anticholinergic action may potentiate the actions of these drugs.
- are receiving guanethidine (Ismelin®) pharmacotherapy or pharmacotherapy with other related drugs that have antihypertensive action. The actions of these drugs may be blocked by nortriptyline. Concurrent pharmacotherapy may require an adjustment to the dosage of the antihypertensive. Patients also require close monitoring for hypertension. Collaboration with the prescriber of the antihypertensive is indicated.
- have cardiovascular disorders. The associated tendency for tachycardia and prolonged conduction time place these patients at risk. Myocardial infarction, dysrhythmias, and strokes have been reported. Closely monitor these patients for cardiovascular effects. Collaboration with the patient's cardiologist is required.
- have histories of bipolar disorder. Patients who have manic depression may display signs and symptoms of the manic phase of their bipolar disorder.
- have histories of psychotic disorders. Patients who have schizophrenia may display an exacerbation of the signs and symptoms of their disorder. Nortriptyline also may activate latent schizophrenia. Agitated or overactive patients may develop increased agitation and anxiety. Troublesome patient hostility also has been associated with nortriptyline pharmacotherapy.
- have histories of seizure disorders. Nortriptyline reportedly lowers the seizure threshold. Monitor these patients closely for seizures. Epileptiform seizures have been associated with nortriptyline pharmacotherapy.
- have hyperthyroidism or are receiving thyroid pharmacotherapy. The potential for cardiac dysrhythmias is increased among these patients. Collaboration with the patient's family physician or a specialist (e.g., cardiologist) is indicated.
- have non-insulin-dependent diabetes mellitus controlled with the oral antidiabetic, chlorpropamide (Diabinese®). Nortriptyline may raise or lower blood sugar concentrations. Although rare, hypoglycemia has been reported among these patients.
- require ECT. Nortriptyline pharmacotherapy may be concurrently prescribed with ECT, although associated risks (e.g., seizures) may be increased.

Caution patients who are receiving nortriptyline pharmacotherapy against

- drinking alcohol. Advise them that their response to usual amounts of alcohol may be exaggerated. Excessive use of alcohol in combination with nortriptyline pharmacotherapy also may potentiate the CNS depression associated with both drugs. This additive action may lead to an increased risk for suicide attempts, including overdosage, especially among patients who have histories of mood disorders, suicidal ideation, or suicide attempts. Suicide precautions may be indicated.

- performing activities that require alertness, judgment, or physical coordination (e.g., driving an automobile, operating dangerous equipment, supervising children) until their response to nortriptyline pharmacotherapy is known. Nortriptyline pharmacotherapy may affect these mental and physical functions.

In addition to these general precautions, caution patients to inform their prescribing psychologist if they begin or discontinue any other pharmacotherapy while receiving nortriptyline pharmacotherapy.

CLINICALLY SIGNIFICANT DRUG INTERACTIONS

Concurrent nortriptyline pharmacotherapy and the following may result in clinically significant drug interactions:

Clonidine Pharmacotherapy

Concurrent nortriptyline pharmacotherapy may decrease the antihypertensive action of clonidine (Catapres®). An adjustment to the dosage of the hypertensive may be required. Collaboration with the prescriber of the antihypertensive is indicated.

Guanethidine Pharmacotherapy

Concurrent nortriptyline pharmacotherapy may decrease the neuronal uptake of guanethidine (Ismelin®) and, thus, decrease its antihypertensive action. These patients may require an adjustment in their guanethidine dosage. Collaboration with the prescriber of the antihypertensive is indicated.

Monoamine Oxidase Inhibitor Pharmacotherapy

Concurrent nortriptyline and MAOI pharmacotherapy may result in an increase in the therapeutic action and toxic effects of both drugs. This combination of pharmacotherapy also has been associated with increased risk for the hypertensive crisis. Concurrent nortriptyline and MAOI pharmacotherapy is *contraindicated.*

ADVERSE DRUG REACTIONS

Nortriptyline pharmacotherapy commonly has been associated with drowsiness and dry mouth. Other ADRs include blurred vision, confusion, constipation, dizziness, restlessness, and weakness.
See also Tricyclic Antidepressants General Monograph

OVERDOSAGE

Signs and symptoms of nortriptyline overdosage are similar to those observed with overdosages involving other TCAs (see Tricyclic Antidepressants General Monograph). As with other TCA overdosage, emergency symptomatic medical support of body systems is required with attention to increasing nortriptyline elimination. There is no known antidote.

OLANZAPINE

(oh lan′za peen)

TRADE NAME

Zyprexa®

CLASSIFICATION

Antipsychotic (atypical, thienobenzodiazepine derivative)

APPROVED INDICATIONS FOR PSYCHOLOGICAL DISORDERS

Adjunctive pharmacotherapy for the symptomatic management of:

Psychotic Disorders: Schizophrenia and Other Psychotic Disorders

USUAL DOSAGE AND ADMINISTRATION

Schizophrenia and Other Psychotic Disorders

Adults: Initially, 5 to 10 mg daily orally in a single dose. Increase the dosage over the next several days to 10 mg daily, as needed, according to the severity of signs and symptoms and individual patient response.

MAXIMUM: 20 mg daily orally

Women who are, or who may become, pregnant: FDA Pregnancy Category C. Safety and efficacy of olanzapine pharmacotherapy for women who are pregnant have not been established. Avoid prescribing olanzapine pharmacotherapy to women who are pregnant. If olanzapine pharmacotherapy is required, advise patients of potential benefits and possible risks to themselves and the embryo, fetus, or neonate. Collaboration with the patient's obstetrician is indicated.

Women who are breast-feeding: Safety and efficacy of olanzapine pharmacotherapy for women who are breast-feeding and their neonates and infants have not been established. Avoid prescribing olanzapine pharmacotherapy to women who are breast-feeding. If olanzapine pharmacotherapy is required, breast-feeding probably should be discontinued. Collaboration with the patient's pediatrician may be indicated.

Elderly, frail, or debilitated patients: Initially, 5 mg daily orally in a single dose. Increase the dosage gradually, if needed, according to individual patient response. Generally prescribe lower dosages for elderly, frail, or debilitated patients. These patients may be more sensitive to the pharmacologic actions of olanzapine, including postural hypotension, than are younger or healthier adult patients.

Children and adolescents younger than 18 years of age: Safety and efficacy of olanzapine pharmacotherapy for children and adolescents have not been established. Olanzapine pharmacotherapy is *not* recommended for this age group.

Notes, Schizophrenia and Other Psychotic Disorders

Olanzapine pharmacotherapy can improve both positive and negative symptoms of schizophrenia. The dosage is determined by the severity and duration of signs and symptoms of the psychotic disorder and individual patient response. Prescribe the lowest effective dosage possible to reduce the risk for the development of tardive dyskinesia.

Esophageal dysmotility and resultant potentially fatal aspiration pneumonia have been associated with olanzapine pharmacotherapy. Elderly patients, particularly those who have Alzheimer's dementia, are at increased risk for esophageal dysmotility and potentially fatal aspiration pneumonia. Monitor these patients carefully for difficulty swallowing (dysphagia). If esophageal dysmotility is suspected, immediately discontinue olanzapine pharmacotherapy and refer the patient for medical evaluation and management. If continued antipsychotic pharmacotherapy is required, prescribe injectable pharmacotherapy.

AVAILABLE DOSAGE FORMS, STORAGE, AND COMPATIBILITY

Tablets, oral: 2.5, 5, 7.5, 10 mg

Notes

General Instructions for Patients   Instruct patients who are receiving olanzapine pharmacotherapy to

- safely store olanzapine tablets in tightly closed light- and child-resistant containers at controlled room temperature (20° to 25°C; 68° to 77°F) out of the reach of children.
- obtain an available patient information sheet regarding olanzapine pharmacotherapy from their pharmacist at the time that their prescription is dispensed. Encourage patients to clarify any questions that they may have concerning olanzapine pharmacotherapy with their pharmacist or, if needed, to consult their prescribing psychologist.

PROPOSED MECHANISM OF ACTION

The exact mechanism of action of olanzapine is complex and has not yet been fully determined. Its antipsychotic action appears primarily to be related to its interaction with neurotransmitter-containing neurons and, specifically, the blockade of adrenergic (α-1) receptors. Olanzapine also has a high affinity for serotonin (5HT$_2$) receptors. Olanzapine, similar to the other atypical antipsychotics, binds with low affinity to the dopamine (D2) receptor. This low affinity for binding to the D2 receptor is thought to be the reason for its relatively low associated incidence of EPRs when compared to the standard antipsychotics (e.g., chlorpromazine, haloperidol).

PHARMACOKINETICS/PHARMACODYNAMICS

Olanzapine is well absorbed following oral ingestion, reaching peak blood concentrations within 5 to 8 hours. It is subject to extensive first-pass hepatic metabolism (F = 0.6). Olanzapine is moderately (i.e., 93%) bound to plasma proteins. It has an apparent volume of distribution of ~1000 L. Olanzapine is significantly metabolized in the liver to several inactive metabolites. Total body clearance ranges from 12 to 47 L/hour (mean 25 L/hour), and the half-life of elimination ranges from 21 to 54 hours (mean 35 hours). The mean half-life of elimination is longer for women (i.e., 39 hours) than for men (i.e., 29 hours). It also is longer for elderly adults (i.e., men 49 hours, women 55 hours) than for younger adults. Approximately 7% of the olanzapine dose is excreted in unchanged form in the urine.

RELATIVE CONTRAINDICATIONS

Hypersensitivity to olanzapine

CAUTIONS AND COMMENTS

Prescribe olanzapine pharmacotherapy cautiously to patients who

- have histories of breast cancer. Tissue culture experiments have provided evidence that approximately one-third of breast cancers are prolactin dependent. Olanzapine elevates prolactin levels and, thus, may increase the risk for breast cancer among susceptible patients. If olanzapine pharmacotherapy is required for these patients, collaboration with their oncologist is indicated.
- have histories of seizure disorders. Seizures have been reported among ~1% of patients who were receiving olanzapine pharmacotherapy. The incidence of seizures may be increased significantly among patients who have histories of seizure disorders or have a lowered seizure threshold for any other reason (e.g., pharmacotherapy).

Caution patients who are receiving olanzapine pharmacotherapy against performing activities that require alertness, judgment, and physical coordination (e.g., driving an automobile, operating dangerous equipment, supervising children) until their response to olanzapine pharmacotherapy is known. Olanzapine's CNS depressant, extrapyramidal, hypotensive, and seizure-inducing actions may adversely affect these mental and physical functions.

In addition to this general precaution, caution patients to inform their prescribing psychologist if they begin or discontinue any other pharmacotherapy while receiving olanzapine pharmacotherapy.

CLINICALLY SIGNIFICANT DRUG INTERACTIONS

Concurrent olanzapine pharmacotherapy and the following may result in clinically significant drug interactions:

Alcohol Use

Concurrent alcohol use may increase the CNS depressant action of olanzapine. Advise patients to avoid, or limit, their use of alcohol while receiving olanzapine pharmacotherapy.

Antihypertensive Pharmacotherapy

Concurrent olanzapine pharmacotherapy and antihypertensive pharmacotherapy may result in additive hypotensive action. This action may result in postural (orthostatic) hypotension and dizziness, fainting (syncope), or tachycardia.

Pharmacotherapy With Central Nervous System Depressants and Other Drugs That Produce Central Nervous System Depression

Concurrent olanzapine pharmacotherapy with opiate analgesics, sedative-hypnotics, or other drugs that produce CNS depression (e.g., antihistamines, TCAs) may result in additive CNS depression.

Pharmacotherapy With Levodopa and Other Dopamine Agonists

Olanzapine may antagonize the actions of levodopa (Dopar®) and other dopamine agonists.

Tobacco Smoking

The total body clearance of olanzapine is ~40% higher among tobacco smokers than non-smokers. Dosage modification generally is not required unless the smoker is a young man (see Pharmacokinetics/Pharmacodynamics). The total body clearance may be 300% higher among young men who smoke tobacco when compared to elderly women who do not smoke tobacco. Monitor patients carefully, and adjust the dosage, as needed, according to individual patient response. Pharmacokinetic analysis may be warranted.

ADVERSE DRUG REACTIONS

Olanzapine pharmacotherapy reportedly has been associated with a lower incidence of EPRs when compared to other available antipsychotics. Olanzapine pharmacotherapy commonly has been associated with constipation, dizziness, non-aggressive objectionable behavior (e.g., masturbation), postural hypotension, restlessness (akathisia), somnolence, and weight gain. Olanzapine pharmacotherapy also has been associated with the following ADRs, listed according to body system:

Cardiovascular: hypotension, palpitations, and tachycardia
CNS: abnormal dreams, agitation, anxiety, headache, hostility, insomnia, migraine, nervousness, seizures, and tardive dyskinesia

Cutaneous: edema, dry skin, hair loss (alopecia), photosensitivity, and rash

Genitourinary: blood in the urine (hematuria), breast pain, excessive menstrual bleeding or prolonged menses (menorrhagia), impotence, premenstrual syndrome, urinary incontinence, and urinary retention

GI: abdominal pain, dry mouth, increased appetite, nausea, salivation (excessive), thirst (excessive), and vomiting

Metabolic/Endocrine: diabetes mellitus and goiter

Musculoskeletal: arthritis, back pain, joint pain, loss of strength and weakness (asthenia), neck rigidity, tremor, and twitching (see also CNS)

Ocular: dimness or reduction of vision (amblyopia) and inflammation of the edges of the eyelids (blepharitis)

Respiratory: asthma, cough, difficult or labored breathing (dyspnea), inflammation of the pharynx (pharyngitis), and runny nose (rhinitis)

Miscellaneous: fever, intentional injury, and attempted suicide

OVERDOSAGE

Signs and symptoms of acute olanzapine overdosage include drowsiness and slurred speech. There have been no reported deaths associated with olanzapine overdosage. Regardless, olanzapine overdosage requires emergency symptomatic medical support of body systems with attention to increasing olanzapine elimination. There is no known antidote.

OPIATE ANALGESICS

(oh'pee ate)

GENERIC NAMES

(for trade names, see individual drug monographs)

Anileridine * (phenylpiperidine derivative)
Buprenorphine * (phenanthrene derivative) (mixed agonist/antagonist)
Butorphanol (phenanthrene derivative) (mixed agonist/antagonist)
Codeine (methylmorphine) (phenanthrene derivative)
Dezocine * (aminotetralin derivative) (mixed agonist/antagonist)
Fentanyl (phenylpiperidine derivative)
Heroin (diacetylmorphine, diamorphine) (phenanthrene derivative)
Hydrocodone (phenanthrene derivative)
Hydromorphone (phenanthrene derivative)
Levorphanol (phenanthrene derivative)
Meperidine (pethidine) (phenylpiperidine derivative)
Methadone (diphenylheptane derivative)
Morphine (phenanthrene derivative)
Nalbuphine (phenanthrene derivative) (mixed agonist/antagonist)
Oxycodone (phenanthrene derivative)

Oxymorphone (phenanthrene derivative)
Pentazocine (phenanthrene derivative) (mixed agonist/antagonist)
Propoxyphene (dextropropoxyphene) (diphenylheptane derivative)

CLASSIFICATION

Opiate analgesic (C-II)

See also individual opiate analgesic monographs

APPROVED INDICATIONS FOR PSYCHOLOGICAL DISORDERS

Adjunctive pharmacotherapy for the symptomatic management of:

- Pain Disorders: Acute Pain, Moderate to Severe
- Pain Disorders: Chronic Cancer Pain, Moderate to Severe

Opiate analgesic	Pain severity
Codeine (methylmorphine)	mild to moderate
Propoxyphene	mild to moderate
Anileridine	moderate to severe
Butorphanol	moderate to severe
Fentanyl	moderate to severe
Hydromorphone	moderate to severe
Meperidine (pethidine)	moderate to severe
Methadone	moderate to severe
Nalbuphine	moderate to severe
Oxycodone	moderate to severe
Oxymorphone	moderate to severe
Pentazocine	moderate to severe
Heroin (diacetylmorphine, diamorphine)	severe
Levorphanol	severe
Morphine	severe

USUAL DOSAGE AND ADMINISTRATION

Pain Disorders

Adults: See the following table (Approximate analgesic equivalents of opiate analgesics) and individual opiate analgesic monographs. *Note:* Butorphanol, nalbuphine, and pentazocine are mixed opiate agonist/antagonist analgesics. Mixed opiate agonist/antagonist analgesics may precipitate the opiate analgesic withdrawal syndrome among patients who are addicted to pure opiate agonist analgesics (e.g., heroin, morphine).

Approximate analgesic equivalents of opiate analgesics.

Opiate analgesic	Intramuscular or subcutaneous formulation (mg)	Oral formulation (mg)
anileridine	25	75
butorphanol	2	2 (intranasal)
codeine	120	200
fentanyl	0.2	—
heroin	5	20
hydromorphone	1.5	7.5
levorphanol	2	4
meperidine	75	300
methadone	10	20
morphine	**10**	**30**
nalbuphine	10	—
oxycodone	15	30
oxymorphone	1.5	10 (rectal)
pentazocine	60	180
propoxyphene	50	100

Women who are, or who may become, pregnant: FDA Pregnancy Category C. Safety and efficacy of opiate analgesic pharmacotherapy for women who are pregnant have not been established. Some opiate analgesics may be used to relieve pain during labor and delivery. Opiate analgesics cross the placental barrier. Thus, their use during labor and delivery may result in drowsiness, lethargy, or other expected pharmacologic actions (e.g., respiratory depression, constipation) among neonates. Although opiate analgesic pharmacotherapy during pregnancy has not been associated with congenital malformations (i.e., birth defects), long-term maternal opiate analgesic pharmacotherapy, or regular personal use, may result in the opiate analgesic withdrawal syndrome among neonates as their opiate analgesic blood concentrations decrease following birth.

The signs and symptoms of the neonatal opiate analgesic withdrawal syndrome include excessive crying and irritability, fever, hyperactive reflexes, increased respiratory rate, increased number of stools, sneezing, tremors, vomiting, and yawning. The intensity of these signs and symptoms does not always reflect the amount or duration of maternal opiate analgesic pharmacotherapy, or regular personal use. There is no general consensus regarding the best approach for the medical management of the neonatal opiate analgesic withdrawal syndrome.

Avoid prescribing opiate analgesic pharmacotherapy to women who are pregnant. If opiate analgesic pharmacotherapy is required, advise patients of potential benefits and possible risks to themselves and the embryo, fetus, or neonate. Collaboration with the patient's obstetrician is required. Opiate analgesic pharmacotherapy is *not* recommended for women prior to labor unless potential benefits outweigh possible risks to the fetus or neonate. Opiate analgesic pharmacotherapy during labor may result in drowsiness, lethargy, and other expected pharmacologic actions (e.g., constipation, respiratory depression) among neonates.

Women who are breast-feeding: Safety and efficacy of opiate analgesic pharmacotherapy for women who are breast-feeding and their neonates and infants have not been established. Opiate analgesics have been detected in breast milk in amounts that can result in expected pharmacologic actions (e.g., CNS or respiratory depression, constipation) and addiction among breast-fed infants. These infants will experience the opiate withdrawal syndrome when maternal opiate analgesic use or breast-feeding is discontinued. Avoid prescribing opiate analgesic pharmacotherapy to women who are breast-feeding. If opiate analgesic pharmacotherapy is required, breast-feeding probably should be discontinued. If desired, lactation may be maintained and breast-feeding resumed following the discontinuation of short-term opiate analgesic pharmacotherapy. Collaboration with the patient's pediatrician is indicated.

Elderly, frail, or debilitated patients and those who have kidney or liver dysfunction: Initially prescribe lower dosages of opiate analgesics, or longer dosing intervals, for elderly, frail, or debilitated patients. Increase the dosage gradually according to individual patient response. These patients may be more sensitive to the pharmacologic actions of opiate analgesics, especially CNS depression, respiratory depression, and constipation, than would be younger or healthier adult patients. The metabolism and elimination of opiate analgesics also may be slowed among these patients. Also initially prescribe lower dosages and increase the dosage gradually, according to individual patient response, for patients who have liver or kidney dysfunction. See individual opiate analgesic monographs.

Children younger than 2 years of age: The safety and efficacy of opiate analgesic pharmacotherapy for children younger than 2 years of age have not been established. Children younger than 2 years of age may be sensitive to the pharmacologic actions of opiate analgesics, particularly CNS depression, respiratory depression, and constipation. Paradoxical excitement also is particularly likely to occur among young children. Thus, opiate analgesic pharmacotherapy is *not* recommended for this age group.

Children 2 years of age and older: See individual opiate analgesic monographs

Notes, Pain Disorders: Acute Pain, Moderate to Severe, and Chronic Cancer Pain, Moderate to Severe

Initiating and Maintaining Opiate Analgesic Pharmacotherapy The prescription of opiate analgesics for the symptomatic management of acute pain, moderate to severe, and chronic cancer pain, moderate to severe, requires a thorough psychological assessment and diagnosis of the pain disorder and its cause. Collaboration with the patient's advanced practice nurse, family physician, or other specialist (e.g., oncologist) may be required in order to provide optimal adjunctive pharmacotherapy with a minimum of adverse effects. Generally prescribe the lowest effective dosage as infrequently as possible with the therapeutic goal of optimal pain management with a minimum of ADRs. Individualize the daily dosage and method of administration for each patient according to such factors as the nature and severity of the pain; heart, kidney, liver, and renal function; daily dosage of other pharmacotherapy, including opiate analgesic pharmacotherapy prescribed previously or concurrently; and history of addiction and habituation to opiate analgesics and other abusable psychotropics with attention to the associated degree of tolerance. Adjust the initial dosage to individual patient response. It may occasionally be necessary to exceed the usual recommended dosage for patients who have severe pain or have developed tolerance to the analgesic action of opiate analgesics.

INTRAVENOUS PHARMACOTHERAPY Opiate analgesics should *not* be injected intravenously unless the opiate antagonist naloxone (Narcan®) and medical personnel and equipment, including that needed for assisted or controlled respirations, are immediately available for the emergency management of the ADRs associated with intravenous opiate analgesic pharmacotherapy. Rapid intravenous injection of opiate analgesics increases the incidence and severity of ADRs, including severe respiratory depression, apnea, hypotension, peripheral circulatory collapse, and cardiac arrest. Patients should be lying down during intravenous injection, and individual response to intravenous pharmacotherapy should be closely monitored.

During the first two to three days of effective pain management, patients may sleep for several hours. This somnolence may be incorrectly attributed to excessive CNS depression rather than effective pain management among exhausted patients who previously had ineffective pain management. Following the relief of severe pain, attempt periodically to reduce the dosage of the opiate analgesic or to replace injectable pharmacotherapy with oral, transdermal, or other dosage forms (see Available Dosage Forms, Storage, and Compatibility). The prescription of lower dosages and alternate dosage forms and methods of administration, or the complete discontinuation of opiate analgesic pharmacotherapy, may become possible as a result of optimal pain management, physiological change, and associated improved psychological health among patients who have pain disorders that require opiate analgesic pharmacotherapy.

AVAILABLE DOSAGE FORMS, STORAGE, AND COMPATIBILITY

A wide variety of dosage forms are available to individualize opiate analgesic pharmacotherapy. These dosage forms include oral tablets (both regular and extended- release tablets); injectables for intramuscular, intravenous, and subcutaneous use; rectal suppositories; nasal sprays; and transdermal drug delivery systems.

See individual opiate analgesic monographs

Notes

General Instructions for Patients   Instruct patients who are receiving opiate analgesic pharmacotherapy to

- safely store opiate analgesic dosage forms out of the reach of children. See individual opiate analgesic monographs for additional storage requirements.
- obtain an available patient information sheet regarding opiate analgesic pharmacotherapy from their pharmacist at the time that their prescription is dispensed. Encourage patients to clarify any questions that they may have concerning opiate analgesic pharmacotherapy with their pharmacist or, if needed, to consult their prescribing psychologist.

PROPOSED MECHANISM OF ACTION

The opiate analgesics act primarily on the CNS. The perception of, and emotional response to, pain is modified when opiate analgesics bind with stereospecific receptors in the CNS. Five major groups of opiate receptors have been identified: delta, epsilon, kappa, mu, and sigma. Opiate analgesic activity occurs at the mu, kappa, and sigma receptors. These receptors are found in the highest concentrations in the hypothalamus, limbic system, midbrain, spinal cord, and thalamus. Pure opiate analgesic agonists (e.g., morphine) exert their activity mainly at the mu receptor. In addition to analgesia, opiate agonists suppress the cough reflex, alter mood (e.g., produce euphoria or dysphoria), and cause mental clouding, nausea, vomiting, and respiratory depression. Nausea and vomiting probably are caused by the stimulation of the CTZ. Mixed agonist/antagonists (e.g., butorphanol, nalbuphine, pentazocine) act primarily at the kappa receptors.

Peripheral vasodilation, reduced peripheral resistance, and the inhibition of baroreceptors can result in postural hypotension and fainting (syncope). The inhibition of GI peristalsis can result in constipation. Increased bladder sphincter tone may cause urinary retention. High dosages have been associated with excitation or seizures. Morphine and its congeners cause abnormal contraction of the pupils or "pin-point" pupils (miosis). Therapeutic dosages also increase accommodation and sensitivity to light and may decrease intraocular pressure.

PHARMACOKINETICS/PHARMACODYNAMICS

Opiate analgesics are rapidly absorbed after oral, rectal, intramuscular, intranasal, subcutaneous, or transdermal administration. Following oral ingestion, most opiate analgesics undergo significant first-pass hepatic metabolism. They are metabolized by the liver and excreted primarily in the urine after conjugation with glucuronic acid in the kidneys. Morphine is the prototype to which all other opiate analgesics generally are compared.

See the Morphine Monograph and other individual opiate analgesic monographs

RELATIVE CONTRAINDICATIONS

CNS depression, severe
Coma
Diarrhea associated with poisoning. Opiate analgesics may slow GI tract motility and, thus, slow the elimination of the toxic substance involved in the poisoning. Opiate analgesic pharmacotherapy is contraindicated for these patients until the toxic substance has been eliminated from the GI tract.
Hypersensitivity to opiate analgesics, history of. Patients who report a history of a hypersensitivity reaction to morphine (e.g., generalized rash, shortness of breath) should *not* be prescribed codeine, hydromorphone, oxycodone, or oxymorphone.
MAOI pharmacotherapy, concurrent or within 14 days. Fentanyl, heroin, meperidine, or morphine pharmacotherapy and MAOI pharmacotherapy, concurrent or within 14 days, is relatively contraindicated. Concurrent pharmacotherapy may result in toxic reactions with varied signs and symptoms. These signs and symptoms include coma, cyanosis, hyperexcitability, hypertension, hypotension, and severe respiratory depression (see Clinically Significant Drug Interactions).
Respiratory depression, acute
Respiratory dysfunction, including any condition where there is a significant decrease in respiratory reserve (e.g., bronchial asthma, cor pulmonale, emphysema, or kyphoscoliosis). Opiate analgesic pharmacotherapy may further compromise respiratory function among these patients.
Upper airway obstruction

CAUTIONS AND COMMENTS

Opiate analgesics are addicting and habituating. Long-term opiate analgesic pharmacotherapy, or regular personal use, is associated with addiction and habituation. Abrupt discontinuation of long-term opiate analgesic pharmacotherapy, or regular personal use, may result in the opiate analgesic withdrawal syndrome. The opiate analgesic withdrawal syndrome also may occur among patients who are addicted to pure opiate agonist analgesics (e.g., morphine) when an opiate antagonist (e.g., naloxone [Narcan®]) or a mixed opiate analgesic agonist/antagonist (e.g., pentazocine [Talwin®]) is administered.

Signs and symptoms of the acute opiate analgesic withdrawal syndrome include abdominal pain, body aches, chills, diarrhea, difficulty sleeping, gooseflesh (piloerection), loss of appetite (anorexia), nervousness, restlessness, runny nose (rhinitis), shivering, sneezing, stomach cramps, sweating (excessive), tachycardia, tremors, unexplained fever, weakness, and yawning. Although the opiate analgesic withdrawal syndrome generally is not life-threatening, the appropriate prescription and monitoring of opiate analgesic pharmacotherapy and the gradual discontinuation of long-term pharmacotherapy will prevent or minimize these signs and symptoms.

Prescribe opiate analgesic pharmacotherapy cautiously to patients who

- have abdominal disorders (e.g., acute appendicitis). Opiate analgesics may obscure the diagnosis or clinical management of these medical disorders.
- have Addison's disease or adrenocortical insufficiency. Opiate analgesics inhibit the release of corticotropin.
- are elderly, frail, or debilitated. These patients may be at risk for CNS or respiratory depression (see also Respiratory dysfunction).
- have CNS depression, including that associated with acute alcohol intoxication
- have gallbladder disease. Opiate analgesics increase biliary tract pressure and cause smooth muscle spasms. These actions may result in biliary spasm or colic.
- have head injuries or other conditions associated with increased intracranial pressure. The respiratory depressant action of the opiate analgesics and their ability to elevate cerebrospinal fluid pressure may be markedly exaggerated among these patients. Opiate analgesic pharmacotherapy may also obscure the clinical course of these conditions.
- have histories of problematic patterns of opiate analgesic or other abusable psychotropic use. These patients may be at increased risk for the development of problematic patterns of opiate analgesic use, including addiction and habituation.
- have hypertrophy of the prostate or urethral stricture. Opiate analgesics may increase vesical sphincter tone. This action may exacerbate this condition and make urination difficult for these patients.
- have hypotension, including that associated with blood loss, shock, antihypertensive pharmacotherapy and other pharmacotherapy, or other conditions that interfere with the maintenance of normal blood pressure. The action of opiate analgesics on the smooth muscles of the blood vessels may cause severe hypotension among these patients. Opiate analgesic pharmacotherapy also has been associated with postural (orthostatic) hypotension among elderly and other susceptible patients.
- have liver dysfunction (severe)
- have myxedema or hypothyroidism. Opiate analgesic pharmacotherapy may place these patients at increased risk for CNS and respiratory depression.
- have respiratory dysfunction, including chronic obstructive pulmonary disease, cor pulmonale, hypoxia or hypercapnia, pre-existing respiratory depression, substantially decreased respiratory reserve, or other conditions that may compromise respiratory function (e.g., kyphoscoliosis)

Caution patients who are receiving opiate analgesic pharmacotherapy against performing activities that require alertness, judgment, or physical coordination (e.g., driving an automobile, operating dangerous equipment, supervising children) until their response to opiate analgesics is known. Opiate analgesic pharmacotherapy may adversely affect these mental and physical functions.

In addition to this general precaution, caution patients to

- avoid or limit the concurrent use of other CNS depressants, including alcohol, other opiate analgesics, sedative-hypnotics, or other drugs that depress the CNS (e.g., cough and cold products containing antihistamines, such as diphenhydramine [Benadryl®] or triprolidine [found in combination with other active ingredients in Actifed® cough and cold products]). Concurrent use may result in severe CNS and respiratory depression. Family members or others involved with the patient's care should be cautioned to observe for over-sedation and other CNS depressant actions. They also should be advised to implement safety precautions, as needed (e.g., supervised ambulation or tobacco smoking). Hospitalization or supervised home care may be required for patients who require opiate analgesic pharmacotherapy (see also monitor respiratory rate, below).
- be aware of the addiction potential of opiate analgesics. Instruct patients, family members, and others involved with their care, regarding the safe storage of opiate analgesics in the home to prevent possible misuse or accidental poisoning, which may be fatal.
- inform their prescribing psychologist if they begin or discontinue any other pharmacotherapy while receiving opiate analgesic pharmacotherapy.
- monitor respiratory rate. An emergency protocol, including the placement by the telephone of emergency telephone numbers, should be in place in the event of significant respiratory depression or overdosage. Family members or others involved with the patient's care should be cautioned to observe for changes in respiratory function. Hospitalization or supervised home care may be required for patients who require opiate analgesic pharmacotherapy (see also avoid or limit the concurrent use of other CNS depressants, above).

CLINICALLY SIGNIFICANT DRUG INTERACTIONS

Concurrent opiate analgesic pharmacotherapy and the following may result in clinically significant drug interactions:

Alcohol Use

Concurrent use of alcohol among patients who are receiving opiate analgesic pharmacotherapy may result in additive CNS depression. Advise patients to avoid, or limit, their use of alcohol while receiving opiate analgesic pharmacotherapy.

Anticholinergic Pharmacotherapy and Pharmacotherapy With Other Drugs That Produce Anticholinergic Actions

Concurrent opiate analgesic and anticholinergic (e.g., atropine) pharmacotherapy, or pharmacotherapy with other drugs that produce anticholinergic actions (e.g., phenothiazines, TCAs), may increase constipation, drowsiness, and urinary retention among susceptible patients (e.g., elderly, frail, or debilitated patients).

Cimetidine Pharmacotherapy

Concurrent opiate analgesic and cimetidine (Tagamet®) pharmacotherapy may result in opiate analgesic toxicity (e.g., respiratory depression). The mechanism for this interaction has not been clearly established. However, it is most likely associated with a decrease in the metabolism of the opiate analgesics by cimetidine.

Monoamine Oxidase Inhibitor Pharmacotherapy

Concurrent fentanyl (Sublimaze®), meperidine (pethidine, Demerol®), or morphine (M.O.S.®) and MAOI pharmacotherapy (including selegiline) has been associated with serious ADRs. The mechanism of this interaction has not been clearly established. Fentanyl, meperidine, or morphine pharmacotherapy should be prescribed with extreme caution, if at all, to patients who are receiving MAOI pharmacotherapy (including selegiline) or within 14 days of such pharmacotherapy (see Relative Contraindications).

Pharmacotherapy With Central Nervous System Depressants and Other Drugs That Produce Central Nervous System Depression

Concurrent opiate analgesic pharmacotherapy with other opiate analgesics, sedative-hypnotics, or other drugs that produce CNS depression (e.g., antihistamines, phenothiazines, TCAs) may result in additive CNS depression. If concurrent pharmacotherapy is required, reduce the dosages of one or both drugs accordingly (see also Clinically Significant Drug Interactions, Pharmacotherapy With Other Opiate Analgesics, Including Opiate Agonist Analgesics and Mixed Opiate Agonist/Antagonist Analgesics).

Pharmacotherapy With Other Opiate Analgesics, Including Opiate Agonist Analgesics and Mixed Opiate Agonist/Antagonist Analgesics

Concurrent pharmacotherapy with two or more opiate agonist analgesics may produce additive actions. These actions may result in severe CNS depression, respiratory depression, and hypotension. Avoid prescribing concurrent opiate agonist pharmacotherapy. Concurrent pharmacotherapy with a mixed opiate agonist/antagonist analgesic (i.e., butorphanol [Stadol NS®], nalbuphine [Nubain®], pentazocine [Talwin®]) and a pure opiate agonist analgesic may reduce the analgesic action of both drugs. This combination of pharmacotherapy also may precipitate the opiate withdrawal syndrome among patients who are addicted to opiate agonist analgesics. Avoid concurrent opiate agonist and opiate agonist/antagonist analgesic pharmacotherapy (see also Clinically Significant Drug Interactions, Pharmacotherapy with CNS Depressants and Other Drugs That Produce CNS Depression).

Tricyclic Antidepressant Pharmacotherapy

Concurrent opiate analgesic and TCA pharmacotherapy may potentiate the respiratory depressant action of the opiate analgesic (see also Clinically Significant Drug Interactions, Pharmacotherapy with CNS Depressants and Other Drugs That Produce CNS Depression).

ADVERSE DRUG REACTIONS

The major ADRs associated with opiate analgesic pharmacotherapy are respiratory depression and respiratory arrest. To a lesser extent, circulatory depression, shock, and cardiac arrest also may occur. Other ADRs associated with opiate analgesic pharmacotherapy, listed according to body system, include:

Cardiovascular

Bradycardia, fainting (syncope), hypertension, palpitations, phlebitis following intravenous injection, postural hypotension, and supraventricular tachycardia

Central Nervous System

Agitation, alterations of mood, disorientation, dreams, drowsiness, euphoria, dysphoria, headache, hallucinations, insomnia, sedation, seizures, and toxic psychosis. Patients who have migraine headaches reportedly may be more susceptible to the ADRs associated with butorphanol pharmacotherapy.
See Butorphanol Monograph

Cutaneous

Edema; excessive sweating; flushing or feelings of warmth; hives (urticaria); local tissue irritation and induration following subcutaneous injection, particularly when repeated injections are required; pain at the injection site; severe itching (pruritus); skin rashes; and wheal and flare over the vein following intravenous injection

Gastrointestinal

Biliary tract spasm, constipation, cramps, diarrhea, dry mouth, dyspepsia, loss of appetite (anorexia), nausea, taste alterations, and vomiting. Constipation, nausea, and vomiting seem to be more prominent among non-hospitalized patients and those who are not experiencing severe pain.

Constipation   Lower dosages are recommended for these patients. Elderly, frail, or debilitated patients, particularly those who are bedridden, may become impacted. Caution patients to maintain a balanced diet and an adequate intake of water. An appropriate regimen of bowel management and exercise may be required, particularly when initiating long-term opiate analgesic pharmacotherapy. Collaboration with the patient's advanced practice nurse, physician, oncologist, or community health nurse may be indicated.

Nausea and Vomiting   Nausea and vomiting often occur following a single dose of an opiate analgesic. Nausea and vomiting also may be troublesome when long-term opiate analgesic pharmacotherapy is initiated. When initiating long-term pharmacotherapy for the symptomatic management of chronic cancer pain, consider the prescription of an antiemetic. Collaboration with the patient's advanced practice nurse, family physician, or a specialist (e.g., oncologist) may be required.

Genitourinary

Impotence, reduced sex drive, and urinary hesitancy or retention

Musculoskeletal

Incoordinated muscle movements and weakness

Ocular

Abnormal contraction of the pupils (miosis) and visual disturbances

Miscellaneous

Spasm of the larynx (laryngospasm)

OVERDOSAGE

Signs and symptoms of opiate overdosage include respiratory depression with reduced respiratory rate and tidal volume, Cheyne-Stokes respirations, cyanosis, extreme somnolence progressing to stupor or coma, skeletal muscle flaccidity, cold clammy skin, and sometimes, hypotension and bradycardia. Severe overdosage may result in apnea, circulatory collapse, cardiac arrest, and death. Abnormal dilation of the pupils (mydriasis) may occur with terminal narcosis, severe hypoxia, or as a toxic reaction associated with meperidine or its congeners. The signs and symptoms of severe propoxyphene overdosage include focal and generalized seizures. Nephrogenic diabetes insipidus and ECG abnormalities also may occur.

Opiate analgesic overdosage requires emergency symptomatic medical support of body systems, particularly respiratory function, with attention to increasing opiate analgesic elimination. Naloxone (Narcan®), a pure opiate analgesic antagonist, is a specific antidote against the respiratory depression associated with opiate agonist and mixed opiate agonist/antagonist analgesic overdosages. However, the usual dosage of the opiate analgesic antagonist will precipitate the opiate analgesic withdrawal syndrome among patients who are addicted to opiate analgesics. The severity of the withdrawal syndrome depends on the severity of the patient's addiction and the dose of the antagonist administered. The use of opiate analgesic antagonists among patients who are addicted to opiates should be avoided if possible. If an opiate analgesic antagonist is required for the medical management of serious respiratory depression and other signs and symptoms of overdosage among these patients, lower dosages and cautious dosage titration are recommended.

See also Naloxone Monograph

OXAZEPAM

(ox a′ze pam)

TRADE NAME

Serax®

CLASSIFICATION

Sedative-hypnotic (benzodiazepine) (C-IV)

See also Benzodiazepines General Monograph

APPROVED INDICATIONS FOR PSYCHOLOGICAL DISORDERS

Adjunctive pharmacotherapy for the short-term symptomatic management of:

Anxiety Disorders. Oxazepam pharmacotherapy is *not* indicated for the management of everyday anxiety or tension, or that anxiety that can be managed with psychotherapy alone. Oxazepam also is *not* recommended for the management of anxiety associated with depression because it has the potential to exacerbate the depression while alleviating the anxiety. The depression associated with anxiety generally resolves with appropriate adjunctive pharmacotherapy (i.e., antidepressant pharmacotherapy) and psychotherapy.

USUAL DOSAGE AND ADMINISTRATION

Anxiety

Adults: 30 to 120 mg daily orally in three or four divided doses

Women who are, or who may become, pregnant: FDA Pregnancy Category C. Safety and efficacy of oxazepam pharmacotherapy for women who are pregnant have not been established. Oxazepam pharmacotherapy during pregnancy has been associated with cleft lip and palate among neonates. In addition, an increased risk for congenital malformations (i.e., birth defects) has been associated with other benzodiazepine pharmacotherapy, including chlordiazepoxide and diazepam pharmacotherapy. Long-term oxazepam pharmacotherapy during pregnancy, or regular personal use, also may result in the neonatal benzodiazepine withdrawal syndrome. Avoid prescribing oxazepam pharmacotherapy to women who are pregnant. If oxazepam pharmacotherapy is required, advise patients of potential benefits and possible risks to themselves and the embryo, fetus, or neonate. Collaboration with the patient's obstetrician is indicated.
See also Benzodiazepines General Monograph

Women who are breast-feeding: Safety and efficacy of oxazepam pharmacotherapy for women who are breast-feeding and their neonates and infants have not been established. Oxazepam is excreted in low concentrations in breast milk. Although concentrations are low, the half-life of oxazepam will be significantly prolonged among breast-fed neonates during the first week following birth because of their immature kidney and liver function. Neonates and infants may display expected pharmacologic effects (e.g., drowsiness, lethargy). Avoid prescribing oxazepam pharmacotherapy to women who are breast-feeding, particularly during the first week following delivery. If oxazepam pharmacotherapy is required, advise patients of the potential benefits and possible risks to themselves and their neonates and infants. If desired, lactation may be maintained and breast-feeding resumed following the discontinuation of short-term oxazepam pharmacotherapy. Collaboration with the patient's pediatrician is indicated.

Elderly, frail, or debilitated patients: 30 mg daily orally in three divided doses. Increase the dosage gradually, as needed, according to individual patient response. Elderly, frail, or debilitated patients may be more sensitive to the pharmacologic actions of oxazepam than are younger or healthier adult patients.

Children younger than 12 years of age: The safety and efficacy of oxazepam pharmacotherapy for children younger than 12 years of age have not been established. Oxazepam pharmacotherapy is *not* recommended for this age group.

Notes, Anxiety

The safety and efficacy of oxazepam pharmacotherapy for longer than 4 months have not been established. Reevaluate patients who appear to require long-term oxazepam pharmacotherapy.

AVAILABLE DOSAGE FORMS, STORAGE, AND COMPATIBILITY

Capsules, oral: 10, 15, 30 mg
Tablets, oral: 10, 15, 30 mg

Notes

The 15 mg oral tablet contains tartrazine (FD&C Yellow No. 5). Tartrazine has been associated with hypersensitivity reactions, including bronchial asthma, among susceptible patients. Patients who have a hypersensitivity to aspirin appear to be at particular risk.

General Instructions for Patients Instruct patients who are receiving oxazepam pharmacotherapy to

- safely store oxazepam oral capsules or tablets out of the reach of children in tightly closed child-resistant containers at controlled room temperature (15° to 30°C; 59° to 86°F).
- obtain an available patient information sheet regarding oxazepam pharmacotherapy from their pharmacist at the time that their prescription is dispensed. Encourage patients to clarify any questions that they may have concerning oxazepam pharmacotherapy with their pharmacist or, if needed, to consult their prescribing psychologist.

PROPOSED MECHANISM OF ACTION

The exact mechanism of action of oxazepam has not yet been fully determined. However, it appears to be mediated or work in concert with the inhibitory neurotransmitter GABA.

See Benzodiazepines General Monograph

PHARMACOKINETICS/PHARMACODYNAMICS

Oxazepam is completely absorbed (~95%) after oral ingestion. Peak blood levels are achieved in approximately 3 hours. Oxazepam is highly plasma protein-bound (~98%) and has an apparent volume of distribution of 0.6 L/kg. The mean half-life of elimination is approximately 8 hours (range 6 to 11 hours). Its mean total body clearance is ~70 ml/minute.

RELATIVE CONTRAINDICATIONS

Glaucoma, acute narrow-angle
Hypersensitivity to oxazepam or other benzodiazepines
Myasthenia gravis

CAUTIONS AND COMMENTS

Oxazepam is addicting and habituating. Long-term oxazepam pharmacotherapy, or regular personal use, may result in addiction and habituation. Abrupt discontinuation of long-term pharmacotherapy (i.e., longer than four months), or regular personal use, will result in the benzodiazepine withdrawal syndrome.

See also Benzodiazepines General Monograph

Prescribe oxazepam pharmacotherapy cautiously to patients who

- have histories of problematic patterns of alcohol or other abusable psychotropic use. Monitor these patients carefully for the development of problematic patterns of oxazepam use, including addiction and habituation.
- have kidney dysfunction. Oxazepam is excreted primarily by the kidneys. The half-life of elimination may be prolonged among these patients.
- have low blood pressure (hypotension), particularly if they are elderly. Hypotension rarely has been associated with oxazepam pharmacotherapy. Oxazepam's hypotensive action may lead to serious cardiac complications and other sequelae (e.g., injury associated with a fall) among these patients.

Caution patients who are receiving oxazepam pharmacotherapy against performing activities that require alertness, judgment, or physical coordination (e.g., driving an automobile, operating dangerous equipment, supervising children) until their response to oxazepam is known. Oxazepam may adversely affect these mental and physical functions.

In addition to this general precaution, caution patients to inform their prescribing psychologist if they begin or discontinue any other pharmacotherapy while receiving oxazepam pharmacotherapy.

CLINICALLY SIGNIFICANT DRUG INTERACTIONS

Concurrent oxazepam pharmacotherapy and the following may result in clinically significant drug interactions:

Alcohol Use

The concurrent use of alcohol may increase the CNS depressant action of both drugs. Advise patients to avoid, or limit, their use of alcohol while receiving oxazepam pharmacotherapy.

Pharmacotherapy With Central Nervous System Depressants and Other Drugs That Produce Central Nervous System Depression

Concurrent oxazepam pharmacotherapy with opiate analgesics, other sedative-hypnotics, or other drugs that produce CNS depression (e.g., antihistamines, phenothiazines, TCAs) may result in additive CNS depression.

ADVERSE DRUG REACTIONS

Oxazepam pharmacotherapy has been associated with drowsiness, dizziness, headache, and vertigo. These ADRs generally can be managed by a reduction in dosage. Oxazepam pharmacotherapy also has been associated with mild paradoxical reactions (e.g., excitement). These reactions usually occur during the first two weeks of pharmacotherapy. Other ADRs *rarely* associated with oxazepam pharmacotherapy include the following, listed according to body system:

Cardiovascular: fainting (syncope), occurring alone or with drowsiness
CNS: incoordination (ataxia), which appears unrelated to dosage or patient's age; lethargy; and slurred speech
Cutaneous: diffuse skin rashes, including maculopapular, morbilliform, and urticarial rashes; and edema
Genitourinary: changes in sex drive
GI: nausea
Hematologic: a reduction in white blood cells, particularly lymphocytes, but also basophils, eosinophils, and monocytes (leukopenia). Monitor blood counts periodically. Collaboration with the patient's family physician or a specialist (e.g., hematologist) is indicated.
Hepatic: liver dysfunction, including jaundice. Obtain liver function tests periodically. Collaboration with the patient's family physician or a specialist (e.g., internist) is indicated.
Musculoskeletal: tremor

See also Benzodiazepines General Monograph

OVERDOSAGE

The signs and symptoms of oxazepam overdosage resemble those associated with other benzodiazepine overdosage (see Benzodiazepines General Monograph). Oxazepam overdosage requires emergency symptomatic medical support of body systems with attention to increasing oxazepam elimination. The benzodiazepine antagonist flumazenil (Anexate®, Romazicon®) may be required.

OXYCODONE [Dihydrohydroxycodeinone]

(ox i koe'done)

TRADE NAMES

OxyContin®
OxyIR®
Roxicodone®
Supeudol®

CLASSIFICATION

Opiate analgesic (C-II)

See also Opiate Analgesics General Monograph

APPROVED INDICATIONS FOR PSYCHOLOGICAL DISORDERS

Adjunctive pharmacotherapy for the symptomatic management of:

- Pain Disorders: Acute Pain, Moderate to Severe
- Pain Disorders: Chronic Cancer Pain, Moderate to Severe

USUAL DOSAGE AND ADMINISTRATION

Acute Pain, Moderate to Severe, and Chronic Cancer Pain, Moderate to Severe

Adults: 5 to 10 mg regular tablets orally every six hours, as needed; *or* 10 to 20 mg rectally every 6 to 8 hours, as needed; *or* 10 to 80 mg extended-release tablets orally every 12 hours, as needed (see Notes, Acute Pain, Moderate to Severe and Chronic Cancer Pain, Moderate to Severe).

Women who are, or who may become, pregnant: FDA Pregnancy Category B. Safety and efficacy of oxycodone pharmacotherapy for women who are pregnant have not been established. Long-term oxycodone pharmacotherapy during pregnancy, or regular personal use, may result in the neonatal opiate withdrawal syndrome (see Opiate Analgesics General Monograph). Avoid prescribing oxycodone pharmacotherapy to women who are pregnant. If oxycodone pharmacotherapy is required, advise patients of potential benefits and possible risks to themselves and the embryo, fetus, or neonate. Collaboration with the patient's obstetrician is indicated.

Women who are breast-feeding: Safety and efficacy of oxycodone pharmacotherapy for women who are breast-feeding and their neonates and infants have not been established. Oxycodone is excreted in breast milk in concentrations higher than maternal blood concentrations. Expected pharmacologic actions (e.g., drowsiness, lethargy) may be observed among breast-fed neonates and infants who also may become addicted. Avoid prescribing oxycodone pharmacotherapy to women who are breast-feeding. If oxycodone pharmacotherapy is required, breast-feeding probably should be discontinued. If desired, lactation may be maintained and breast-feeding resumed following the discontinuation of short-term oxycodone pharmacotherapy. Collaboration with the patient's pediatrician may be indicated.

Elderly, frail, or debilitated patients: Generally prescribe lower dosages for elderly, frail, or debilitated patients. Increase the dosage gradually, if needed, according to individual patient response. These patients may be more sensitive to the pharmacologic actions of oxycodone than are younger or healthier adult patients.

Children and adolescents younger than 18 years of age: Safety and efficacy of oxycodone pharmacotherapy for children and adolescents have not been established. Oxycodone pharmacotherapy is *not* recommended for this age group.

Notes, Acute Pain, Moderate to Severe, and Chronic Cancer Pain, Moderate to Severe

The difference in the recommended dosages for oxycodone oral and rectal pharmacotherapy is due to the effects of first-pass hepatic metabolism on the oral dosage forms. Adjust the dosage to the type and severity of pain and individual patient response. It may be necessary to occasionally exceed the usual recommended dosage for patients who have severe pain or who have developed tolerance to oxycodone's analgesic action. Oral pharmacotherapy is usually adequate for the management of moderate to severe pain of short duration or for severe chronic cancer pain. Oral pharmacotherapy should *not* be prescribed for the symptomatic management of chronic benign pain.

Oxycodone Oral Extended-Release Tablet Pharmacotherapy for the Symptomatic Management of Chronic, Severe Cancer Pain   Experience with and use of oxycodone oral extended-release tablet pharmacotherapy for the *initial* symptomatic management of severe chronic cancer pain are generally limited and not recommended. The extended-release tablets are formulated in high dosages (i.e., 10, 20, 40, 80 mg). They also are formulated to have a prolonged duration of action (i.e., 12 hours). Although these features prevent their use for the initial management of severe chronic cancer pain because of the associated difficulty establishing adequate analgesia, these same features can be used to provide effective and convenient oral opiate analgesic pharmacotherapy once adequate analgesia with the regular formulations has been achieved. In this regard, prescribe oxycodone extended-release pharmacotherapy only for patients whose moderate to severe cancer pain has been adequately managed with regular oral dosage forms of oxycodone or other opiate analgesics. For these patients, calculate their total current daily opiate analgesic requirement to determine the oral oxycodone equivalent daily dosage (see Opiate Analgesics General Monograph, Usual Dosage and Administration).

Initially prescribe the equivalent daily dosage in two equally divided doses at 12-hour intervals using the extended-release tablets. This initial recommended equivalent daily dosage generally is a conservative estimate of the required daily dosage. Most patients will need an adjustment (i.e., increase) in their dosage. For these patients, increase the dosage at 24-hour intervals, as needed, according to individual patient response. Breakthrough pain during the 24 hours following the initiation of oxycodone oral extended-release tablet pharmacotherapy generally requires an increase in dosage rather than a decrease in dosing interval. Once therapeutic benefit has been achieved, maintain oxycodone oral extended-release tablet pharmacotherapy with the lowest effective dosage. Attempt to reduce the dosage or discontinue pharmacotherapy periodically.

See also Opiate Analgesics General Monograph

AVAILABLE DOSAGE FORMS, STORAGE, AND COMPATIBILITY

Capsules, oral: 5 mg
Solution, concentrated oral (Roxicodone Intensol®): 20 mg/ml
Solution, oral (unit dose Patient Cups®): 5 mg/5 ml (contains 0.4% or 8% alcohol, depending upon the manufacturer)
Suppositories, rectal: 10, 20 mg
Tablets, oral: 5, 10 mg
Tablets, oral extended-release: 10, 20, 40, 80 mg

Notes

Caution is required when prescribing oxycodone oral formulations. Do not confuse the concentrated oral solution (Intensol®, 20 mg/ml) with the regular oral solution (1 mg/ml). Do not confuse the extended-release oral tablets (10, 20, 40, 80 mg) with the regular oral tablets (5, 10 mg).

General Instructions for Patients   Instruct patients who are receiving oxycodone pharmacotherapy to

- measure each dose of the oxycodone concentrated oral solution (Roxicodone Intensol®) with the calibrated dropper supplied with the product to assure that an accurate dose is measured and ingested.
- swallow whole each dose of the oxycodone oral extended-release tablets without breaking, crushing, or chewing. Breaking, crushing, or chewing the oral extended-release tablets may result in the absorption of a potentially toxic dose of oxycodone. Also instruct them to ingest each dose with an adequate amount of liquid chaser (i.e., 60 to 120 ml).
- safely store oxycodone capsules, tablets, or oral solution out of the reach of children. Oral capsules and tablets should also be stored in tightly closed child- and light-resistant containers at controlled room temperature (15° to 30°C; 59° to 86°F).
- safely store oxycodone rectal suppositories under refrigeration (2° to 8°C; 36° to 46°F) out of the reach of children.
- obtain an available patient information sheet regarding oxycodone pharmacotherapy from their pharmacist at the time that their prescription is dispensed. Encourage patients to clarify any questions that they may have concerning oxycodone pharmacotherapy with their pharmacist or, if needed, to consult their prescribing psychologist.

PROPOSED MECHANISM OF ACTION

Oxycodone is a semi-synthetic opiate with several actions qualitatively similar to morphine. It appears to elicit its analgesic and CNS depressant actions primarily by binding to the endorphin receptors in the CNS. However, the exact mechanism of action has not yet been fully determined.

See Opiate Analgesics General Monograph

PHARMACOKINETICS/PHARMACODYNAMICS

Approximately 60% to 90% of oxycodone is absorbed following oral ingestion. Although oxycodone undergoes extensive first-pass hepatic metabolism, it is similar to codeine and methadone in that it retains at least half of its analgesic action when orally ingested. Oxycodone's apparent volume of distribution is approximately 2.6 L/kg. Its plasma protein binding is low (~45%), and its duration of analgesic action generally is 4 to 5 hours. Oxycodone is extensively metabolized, primarily to inactive metabolites. However, low concentrations of an active metabolite, oxymorphone, have been identified. Oxycodone and its metabolites are excreted primarily by the kidneys, with up to 20% being eliminated in unchanged form. The total plasma clearance of oxycodone among adults is approximately 0.8 L/minute. The mean half-life of elimination is approximately 4 hours.

RELATIVE CONTRAINDICATIONS

Head injury or any other medical disorder associated with increased intracranial or cerebrospinal fluid pressure
Hypersensitivity to oxycodone
Respiratory dysfunction, including any medical disorder where there is a significant decrease of respiratory reserve (e.g., bronchial asthma, cor pulmonale, emphysema, or kyphosis)

CAUTIONS AND COMMENTS

Oxycodone is addicting and habituating. It has a high addiction potential and is a commonly abused oral opiate analgesic.

For cautions in prescribing, see Opiate Analgesics General Monograph.

Caution patients who are receiving oxycodone pharmacotherapy against

- drinking alcohol or using other drugs that produce CNS depression. Concurrent use of these drugs with oxycodone can result in excessive CNS depression.
- performing activities that require alertness, judgment, and physical coordination (e.g., driving an automobile, operating dangerous equipment, supervising children) until their response to oxycodone pharmacotherapy is known. Oxycodone may adversely affect these mental and physical functions.

In addition to these general precautions, caution patients to inform their prescribing psychologist if they begin or discontinue any other pharmacotherapy while receiving oxycodone pharmacotherapy.

CLINICALLY SIGNIFICANT DRUG INTERACTIONS

Concurrent oxycodone pharmacotherapy and the following may result in clinically significant drug interactions:

Alcohol Use

Concurrent alcohol use may increase the CNS depressant action of oxycodone. Advise patients to avoid, or limit, their use of alcohol while receiving oxycodone pharmacotherapy.

Pharmacotherapy With Central Nervous System Depressants and Other Drugs That Produce Central Nervous System Depression

Concurrent oxycodone pharmacotherapy with other opiate analgesics, sedative-hypnotics, or other drugs that produce CNS depression (e.g., antihistamines, phenothiazines, TCAs) may result in additive CNS depression.

ADVERSE DRUG REACTIONS

Oxycodone pharmacotherapy commonly has been associated with dizziness, light-headedness, nausea, and vomiting. It also has been associated with constipation, dry mouth, euphoria or dysphoria, severe itching (pruritus), and skin rash.

See also Opiate Analgesics General Monograph

OVERDOSAGE

The signs and symptoms of oxycodone overdosage resemble those associated with other opiate analgesic overdosage (see Opiate Analgesics General Monograph). Oxycodone overdosage requires emergency symptomatic medical support of body systems with attention to increasing oxycodone elimination. The opiate antagonist naloxone (Narcan®) is usually required to reverse the respiratory depression associated with oxycodone and other opiate analgesic overdosage.

OXYMORPHONE

(ox i mor'fone)

TRADE NAME

Numorphan®

CLASSIFICATION

Opiate analgesic (C-II)

See also Opiate Analgesics General Monograph

APPROVED INDICATIONS FOR PSYCHOLOGICAL DISORDERS

Adjunctive pharmacotherapy for the symptomatic management of:

Pain Disorders: Acute Pain, Moderate to Severe

USUAL DOSAGE AND ADMINISTRATION

Acute Pain, Moderate to Severe

Adults: Initially, 1 to 1.5 mg intramuscularly or subcutaneously; *or* 5 mg rectally; *or* 0.5 mg intravenously slowly every 4 to 6 hours, as needed.

Women who are, or who may become, pregnant: FDA Pregnancy Category "not established." Safety and efficacy of oxymorphone pharmacotherapy for women who are pregnant have not been established. Long-term pharmacotherapy during pregnancy, or regular personal use, may result in the neonatal opiate withdrawal syndrome (see Opiate Analgesics General Monograph). Avoid prescribing oxymorphone pharmacotherapy to women who are pregnant. If oxymorphone pharmacotherapy is required, advise patients of potential benefits and possible risks to themselves and the embryo, fetus, or neonate. Collaboration with the patient's obstetrician is indicated.

Women who are breast-feeding: Safety and efficacy of oxymorphone pharmacotherapy for women who are breast-feeding and their neonates and infants have not been established (see Opiate Analgesics General Monograph). Avoid prescribing oxymorphone pharmacotherapy to women who are breast-feeding. If oxymorphone pharmacotherapy is required, breast-feeding probably should be discontinued. If desired, lactation may be maintained and breast-feeding resumed following the discontinuation of short-term oxymorphone pharmacotherapy. Collaboration with the patient's pediatrician may be indicated.

Elderly, frail, or debilitated patients: Generally prescribe lower dosages of oxymorphone for elderly, frail, or debilitated patients. Increase the dosage gradually according to individual patient response. These patients may be more sensitive to the pharmacologic actions of oxymorphone than are younger or healthier adult patients.

Children younger than 12 years of age: The safety and efficacy of oxymorphone pharmacotherapy for children younger than 12 years of age have not been established. Oxymorphone pharmacotherapy is *not* recommended for this age group.

Notes, Acute Pain, Moderate to Severe

Initiate oxymorphone pharmacotherapy with lower dosages. Increase the dosage gradually according to individual patient response until pain is adequately managed. Oxymorphone pharmacotherapy with the rectal suppositories may be prescribed when oral opiate analgesic pharmacotherapy is not feasible (e.g., patients are nauseated or vomiting) and injectable pharmacotherapy is not desired. Oxymorphone pharmacotherapy with the rectal suppositories also may be of benefit for elderly, frail, or debilitated patients who may require a potent, rapid acting analgesic and generally are unable to tolerate oral or injectable opiate analgesic pharmacotherapy.

AVAILABLE DOSAGE FORMS, STORAGE, AND COMPATIBILITY

Injectables, intramuscular, intravenous, or subcutaneous: 1, 1.5 mg/ml
Suppository, rectal: 5 mg

Notes

The oxymorphone injectable formulation contains sodium dithionite, a sulfite. Sulfites may cause hypersensitivity reactions, including anaphylactic reactions, among susceptible patients. Although relatively uncommon, these reactions appear to occur with a higher incidence among patients who have asthma.

General Instructions for Patients   Instruct patients who are receiving oxymorphone pharmacotherapy, or those assisting them with their pharmacotherapy, to

- safely store oxymorphone injectables protected from light at controlled room temperature (15° to 30°C; 59° to 86°F) out of the reach of children.
- safely store oxymorphone rectal suppositories under refrigeration (2° to 8°C; 36° to 46°F) out of the reach of children.
- obtain an available patient information sheet regarding oxymorphone pharmacotherapy from their pharmacist at the time that their prescription is dispensed. Encourage patients to clarify any questions that they may have concerning oxymorphone pharmacotherapy with their pharmacist or, if needed, to consult their prescribing psychologist.

PROPOSED MECHANISM OF ACTION

Oxymorphone is a potent opiate analgesic that appears to elicit its analgesic action primarily by binding to the endorphin receptors in the CNS. However, the exact mechanism of action has not yet been fully determined.

See also Opiate Analgesics General Monograph

PHARMACOKINETICS/PHARMACODYNAMICS

When injected, 1 mg of oxymorphone is equivalent to 10 mg of morphine. When compared to morphine, oxymorphone reportedly produces equal analgesia with less respiratory depression. The onset of action is rapid and generally occurs within 5 to 10 minutes after intravenous injection, 10 to 15 minutes after intramuscular or subcutaneous injection, and 15 to 30 minutes after rectal insertion. Analgesia persists for 3 to 6 hours. Oxymorphone is conjugated with glucuronic acid in the liver and is excreted in the urine. Additional data are unavailable.

RELATIVE CONTRAINDICATIONS

Hypersensitivity to oxymorphone, morphine, or other opiate analgesics
Respiratory depression
Seizure disorders

CAUTIONS AND COMMENTS

Addiction and habituation are associated with long-term oxymorphone pharmacotherapy, or regular personal use.

Prescribe oxymorphone pharmacotherapy cautiously for patients who are receiving concurrent pharmacotherapy with other opiate analgesics or other drugs that depress CNS or respiratory function.

Caution patients who are receiving oxymorphone pharmacotherapy against performing activities that require alertness, judgment, and physical coordination (e.g., driving an automobile, operating dangerous equipment, supervising children) until their response to oxymorphone is known. The CNS depressant action of oxymorphone may adversely affect these mental and physical functions.

CLINICALLY SIGNIFICANT DRUG INTERACTIONS

Concurrent oxymorphone pharmacotherapy and the following may result in clinically significant drug interactions:

Alcohol Use

Concurrent alcohol use may increase the CNS depressant action of oxymorphone. Advise patients to avoid, or limit, their use of alcohol while receiving oxymorphone pharmacotherapy.

Pharmacotherapy With Central Nervous System Depressants and Other Drugs That Produce Central Nervous System Depression

Concurrent oxymorphone pharmacotherapy with other opiate analgesics, sedative-hypnotics, or other drugs that produce CNS depression (e.g., antihistamines, phenothiazines, TCAs) may result in additive CNS depression.

ADVERSE DRUG REACTIONS

Oxymorphone pharmacotherapy has been associated with abnormal contraction of the pupils or "pin-point pupils" (miosis), drowsiness, dysphoria, GI upset, headache, itching, light-headedness, nausea, respiratory depression, and vomiting.

See also Opiate Analgesics General Monograph

OVERDOSAGE

The signs and symptoms of oxymorphone overdosage resemble those associated with other opiate analgesic overdosage (see Opiate Analgesics General Monograph). Oxymorphone overdosage requires emergency symptomatic medical support of body systems with attention to increasing oxymorphone elimination. The opiate antagonist naloxone (Narcan®) is usually required to reverse the respiratory depression associated with oxymorphone and other opiate overdosage.

PAROXETINE

(pa rox'e teen)

TRADE NAME

Paxil®

CLASSIFICATION

Antidepressant (SSRI)

See also Selective Serotonin Re-Uptake Inhibitors General Monograph

APPROVED INDICATIONS FOR PSYCHOLOGICAL DISORDERS

Adjunctive pharmacotherapy for the symptomatic management of:

- Mood Disorders, Depressive Disorders: Major Depressive Disorder
- Anxiety Disorders: Obsessive-Compulsive Disorder
- Anxiety Disorders: Panic Disorder

USUAL DOSAGE AND ADMINISTRATION

Depressive Disorders: Major Depressive Disorder

Adults: Initially, 20 mg daily orally in a single morning dose. Increase the daily dosage weekly by 10 mg increments according to individual patient response.

MAXIMUM: 50 mg daily orally

Women who are, or who may become, pregnant: FDA Pregnancy Category C. Safety and efficacy of paroxetine pharmacotherapy for women who are pregnant have not been established. Paroxetine pharmacotherapy during pregnancy has been associated with uterine spasms (rare), vaginal hemorrhage (rare), and spontaneous abortion (see Adverse Drug Reactions; see also Selective Serotonin Re-Uptake Inhibitors General Monograph). Avoid prescribing paroxetine pharmacotherapy to women who are pregnant. If paroxetine pharmacotherapy is required, advise patients of potential benefits and possible risks to themselves and the embryo, fetus, or neonate. Collaboration with the patient's obstetrician is indicated.

Women who are breast-feeding: Safety and efficacy of paroxetine pharmacotherapy for women who are breast-feeding and their neonates and infants have not been established. Paroxetine is excreted in breast milk in concentrations equal to those found in maternal blood (see Selective Serotonin Re-Uptake Inhibitors General Monograph). Avoid prescribing paroxetine pharmacotherapy to women who are breast-feeding. If paroxetine pharmacotherapy is required, breast-feeding probably should be discontinued. Collaboration with the patient's pediatrician is indicated.

Elderly, frail, or debilitated patients and those who have significant kidney or liver dysfunction: Generally prescribe lower dosages of paroxetine for elderly, frail, or debilitated patients and those who have significant kidney or liver dysfunction. Increase the dosage gradually, if needed, according to individual patient response. These patients may be more sensitive to the pharmacologic actions of paroxetine than are younger or healthier adult patients.

MAXIMUM: 40 mg daily orally

Children and adolescents younger than 18 years of age: Safety and efficacy of paroxetine pharmacotherapy for children and adolescents have not been established. Paroxetine pharmacotherapy is *not* recommended for this age group.

Anxiety Disorders: Obsessive-Compulsive Disorder

Adults: Initially, 20 mg daily orally in a single morning dose. Increase the daily dosage weekly by 10 mg increments, as needed, according to individual patient response.

MAINTENANCE: The usual maintenance dosage is 40 mg daily orally

MAXIMUM: 60 mg daily orally

Women who are, or who may become, pregnant: See Usual Dosage and Administration, Major Depressive Disorder

Women who are breast-feeding: See Usual Dosage and Administration, Major Depressive Disorder

Elderly, frail, or debilitated patients: See Usual Dosage and Administration, Major Depressive Disorder

Children and adolescents younger than 18 years of age: See Usual Dosage and Administration, Major Depressive Disorder

Anxiety Disorders: Panic Disorder

Adults: Initially, 10 mg daily orally in a single morning dose. Increase the daily dosage weekly by 10 mg increments, as needed, according to individual patient response.

MAINTENANCE: The usual maintenance dosage is 40 mg daily orally

MAXIMUM: 60 mg daily orally

Women who are, or who may become, pregnant: See Usual Dosage and Administration, Major Depressive Disorder

Women who are breast-feeding: See Usual Dosage and Administration, Major Depressive Disorder

Elderly, frail, or debilitated patients: See Usual Dosage and Administration, Major Depressive Disorder

Children and adolescents younger than 18 years of age: See Usual Dosage and Administration, Major Depressive Disorder

AVAILABLE DOSAGE FORMS, STORAGE, AND COMPATIBILITY

Tablets, oral: 10, 20, 30, 40 mg

Notes

General Instructions for Patients Instruct patients who are receiving paroxetine pharmacotherapy to

- safely store paroxetine oral tablets in child-resistant containers out of the reach of children at controlled room temperature (15° to 30°C; 59° to 86°F).
- obtain an available patient information sheet regarding paroxetine pharmacotherapy from their pharmacist at the time that their prescription is dispensed. Encourage patients to clarify any questions that they may have concerning paroxetine pharmacotherapy with their pharmacist or, if needed, to consult their prescribing psychologist.

PROPOSED MECHANISM OF ACTION

The exact mechanism of paroxetine's antidepressant and other related actions has not yet been fully determined. These actions appear to be directly related to paroxetine's ability to inhibit selectively the neuronal re-uptake of serotonin.

See also Selective Serotonin Re-Uptake Inhibitors General Monograph

PHARMACOKINETICS/PHARMACODYNAMICS

Paroxetine is well absorbed following oral ingestion. However, it is subject to extensive first-pass hepatic metabolism. The ingestion of food does not appear to affect paroxetine's bioavailability. It is highly plasma protein-bound (~95%). Paroxetine is metabolized extensively in the liver to several inactive metabolites. Its metabolism is subject to genetic polymorphism (i.e., variation in metabolism by patients who are "extensive" or "poor" metabolizers). Less than 2% of paroxetine is excreted in unchanged form in the urine. The mean half-life of elimination is ~17 hours for extensive metabolizers and ~41 hours for poor metabolizers (range 3 to 64 hours). The mean total body clearance is ~630 ml/minute for extensive metabolizers and ~350 ml/minute for poor metabolizers.

RELATIVE CONTRAINDICATIONS

Hypersensitivity to paroxetine

MAOI pharmacotherapy, concurrent or within 14 days. This combination of pharmacotherapy, concurrent or within 14 days, may result in the potentially fatal serotonin syndrome (see Selective Serotonin Re-uptake Inhibitors General Monograph).

CAUTIONS AND COMMENTS

Paroxetine pharmacotherapy has been associated with a lower incidence of seizures (~0.1%) and mania (~1%) than most of the other SSRIs. In addition, paroxetine does not appear to cause significant sedation or to interfere with cognitive or psychomotor performance.

Caution patients who are receiving paroxetine pharmacotherapy to inform their prescribing psychologist if they begin or discontinue any other pharmacotherapy while receiving paroxetine pharmacotherapy.

See also Selective Serotonin Re-Uptake Inhibitors General Monograph

CLINICALLY SIGNIFICANT DRUG INTERACTIONS

Concurrent paroxetine pharmacotherapy and the following may result in clinically significant drug interactions:

Pharmacotherapy With Drugs That Are Highly Bound to Plasma Proteins

Paroxetine may displace from their binding sites other drugs that are highly bound to plasma proteins (e.g., digitoxin [Digitaline®], warfarin [Coumadin®]). This interaction results in significantly higher concentrations of free drug and associated actions, including ADRs. Conversely, paroxetine may be displaced from its binding sites by other drugs, depending upon their relative affinity for the plasma protein binding sites.

Pharmacotherapy With Drugs That Are Metabolized by the Hepatic Cytochrome P450 Enzyme System, Particularly Isoenzyme CYP2D6

Paroxetine inhibits this particular hepatic isoenzyme and, consequently, reduces the rate and extent of metabolism of a number of different drugs. These drugs include amitriptyline, clomipramine, clozapine, codeine, desipramine, diazepam, flecainide [Tambocor®], fluoxetine, haloperidol, imipramine, nortriptyline, perphenazine, propafenone [Rythmol®], propranolol [Inderal®], risperidone, sertraline, thioridazine, and venlafaxine.

See also Selective Serotonin Re-uptake Inhibitors General Monograph

ADVERSE DRUG REACTIONS

Paroxetine pharmacotherapy commonly has been associated with delayed ejaculation, dizziness, dry mouth, insomnia, lack of strength or weakness (asthenia), loss of appetite (anorexia), nausea, nervousness, somnolence, sweating (excessive), and tremor. Other ADRs associated with paroxetine pharmacotherapy, listed according to body system, include:

Cardiovascular: blood pressure changes, increased (hypertension) or decreased (hypotension), fainting (syncope), increase in the caliber of blood vessels (vasodilation), postural (orthostatic) hypotension, rapid or slow heart beat (tachycardia or bradycardia), rapid throbbing or fluttering of the heart (palpitations)

CNS: agitation, amnesia, anxiety, headache, impaired concentration, and vertigo

Cutaneous: acne, hair loss (alopecia), dry skin, itching (severe), rash, and sweating (excessive)

Endocrine: breast pain, diabetes mellitus (rare), excessive secretion of the thyroid gland (hyperthyroidism, rare), and inflammation of the thyroid gland (thyroiditis)

Genitourinary: absent or missed menses (amenorrhea), decreased sex drive, excessive bleeding during menses (menorrhagia), excessive urination (polyuria), excessive urination during the night (nocturia), inflammation of the urinary bladder (cystitis), impotence, involuntary urination (urinary incontinence), painful menstruation (dysmenorrhea), painful urination (dysuria), spontaneous abortion, urinary retention, uterine spasm (rare), vaginal hemorrhage (rare), and vaginitis (inflammation of the vagina)

GI: abnormal taste, constipation, diarrhea, difficulty swallowing (dysphagia), excessive gas in the stomach and intestines (flatulence), grinding of the teeth (bruxism), inflammation of the tongue (glossitis), salivation (excessive), and vomiting

Hematologic: abnormal reduction in circulating white blood cells, including basophils, eosinophils, monocytes, and, in particular, lymphocytes (leukopenia); anemia; bleeding associated with impaired platelet aggregation (rare); disease of the lymph node (lymphadenopathy); and hemorrhages into the skin and other body tissues (purpura)

Musculoskeletal: abnormal striated muscle (myopathy), arthritis, back pain, joint pain (arthralgia), muscle pain (myalgia), and muscular weakness or abnormal fatigue (myasthenia)

Ocular: abnormal accommodation, blurred vision, conjunctivitis, and eye pain

Otic: ear pain and ringing in the ears (tinnitus)

Respiratory: asthma, bronchitis, cough (increased), difficult or labored breathing (dyspnea), excessive yawning, and runny nose (rhinitis)

Miscellaneous: chills, fever, low blood sodium concentration (hyponatremia, rare), and malaise

See also Selective Serotonin Re-Uptake Inhibitors General Monograph

OVERDOSAGE

Signs and symptoms of paroxetine overdosage include dilated pupils (mydriasis), drowsiness, dry mouth, irritability, nausea, tachycardia, tremor, and vomiting. No deaths have been reported involving paroxetine overdosage alone. Regardless, paroxetine overdosage requires emergency symptomatic medical support of body systems with attention to increasing paroxetine elimination. There is no known antidote.

PEMOLINE [Phenylisohydantoin]

(pem oh'leen)

TRADE NAME

Cylert®

CLASSIFICATION

CNS Stimulant (amphetamine-like) (oxazolidine derivative) (C-IV)

APPROVED INDICATIONS FOR PSYCHOLOGICAL DISORDERS

Adjunctive pharmacotherapy for the symptomatic management of:

Attention-Deficit/Hyperactivity Disorder

USUAL DOSAGE AND ADMINISTRATION

Attention-Deficit/Hyperactivity Disorder

Adults: Safety and efficacy of pemoline pharmacotherapy for adults who have A-D/HD have not been established. Pemoline pharmacotherapy is *not* recommended for this age group.

Women who are, or who may become, pregnant: FDA Pregnancy Category B. Safety and efficacy of pemoline pharmacotherapy for women who are pregnant have not been established. Avoid prescribing pemoline pharmacotherapy to women who are pregnant.
See Amphetamines General Monograph

Women who are breast-feeding: Safety and efficacy of pemoline pharmacotherapy for women who are breast-feeding and their neonates and infants have not been established. Avoid prescribing pemoline pharmacotherapy to women who are breast-feeding.
See Amphetamines General Monograph

Children younger than 6 years of age: Safety and efficacy of pemoline pharmacotherapy for children younger than 6 years of age have not been established. Pemoline pharmacotherapy is *not* recommended for this age group.

Children 6 years of age and older: 37.5 mg daily orally in a single dose each morning. Increase the daily dosage weekly by 18.75 mg increments until optimal therapeutic response is achieved. Most patients benefit from daily dosages between 56.25 to 75 mg. Therapeutic response is gradual. Significant benefit may not be observed until the third or fourth week of pemoline pharmacotherapy. Children who have kidney dysfunction may require lower dosages.

MAXIMUM: 3 mg/kg daily orally *or* 112.5 mg daily orally, whichever dosage is lower

Notes, Attention-Deficit/Hyperactivity Disorder

Pemoline pharmacotherapy is *not* indicated for all children who are diagnosed with A-D/HD. Prescribe pemoline pharmacotherapy only after a comprehensive psychological assessment of the child supports its prescription. *Pemoline pharmacotherapy should not be considered the pharmacotherapy of first choice for the symptomatic management of A-D/HD because of its association with life-threatening hepatic failure.*

Long-Term Pemoline Pharmacotherapy The safety and efficacy of long-term pemoline pharmacotherapy for children who are 6 years of age and older have not been established. Data are inconclusive regarding the effects of long-term pemoline pharmacotherapy on normal growth. Liver function also may be affected. Monitor height and liver function prior to and periodically during long-term pemoline pharmacotherapy. Discontinue pemoline pharmacotherapy if noted abnormalities are medically confirmed with follow-up diagnostic tests. Collaboration with the patient's pediatrician or a specialist (e.g., internist) may be indicated (see Adverse Drug Reactions).

Whenever possible, occasionally interrupt long-term pemoline pharmacotherapy to determine if there is a recurrence of the signs and symptoms of A-D/HD. Evaluate these signs and symptoms in order to determine if they are sufficient to continue pharmacotherapy. The A-D/HD appears to remit with increasing age among most children who have been diagnosed with this disorder. By puberty, pemoline pharmacotherapy may not be required.

AVAILABLE DOSAGE FORMS, STORAGE, AND COMPATIBILITY

Tablets, oral: 18.75, 37.5, 75 mg
Tablets, oral chewable: 37.5 mg

Notes

General Instructions for Patients Instruct patients (and their parents in regard to the patient) to

- thoroughly chew, or allow to dissolve in the mouth, each dose of the chewable tablets before swallowing. Chewing the tablets or allowing them to dissolve in the mouth before swallowing will help to achieve optimal therapeutic benefit.
- safely store pemoline tablets out of the reach of children in tightly closed child-resistant containers at controlled room temperature (15° to 30°C; 59° to 86°F).

- obtain an available patient information sheet regarding pemoline pharmacotherapy from their pharmacist at the time that their prescription is dispensed. Encourage patients (and their parents) to clarify any questions that they may have concerning pemoline pharmacotherapy with their pharmacist or, if needed, to consult their prescribing psychologist.

PROPOSED MECHANISM OF ACTION

Pemoline is a CNS stimulant that is structurally different from the amphetamines and methylphenidate (Ritalin®). Although it possesses similar stimulant actions, pemoline has minimal sympathomimetic actions. The exact mechanism of action of pemoline for the symptomatic management of A-D/HD has not yet been fully determined. However, it appears primarily to involve the stimulation of the CNS.

PHARMACOKINETICS/PHARMACODYNAMICS

Pemoline is rapidly absorbed following oral ingestion. Peak blood levels generally are achieved within 4 hours. Pemoline is moderately plasma protein-bound (i.e., ~50%). It achieves steady-state in two to three days. Pemoline is metabolized primarily by the liver. Approximately 50% of pemoline is excreted in unchanged form in the urine. The mean half-life of elimination is approximately 12 hours (range 9 to 14 hours).

RELATIVE CONTRAINDICATIONS

Hypersensitivity to pemoline
Liver dysfunction (see Adverse Drug Reactions)

CAUTIONS AND COMMENTS

The pharmacological similarity of pemoline to other CNS stimulants known to be addicting and habituating suggests that addiction and habituation also may occur with pemoline pharmacotherapy, particularly long-term pharmacotherapy.

Prescribe pemoline pharmacotherapy cautiously to patients who

- are concurrently receiving pharmacotherapy with drugs that also stimulate the CNS. When concurrent pharmacotherapy is required, monitor patients carefully for excessive CNS stimulation. Also monitor these patients for problematic patterns of stimulant use.
- have histories of Tourette's disorder (Gilles de la Tourette's syndrome). Although not directly associated with pemoline pharmacotherapy, the precipitation of Tourette's syndrome among susceptible patients has been associated with CNS stimulant pharmacotherapy.
- have histories of problematic patterns of abusable psychotropic use, particularly CNS stimulant use. These patients may increase their pemoline dosage on their own initiative. They also may crave pemoline when long-term pharmacotherapy has been abruptly discontinued. Signs and symptoms of psychoses, although usually brief in duration, also rarely have been reported among these patients.
- have kidney dysfunction (significant). Pemoline is excreted in the urine. Toxicity may occur among these patients because of their decreased kidney function.
- have psychotic disorders. Signs and symptoms of psychoses, including behavior disturbances and thought disorders, may be exacerbated among these patients.

Caution patients who are receiving pemoline pharmacotherapy (or their parents in regard to the patient) against performing activities that require alertness, judgment, and physical coordination (e.g., operating dangerous equipment, sports and recreational activities) until their response to pemoline pharmacotherapy is known.

CLINICALLY SIGNIFICANT DRUG INTERACTIONS

None commonly identified at present

ADVERSE DRUG REACTIONS

Pemoline pharmacotherapy has been associated with insomnia prior to the achievement of an optimal therapeutic dosage. The insomnia usually remits with continued pharmacotherapy or with a reduction in dosage. Pemoline pharmacotherapy also has been associated with a loss of appetite (anorexia) and resultant weight loss during the first weeks of pharmacotherapy. However, patients generally regain their lost weight within three to six months. In addition to these ADRs, pemoline pharmacotherapy has been associated with the following ADRs, listed according to body system:

CNS: convulsions; depression (mild); dizziness; drowsiness; dyskinetic movements of the tongue, lips, face, and extremities; hallucinations; and irritability (increased)

Cutaneous: skin rashes

Hepatic: Pemoline pharmacotherapy over several months has been associated with liver dysfunction and abnormal changes in liver function tests. These abnormal changes in liver function are thought to be associated with a delayed hypersensitivity reaction and appear to be reversible upon discontinuation of pemoline pharmacotherapy. Jaundice also has been reported.

Pemoline pharmacotherapy also has been associated with potentially fatal acute liver failure. Acute liver failure, which may require a liver transplantation, may occur suddenly or following years of pemoline pharmacotherapy. Patients, as appropriate for their age and cognitive abilities, and their parents or legal guardians, must be advised of the risk for this serious ADR. They also must be instructed to recognize and report to the prescribing psychologist any signs and symptoms of liver toxicity (e.g., dark amber urine, fatigue, yellowing of the eyes and skin [jaundice], nausea). Monitor patients for liver dysfunction periodically. Collaboration with the patient's pediatrician, family physician, or a specialist (e.g., internist) is required. In the event that any signs and symptoms suggestive of liver dysfunction are noted, immediately discontinue pemoline pharmacotherapy and refer patients for emergency medical evaluation and appropriate treatment.

Musculoskeletal: (see CNS)

Ocular: constant, involuntary, cyclical movement of the eyeball (nystagmus)

OVERDOSAGE

Signs and symptoms of acute pemoline overdosage include abnormal dilation of the pupils (mydriasis), agitation, dyskinetic movements, euphoria, hallucinations, hyperreflexia, restlessness, seizures, sweating, and tachycardia. Pemoline overdosage requires emergency symptomatic medical support of body systems with attention to increasing pemoline elimination. There is no known antidote.

PENTAZOCINE

(pen taz'oh seen)

TRADE NAMES

Talwin®
Talwin Nx® (see Available Dosage Forms, Storage, and Compatibility, Notes)

CLASSIFICATION

Opiate analgesic (mixed agonist/antagonist) (C-IV)

See also Opiate Analgesics General Monograph

APPROVED INDICATIONS FOR PSYCHOLOGICAL DISORDERS

Adjunctive pharmacotherapy for the symptomatic management of:

- Pain Disorders: Acute Pain, Moderate to Severe
- Pain Disorders: Chronic Cancer Pain, Moderate to Severe

USUAL DOSAGE AND ADMINISTRATION

Acute Pain, Moderate to Severe, and Chronic Cancer Pain, Moderate to Severe

Adults: 30 to 60 mg intramuscularly or intravenously every three to four hours, as needed; *or* 50 to 100 mg orally every three to four hours, as needed

MAXIMUM: 360 mg daily intramuscularly or intravenously; *or* 600 mg daily orally

Women who are, or who may become, pregnant: FDA Pregnancy Category C. Safety and efficacy of pentazocine pharmacotherapy for women who are pregnant have not been established. Pentazocine crosses the placenta. Blood concentrations among neonates at delivery are equal to approximately 65% of maternal blood concentrations. Neonates born to women who have received pentazocine pharmacotherapy, or regularly used pentazocine, during pregnancy or near term may display expected pharmacologic actions (e.g., drowsiness, lethargy, respiratory depression). They also may display signs and symptoms of the neonatal opiate withdrawal syndrome (see Opiate Analgesics General Monograph). Avoid prescribing pentazocine pharmacotherapy to women who are pregnant. If pentazocine pharmacotherapy is required, advise patients of potential benefits and possible risk to themselves and the embryo, fetus, or neonate. Collaboration with the patient's obstetrician is indicated.

Women who are breast-feeding: Safety and efficacy of pentazocine pharmacotherapy for women who are breast-feeding and their neonates and infants have not been established. Avoid prescribing pentazocine pharmacotherapy to women who are breast-feeding. If pentazocine pharmacotherapy is required, breast-feeding probably should be discontinued. If desired, lactation may be maintained and breast-feeding resumed following the discontinuation of short-term pentazocine pharmacotherapy.

See Opiate Analgesics General Monograph

Elderly, frail, or debilitated patients and those who have liver dysfunction: Generally prescribe lower dosages of pentazocine for elderly, frail, or debilitated patients and those who have liver dysfunction. Increase the dosage gradually according to individual patient response. These patients may be more sensitive to the pharmacologic actions of pentazocine than are younger or healthier adult patients. Pentazocine pharmacotherapy may produce marked sedation among these patients. Avoid also injectable use among these patients because of the potential for serious CNS and respiratory depression.

Children younger than 12 years of age: Safety and efficacy of pentazocine pharmacotherapy for children younger than 12 years of age have not been established. Pentazocine pharmacotherapy is *not* recommended for this age group.

Notes, Acute Pain, Moderate to Severe, and Chronic Cancer Pain, Moderate to Severe

Note the differences in recommended dosages for oral and injectable pharmacotherapy. An oral dosage of pentazocine is about one-fourth to one-third as effective as an equal injectable dosage.

Multiple intramuscular injections of the pentazocine lactate injectable formulation have been associated with severe sclerosis of the skin, subcutaneous tissues, and underlying muscle at injection sites. When more than one injection is required, rotate injection sites carefully. When long-term pentazocine pharmacotherapy is required, replace injectable pharmacotherapy as soon as possible with oral pharmacotherapy. Avoid subcutaneous injection because of pentazocine's potential to seriously damage subcutaneous tissues.

AVAILABLE DOSAGE FORMS, STORAGE, AND COMPATIBILITY

Injectable, intramuscular and intravenous: 30 mg/ml
Tablets, oral: 50 mg (see Notes)

Notes

Injectable Pentazocine Formulations   Pentazocine injectable formulations are available in both single-unit dose ampules and cartridge-needle injection delivery systems (Carpuject®). Do *not* mix the injectable pentazocine in the same syringe with injectable formulations of barbiturates, chlordiazepoxide, or diazepam. A precipitate will form. The Carpuject® system contains sodium bisulfite, which may cause hypersensitivity reactions, including anaphylactic reactions, among susceptible patients. Although relatively uncommon, these reactions appear to occur with a higher incidence among patients who have asthma.

Oral Pentazocine Formulations The pentazocine oral tablet formulations are different for the United States and Canada. The Talwin Nx® tablets are available in the United States, whereas the Talwin® tablets are available in Canada.

TALWIN Nx® TABLETS.   In the United States, the oral pentazocine tablets have been formulated with 0.5 mg of naloxone, an opiate analgesic antagonist (i.e., Talwin Nx®). The naloxone was added to the pentazocine tablet formulation to prevent its illicit intravenous use as "poor man's heroin." The naloxone is poorly absorbed from the GI tract following oral ingestion (see the Naloxone Monograph) and, thus, has virtually no effect on the analgesic action of pentazocine. However, if the Talwin Nx® tablet is illicitly crushed, dissolved, and injected intravenously, the naloxone is immediately absorbed, blocking the desired action of the pentazocine.

TALWIN® TABLETS.   In Canada, Talwin® tablets contain sodium metabisulfite. Sulfites may cause hypersensitivity reactions, including anaphylactic reactions, among susceptible patients. Although relatively uncommon, these reactions appear to occur with a higher incidence among patients who have asthma. These tablets are used illicitly by intravenous drug users for their opiate agonist/antagonist actions. The Talwin® tablets do not contain naloxone.

General Instructions for Patients Instruct patients who are receiving pentazocine pharmacotherapy to

- safely store pentazocine tablets out of the reach of children in tightly closed light- and child-resistant containers at controlled room temperature (15° to 30°C; 59° to 86°F).
- obtain an available patient information sheet regarding pentazocine pharmacotherapy from their pharmacist at the time that their prescription is dispensed. Encourage patients to clarify any questions that they may have concerning pentazocine pharmacotherapy with their pharmacist or, if needed, to consult their prescribing psychologist.

PROPOSED MECHANISM OF ACTION

Pentazocine elicits its analgesic, CNS depressant, and respiratory depressant actions primarily by binding to the endorphin receptors in the CNS. However, its exact mechanism of action has not yet been fully determined.

See also Opiate Analgesics General Monograph

PHARMACOKINETICS/PHARMACODYNAMICS

The pharmacokinetics and pharmacodynamics of pentazocine depend upon its formulation for injectable or oral pharmacotherapy.

Injectable Formulations

Pentazocine's analgesic action occurs within three minutes after intravenous injection and within 30 minutes after intramuscular or subcutaneous injection. The duration of analgesia lasts for three to four hours. A dose of 30 mg by injection is approximately equal in analgesic action to 10 mg of morphine or 75 to 100 mg of meperidine (pethidine, Demerol®). Pentazocine weakly antagonizes the analgesic action of morphine and meperidine (pethidine, Demerol®). It also produces incomplete reversal of the cardiovascular, respiratory, and CNS depression induced by morphine and meperidine (pethidine, Demerol®). Pentazocine has approximately 1/50 the antagonistic action of naloxone. The respiratory depressant action of pentazocine is equal to, or less than, that observed after a single dose of other opiate analgesics. Pentazocine's respiratory depression appears to have a ceiling effect with repeated doses of 30 to 60 mg.

Oral Formulations

The analgesic action of 50 mg of orally ingested pentazocine is approximately equivalent to 60 mg of orally ingested codeine. Pentazocine is well absorbed following oral ingestion. However, only ~20% of the oral dose reaches the systemic circulation because of extensive first-pass hepatic metabolism. The onset of action following oral ingestion is within 30 minutes. Its duration of action is three hours or longer. The onset and duration of action are, in part, related to the dose ingested and the severity of the patient's pain. Peak blood concentrations of orally ingested pentazocine generally are achieved within 1 to 3 hours. Pentazocine is ~60% bound to plasma proteins. The half-life of elimination is approximately 2 to 3 hours, and the clearance is ~1.4 L/minute. The half-life of elimination may be significantly prolonged among patients who have liver dysfunction.

RELATIVE CONTRAINDICATIONS

Addiction and habituation to opiate analgesics, history of
Hypersensitivity to pentazocine
Opiate agonist analgesic pharmacotherapy (e.g., morphine pharmacotherapy), concurrent

CAUTIONS AND COMMENTS

Pentazocine is addicting and habituating. Long-term pentazocine pharmacotherapy, or regular personal use, may result in addiction and habituation. Pentazocine has mixed opiate agonist/antagonist analgesic actions. Thus, it also may cause signs and symptoms of the opiate withdrawal syndrome among patients who are receiving long-term opiate analgesic pharmacotherapy with pure opiate agonist analgesics (e.g., morphine). The tablet formulation of pentazocine (Talwin Nx®) contains both pentazocine and naloxone in an attempt to discourage the widespread illicit intravenous injection of pentazocine. Abrupt discontinuation after long-term pharmacotherapy, or regular personal use, may result in a reportedly mild form of the opiate analgesic withdrawal syndrome. Signs and symptoms of this withdrawal syndrome include abdominal cramps, anxiety, fever, restlessness, runny nose (rhinorrhea), and tears.

Although further study is needed, pentazocine reportedly does not generally produce addiction among patients who require long-term (300 days) pentazocine pharmacotherapy for the symptomatic management of chronic pain. Signs and symptoms of the opiate analgesic withdrawal syndrome were not observed among a sample of patients even upon abrupt discontinuation of pentazocine pharmacotherapy. However, a pentazocine withdrawal syndrome has been reported for a few patients after the discontinuation of regular long-term use. To avoid the possibility of precipitating the signs and symptoms of the opiate analgesic withdrawal syndrome, gradually reduce the dosage when discontinuing long-term pentazocine pharmacotherapy.

Prescribe pentazocine pharmacotherapy cautiously for patients who

- have acute inflammation of the gallbladder (cholecystitis) or pancreas (pancreatitis) or will be undergoing surgery of the biliary tract. Opiate analgesics generally increase biliary tract pressure. Although pentazocine reportedly may cause little or no elevation of biliary pressure, caution is advised.
- have head injuries, intracranial lesions, or other conditions associated with increased intracranial pressure. The respiratory depressant action associated with pentazocine and its potential for elevating cerebrospinal fluid pressure may markedly increase intracranial pressure among these patients. Pentazocine's analgesic and sedative actions also may obscure the clinical course of these patients.
- have histories of problematic patterns of opiate analgesic or other abusable psychotropic use. Prescribe for dispensing the least quantity of pentazocine feasible to help to avoid the development of problematic patterns of use, including unadvised patient increases in dosage or frequency of use. Pentazocine, a mixed agonist/antagonist opiate analgesic, has weak opiate antagonist action. Patients who are addicted to pure opiate agonist analgesics may experience signs and symptoms of the opiate analgesic withdrawal syndrome.
- have kidney dysfunction, including obstructive uropathy. Urinary retention rarely has been associated with pentazocine pharmacotherapy.
- have liver dysfunction. Serious liver dysfunction appears to predispose patients to a higher incidence of ADRs (e.g., anxiety; apprehension, marked; dizziness; drowsiness) even when usual recommended dosages of pentazocine are prescribed. These ADRs may be related to the accumulation of pentazocine, which is associated with its decreased metabolism by the liver.
- have respiratory depression, limited respiratory function (e.g., severely limited respiratory reserve, severe bronchial asthma, other obstructive respiratory conditions), or cyanosis. The respiratory depressant action of pentazocine may further compromise respiratory function among these patients.

Caution patients who are receiving pentazocine pharmacotherapy against performing activities that require alertness, judgment, and physical coordination (e.g., driving an automobile, operating dangerous equipment, supervising children) until their response to pentazocine pharmacotherapy is known. The CNS depressant action of pentazocine may affect these mental and physical functions.

In addition to this general precaution, caution patients to inform their prescribing psychologist if they begin or discontinue any other pharmacotherapy while receiving pentazocine pharmacotherapy.

CLINICALLY SIGNIFICANT DRUG INTERACTIONS

Concurrent pentazocine pharmacotherapy and the following may result in clinically significant drug interactions:

Alcohol Use

Concurrent alcohol use may increase the CNS depressant action of pentazocine. Advise patients to avoid, or limit, their use of alcohol while receiving pentazocine pharmacotherapy.

Pharmacotherapy With Central Nervous System Depressants and Other Drugs That Produce Central Nervous System Depression

Concurrent pentazocine pharmacotherapy with other opiate analgesics, sedative-hypnotics, or other drugs that produce CNS depression (e.g., antihistamines, phenothiazines, TCAs) may result in additive CNS depression.

Tobacco Smoking

Concurrent tobacco smoking may increase the metabolism of pentazocine. Higher dosages of pentazocine may be required for patients who smoke tobacco.

See also Opiate Analgesics General Monograph

ADVERSE DRUG REACTIONS

Acute onset of confusion, disorientation, and hallucinations (usually visual) has been reported among patients who were receiving recommended dosages of pentazocine. These ADRs usually resolve spontaneously within hours of the discontinuation of pentazocine pharmacotherapy. The cause of these ADRs is unknown. Cautiously resume pentazocine pharmacotherapy for these patients, and monitor for the recurrence of these ADRs carefully. If these ADRs recur, discontinue pentazocine pharmacotherapy. Further pentazocine pharmacotherapy is not advised.

Oral pentazocine pharmacotherapy commonly has been associated with nausea, sedation, somnolence, vertigo, and vomiting. Sedation may be more marked among elderly, frail, or debilitated patients. Injectable pentazocine pharmacotherapy commonly has been associated with dizziness, euphoria, light-headedness, nausea, stinging upon injection, and vomiting. Ulceration (sloughing) and severe sclerosis of the skin and subcutaneous tissues, and, rarely, underlying muscles have been reported with repeated multiple injections at one site. Avoid prescribing injectable pharmacotherapy whenever possible. If injections are required, carefully rotate injection sites. In addition to these ADRs, pentazocine pharmacotherapy has been associated with the following ADRs, listed according to body system:

Cardiovascular: circulatory depression and shock, hypertension, syncope (fainting), and tachycardia

CNS: confusion, depression, disorientation, disturbed dreams, excitement, hallucinations, headache, insomnia, irritability, and sedation

Cutaneous: dermatitis, including severe itching (pruritus); edema of the face; flushed skin, including congestion and distention of blood vessels (plethora); nodules and soft tissue induration or cutaneous depression at injection sites; and toxic epidermal necrolysis

GI: constipation, cramps, diarrhea, dry mouth, and taste alteration

Hematologic: depression of white blood cells, particularly granulocytes (reversible), and eosinophilia (moderate, transient)

Musculoskeletal: weakness, and, rarely, tremor

Ocular: abnormal contraction of the pupils (miosis); blurred vision; constant, involuntary cyclical movement of the eyeballs (nystagmus); double vision (diplopia); and difficulty focusing

Otic: ringing in the ears (tinnitus)

Miscellaneous: chills

See also Opiate Analgesics General Monograph

OVERDOSAGE

Signs and symptoms of pentazocine overdosage are similar to the signs and symptoms associated with other opiate analgesic overdosage (see Opiate Analgesics General Monograph). However, pentazocine does not appear to produce the severe respiratory depression usually associated with opiate agonist overdosage. Regardless, pentazocine overdosage requires emergency symptomatic medical support of body systems with attention to increasing pentazocine elimination. Naloxone (Narcan®) is the specific and effective antagonist for the respiratory depression associated with pentazocine overdosage.

PENTOBARBITAL

(pen toe bar'bi tal)

TRADE NAMES

Nembutal®
Nova Rectal®
Novo-Pentobarb®

CLASSIFICATION

Sedative-Hypnotic (Barbiturate) (C-II, C-III)

See also Barbiturates General Monograph

APPROVED INDICATIONS FOR PSYCHOLOGICAL DISORDERS

Adjunctive pharmacotherapy for the short-term symptomatic management of:

- Anxiety Disorders. Pentobarbital pharmacotherapy is *not* indicated for the management of everyday anxiety or tension, or anxiety that can be managed with psychotherapy alone. Pentobarbital also is *not* recommended for the management of anxiety associated with depression because it has the potential to exacerbate the depression while alleviating the anxiety. The depression associated with anxiety generally resolves with appropriate adjunctive pharmacotherapy (i.e., antidepressant pharmacotherapy) and psychotherapy.
- Sleep Disorders: Insomnia

USUAL DOSAGE AND ADMINISTRATION

Anxiety Disorders

Although approved for the symptomatic management of acute anxiety, the barbiturates, including pentobarbital, generally have been replaced by the benzodiazepines for this indication because of their greater efficacy and lower toxicity (i.e., better ADR profile and significantly lower rates of morbidity and mortality with overdosage) (see Benzodiazepines General Monograph). For patients who are hypersensitive to the benzodiazepines, or when benzodiazepine pharmacotherapy is contraindicated for any other reason, mephobarbital pharmacotherapy is the barbiturate recommended for the symptomatic management of acute anxiety (see Mephobarbital Monograph).

Insomnia

Adults: 100 to 200 mg daily intramuscularly, orally, or rectally 30 minutes before retiring for bed in the evening. For most patients this dosage range usually induces sedation, followed by sleep.

Women who are, or who may become, pregnant: FDA Pregnancy Category D. Safety and efficacy of pentobarbital pharmacotherapy for women who are pregnant have not been established with regard to teratogenic effects. Pentobarbital pharmacotherapy near term may result in respiratory depression among neonates and signs and symptoms of the neonatal barbiturate withdrawal syndrome (see Barbiturates General Monograph). Avoid prescribing pentobarbital pharmacotherapy to women who are pregnant. If pentobarbital pharmacotherapy is required, advise patients of potential benefits and possible risks to themselves and the embryo, fetus, or neonate. Collaboration with the patient's obstetrician is indicated.

Women who are breast-feeding: Safety and efficacy of pentobarbital pharmacotherapy for women who are breast-feeding and their neonates and infants have not been established. Pentobarbital is excreted in breast milk. Breast-fed neonates and infants may display expected pharmacologic actions (e.g., drowsiness). They also may become addicted (see Barbiturates General Monograph). Avoid prescribing pentobarbital pharmacotherapy to women who are breast-feeding. If pentobarbital pharmacotherapy is required, breast-feeding probably should be discontinued. If desired, lactation may be maintained and breast-feeding resumed following the discontinuation of short-term pentobarbital pharmacotherapy. Collaboration with the patient's pediatrician is required.

Elderly, frail, or debilitated patients and those who have kidney dysfunction: Generally prescribe lower dosages for elderly, frail, and debilitated patients or those who have kidney dysfunction. Increase the dosage gradually, if needed, according to individual patient response. These patients may be more sensitive to the pharmacologic actions of pentobarbital than are younger or healthier adult patients.

Children: 30 to 120 mg daily orally or rectally 30 minutes before bedtime

Notes, Insomnia

Intramuscular, oral, and rectal pentobarbital pharmacotherapy may be prescribed according to individual patient needs. Intramuscular pharmacotherapy provides a precise dosage and a rapid onset of hypnotic action. It may be prescribed when other methods of administration are impractical. Intravenous pharmacotherapy generally is not recommended because of associated risks to respiratory function. Rectal suppositories provide mild sedation and sleep when oral pharmacotherapy is not feasible. Prescribe the correct dosage of the rectal suppository. Do not cut (e.g., halve or quarter) suppositories in an attempt to obtain desired dosages.

Intramuscular Pentobarbital Pharmacotherapy   For adults, do not inject more than 5 ml per healthy intramuscular injection site. Inject deeply into a healthy muscle site to minimize tissue irritation and associated tissue necrosis. Monitor patients for at least 20 to 30 minutes following intramuscular injection. Excessive hypnosis has been associated with intramuscular pentobarbital pharmacotherapy.

Intravenous Pentobarbital Pharmacotherapy   Intravenous pentobarbital pharmacotherapy is *not* recommended for the symptomatic management of insomnia because of the associated danger of respiratory arrest and laryngospasm. In addition, this indication does not usually require immediate pharmacologic action. Pentobarbital is a potent CNS depressant. Too rapid injection may result in fatal circulatory and respiratory depression. Emergency respiratory supportive equipment and medical personnel must be immediately available for patients who require intravenous pentobarbital pharmacotherapy.

AVAILABLE DOSAGE FORMS, STORAGE, AND COMPATIBILITY

Capsules, oral: 30, 50, 100 mg
Elixir, oral: 18.2 mg/5 ml (contains 18% alcohol)
Injectables, intramuscular, intravenous: 50, 125, 300 mg/ml (contains 10% alcohol)
Suppositories, rectal: 15, 25, 30, 50, 60, 100, 120, 200 mg
Tablets, oral: 30 mg

Notes

Injectable Formulations   Inspect pentobarbital injectable formulations carefully prior to use. Discard cloudy or discolored injectable solutions appropriately.

Oral Formulations   The pentobarbital oral capsules may contain tartrazine (FD&C Yellow No. 5). Tartrazine has been associated with hypersensitivity reactions (e.g., bronchial asthma) among susceptible patients, particularly those who are hypersensitive to aspirin.

General Instructions for Patients   Instruct patients who are receiving pentobarbital pharmacotherapy to

- safely store pentobarbital oral dosage forms out of the reach of children in tightly closed child-resistant containers at room temperature below 30°C (86°F).

- safely store pentobarbital rectal suppositories under refrigeration (2° to 8°C; 36° to 46°F) and out of the reach of children.
- obtain an available patient information sheet regarding pentobarbital pharmacotherapy from their pharmacist at the time that their prescription is dispensed. Encourage patients to clarify any questions that they may have concerning pentobarbital pharmacotherapy with their pharmacist or, if needed, to consult their prescribing psychologist.

PROPOSED MECHANISM OF ACTION

Pentobarbital is a short-acting barbiturate with sedative-hypnotic action. The exact mechanism of pentobarbital's sedative-hypnotic action has not yet been fully determined. Pentobarbital appears to act primarily at the level of the thalamus, where it interferes with impulse transmission to the cortex.

See also Barbiturates General Monograph

PHARMACOKINETICS/PHARMACODYNAMICS

Pentobarbital is rapidly and completely absorbed following oral or rectal administration and generally has an onset of action within 15 to 30 minutes. Pentobarbital is ~40% plasma protein-bound. It is extensively metabolized in the liver, with less than 5% excreted in unchanged form in the urine. Changes in the volume of urine flow or pH do not significantly affect urinary excretion of pentobarbital. The half-life of elimination ranges from 15 to 50 hours and appears to be dose dependent. Additional data are unavailable.

RELATIVE CONTRAINDICATIONS

Hypersensitivity to pentobarbital or other barbiturates
Liver dysfunction, severe
Porphyria, active or latent
Respiratory depression, severe

CAUTIONS AND COMMENTS

Pentobarbital, once a popular street drug, has been commonly known as "yellows" or "yellow jackets." Long-term pentobarbital pharmacotherapy, or regular personal use, may result in addiction and habituation. Addiction and habituation also have been associated with therapeutic dosages. Abrupt discontinuation of long-term pentobarbital pharmacotherapy, or regular personal use, may result in the barbiturate withdrawal syndrome. Signs and symptoms of this withdrawal syndrome include delirium and convulsions, which may culminate in death. Thus, the barbiturate withdrawal syndrome is a medical emergency that may be fatal if not appropriately treated. Avoid abruptly discontinuing pentobarbital pharmacotherapy, particularly among patients who have received long-term high-dosage pharmacotherapy or have personally regularly used pentobarbital.

Prescribe pentobarbital pharmacotherapy cautiously to patients who

- are in shock, have severe liver dysfunction, have uremia, or are receiving pharmacotherapy with other drugs that produce respiratory depression (e.g., opiate analgesics). These patients may experience a prolonged or intensified hypnotic effect.

- are receiving oral anticoagulant pharmacotherapy. Concurrent pentobarbital pharmacotherapy makes it difficult to stabilize prothrombin times for these patients.
- have histories of problematic patterns of alcohol or other abusable psychotropic use. These patients may be at risk for developing problematic patterns of pentobarbital use.
- have nocturnal confusion or restlessness associated with sedative-hypnotic pharmacotherapy. Pentobarbital pharmacotherapy also may cause these reactions among these patients. Elderly, frail, or debilitated patients may be especially susceptible.
- have pain disorders that are inadequately managed. Pentobarbital pharmacotherapy may produce delirium among these patients.
- have respiratory dysfunction, particularly status asthmaticus. Pentobarbital pharmacotherapy may exacerbate respiratory dysfunction.

Caution patients who are receiving pentobarbital pharmacotherapy against performing activities that require alertness, judgment, and physical coordination (e.g., driving an automobile, operating dangerous equipment, supervising children) until their response to pentobarbital pharmacotherapy is known. Pentobarbital may adversely affect these mental and physical functions.

In addition to this general precaution, caution patients to inform their prescribing psychologist if they begin or discontinue any other pharmacotherapy while receiving pentobarbital pharmacotherapy.

CLINICALLY SIGNIFICANT DRUG INTERACTIONS

Concurrent pentobarbital pharmacotherapy and the following may result in clinically significant drug interactions:

Alcohol Use

Concurrent alcohol use may increase the CNS depressant action of pentobarbital. Advise patients to avoid, or limit, their use of alcohol while receiving pentobarbital pharmacotherapy.

Pharmacotherapy With Central Nervous System Depressants and Other Drugs That Produce Central Nervous System Depression

Concurrent pentobarbital pharmacotherapy with opiate analgesics, other sedative-hypnotics, and other drugs that produce CNS depression (e.g., antihistamines, phenothiazines, TCAs) may result in additive CNS depression.

Pharmacotherapy With Drugs That Are Metabolized by the Liver

Pentobarbital may stimulate the production of hepatic microsomal enzymes, which are responsible for the metabolism of many different classes of drugs (e.g., corticosteroids, oral anticoagulants, oral contraceptives, quinidine [Biquin®]). Whenever pentobarbital is prescribed or discontinued, attention must be given to the effect on the patient's overall pharmacotherapy. Collaboration with other prescribers is required.

See also Barbiturates General Monograph

ADVERSE DRUG REACTIONS

Pentobarbital pharmacotherapy has been associated with the following ADRs, listed according to body system:

Cardiovascular: circulatory collapse and low blood pressure (hypotension)

CNS: CNS depression, severe; paradoxical excitement; and residual sedation ("hangover effect"). The residual sedation is thought to be associated with pentobarbital's suppression of REM sleep.

Cutaneous: pain at the injection site

GI: hiccuping, nausea, and vomiting

Musculoskeletal: pain at the injection site following intramuscular injection

Respiratory: bronchial spasm, chest-wall spasm, coughing, and temporary cessation of breathing (apnea). Spasm of the laryngeal muscles (laryngospasm) and respiratory depression have been associated with higher oral dosages or rapid intravenous injection.

See also Barbiturates General Monograph

OVERDOSAGE

Signs and symptoms of pentobarbital overdosage include coma, hypothermia (early), fever (late), sluggish or absent reflexes, respiratory depression, gradual circulatory collapse, and pulmonary edema. Pentobarbital overdosage requires emergency symptomatic medical support of body systems with attention to increasing pentobarbital elimination. There is no known antidote.

PERICYAZINE * [Propericyazine]

(per ee si'a zeen)

TRADE NAME

Neuleptil®

CLASSIFICATION

Antipsychotic (phenothiazine, piperidine derivative)

See also Phenothiazines General Monograph

APPROVED INDICATIONS FOR PSYCHOLOGICAL DISORDERS

Adjunctive pharmacotherapy for the symptomatic management of:

Psychotic Disorders, Particularly Those Associated With Aggressiveness, Hostility, and Impulsiveness

USUAL DOSAGE AND ADMINISTRATION

Psychotic Disorders, Particularly Those Associated With Aggressiveness, Hostility, and Impulsiveness

Adults: Initially, 15 to 60 mg daily orally. Prescribe the daily oral dosage in two divided doses, 5 to 20 mg orally in the morning and 10 to 40 mg orally in the evening.

MAINTENANCE: Prescribe the lowest effective dosage. This dosage is usually half the initial daily dosage. A maintenance dosage exceeding 30 mg daily is rarely needed.

Women who are, or who may become, pregnant: FDA Pregnancy Category "not established." Safety and efficacy of pericyazine pharmacotherapy for women who are pregnant have not been established (see Phenothiazines General Monograph). Avoid prescribing pericyazine pharmacotherapy to women who are pregnant. If pericyazine pharmacotherapy is required, advise patients of potential benefits and possible risks to themselves and the embryo, fetus, or neonate. Collaboration with the patient's obstetrician is indicated.

Women who are breast-feeding: Safety and efficacy of pericyazine pharmacotherapy for women who are breast-feeding and their neonates and infants have not been established (see Phenothiazines General Monograph). Avoid prescribing pericyazine pharmacotherapy to women who are breast-feeding. If pericyazine pharmacotherapy is required, breast-feeding probably should be discontinued. Collaboration with the patient's pediatrician is required.

Elderly, frail, and debilitated patients: Initially, 5 mg daily orally in two divided doses. Increase the dosage gradually, as needed, according to individual patient response. Generally prescribe lower dosages for elderly, frail, or debilitated patients. These patients may be more sensitive to the pharmacologic actions of pericyazine than are younger or healthier adult patients.

Children younger than 5 years of age: Safety and efficacy of pericyazine pharmacotherapy for children younger than 5 years of age have not been established. Pericyazine pharmacotherapy is *not* recommended for this age group.

Children 5 years of age and older: Initially, 7.5 to 40 mg daily orally. Prescribe the daily oral dosage in two divided doses, 2.5 to 10 mg orally in the morning and 5 to 30 mg orally in the evening. Adjust dosage according to individual patient response.

AVAILABLE DOSAGE FORMS, STORAGE, AND COMPATIBILITY

Capsules, oral: 5, 10, 20 mg
Drops, oral (with calibrated dropper): 10 mg/ml (contains 12% alcohol)

Notes

General Instructions for Patients Instruct patients who are receiving pericyazine pharmacotherapy to

- measure each dose of the pericyazine oral drops with the calibrated dropper supplied with the product to assure an accurate dose is measured.
- safely store pericyazine oral formulations out of the reach of children in child-resistant containers at room temperature below 30°C (86°F).
- obtain an available patient information sheet regarding pericyazine pharmacotherapy from their pharmacist at the time that their prescription is dispensed. Encourage patients to clarify any questions that they may have concerning pericyazine pharmacotherapy with their pharmacist or, if needed, to consult their prescribing psychologist.

PROPOSED MECHANISM OF ACTION

Pericyazine is a piperidine phenothiazine related to thioridazine. It reduces pathologic arousal and affective tension among selected patients who have psychotic disorders. In so doing, it affects normal mental integration minimally. A sedative phenothiazine with weak antipsychotic properties, pericyazine also has adrenolytic, anticholinergic, endocrine, extrapyramidal, and metabolic actions. Like other phenothiazines, pericyazine is thought to act primarily in the subcortical areas, where it produces a central adrenergic blockade.

See also Phenothiazines General Monograph

PHARMACOKINETICS/PHARMACODYNAMICS

Peak blood concentrations are generally obtained within 2 hours following oral ingestion. The mean half-life of elimination is approximately 12 hours. Additional data are unavailable.

RELATIVE CONTRAINDICATIONS

Anesthetic pharmacotherapy, regional or spinal
Blood disorders
Circulatory collapse
Coma, particularly that associated with the use of CNS depressants
Liver dysfunction
Hypersensitivity to pericyazine or other phenothiazines

CAUTIONS AND COMMENTS

Prescribe pericyazine pharmacotherapy cautiously to patients who

- are receiving pharmacotherapy with anticholinergics (e.g., atropine) or other drugs that produce anticholinergic actions (e.g., TCAs). Pharmacotherapy with one or more drugs that have anticholinergic actions has been associated with paralytic ileus. Elderly, frail, or debilitated patients, particularly those who are receiving long-term pharmacotherapy, are at particular risk. Plan to maintain normal bowel function, and monitor these patients carefully for constipation, an early sign of paralytic ileus. Collaboration with the patient's advanced practice nurse, family physician, or a specialist (e.g., gerontologist) may be required.

- are receiving pharmacotherapy with antihistamines, barbiturates, opiate analgesics, or other drugs that depress the CNS. The usual dosages of these drugs probably should be reduced by at least one-half while pericyazine pharmacotherapy is initiated gradually.
- have glaucoma or prostatic hypertrophy. Pericyazine's anticholinergic actions may exacerbate these medical disorders.
- have histories of seizure disorders and who are not receiving appropriate anticonvulsant pharmacotherapy. Pericyazine generally is well tolerated by patients who are receiving appropriate anticonvulsant pharmacotherapy for the symptomatic management of seizure disorders, including epilepsy. However, epileptic seizures have been associated with pericyazine pharmacotherapy. It has not been established whether pericyazine pharmacotherapy effectively controls arousal or affective tension among these patients.
- regularly drink alcohol. Caution patients to avoid, or limit, their use of alcohol during pericyazine pharmacotherapy (see Clinically Significant Drug Interactions).

Caution patients who are receiving pericyazine pharmacotherapy against performing activities that require alertness, judgment, and physical coordination (e.g., driving an automobile, operating dangerous equipment, supervising children) until their response to pericyazine is known.

In addition to this general precaution, caution patients to inform their prescribing psychologist if they begin or discontinue any other pharmacotherapy while receiving pericyazine pharmacotherapy.

CLINICALLY SIGNIFICANT DRUG INTERACTIONS

Concurrent pericyazine pharmacotherapy and the following may result in clinically significant drug interactions:

Alcohol Use

Concurrent alcohol use may increase the CNS depressant action of pericyazine. Advise patients to avoid, or limit, their use of alcohol while receiving pericyazine pharmacotherapy.

Pharmacotherapy With Central Nervous System Depressants and Other Drugs That Produce Central Nervous System Depression

Concurrent pericyazine pharmacotherapy with opiate analgesics, sedative-hypnotics, or other drugs that produce CNS depression (e.g., antihistamines, TCAs) may result in additive CNS depression.

See also Phenothiazines General Monograph

ADVERSE DRUG REACTIONS

The ADRs associated with phenothiazine pharmacotherapy vary in type, frequency, and cause (e.g., some are dose-related, while others involve individual patient susceptibility). Some ADRs may be more likely to occur, or occur with a greater intensity, among patients who have concurrent medical disorders. For example, patients who have mitral insufficiency or pheochromocytoma (i.e., a tumor of the sympathoadrenal system that produces the catecholamines epinephrine and norepinephrine) have experienced severe hypertension and other ADRs when prescribed recommended dosages of certain phenothiazines. While all phenothiazine-related ADRs may not occur with pericyazine pharmacotherapy, prescribing psychologists should monitor patients for these ADRs because of pericyazine's chemical and pharmacological similarity to the other phenothiazines (see also Phenothiazines General Monograph).

Pericyazine pharmacotherapy commonly has been associated with drowsiness, EPRs, and hypotension. Anticholinergic and psychomotor ADRs usually occur initially during pericyazine pharmacotherapy. These ADRs generally remit with continued pharmacotherapy or with a reduction in dosage. EPRs usually occur later during pericyazine pharmacotherapy. These ADRs generally are associated with higher dosages. Pericyazine pharmacotherapy also has been associated with a voracious appetite and weight gain. Other ADRs reflect its anticholinergic and other actions. These include the following ADRs, listed according to body system:

Cardiovascular: rapid heart beat (tachycardia)

CNS: dystonic reactions, feeling of restlessness or an inability to sit down (akathisia), and Parkinsonism. These ADRs usually can be managed by reducing the dosage or by temporarily withholding pericyazine pharmacotherapy. The dystonic reactions usually include contraction of the muscles of the neck and face, hyperextension of the neck and trunk, myelonic twitches, oculogyric crisis, protrusion of the tongue, and spasms of the hands and feet. The dystonic reactions associated with pericyazine pharmacotherapy usually are not dose-related. They may be quite dramatic and may require immediate attention. Parkinsonism may occur more commonly among patients who are receiving higher dosages of pericyazine. Concurrent anti-parkinsonian pharmacotherapy may be required for some patients.

Cutaneous: sweating (excessive)

GI: constipation, diarrhea, dry mouth, fecal impaction, paralytic ileus, and vomiting

Musculoskeletal: see CNS

Ocular: aggravation of glaucoma and blurred vision

Respiratory: nasal congestion

See also Phenothiazines General Monograph

OVERDOSAGE

Signs and symptoms of pericyazine overdosage resemble those associated with other phenothiazine overdosage and include agitation, confusion, delirium, lethargy, and coma. Twitching, dystonic movements, or seizures may occur with hypotension, cardiovascular collapse, dysrhythmias, and hypothermia. Pericyazine overdosage requires emergency symptomatic medical support of body systems with attention to increasing pericyazine elimination. There is no known antidote.

PERPHENAZINE

(per fen'a zeen)

TRADE NAMES

Phenazine®
Trilafon®

CLASSIFICATION

Antipsychotic (phenothiazine)

See also Phenothiazines General Monograph

APPROVED INDICATIONS FOR PSYCHOLOGICAL DISORDERS

Adjunctive pharmacotherapy for the symptomatic management of:

Psychotic Disorders: Schizophrenia and Other Psychotic Disorders

USUAL DOSAGE AND ADMINISTRATION

Schizophrenia and Other Psychotic Disorders

Adults: Generally, 12 to 24 mg daily orally in three divided doses; *or* 1 to 10 mg intramuscularly, repeated in 6 hours, if needed. Dosage is determined by the dosage form, the severity of the signs and symptoms of the psychotic disorder, and individual patient response (see Notes, Schizophrenia and Other Psychotic Disorders).

MAXIMUM: 15 mg daily intramuscularly or 24 mg daily orally for non-hospitalized patients; and 30 mg daily intramuscularly or 64 mg daily orally for hospitalized patients

Women who are, or who may become, pregnant: FDA Pregnancy Category C. Safety and efficacy of perphenazine pharmacotherapy for women who are pregnant have not been established. Perphenazine and other phenothiazine pharmacotherapy has been associated with a neonatal extrapyramidal-related syndrome. The signs and symptoms of this syndrome include hypertonus, poor sucking, and weakness among neonates (see Phenothiazines General Monograph). Avoid prescribing perphenazine pharmacotherapy to women who are pregnant. If perphenazine pharmacotherapy is required, advise patients (or their legal guardians in regard to the patient) of the potential benefits and possible risks to themselves and the embryo, fetus, or neonate. Collaboration with the patient's obstetrician is required.

Women who are breast-feeding: Safety and efficacy of perphenazine pharmacotherapy for women who are breast-feeding and their neonates and infants have not been established. Perphenazine is rapidly excreted in breast milk and may cause unwanted effects among breast-fed neonates and infants (see Phenothiazines General Monograph). Avoid prescribing perphenazine pharmacotherapy to women who are breast-feeding. If perphenazine pharmacotherapy is required, breast-feeding should be discontinued. Collaboration with the patient's pediatrician is indicated.

Elderly, frail, or debilitated patients: Generally prescribe lower dosages of perphenazine for elderly, frail, or debilitated patients. Increase the dosage gradually, as needed, according to individual patient response. These patients may be more sensitive to perphenazine's pharmacologic actions than are younger or healthier adult patients.

Children younger than 12 years of age: Safety and efficacy of perphenazine pharmacotherapy for children younger than 12 years of age have not been established. Perphenazine pharmacotherapy is *not* recommended for this age group.

Children and adolescents 12 years of age and older: Initially prescribe the lower range of the recommended adult dosage. Increase the dosage gradually, as needed, according to individual patient response.

Notes, Schizophrenia and Other Psychotic Disorders

Initially select the dosage form and daily dosage according to the severity of the patient's signs and symptoms of psychosis. Adjust the dosage gradually according to individual patient response. The lowest effective dosage should be prescribed. EPRs increase in frequency and severity with higher dosages. These reactions generally remit upon a reduction of dosage, upon discontinuation of perphenazine pharmacotherapy, or with concurrent anti-parkinsonian pharmacotherapy. When maximal therapeutic benefit has been achieved, decrease the dosage gradually to the lowest effective maintenance dosage. Hospitalization with continued monitoring is usually recommended for patients who require long-term perphenazine pharmacotherapy exceeding 24 mg daily orally.

Injectable Perphenazine Pharmacotherapy

INTRAMUSCULAR PHARMACOTHERAPY   Initially, 5 mg intramuscularly every six hours, as needed. For severe signs and symptoms, some patients may initially require 10 mg intramuscularly. Inject perphenazine deeply into healthy muscle sites while the patient is seated or lying down. The injectable formulation is associated with more rapid and greater pharmacologic action than the oral formulations. Infrequent and transient dizziness and significant hypotension rarely have occurred with intramuscular injection. Monitor patients for a short time after the injection for the possible occurrence of these ADRs. Therapeutic response usually occurs within 10 minutes and is maximal by 2 hours. The duration of action ranges from 12 to 24 hours.

Replace perphenazine injectable pharmacotherapy with oral pharmacotherapy as soon as possible, usually within 24 to 48 hours. Prescribe equal or higher oral dosages when replacing intramuscular pharmacotherapy. Once the desired therapeutic response is achieved, reduce the dosage gradually to the minimum effective oral maintenance dosage. Patients who have acute signs and symptoms often respond well to a single injection. Those who have chronic signs and symptoms may require several injections before the injectable pharmacotherapy can be replaced with oral pharmacotherapy. Some patients may require injectable pharmacotherapy for several months.

INTRAVENOUS PHARMACOTHERAPY   Do *not* prescribe intravenous perphenazine pharmacotherapy for the symptomatic management of psychotic disorders. Although perphenazine may be injected intravenously, intravenous pharmacotherapy is generally not recommended except to counteract retching or hiccups among patients during surgery. Intravenous pharmacotherapy is *not* recommended for children.

Oral Perphenazine Pharmacotherapy

ORAL TABLETS   Moderately disturbed non-hospitalized patients may initially require 12 to 24 mg daily orally in three divided doses. Reduce the dosage as soon as possible to the minimum effective dosage. Some patients require, rarely, dosages of up to 32 mg daily. Severely disturbed hospitalized patients, or those who have clinically resistant disorders, may require higher dosages initially. Adjust dosage to the lowest effective dosage. Extrapyramidal reactions increase in frequency and severity with higher dosages.

ORAL CONCENTRATE   16 to 64 mg daily orally in two to four divided doses according to severity of signs and symptoms of the psychotic disorder and individual patient response. A total daily dosage exceeding 64 mg is not usually required.

Shake the oral concentrate well before measuring each dose. Prior to administration, dilute the concentrate with water, saline, Seven-Up®, homogenized milk, carbonated orange drink, or pineapple, prune, apricot, orange, grapefruit, V-8®, or tomato juice. The suggested ratio for dilution is 60 ml of water or a compatible beverage for each 5 ml of oral concentrate. Do *not* dilute the concentrate with beverages containing caffeine, such as coffee and cola drinks; tannics, such as tea; or pectinates, such as apple juice because of physical incompatibility.

AVAILABLE DOSAGE FORMS, STORAGE, AND COMPATIBILITY

Concentrated solution, oral: 16 mg/5 ml (raspberry odor, contains 0.1% alcohol)
Injectable, intramuscular or intravenous: 5 mg/ml
Suppositories, rectal: 2, 4, 8 mg (generally used for the medical management of severe nausea and vomiting)
Syrup, oral: 2 mg/5 ml (lemon flavored, contains alcohol)
Tablets, oral: 2, 4, 8, 16 mg

Notes

Injectable Formulation   The perphenazine injectable formulation (i.e., Tilafon®) contains sodium bisulfite as a preservative. Sulfites have been associated with hypersensitivity reactions. These reactions include anaphylaxis and life-threatening, or less severe, asthmatic reactions among susceptible patients. Although relatively uncommon, these reactions appear to occur with a higher incidence among patients who have asthma.

Intravenous perphenazine pharmacotherapy rarely is prescribed. When prescribed, it is generally only for the medical management of severe nausea and vomiting among adults.

Oral Formulations   When preparing oral formulations for administration, avoid getting the oral solution on the skin, clothes, or in the eyes because of associated contact dermatitis. To increase palatability, dilute each 5 ml of the oral concentrate with 60 ml of carbonated beverage, fruit juice (e.g., apricot, grapefruit, orange, pineapple, or prune), tomato juice, milk, Seven-Up®, or water immediately before administration. Do *not* dilute the oral concentrate with apple juice, black coffee, cola drinks, grape juice, or tea because a color change or precipitation may occur.

General Instructions for Patients   Instruct patients who are receiving perphenazine pharmacotherapy to

- swallow whole each dose of the perphenazine oral tablets without breaking, chewing, or crushing. Also instruct them to ingest each dose of the oral tablets with adequate liquid chaser (e.g., 60 to 120 ml of water).

- avoid ingesting perphenazine oral tablets with antacids or antidiarrheals. If antacids or antidiarrheals are required, advise patients to ingest each dose of these drugs one hour before or one hour after ingesting the perphenazine dose.
- shake the perphenazine oral concentrate well before measuring each dose to assure an accurate dose is measured.
- dilute each 5 ml of the perphenazine oral concentrate with 60 ml of carbonated beverage, fruit juice (e.g., apricot, grapefruit, orange, pineapple, or prune), tomato juice, milk, Seven-Up®, or water immediately before ingestion in order to increase palatability. Advise patients not to dilute their doses with apple juice, black coffee, cola drinks, grape juice, or tea because a color change or precipitation may occur.
- avoid getting the perphenazine oral solution on the skin, clothes, or in the eyes because of associated contact dermatitis.
- safely store perphenazine oral formulations out of the reach of children in tightly closed child- and light-resistant containers (2° to 25°C; 36° to 77°F).
- obtain an available patient information sheet regarding perphenazine pharmacotherapy from their pharmacist at the time that their prescription is dispensed. Encourage patients to clarify any questions that they may have concerning perphenazine pharmacotherapy with their pharmacist or, if needed, to consult their prescribing psychologist.

PROPOSED MECHANISM OF ACTION

The exact mechanism of action of perphenazine is complex and has not yet been fully determined. Its antipsychotic activity appears to be primarily related to an interaction with dopamine-containing neurons, specifically the blockade of dopamine receptors both pre- and post-synaptically. Perphenazine also has antiemetic actions. It appears to inhibit vomiting primarily by directly affecting the medullary CTZ.

See also Phenothiazines General Monograph

PHARMACOKINETICS/PHARMACODYNAMICS

Data are unavailable

RELATIVE CONTRAINDICATIONS

Alcohol use, excessive or concurrent
Blood disorders
Bone marrow depression
Cardiac dysfunction, severe
Coma
Hypersensitivity to perphenazine or other phenothiazines
Liver dysfunction, severe
Parkinson's disease
Pharmacotherapy with drugs that produce CNS depression (e.g., antihistamines, opiate analgesics, sedative-hypnotics, TCAs), concurrent
Subcortical brain injury, with or without hypothalamic damage, suspected or established. A hyperthermic reaction with an elevated body temperature in excess of 40°C (104°F) may occur up to 16 hours following the administration of perphenazine to these patients.

CAUTIONS AND COMMENTS

Prescribe perphenazine pharmacotherapy cautiously to patients who

- have depression
- have histories of seizure disorders. Perphenazine can lower the seizure threshold. Patients who are receiving anticonvulsant pharmacotherapy may require an increase in the dosage of the anticonvulsant when concurrent perphenazine pharmacotherapy is prescribed. Collaboration with the prescriber of the anticonvulsant is required.

CLINICALLY SIGNIFICANT DRUG INTERACTIONS

Concurrent perphenazine pharmacotherapy and the following may result in clinically significant drug interactions:

Paroxetine Pharmacotherapy

Paroxetine (Paxil®) is an inhibitor of cytochrome P450 isoenzyme 2D6 (i.e., CYP2D6). Concurrent perphenazine and paroxetine pharmacotherapy may result in a severalfold (range 2- to 13-fold) increase in perphenazine blood concentrations and associated ADRs and toxicity. Avoid prescribing concurrent perphenazine and paroxetine pharmacotherapy. If perphenazine pharmacotherapy is required among patients who are receiving paroxetine pharmacotherapy, initiate the perphenazine pharmacotherapy with a lower dosage. If paroxetine pharmacotherapy is prescribed to patients who are already receiving perphenazine pharmacotherapy, reduce the dosage of the perphenazine. Monitor these patients carefully, and further adjust the perphenazine dosage according to individual patient response.

Guanethidine Pharmacotherapy

Perphenazine may decrease the neuronal uptake of guanethidine (Ismelin®) and, thus, decrease its antihypertensive action.

Pharmacotherapy With Anticholinergics and Other Drugs That Produce Anticholinergic Actions

Concurrent perphenazine pharmacotherapy with anticholinergics (e.g., atropine) or other drugs that produce anticholinergic actions (e.g., TCAs) may result in additive anticholinergic actions (see Adverse Drug Reactions).

See also Phenothiazines General Monograph

ADVERSE DRUG REACTIONS

Perphenazine pharmacotherapy has been commonly associated with EPRs, particularly when higher dosages are prescribed. It also has been associated with drowsiness and photosensitivity. Although not directly associated with perphenazine pharmacotherapy, several ADRs generally have been associated with phenothiazine pharmacotherapy. Attention to these ADRs is required because of perphenazine's chemical and pharmacological similarities to the other phenothiazines (see Phenothiazines General Monograph).

EPRs are commonly associated with the piperazine group, to which perphenazine belongs. Other ADRs (e.g., blood disorders, jaundice, sedation) have been less commonly associated with perphenazine pharmacotherapy. Although significant anticholinergic reactions (e.g., blurred vision, dry mouth, dynamic or paralytic ileus, sweating, urinary retention) commonly occur with phenothiazine pharmacotherapy, they occur infrequently among patients who are receiving less than 24 mg daily of perphenazine. However, dynamic ileus may occur among patients regardless of the daily dosage. If severe, this ADR may result in serious complications and death. Patients who have schizophrenia or other psychotic disorders may not recognize the signs and symptoms of this medical disorder and fail to seek appropriate medical evaluation and treatment. Monitor these patients carefully for changes in bowel elimination patterns, particularly constipation. Collaboration with the patient's advanced practice nurse or family physician may be indicated.

See also Phenothiazines General Monograph

OVERDOSAGE

Signs and symptoms of perphenazine overdosage are generally extensions of its pharmacologic actions and involve the extrapyramidal system. These signs and symptoms include CNS depression progressing from drowsiness to stupor or coma with areflexia. Patients who have a mild overdosage may display restlessness, confusion, and excitement. Other signs and symptoms include abnormal contraction of the pupils (miosis), convulsions, cyanosis, difficulty swallowing and breathing, hypotension, hypothermia, muscle twitching, respiratory collapse, rigidity or hypotonia, spasm, tachycardia, tremor and vasomotor collapse, possibly with sudden apnea. Perphenazine overdosage requires emergency symptomatic medical support of body systems with attention to increasing perphenazine elimination. There is no known antidote.

PHENDIMETRAZINE *

(fen dye me′tra zeen)

TRADE NAMES

Adipost®
Bontril PDM®, Bontril® Slow-Release
Plegine®
Prelu-2®

CLASSIFICATION

Anorexiant (CNS stimulant, amphetamine-related) (sympathomimetic) (C-III)

APPROVED INDICATIONS FOR PSYCHOLOGICAL DISORDERS

Adjunctive pharmacotherapy for the short-term symptomatic management of:

Eating Disorders: Exogenous Obesity

USUAL DOSAGE AND ADMINISTRATION

Eating Disorders: Exogenous Obesity

Adults: 70 to 105 mg regular capsule or tablet daily orally in two or three divided doses one hour before meals; *or* 105 mg extended-release capsule daily orally thirty to sixty minutes before breakfast. Prescribe the lowest effective dosage adjusted to individual patient response. Some patients may benefit from 30 to 52.5 mg daily orally in two or three divided doses. Dosage should not exceed 210 mg daily orally in three divided doses. Tolerance to phendimetrazine's anorexiant action usually develops within a few weeks. When tolerance is noted, discontinue phendimetrazine pharmacotherapy. Do *not* exceed the recommended dosage in an attempt to maintain phendimetrazine's anorexiant action.

MAXIMUM: 210 mg daily

Women who are, or who may become, pregnant: FDA Pregnancy Category "not established." Safety and efficacy of phendimetrazine pharmacotherapy for women who are pregnant have not been established. Avoid prescribing phendimetrazine pharmacotherapy to women who are pregnant. If phendimetrazine pharmacotherapy is required, advise patients of potential benefits and possible risks to themselves and the embryo, fetus, or neonate. Collaboration with the patient's obstetrician is required.

Women who are breast-feeding: Safety and efficacy of phendimetrazine pharmacotherapy for women who are breast-feeding and their neonates and infants have not been established. Avoid prescribing phendimetrazine pharmacotherapy to women who are breast-feeding. If phendimetrazine pharmacotherapy is required, breast-feeding probably should be discontinued. If desired, lactation may be maintained and breast-feeding resumed following the discontinuation of short-term phendimetrazine pharmacotherapy. Collaboration with the patient's pediatrician is indicated.

Children younger than 12 years of age: The safety and efficacy of phendimetrazine pharmacotherapy for children who are younger than 12 years of age have not been established. Phendimetrazine pharmacotherapy is *not* recommended for this age group.

Notes, Eating Disorders: Exogenous Obesity

Phendimetrazine pharmacotherapy is only indicated for the short-term (a maximum of 12 weeks) symptomatic management of exogenous obesity for patients who also are receiving caloric restriction, a medically supervised or otherwise individualized exercise program, and appropriate psychotherapy. The reportedly limited therapeutic effectiveness of phendimetrazine pharmacotherapy for this indication must be weighed against potential risks, including addiction and habituation (see also ADRs). If addiction and habituation to phendimetrazine are identified, discontinue phendimetrazine pharmacotherapy or regular personal use gradually. Abrupt discontinuation after regular long-term high-dosage use may result in such signs and symptoms as fatigue and mental depression.

AVAILABLE DOSAGE FORMS, STORAGE, AND COMPATIBILITY

Capsules, oral: 35 mg
Capsules, oral extended-release: 105 mg
Tablets, oral: 35 mg

Notes

General Instructions for Patients   Instruct patients who are receiving phendimetrazine pharmacotherapy to

- swallow whole each dose of the phendimetrazine oral extended-release capsules without breaking, chewing, or crushing. Also instruct them to ingest each dose with an adequate amount of water or other compatible liquid chaser (e.g., 60 to 120 ml).
- safely store their phendimetrazine oral dosage forms out of the reach of children in tightly closed child-resistant containers at controlled room temperature (15° to 30°C; 59° to 86°F).
- obtain an available patient information sheet regarding phendimetrazine pharmacotherapy from their pharmacist at the time that their prescription is dispensed. Encourage patients to clarify any questions that they may have concerning phendimetrazine pharmacotherapy with their pharmacist or, if needed, to consult their prescribing psychologist.

PROPOSED MECHANISM OF ACTION

Phendimetrazine is a CNS stimulant sympathomimetic amine pharmacologically similar to the amphetamines. Phendimetrazine pharmacotherapy has been associated with tachyphylaxis and tolerance. Phendimetrazine's actions include CNS stimulation and increased blood pressure. The exact mechanism of its anorexiant action, including appetite suppression, has not yet been fully determined. However, it appears to be associated with its direct stimulation of the CNS. Metabolic or other actions also may be involved.

PHARMACOKINETICS/PHARMACODYNAMICS

Phendimetrazine is readily absorbed following oral ingestion. Phendimetrazine is excreted by the kidneys. The mean half-life of elimination is approximately 4 hours. Additional data are unavailable.

RELATIVE CONTRAINDICATIONS

Agitation

Arteriosclerosis, advanced

Cardiovascular disorders, severe

Glaucoma

Hypersensitivity to phendimetrazine or sympathomimetic amines (e.g., epinephrine, norepinephrine)

Hypertension, moderate to severe

Hyperthyroidism

MAOI pharmacotherapy, concurrent or within 14 days. Phendimetrazine and MAOI pharmacotherapy, concurrent or within 14 days, may result in hypertensive crisis. Hypertensive crisis is characterized by hypertension and severe headache.

Problematic patterns of amphetamine or other abusable psychotropic use, history of

CAUTIONS AND COMMENTS

Long-term phendimetrazine pharmacotherapy, or regular personal use, may result in addiction and habituation. Phendimetrazine is related chemically and pharmacologically to the amphetamines, which have high abuse potential. Patients may increase their dosages to many times those recommended. Monitor patients for problematic patterns of use and signs and symptoms of toxicity, which may include dermatoses (severe), hyperactivity, irritability, insomnia, and personality changes. One of the most serious signs and symptoms of toxicity is psychosis. Phendimetrazine-induced psychosis is often clinically indistinguishable from schizophrenia. Prescribe short-term pharmacotherapy and the least amount of phendimetrazine feasible for dispensing at one time to minimize the possible development of problematic patterns of use.

Abrupt discontinuation of long-term phendimetrazine pharmacotherapy, or regular personal use, has been associated with an amphetamine-like withdrawal syndrome, including signs and symptoms of extreme fatigue and mental depression. EEG changes also have been reported. Avoid abrupt discontinuation of phendimetrazine pharmacotherapy.

Prescribe phendimetrazine pharmacotherapy cautiously to patients who

- have hypertension, even mild hypertension. Phendimetrazine may exacerbate hypertension among these patients.
- have insulin-dependent diabetes mellitus. Phendimetrazine, particularly when prescribed with concurrent caloric restrictions, may alter insulin requirements.

Caution patients who are receiving phendimetrazine pharmacotherapy against performing activities that require alertness, judgment, and physical coordination (e.g., driving an automobile, operating dangerous equipment, supervising children) until their response to phendimetrazine is known.

In addition to this general precaution, caution patients to inform their prescribing psychologist if they begin or discontinue any other pharmacotherapy while receiving phendimetrazine pharmacotherapy.

CLINICALLY SIGNIFICANT DRUG INTERACTIONS

Concurrent phendimetrazine pharmacotherapy and the following may result in clinically significant drug interactions:

Guanethidine Pharmacotherapy

Concurrent phendimetrazine and guanethidine (Ismelin®) pharmacotherapy may result in a decrease in the neuronal uptake of guanethidine and a decrease in its associated antihypertensive action. An adjustment in the guanethidine dosage may be required. Collaboration with the prescriber of the guanethidine is indicated.

Monoamine Oxidase Inhibitor Pharmacotherapy

Phendimetrazine may interact with MAOIs (e.g., phenelzine, tranylcypromine). This interaction may cause the release of large amounts of catecholamines, particularly epinephrine and norepinephrine, and associated hypertensive crisis. Thus, this combination of pharmacotherapy, concurrent or within 14 days, is *contraindicated*.

See also Amphetamines General Monograph

ADVERSE DRUG REACTIONS

Phendimetrazine pharmacotherapy has been associated with the following ADRs, listed according to body system:

Cardiovascular: hypertension, palpitations, and tachycardia
CNS: dizziness, dysphoria, euphoria, headache, insomnia, overstimulation, restlessness, and, rarely, psychotic episodes at recommended dosages
Cutaneous: hives (urticaria)
Genitourinary: impotence and changes in sex drive
GI: constipation, diarrhea, dry mouth, GI complaints, and unpleasant taste
Musculoskeletal: tremor

See also Amphetamines General Monograph

OVERDOSAGE

Signs and symptoms of acute phendimetrazine overdosage include assaultiveness, belligerence, confusion, hallucinations, hyperreflexia, hyperventilation, panic, restlessness, and tremor. Depression and fatigue usually follow the CNS stimulation. Cardiovascular signs and symptoms include dysrhythmias, hypertension or hypotension, and circulatory collapse. GI signs and symptoms include abdominal cramps, diarrhea, nausea, and vomiting. Fatal overdosage usually terminates in convulsions and coma. Acute phendimetrazine overdosage requires emergency symptomatic medical support of body systems with attention to increasing phendimetrazine elimination. There is no known antidote.

PHENELZINE

(fen'el zeen)

TRADE NAME

Nardil®

CLASSIFICATION

Antidepressant (MAOI)

APPROVED INDICATIONS FOR PSYCHOLOGICAL DISORDERS

Adjunctive pharmacotherapy for the symptomatic management of:

Mood Disorders: Depressive Disorders: Atypical, Reactive, or Neurotic Depression. Phenelzine is indicated particularly for patients who have histories of poor response to pharmacotherapy with other classes of antidepressants.

USUAL DOSAGE AND ADMINISTRATION

Depressive Disorders: Atypical, Reactive, or Neurotic Depression

Adults: Initially, 45 mg daily orally in three divided doses. Increase the daily dosage relatively rapidly over two weeks to a maximum of 90 mg daily orally.

MAINTENANCE: 15 mg daily or every other day orally

MAXIMUM: 90 mg daily orally

Women who are, or who may become, pregnant: FDA Pregnancy Category "not established." Safety and efficacy of phenelzine pharmacotherapy for women who are pregnant have not been established. Avoid prescribing phenelzine pharmacotherapy to women who are pregnant. If phenelzine pharmacotherapy is required, advise patients of potential benefits and possible risks to themselves and the embryo, fetus, or neonate. Collaboration with the patient's obstetrician is indicated.

Women who are breast-feeding: Safety and efficacy of phenelzine pharmacotherapy for women who are breast-feeding and their neonates and infants have not been established. Avoid prescribing phenelzine pharmacotherapy to women who are breast-feeding. If phenelzine pharmacotherapy is required, breast-feeding probably should be discontinued. Collaboration with the patient's pediatrician is indicated.

Children and adolescents younger than 16 years of age: Safety and efficacy of phenelzine pharmacotherapy for children and adolescents who are younger than 16 years of age have not been established. Phenelzine pharmacotherapy is *not* recommended for this age group.

Notes, Depressive Disorders: Atypical, Reactive, or Neurotic Depression

Depressed patients are at increased risk for suicide. Prescribe the smallest quantity of phenelzine feasible for dispensing (i.e., do not exceed a two-week supply). Other suicide precautions may be indicated. In addition to phenelzine pharmacotherapy as an adjunct to appropriate psychotherapy, ECT, hospitalization, or other therapy may be required.

Initiating Phenelzine Pharmacotherapy   During the early initiation of pharmacotherapy, increase dosages relatively rapidly to at least 60 mg daily according to individual patient response. Some patients may require 90 mg daily to obtain desired monoamine oxidase inhibition. Therapeutic benefit may not be observed among some patients until they have received 60 mg daily for at least one month. After maximum therapeutic response is achieved, reduce the dosage slowly over several weeks to achieve an optimal maintenance dosage of 15 mg daily or 15 mg every other day.

Maintaining Phenelzine Pharmacotherapy   Monitor all patients who are receiving phenelzine pharmacotherapy for postural (orthostatic) hypotension, including patients who usually have normal blood pressure, hypertension, or hypotension. Blood pressure generally returns to measurements obtained prior to phenelzine pharmacotherapy when the phenelzine dosage is reduced or when phenelzine pharmacotherapy is discontinued. Discontinue phenelzine pharmacotherapy immediately if frequent headaches or palpitations are reported. Collaboration with the patient's family physician or a specialist (e.g., cardiologist) may be indicated. Continue phenelzine pharmacotherapy for as long as needed.

Discontinuing Phenelzine Pharmacotherapy   The discontinuation of long-term phenelzine pharmacotherapy has been associated with a phenelzine withdrawal syndrome. The signs and symptoms of this withdrawal syndrome occur generally within 72 hours of discontinuing phenelzine pharmacotherapy and include malaise, nausea, and vomiting. Other signs and symptoms include agitation with vivid nightmares, convulsions, and psychosis. This withdrawal syndrome generally can be managed by reinstituting low-dosage phenelzine pharmacotherapy followed by a cautious and gradual reduction of dosage until phenelzine pharmacotherapy is completely discontinued.

AVAILABLE DOSAGE FORMS, STORAGE, AND COMPATIBILITY

Tablets, oral: 15 mg

Notes

General Instructions for Patients   Instruct patients who are receiving phenelzine pharmacotherapy to

- safely store phenelzine oral tablets out of the reach of children in child-resistant containers at controlled room temperature (15° to 30°C; 59° to 86°F).
- obtain an available patient information sheet regarding phenelzine pharmacotherapy from their pharmacist at the time that their prescription is dispensed. Encourage patients to clarify any questions that they may have concerning phenelzine pharmacotherapy with their pharmacist or, if needed, to consult their prescribing psychologist.

PROPOSED MECHANISM OF ACTION

Phenelzine, a potent MAOI, appears to produce its antidepressant action primarily by potentiating the actions of various amines, specifically dopamine, epinephrine, norepinephrine, and serotonin.

Phenelzine potentiates the actions of these amines by inhibiting the enzyme that catalyzes their oxidative deamination (i.e., monoamine oxidase). This inhibition of amine metabolism increases the amounts of these amines throughout the body, including the synapses. The result is increased activity at the post-synaptic neuron receptor sites.

PHARMACOKINETICS/PHARMACODYNAMICS

Phenelzine is readily absorbed following oral ingestion. Additional data are unavailable.

RELATIVE CONTRAINDICATIONS

Cardiovascular disorders
Cerebrovascular disorders
Congestive heart failure
Elderly, frail, or debilitated patients
Elective surgery requiring anesthesia. Discontinue phenelzine pharmacotherapy at least 10 days prior to elective surgery.
Headaches, history of frequent or severe
Hypersensitivity to phenelzine
Liver dysfunction
Pheochromocytoma
Sympathomimetic and related pharmacotherapy (e.g., amphetamine, cocaine, methylphenidate, dopamine, epinephrine, norepinephrine), or regular personal use, concurrent

CAUTIONS AND COMMENTS

Hypertensive Crisis

Hypertensive crisis among patients receiving phenelzine pharmacotherapy may occur as a result of concurrent sympathomimetic or related pharmacotherapy (e.g., amphetamine, cocaine, methylphenidate, dopamine, epinephrine, norepinephrine), TCA pharmacotherapy, or the ingestion of beverages and foods that have a high concentration of dopamine or tyramine. Hypertensive crisis may be fatal. The signs and symptoms of hypertensive crisis, include bradycardia or tachycardia, which may be associated with constricting chest pain; dilated pupils; photophobia; nausea; neck stiffness or soreness; occipital headache, which may radiate frontally; palpitations; sweating, sometimes with fever and cold, clammy skin; and vomiting. Intracranial bleeding has been associated with increased blood pressure. Advise patients to report immediately the occurrence of a headache or other unusual signs and symptoms while receiving phenelzine pharmacotherapy. In the event of hypertensive crisis, instruct patients to discontinue immediately phenelzine pharmacotherapy and obtain emergency medical evaluation and treatment. Hypertensive crisis requires symptomatic medical management of associated signs and symptoms with attention to lowering blood pressure.

Prescribe phenelzine pharmacotherapy cautiously to patients who

- are receiving other MAOI pharmacotherapy (e.g., moclobemide [Manerix®], tranylcypromine [Parnate®]) or pharmacotherapy with dibenzazepine derivative drugs (e.g., amitriptyline, amoxapine, carbamazepine, clomipramine, cyclobenzaprine (Flexeril®), desipramine, doxepin, imipramine, maprotiline, nortriptyline, trimipramine). Do *not* prescribe phenelzine pharmacotherapy with, or within 14 days of, other MAOI or dibenzazepine derivative pharmacotherapy. Hypertensive crisis and convulsions, delirium, excitation, fever, sweating (marked), tremor, coma, and circulatory collapse may occur. At least 14 days should elapse between the discontinuation of pharmacotherapy with another MAOI or dibenzazepine derivative and the initiation of phenelzine pharmacotherapy.

- have histories of bipolar disorders. Phenelzine pharmacotherapy may cause a swing from a depressive to a manic phase among these patients.
- have histories of Parkinsonism. Phenelzine pharmacotherapy may increase the incidence and severity of the signs and symptoms associated with Parkinsonism.
- have histories of schizophrenia. Phenelzine pharmacotherapy has been associated with excessive stimulation among these patients.
- have histories of seizure disorders. Phenelzine has varying actions on the seizure threshold. Ensure adequate precautions are implemented when phenelzine is prescribed to patients who have histories of epilepsy or other seizure disorders.
- regularly drink alcohol or are receiving concurrent pharmacotherapy with the cough suppressant dextromethorphan or certain opiate analgesics (e.g., meperidine). Excitation, seizures, delirium, hyperpyrexia, circulatory collapse, coma, and death may result.

Caution patients who are receiving phenelzine pharmacotherapy against performing activities that require alertness, judgment, and physical coordination (e.g., driving an automobile, operating dangerous equipment, supervising children) until their response to phenelzine is known.

In addition to this general precaution, caution patients to inform their prescribing psychologist if they begin or discontinue any other pharmacotherapy while receiving phenelzine pharmacotherapy.

CLINICALLY SIGNIFICANT DRUG INTERACTIONS

Concurrent phenelzine pharmacotherapy and the following may result in clinically significant drug interactions:

Bupropion Pharmacotherapy

Concurrent bupropion (Wellbutrin®) and MAOI pharmacotherapy (e.g., phenelzine [Nardil®], tranylcypromine [Parnate®]) may result in bupropion toxicity. Concurrent bupropion and MAOI pharmacotherapy is *contraindicated*. At least 14 days should elapse between the discontinuation of MAOI pharmacotherapy and the initiation of bupropion pharmacotherapy.

Buspirone Pharmacotherapy

Concurrent buspirone (BuSpar®) and MAOI pharmacotherapy (e.g., phenelzine [Nardil®], tranylcypromine [Parnate®]) has resulted in severe hypertension. Avoid, if possible, concurrent buspirone and MAOI pharmacotherapy. If concurrent pharmacotherapy is unavoidable, carefully monitor the patient's blood pressure. Collaboration with the patient's advanced practice nurse or family physician may be indicated.

Dopamine Containing Beverages and Foods

See Tyramine Containing Beverages and Foods

Sympathomimetic, Tricyclic Antidepressant, and Related Pharmacotherapy

Concurrent phenelzine pharmacotherapy with a sympathomimetic (e.g., certain cough and cold formulations, dopamine, epinephrine, levodopa [Dopar®], methyldopa [Aldomet®], and norepinephrine) or a TCA (e.g., desipramine, imipramine) may result in hypertensive crisis. Thus, concurrent pharmacotherapy is *contraindicated*.

Tyramine Containing Beverages and Foods

Concurrent ingestion of beverages (e.g., beer, caffeine containing beverages [excessive], wine) and foods that contain high concentrations of tyramine (e.g., aged cheeses, broad beans, chicken livers, chocolate (excessive), pickled herring, and yeast extract) may result in hypertensive crisis among patients who are receiving phenelzine pharmacotherapy. Advise patients to avoid these beverages and foods while receiving phenelzine pharmacotherapy.

Caution patients who are receiving phenelzine pharmacotherapy against

- consuming beverages and foods that have high concentrations of dopamine or tyramine. These beverages and foods generally are high protein beverages and foods that have undergone protein breakdown by aging, fermenting, pickling, smoking, or introducing bacteria. Patients should avoid aged cheeses, dry sausage (e.g., Genoa salami, hard salami, pepperoni, Lebanon bologna), liver, liver extract (including brewer's yeast in large amounts), pods of broad beans (fava beans), sauerkraut, and yogurt. Also caution patients against drinking beer and wine, including alcohol-free and reduced-alcohol beers and wines. The ingestion of excessive amounts of caffeine or chocolate also can result in hypertensive crisis and should be avoided.
- pharmacotherapy with TCAs or sympathomimetics, including the following prescription and nonprescription products: anorexiants, appetite suppressants, or weight reducing drugs (e.g., phenylpropanolamine), asthma inhalant drugs (e.g., ephedrine, a component of Bronkotabs® and Primatene Tablets®), cold and cough formulations, including those containing dextromethorphan (dextromethorphan may cause a reaction similar to that reported with meperidine), hay-fever drugs, nasal and sinus decongestant products in drops, liquids, sprays, or tablets (e.g., ephedrine, phenylephedrine [Neo-Synephrine®], pseudoephedrine [Sudafed®], phenylpropanolamine), and L-tryptophan containing products.

Note: These potentially interacting beverages, foods, and drugs need to be avoided during phenelzine pharmacotherapy and for two weeks following the discontinuation of phenelzine pharmacotherapy. The use of these drugs, beverages, and foods during, or within 14 days of, phenelzine pharmacotherapy may result in severe headaches, excessively high blood pressure, and other serious signs and symptoms associated with the hypertensive crisis.

In addition to these general precautions, caution patients to inform their physician, dentist, advanced practice nurse, or other prescribers that they are receiving phenelzine pharmacotherapy.

ADVERSE DRUG REACTIONS

Phenelzine is a potent inhibitor of monoamine oxidase, an enzyme that is widely distributed throughout the body. Thus a diversity of ADRs has been associated with phenelzine pharmacotherapy. These ADRs are listed according to body system. When these ADRs occur, they tend to be mild to moderate in severity and generally may be managed by reducing the phenelzine dosage. It is rarely necessary to prescribe counteracting measures or to discontinue phenelzine pharmacotherapy:

Cardiovascular: edema and postural hypotension. Rarely, cardiac and respiratory depression (transient) following ECT, and shock-like coma

CNS: abnormal repetitious use of words and phrases with increasing rapidity (palilalia), dizziness, drowsiness, fatigue, headache, euphoria, jitteriness, and sleep disorders (e.g., hypersomnia; insomnia). Rarely, anxiety reactions (acute), convulsions, incoordination (ataxia), precipitation of schizophrenia, toxic delirium, and mania. Hypomania and agitation also have been associated with phenelzine pharmacotherapy.

Hypomania is one of the more severe ADRs associated with phenelzine pharmacotherapy. This ADR occurs mainly among patients who have disorders characterized by hyperkinetic signs and symptoms that may be obscured by depression. Hypomania is usually observed as depression improves. Phenelzine pharmacotherapy also may increase agitation among patients who are agitated. Hypomania and agitation generally are associated with higher than recommended dosages of phenelzine or with long-term phenelzine pharmacotherapy.

Cutaneous: itching (severe), rash, and sweating (excessive). Rarely, a lupus-like syndrome.

Genitourinary: sexual dysfunction (e.g., anorgasmia, ejaculation disturbances) and urinary retention

GI: constipation, dry mouth, and GI upset

Hematologic: rarely, a reduction in the circulating white blood cells, including basophils, eosinophils, monocytes, and, in particular, lymphocytes (leukopenia)

Hepatic: elevated blood transaminases without accompanying signs and symptoms of liver dysfunction. Rarely, fatal progressive necrotizing hepatocellular damage and jaundice (reversible).

Metabolic/Endocrine: excess of sodium in the blood (hypernatremia) and weight gain. Rarely, hypermetabolic syndrome, including, but not limited to, coma, elevated body temperature above 41°C (106°F) (hyperpyrexia), oxygen difficiency (hypoxia), rapid heart rate (tachycardia), rapid respirations (tachypnea), muscle rigidity, and metabolic acidosis (may resemble signs and symptoms of overdosage)

Musculoskeletal: hyperreflexia, myoclonic movements, numbness or tingling of the extremities (paresthesias), tremors, twitching, and weakness

Ocular: blurred vision; glaucoma; and involuntary, continuous cyclical movement of the eyeballs (nystagmus)

Respiratory: edema of the glottis

Miscellaneous: rarely, fever

OVERDOSAGE

Signs and symptoms of phenelzine overdosage are related to the amount of phenelzine ingested and other factors (e.g., the time elapsed since drug ingestion; the concurrent ingestion of other drugs, including alcohol). These signs and symptoms may be absent or minimal during the initial 12 hours following the overdosage and may include cardiovascular and CNS stimulation or depression. However, more serious signs and symptoms may develop slowly over the subsequent 12 hours.

By 24 to 48 hours, signs and symptoms may include agitation; convulsions; coma; cold, clammy skin; dizziness; drowsiness; excessive sweating (diaphoresis); faintness; hallucinations; headache (severe); hyperactivity; hyperpyrexia; hypertension or hypotension and vascular collapse; irregular and rapid pulse; irritability; precordial pain; rigidity; respiratory depression and failure; spasm where the head and heels are bent backward and the body is bowed forward (opisthotonos); and tonic contraction of the muscles of mastication (trismus).

Phenelzine overdosage requires emergency symptomatic medical support of body systems with attention to increasing phenelzine elimination. There is no known antidote.

PHENOBARBITAL [Phenobarbitone]

(fee noe bar'bi tal)

TRADE NAMES

Barbilixir®
Luminal®
Solfoton®

CLASSIFICATION

Sedative-hypnotic (barbiturate) (C-IV)

See Barbiturates General Monograph

APPROVED INDICATIONS FOR PSYCHOLOGICAL DISORDERS

Adjunctive pharmacotherapy for the short-term symptomatic management of:

- Anxiety Disorders. Phenobarbital pharmacotherapy is *not* indicated for the management of everyday anxiety or tension, or that anxiety that can be managed with psychotherapy alone. Phenobarbital also is *not* recommended for the management of anxiety associated with depression because it has the potential to exacerbate the depression while alleviating the anxiety. The depression associated with anxiety generally resolves with appropriate adjunctive pharmacotherapy (i.e., antidepressant pharmacotherapy) and psychotherapy.
- Sleep Disorders: Insomnia

USUAL DOSAGE AND ADMINISTRATION

Anxiety Disorders

Although approved for the symptomatic management of anxiety disorders, the barbiturates, including phenobarbital, are *not* generally recommended for this indication because of the availability of benzodiazepines (see Benzodiazepines General Monograph). The benzodiazepines possess both greater efficacy for the management of anxiety disorders and lower toxicity (i.e., better ADR profile and significantly less associated morbidity and mortality with overdosage). For patients who are hypersensitive to benzodiazepines, or for whom benzodiazepine pharmacotherapy is contraindicated for any other reason, mephobarbital may be prescribed for the symptomatic management of anxiety disorders (see Mephobarbital Monograph).

Sleep Disorders: Insomnia

Adults: 100 to 300 mg daily orally 60 minutes before retiring for bed in the evening

Women who are, or who may become, pregnant: FDA Pregnancy Category D. Safety and efficacy of phenobarbital pharmacotherapy for women who are pregnant have not been established. Numerous reports in the literature have associated the use of phenobarbital with various fetal and congenital malformations (i.e., birth defects), including cleft lip and palate, congenital dislocated hip, microcephaly, and wide fontanelle. In addition, the neonatal barbiturate withdrawal syndrome, developmental delay, and psychomotor retardation have been noted among neonates and infants born to mothers who had used phenobarbital regularly during pregnancy (see Barbiturates General Monograph). Do *not* prescribe phenobarbital pharmacotherapy to women who are pregnant.

Women who are breast-feeding: Safety and efficacy of phenobarbital pharmacotherapy for women who are breast-feeding and their neonates and infants have not been established. Phenobarbital is excreted in sufficient quantities in breast milk to cause drowsiness and lethargy among nursing neonates and infants. These neonates and infants also may become addicted (see Barbiturates General Monograph). Avoid prescribing phenobarbital pharmacotherapy to women who are breast-feeding. If phenobarbital pharmacotherapy is required, breast-feeding should be discontinued. If desired, lactation may be maintained and breast-feeding resumed following the discontinuation of short-term phenobarbital pharmacotherapy.

Elderly, frail, or debilitated patients: Generally prescribe lower dosages of phenobarbital for elderly, frail, or debilitated patients. These patients may be more sensitive to the pharmacologic actions of phenobarbital, particularly its respiratory depressant action, than are younger or healthier adult patients. Phenobarbital pharmacotherapy also has been associated with increased excitability among these patients.

Children and Adolescents: Phenobarbital pharmacotherapy is *not* recommended for this indication for this age group.

Notes, Insomnia

See Barbiturates General Monograph

AVAILABLE DOSAGE FORMS, STORAGE, AND COMPATIBILITY

Capsules, oral: 16, 65 mg
Drops, oral: 16 mg/ml
Elixir, oral: 3, 4 mg/ml (contains 10% to 13.5% alcohol)
Injectables, intramuscular or intravenous: 30, 60, 65, 120, 130 mg/ml (contains 10% alcohol). Injectables generally are indicated for use among hospitalized patients and those who require anticonvulsant phenobarbital pharmacotherapy.
Suppositories, rectal: 8, 15, 30, 60, 100, 120 mg
Tablets, oral: 8.5, 15, 16, 30, 32, 50, 60, 65, 100 mg

Notes

Phenobarbital is available in a variety of injectable, oral, and rectal formulations.

Injectable Formulations　Some injectable formulations of phenobarbital contain sodium bisulfite. Sulfites may cause hypersensitivity reactions, including anaphylactic reactions, among susceptible patients. Although relatively uncommon, these reactions appear to occur with a higher incidence among patients who have asthma.

Oral Formulations　The oral drops (i.e., Sedadrops®) contain tartrazine. Tartrazine may cause hypersensitivity reactions, including bronchial asthma, among susceptible patients, particularly those who have a hypersensitivity to aspirin.

General Instructions for Patients　Instruct patients who are receiving phenobarbital pharmacotherapy to

- safely store oral dosage forms of phenobarbital out of the reach of children in tightly closed child- and light-resistant containers.
- obtain an available patient information sheet regarding phenobarbital pharmacotherapy from their pharmacist at the time that their prescription is dispensed. Encourage patients to clarify any questions that they may have concerning phenobarbital pharmacotherapy with their pharmacist or, if needed, to consult their prescribing psychologist.

PROPOSED MECHANISM OF ACTION

The exact mechanism of phenobarbital's CNS depressant action has not been fully determined. Phenobarbital appears to act primarily at the level of the thalamus, where it interferes with impulse transmission to the cortex.

See also Barbiturates General Monograph

PHARMACOKINETICS/PHARMACODYNAMICS

Phenobarbital is slowly but well absorbed (90% to 100%) following oral ingestion. Peak blood levels are generally obtained within 12 hours. Onset of action depends on the method of administration, but generally is within 60 minutes. After intravenous injection, onset of action occurs within 5 minutes. The onset of action following intramuscular injection is slightly slower than that following oral ingestion or rectal insertion.

The duration of action is 6 to 12 hours. Phenobarbital is approximately 50% plasma protein-bound and has an apparent volume of distribution of 0.5 L/kg. Of the barbiturates, phenobarbital is the least soluble and has the slowest distribution. Phenobarbital is not as extensively metabolized as other barbiturates because of its lower lipid solubility. Almost 25% is excreted unchanged in the urine. The half-life of elimination is approximately 4 days (range 80 to 120 hours). The total body clearance ranges from 4 to 5 ml/minute, and the half-life of elimination ranges from approximately 2 to 6 days.

Therapeutic Drug Monitoring

Blood samples for periodic therapeutic drug monitoring should be obtained from trough blood concentrations (i.e., just before the next dose). In cases of suspected toxicity, samples may be obtained at any time. Generally, phenobarbital blood concentrations of 10 μg/ml produce sedation, 40 μg/ml produce sleep, 50 μg/ml (215 mmol/L) or higher are toxic and may produce coma, and 80 μg/ml or higher may be fatal.

RELATIVE CONTRAINDICATIONS

Liver dysfunction, severe
Hypersensitivity to phenobarbital or other barbiturates
Kidney dysfunction, severe
Porphyria
Pregnancy
Respiratory depression, severe

CAUTIONS AND COMMENTS

Long-term phenobarbital pharmacotherapy, or regular personal use, may lead to addiction and habituation. Sudden discontinuation of long-term phenobarbital pharmacotherapy, or regular personal use, can result in the barbiturate withdrawal syndrome. This withdrawal syndrome is considered to be a medical emergency that can be fatal if not appropriately treated.

Prescribe phenobarbital pharmacotherapy cautiously to patients who

- are concurrently receiving oral anticoagulant pharmacotherapy because of the associated difficulty in stabilizing prothrombin times for these patients.
- have CNS or respiratory depression. Phenobarbital may increase both CNS and respiratory depression among these patients.
- have kidney or liver dysfunction. The metabolism and elimination of phenobarbital may be prolonged among these patients.

Caution patients who are receiving phenobarbital pharmacotherapy against performing activities that require alertness, judgment, and physical coordination (e.g., driving an automobile, operating dangerous equipment, supervising children). Phenobarbital may adversely affect these mental and physical functions.

In addition to this general precaution, caution patients to inform their prescribing psychologist if they begin or discontinue any other pharmacotherapy while receiving phenobarbital pharmacotherapy.

CLINICALLY SIGNIFICANT DRUG INTERACTIONS

Concurrent phenobarbital pharmacotherapy and the following may result in clinically significant drug interactions:

Alcohol Use

Concurrent alcohol use may increase the CNS depressant action of phenobarbital. Advise patients to avoid, or limit, their use of alcohol while receiving phenobarbital pharmacotherapy.

Pharmacotherapy With Drugs That Are Primarily Metabolized by the Liver

Phenobarbital may stimulate the production of hepatic microsomal enzymes, which are responsible for the metabolism of many different drugs. Whenever phenobarbital is added to or removed from a patient's pharmacotherapy, attention must be given to the effect on concurrently prescribed drugs (e.g., corticosteroids, oral anticoagulants, oral contraceptives, quinidine [Biquin®]). Collaboration with other prescribers may be needed, so that dosages can be appropriately adjusted (i.e., increased or decreased), if necessary.

Pharmacotherapy With Central Nervous System Depressants and Other Drugs That Produce Central Nervous System Depression

Concurrent phenobarbital pharmacotherapy with opiate analgesics, other sedative-hypnotics, and other drugs that produce CNS depression (e.g., antihistamines, phenothiazines, TCAs) may result in additive CNS depression.

See also Barbiturates General Monograph

ADVERSE DRUG REACTIONS

Phenobarbital pharmacotherapy has been associated with mental changes and reduced performance on neurological tests, osteomalacia, respiratory depression, sedation, and skin rashes. Phenobarbital suppresses REM sleep, which may result in a "hang-over" effect the day following the use of phenobarbital for the symptomatic management of insomnia.

See also Barbiturates General Monograph

OVERDOSAGE

See Barbiturates General Monograph

PHENOTHIAZINES

(fee noe thye'a zeens)

GENERIC NAMES

(for trade names, see individual drug monographs)

Chlorpromazine
Fluphenazine

Mesoridazine
Methotrimeprazine
Pericyazine ✴
Perphenazine
Pipotiazine ✴
Prochlorperazine
Promazine *
Thioproperazine ✴
Thioridazine
Trifluoperazine

CLASSIFICATION

Antipsychotic (phenothiazine)

APPROVED INDICATIONS FOR PSYCHOLOGICAL DISORDERS

Adjunctive pharmacotherapy for the symptomatic management of:

- Disruptive Behavior Disorders: Severe Behavioral Problems Among Children Characterized by Uncontrollable Combativeness. *Note:* The phenothiazines have *no* demonstrated efficacy for this indication for children who are mentally retarded.
- Psychotic Disorders: Schizophrenia and Other Psychotic Disorders

USUAL DOSAGE AND ADMINISTRATION

Severe Behavioral Problems Among Children Characterized by Uncontrollable Combativeness

Children: The initiation and maintenance of phenothiazine pharmacotherapy for severe behavioral problems among children require careful prescription and stabilization of the dosage according to each child's signs and symptoms and individual response to pharmacotherapy. Close monitoring by the prescribing psychologist is indicated.
See individual phenothiazine monographs

Notes, Severe Behavioral Problems Among Children Characterized by Uncontrollable Combativeness

See Notes, Schizophrenia and Other Psychotic Disorders

Schizophrenia and Other Psychotic Disorders

Adults: The initiation and maintenance of phenothiazine pharmacotherapy require careful prescription and stabilization of the dosage according to each patient's signs and symptoms of psychosis and individual response to pharmacotherapy. Close monitoring by the prescribing psychologist is indicated.

See individual phenothiazine monographs

Women who are, or who may become, pregnant: FDA Pregnancy Category "not established." Safety and efficacy of phenothiazine pharmacotherapy for women who are pregnant have not been established. Results of teratogenic studies have been mixed. Phenothiazines, such as chlorpromazine and methotrimeprazine, that have a three-carbon side chain (i.e., propylamino derivatives) have been more often associated with congenital malformations (i.e., birth defects), including cleft lip, club hands, hypospadias, and microcephaly, than have other phenothiazines when prescribed during pregnancy. Avoid prescribing phenothiazine pharmacotherapy to women who are pregnant. If phenothiazine pharmacotherapy is required, advise patients (or their parents or legal guardians, as appropriate, in regard to the patient) of potential benefits and possible risks to themselves and the embryo, fetus, or neonate. Collaboration with the patient's obstetrician is indicated.

See also individual phenothiazine monographs

Women who are breast-feeding: Safety and efficacy of phenothiazine pharmacotherapy for women who are breast-feeding and their neonates and infants have not been established. Phenothiazines are excreted in breast milk. Avoid prescribing phenothiazine pharmacotherapy to women who are breast-feeding. If phenothiazine pharmacotherapy is required, breast-feeding probably should be discontinued. Collaboration with the patient's pediatrician is indicated.

Elderly, frail, or debilitated patients: Generally prescribe lower dosages for elderly, frail, or debilitated patients. Increase the dosage gradually, if needed, according to individual patient response. These patients may be more sensitive to the pharmacologic actions of phenothiazines than are younger or healthier adult patients.

Children: Safety and efficacy of phenothiazine pharmacotherapy for the symptomatic management of schizophrenia and other psychotic disorders among children generally have not been established. Phenothiazine pharmacotherapy is *not* recommended for this age group except where specific dosages have been established for children.

See individual phenothiazine monographs

Notes, Schizophrenia and Other Psychotic Disorders

Intramuscular phenothiazine pharmacotherapy has been significantly associated with hypotension, which may be severe enough to cause fainting (syncope) and, rarely, cardiac arrest. Patients should be lying down for intramuscular pharmacotherapy and should remain lying down for at least 30 to 60 minutes following intramuscular pharmacotherapy. They also should be appropriately monitored during this period of time for any ADRs. Each dose of the phenothiazine injectable should be deeply and slowly injected into a large healthy muscle site (e.g., the dorsogluteal site). When more than one injection is required, injection sites should be rotated to avoid associated tissue irritation and damage.

Initiating Phenothiazine Pharmacotherapy *Before* initiating phenothiazine pharmacotherapy, ensure that an accurate diagnosis of the psychotic or behavioral disorder has been properly made and documented. Depending upon the clinical situation, also assure for patients and their parents or legal guardians, as appropriate, that the following are completed as soon as possible:

- assess the patient's perception of his or her mental disorder and the need for adjunctive phenothiazine pharmacotherapy. Include as part of the psychological assessment a family history of mental disorders. Ascertain the presence of any current or active medical disorders (e.g., diabetes mellitus, Wilson's disease), or a history of such disorders, and identify any related pharmacotherapy for their medical management. Note particularly any pharmacotherapy (e.g., CNS stimulant or corticosteroid pharmacotherapy) that has been associated with mimicking the signs and symptoms of psychotic disorders. Also identify any problematic patterns of abusable psychotropic use, including any heavy alcohol, amphetamine, or cocaine use during the previous week. The use of alcohol, amphetamines, and cocaine has been associated with drug-induced psychosis, the signs and symptoms of which may mimic schizophrenia and other psychotic disorders.
- note any previous phenothiazine or other antipsychotic pharmacotherapy and the patient's general response.
- identify possible hypersensitivity to phenothiazines and other potential contraindications and cautions that may require consideration when prescribing phenothiazine pharmacotherapy.
- assess the patient's abilities to manage his or her phenothiazine pharmacotherapy.
- ensure civil liberties in relation to the following:

  - obtain the patient's (or parent's or legal guardian's) informed consent for phenothiazine pharmacotherapy. Patients, commensurate with their intelligence and mental status, and their parents or legal guardians, require an understanding of the benefits (i.e., management of the mental disorder) and risks (e.g., TD, NMS) associated with phenothiazine pharmacotherapy.
  - address patient refusal of pharmacotherapy. Phenothiazine pharmacotherapy should be prescribed for these patients in accordance with provincial and state mental health acts and professional standards of practice. Some patients may require supervised administration of their phenothiazine pharmacotherapy to help ensure that oral doses are swallowed. Such patients may require alternative approaches to drug administration (e.g., contracting) or the prescription of dosage forms (e.g., intramuscular) that will prevent them from "cheeking" or "hoarding" their phenothiazine tablets or spitting out liquid doses until their psychotic disorder is better managed.

- ensure that patients (or their parents or legal guardians) have an understanding of the planned pharmacotherapy and any adjunctive psychotherapy or other related therapy. For example, they should know that a low dosage of the phenothiazine will be initially prescribed and gradually increased until therapeutic benefit is achieved. They should know that it may take several days, weeks, or months before optimal therapeutic benefit is fully achieved. They also should understand that during this time, they will be monitored for common ADRs, such as constipation, dry mouth, and urinary retention, and that they will be helped to manage these ADRs. Any questions that patients or their parents or legal guardians may have regarding phenothiazine pharmacotherapy should be answered honestly.
- ensure that they know the exact name of the required phenothiazine. They also should know its general action, dosage and administration, and storage requirements. They should be aware of associated contraindications and cautions. In addition, they should know how to monitor for therapeutic benefit and identify and manage common ADRs.

They should know the signs and symptoms of toxicity and know when it may be necessary to contact the prescribing psychologist immediately.

- advise patients and their parents or legal guardians, as appropriate, that many of the ADRs associated with phenothiazine pharmacotherapy usually diminish over the first few weeks of pharmacotherapy and that these ADRs do not necessarily mean that the patient has a more severe mental disorder or has relapsed. They should be encouraged to continue phenothiazine pharmacotherapy despite mild ADRs and be assisted with the management of these ADRs. More troublesome ADRs may require a reduction of the dosage, other concurrent pharmacotherapy (e.g., anti-parkinsonian pharmacotherapy), or changes in dosage schedule (e.g., ingesting oral dosage forms before retiring for bed in the evening). Explore these and other possible countermeasures (see following discussion) with patients, as needed.
- ensure that patients understand that if ADRs occur, they can, for the most part, be treated quickly. It is important to acknowledge how annoying and uncomfortable ADRs can be. Patients should be encouraged to discuss their feelings about ADRs and assist with their management. Special attention should be given to the management of common mild ADRs because the inability to manage or tolerate ADRs is often a major reason for patients to discontinue phenothiazine pharmacotherapy. For patients who want to discontinue their phenothiazine pharmacotherapy because of associated ADRs, it is often helpful to weigh with them and their parents or legal guardians, as appropriate, the discontinuation of pharmacotherapy with expected or actual benefits and the risk for the return of psychotic signs and symptoms.
- assist patients to manage common or troublesome ADRs, such as constipation, contact dermatitis, dry mouth, photosensitivity reactions, urinary retention, and weight gain, by suggesting that patients do the following:

Constipation:

- drink adequate liquids and eat dietary bulk.
- maintain an individualized activity pattern.
- monitor their daily intake of water and other beverages and the amount and color of their urine.

Contact dermatitis: avoid direct skin contact with the oral solution because of associated contact dermatitis.

Dry mouth:

- frequently rinse their mouths with warm water throughout the day.
- chew sugarless gum, or suck on sugarless hard candy (sugarless gum and candy cause less chance of associated oral monilial infections).
- brush their teeth at least twice a day with a soft toothbrush.

Photosensitivity reactions: use sunscreens, wear protective clothing, and avoid prolonged exposure to direct sunlight because of associated photosensitivity reactions.

Urinary retention: monitor their daily intake of water and other beverages and the amount and color of their urine. This is particularly important for elderly men who have histories of prostatic hypertrophy.

Weight gain:

- follow a balanced diet and exercise program to maintain their normal weight.
- monitor their daily caloric intake.
- eat nutritious low-calorie snack foods. Collaboration with the patient's advanced practice nurse or a nutritional consultant may be required.

- provide realistic information regarding phenothiazine pharmacotherapy. Patients and their parents or legal guardians, as appropriate, should have a realistic view of what to expect in relation to phenothiazine pharmacotherapy. They should understand that phenothiazine pharmacotherapy will not solve all of the patient's problems but will help him or her to be better able to work on the problems. They should understand that phenothiazine pharmacotherapy will not improve judgment, poor socialization, and interpersonal skills or change the patient's personality. However, they can expect that adjunctive phenothiazine pharmacotherapy will help the patient to better focus his or her thoughts, concentrate on a wider range of topics, and control hallucinations or other troublesome signs and symptoms of psychosis or severe behavior disorders.
- clarify misconceptions. Patients and their parents or legal guardians, as appropriate, should be aware that phenothiazine antipsychotics are not addicting or habituating. They should also be aware that high dosages do not necessarily indicate a more serious mental disorder. Dosage selection depends on several factors, such as age, gender, weight, metabolism, and response to previous antipsychotic pharmacotherapy. Patients and their parents or legal guardians, as appropriate, should recognize that concurrent participation in other rehabilitative activities and the maintenance of regular appointments with the clinical psychologist are important adjuncts for the symptomatic management of the psychotic or behavioral disorder. Patients and their parents or legal guardians, as appropriate, should be encouraged to ask questions about the individualized therapeutic plan as active consumers of comprehensive psychologic services. They also should be directed to available support groups for additional help.
- involve patients and their parents or legal guardians, as appropriate, in treatment planning, whenever possible. Provide them with frequent evaluations of the patient's progress.
- monitor individual clinical response until the maintenance dosage is stabilized. Observe for signs and symptoms of therapeutic benefit and ADRs, including over-sedation. In addition, avoid concurrent use of interacting drugs. Elderly, frail, or debilitated patients or those who have histories of chronic alcoholism may be particularly sensitive to postural (orthostatic) hypotension and the sedative action associated with the phenothiazines. Excessive sedation among these patients may result in falls and related injuries (e.g., fractured femur). Assure safety precautions (e.g., supervised ambulation, supervised cigarette smoking) are implemented, as needed, for these patients.

Maintaining Phenothiazine Pharmacotherapy   Monitor for continued therapeutic benefit. Therapeutic benefit associated with phenothiazine pharmacotherapy is characterized by improvement in disordered thought; calming or emotional quieting; and decreased hallucinations, paranoid ideation, or other troublesome signs and symptoms (e.g., combativeness).

Continue to monitor for ADRs, particularly those associated with long-term phenothiazine pharmacotherapy (e.g., agranulocytosis; EPRs, including TD; and the NMS) (see also Adverse Drug Reactions)

Discontinuing Phenothiazine Pharmacotherapy   See Cautions and Comments

AVAILABLE DOSAGE FORMS, STORAGE, AND COMPATIBILITY

A variety of oral and injectable formulations are available for individualizing phenothiazine pharmacotherapy.

See individual phenothiazine monographs

Notes

A slight yellowish discoloration of injectable formulations or oral solutions does *not* indicate that an associated loss or change in efficacy or potency has occurred. However, formulations that are significantly discolored or that contain a precipitate should not be used. Return these products to the dispensing pharmacy or manufacturer for safe and appropriate disposal. Avoid skin contact with phenothiazine oral solutions or injectables because these formulations can be irritating to the skin and may cause contact dermatitis (occurs rarely).

General Instructions for Patients   Instruct patients who require phenothiazine pharmacotherapy (or their parents or legal guardians in regard to the patient, as appropriate) to

- ingest each phenothiazine oral dose with food or a glassful (60 to 120 ml) of water to prevent associated stomach upset.
- avoid skin contact with phenothiazine oral solutions because they can be irritating to the skin and may cause contact dermatitis (occurs rarely).
- safely store phenothiazine formulations in tightly closed child- and light-resistant containers at controlled room temperature (15° to 30°C; 59° to 86°F) out of the reach of children.
- obtain an available patient information sheet regarding phenothiazine pharmacotherapy from their pharmacist at the time that their prescription is dispensed. Encourage patients to clarify any questions that they may have concerning phenothiazine pharmacotherapy with their pharmacist or, if needed, to consult their prescribing psychologist.

PROPOSED MECHANISM OF ACTION

The exact mechanism of action of the phenothiazines is complex and has not yet been fully determined. Their antipsychotic activity appears to be primarily related to an interaction with dopamine-containing neurons, specifically the blockade of dopamine receptors (D1 and D2) both pre- and post-synaptically. The D2 receptor interaction appears to be more significant. The D2 receptor activation suppresses the synthesis of dopamine by diminishing the phosphorylation of tyrosine hydroxylase (i.e., the enzyme that stimulates the conversion [oxidation] of the amino acid tyrosine to dopa, which is the immediate precursor of dopamine [dopa is decarboxylated to dopamine]). Tyrosine hydroxylase is the rate-limiting enzyme for the entire intra-neuronal process of conversion of tyrosine to dopa to dopamine. Initially, upon blockade of the D2 receptors by the phenothiazines, the dopamine neurons activate and release increased amounts of dopamine. However, upon continued D2 receptor blockade, the dopamine neurons down-regulate (i.e., enter a state of depolarized inactivation during which production and release of dopamine are significantly reduced).

The phenothiazines also have other actions. They appear to inhibit vomiting primarily by directly affecting the medullary CTZ. The blockade of D2 receptors in the anterior pituitary is thought to be responsible for the increase in prolactin secretion associated with phenothiazine pharmacotherapy. Pharmacologic actions mediated through the autonomic nervous system vary among the phenothiazines and include α-adrenergic receptor and muscarinic blockade. The α-adrenergic receptor blockade can block the pressor effects of norepinephrine and cause hypotension. The muscarinic cholinergic blocking action that produces the anticholinergic reactions often associated with phenothiazine pharmacotherapy occurs with a much higher incidence among the aliphatic phenothiazines (e.g., chlorpromazine, methotrimeprazine, promazine, and triflupromazine) and piperidine phenothiazines (e.g., mesoridazine, pericyazine, and thioridazine) than among the piperazine phenothiazines (e.g., acetophenazine, fluphenazine, perphenazine, prochlorperazine, thioproperazine, and trifluoperazine).

PHARMACOKINETICS/PHARMACODYNAMICS

The phenothiazines generally are erratically and poorly absorbed following oral ingestion but are well absorbed following intramuscular injection. Some (e.g., chlorpromazine) undergo enterohepatic recirculation. The phenothiazines are highly plasma protein-bound. They also are highly lipophilic and are, thus, distributed into most body fluids and tissues, including the fetal circulation and breast milk. They are metabolized extensively in the liver and are excreted primarily as inactive metabolites in the urine.

See individual phenothiazine monographs

RELATIVE CONTRAINDICATIONS

Blood disorders or bone marrow suppression

Cerebral atherosclerosis (severe) or subcortical brain damage, suspected or established, with or without hypothalamic damage. Hyperthermic reactions with body temperatures above 40°C (104°F) have been associated with phenothiazine pharmacotherapy among these patients. These hyperthermic reactions may not occur for 14 to 16 hours after the initiation of phenothiazine pharmacotherapy.

Coma

CNS depression, severe

Hypersensitivity to the phenothiazines

Hypnotic pharmacotherapy, concurrent high dosage. Concurrent phenothiazine pharmacotherapy for patients who are receiving hypnotic pharmacotherapy is contraindicated because of the potential for additive CNS depression.

Liver dysfunction, severe

Metrizamide (Amipaque® contrast media), concurrent use or use within 48 hours (see Clinically Significant Drug Interactions)

CAUTIONS AND COMMENTS

Phenothiazine pharmacotherapy generally is not associated with the development of addiction and habituation. However, dizziness, gastritis, nausea, tremulousness, and vomiting have been reported upon abrupt discontinuation of long-term high-dosage pharmacotherapy. These signs and symptoms can be reduced among patients who are concurrently receiving anti-parkinsonian pharmacotherapy by continuing the anti-parkinsonian pharmacotherapy for several weeks after discontinuing the phenothiazine pharmacotherapy.

Prescribe phenothiazine pharmacotherapy cautiously to patients who

- are exposed to extreme changes in environmental temperature. Phenothiazines depress the hypothalamic control mechanisms for body temperature regulation. Thus, patients exposed to extremes in temperature (i.e., hot or cold climatic or environmental conditions) have increased vulnerability for hypothermia or hyperthermia. Patients should be advised of this potential risk and encouraged to take appropriate precautions (e.g., avoiding extreme environmental temperatures, dressing appropriately for environmental temperature changes).

- have histories of brain damage or seizure disorders. Sudden unexpected and unexplained deaths have been reported among hospitalized patients who were receiving phenothiazine pharmacotherapy. A history of brain damage or seizure disorders may be a predisposing factor. The phenothiazines lower the seizure threshold and, therefore, place patients who have seizure disorders at additional risk. Phenothiazines have the potential to cause seizures in approximately 1% to 2% of patients. Avoid prescribing high-dosage phenothiazine pharmacotherapy for these patients. If phenothiazine pharmacotherapy is unavoidable, cautiously prescribe phenothiazines, particularly long-acting injectable formulations (e.g., fluphenazine decanoate and pipotiazine palmitate), for patients who have histories of seizure disorders. Phenothiazine pharmacotherapy should not be initiated unless these patients are receiving appropriate anticonvulsant pharmacotherapy. Monitor these patients carefully and ensure that adequate anticonvulsant pharmacotherapy is maintained. Collaboration with the prescriber of the anticonvulsant (i.e., the patient's family physician or neurologist) is indicated.
- have histories of breast cancer. Phenothiazines elevate blood prolactin levels (see Adverse Drug Reactions, Metabolic/Endocrine). Approximately one-third of human breast cancers are prolactin dependent. Clozapine (see Clozapine Monograph), an atypical antipsychotic, causes significantly less of an elevation of blood prolactin levels than do the phenothiazines and may be an appropriate alternative for women who require antipsychotic pharmacotherapy and have a history of breast cancer. Collaboration with the patient's oncologist is indicated.
- have histories of severe cardiovascular disorders. Hypotension, including postural (orthostatic) hypotension, has been associated with phenothiazine pharmacotherapy. Referral of the patient to his or her family physician or specialist (e.g., cardiologist) for appropriate medical evaluation and management is indicated. If hypotension occurs and a vasopressor is required, norepinephrine (Levophed®) or phenylephrine (Neo-Synephrine®) is usually recommended. Epinephrine should *not* be used because the phenothiazines cause a reversal of epinephrine's vasopressor action. This action may result in a further lowering of blood pressure.
- require elective surgery. Patients who are receiving phenothiazine pharmacotherapy may be at increased risk for excessive hypotension during surgery because of the hypotensive actions associated with the phenothiazines. In addition, patients who are receiving high-dosage phenothiazine pharmacotherapy when undergoing surgery may require a reduction in the amount of anesthetics or other CNS depressants because of possible additive CNS depression. Advise patients to inform their anesthesiologist and surgeon that they are receiving phenothiazine pharmacotherapy. Collaboration with the patient's surgeon or anesthesiologist is indicated.

Caution patients who require phenothiazine pharmacotherapy against

performing activities that require alertness, judgment, and physical coordination (e.g., driving an automobile, operating dangerous equipment, supervising children) until their response to phenothiazine pharmacotherapy is known. Phenothiazines may adversely affect these mental and physical functions because of their sedative actions.

In addition to these general precautions, caution patients to

- understand that phenothiazine pharmacotherapy is associated with the development of TD. Advise all patients for whom long-term high-dosage pharmacotherapy is required of this potentially serious and irreversible ADR. The decision to inform patients, or their parents or legal guardians, must take into account the clinical circumstances and the competency of the patient to understand the information provided. Assure civil liberties appropriately for these, and all other, patients.

- inform their prescribing psychologist if they begin or discontinue any other pharmacotherapy while receiving phenothiazine pharmacotherapy.
- carry a card for emergency use, indicating that they are receiving phenothiazine pharmacotherapy and other relevant information (e.g., the name and telephone number of the prescribing psychologist and the family member to call in the event of an accident).
- inform their advanced practice nurse, dentist, family physician, and other prescribers that they are receiving phenothiazine pharmacotherapy.

CLINICALLY SIGNIFICANT DRUG INTERACTIONS

Concurrent phenothiazine pharmacotherapy and the following may result in clinically significant drug interactions:

Alcohol Use

Concurrent alcohol use may increase the CNS depressant action of the phenothiazines. Advise patients to avoid, or limit, their use of alcohol while receiving phenothiazine pharmacotherapy.

Guanethidine Pharmacotherapy

Phenothiazines can antagonize the antihypertensive action of guanethidine (Ismelin®) by competitively inhibiting its uptake and that of norepinephrine into the adrenergic neuron. If an antihypertensive is needed by a patient stabilized on phenothiazine pharmacotherapy, it is recommended that an antihypertensive (e.g., methyldopa [Aldomet®]) that does not significantly interact with the phenothiazines be prescribed. Collaboration with the prescriber of the guanethidine pharmacotherapy is required. Conversely, when an antipsychotic is required by a patient stabilized on guanethidine, the prescription of a non-interacting antipsychotic (e.g., a butyrophenone or an atypical antipsychotic) may be prudent. Collaboration with the prescriber of the guanethidine is indicated.

Lithium Pharmacotherapy

Concurrent phenothiazine and lithium pharmacotherapy, particularly when lithium blood concentrations are in the high range, has occasionally resulted in an acute encephalopathic or extrapyramidal syndrome. Signs and symptoms of this syndrome include dyskinesias, Parkinsonism, and irreversible brain damage. If any signs and symptoms of this syndrome are noted, discontinue phenothiazine pharmacotherapy immediately, and refer the patient for emergency medical evaluation and confirmation of the syndrome, which requires appropriate medical management.

Metrizamide Contrast Media

The use of metrizamide (Amipaque®), a radiopaque contrast media, for patients who are receiving phenothiazine pharmacotherapy may result in an increased incidence of seizures. The use of metrizamide is contraindicated among these patients. Metrizamide can induce seizures, and the phenothiazines lower the seizure threshold.

Pharmacotherapy With Central Nervous System Depressants and Other Drugs That Produce Central Nervous System Depression

Concurrent phenothiazine pharmacotherapy with opiate analgesics, sedative-hypnotics, or other drugs that produce CNS depression (e.g., antihistamines, TCAs) may result in additive CNS depression.

Tobacco Smoking

Smoking a package or more of tobacco cigarettes daily can induce the hepatic microsomal enzyme metabolism of the phenothiazines. Thus, patients who are smokers generally require a significantly higher dosage of phenothiazines than do non-smokers. The effects of smoking on phenothiazine metabolism may continue for a month or longer after smoking has been discontinued.

See also individual phenothiazine monographs

ADVERSE DRUG REACTIONS

Phenothiazine pharmacotherapy has been associated with the following ADRs, listed according to body systems. Most of these ADRs can usually be managed by reducing the dosage or temporarily discontinuing phenothiazine pharmacotherapy. However, severe ADRs, including EPRs, TD, and NMS, require collaborative diagnosis and management with the patient's family physician. The NMS requires immediate medical attention. The occurrence of these ADRs is difficult to predict among patients who require phenothiazine pharmacotherapy. Therefore, monitor all patients carefully who are receiving phenothiazine pharmacotherapy.

Cardiovascular

Alterations in ECG tracings (usually, nonspecific reversible Q- and T-wave changes), postural (orthostatic) hypotension, tachycardia, and, rarely, hypotension severe enough to cause fatal cardiac arrest. These ADRs are particularly associated with injectable phenothiazine pharmacotherapy. In addition, patients who have pheochromocytoma, cerebral vascular insufficiency, kidney dysfunction, or severe cardiac reserve deficiency (e.g., mitral insufficiency) appear to be at risk for hypotensive reactions associated with phenothiazine pharmacotherapy. Monitor these patients closely. In the event of severe hypotension, emergency symptomatic medical support of body systems is required with attention to stabilizing blood pressure. An intravenous vasopressor may be required (see Usual Dosage and Administration, Notes). However, for most patients, tolerance to the hypotensive action of the phenothiazines generally develops with continued pharmacotherapy.

Central Nervous System

Agitation, anxiety, bizarre dreams, cerebral edema, changes in sex drive (increase or decrease), depression, drowsiness, EEG tracing changes, excitement, headache, insomnia, restlessness, and seizures. Phenothiazine pharmacotherapy commonly is associated with EPRs, which may include TD and NMS.

Extrapyramidal Reactions EPRs include acute dystonia, akathisia, Parkinsonism, and other signs and symptoms (see table, Phenothiazine-induced extrapyramidal reactions, below). EPRs appear to be mediated by the blockade of the central dopaminergic neurons involved in motor function. Most often, these EPRs are reversible upon dosage reduction or discontinuation of phenothiazine pharmacotherapy. However, they may be persistent.

The frequency and severity of EPRs are related partly to the chemical structure of the phenothiazine and its dosage form. For example, a higher incidence may be associated with fluphenazine decanoate or enanthate formulations than with less potent chlorpromazine formulations. However, individual patient sensitivity, dosage, and patient age may be other factors. EPRs may be alarming. Thus, patients should be forewarned of their possible occurrence. The EPRs can usually be managed with a reduction in dosage or concurrent anti-parkinsonian pharmacotherapy (e.g., benztropine [Cogentin®] or trihexyphenidyl [Artane®] pharmacotherapy).

Phenothiazine-induced extrapyramidal reactions.

EPR	Usual period of maximal risk	Characteristics and comments
Acute dystonia	Upon initiation of phenothiazine pharmacotherapy, particularly during the first week (days 1 to 7).	Muscular contractions (spasms) causing twisting and repetitive movements. Muscles of the head (i.e., face and tongue), neck, and back generally are affected and may occur as facial grimacing, oculogyric crisis, or torticollis. These spasms may resemble or be confused with seizure activity. Acute dystonia generally occurs with the highest incidence with fluphenazine, perphenazine, trifluoperazine, and thioproperazine pharmacotherapy.
Akathisia	After the first week of pharmacotherapy, particularly during the first two months (days 7 to 60).	Motor restlessness with a strong compulsion to be in a state of constant movement (e.g., fidgeting, pacing, and swinging of the foot and leg). May resemble and be confused with agitation and anxiety. The highest incidence of akathisia generally occurs with fluphenazine, mesoridazine, perphenazine, trifluoperazine, and thioproperazine pharmacotherapy.
Parkinsonism	After the first week of pharmacotherapy, particularly during the first month (days 7 to 30).	Phenothiazine-induced Parkinsonism is virtually indistinguishable from idiopathic Parkinsonism. Idiopathic Parkinsonism generally is associated with a significant decrease in the number of dopamine-containing neurons in the substantia nigra region of the CNS. It has been referred to as a paralysis agitans and shaking palsy characterized by a festinating gait; fine, slowly spreading tremor; and muscular rigidity and weakness. A flat facial expression and slowed or reduced psychomotor activity may resemble and be confused with depression. The highest incidence occurs generally with fluphenazine, perphenazine, pipotiazine, thioproperazine, and trifluoperazine pharmacotherapy.

Tardive Dyskinesia　TD is a syndrome of abnormal involuntary movements. This syndrome generally occurs among predisposed patients after months or years of continuous phenothiazine pharmacotherapy, or upon discontinuation of pharmacotherapy, particularly long-term pharmacotherapy. It has also been associated with other antipsychotic pharmacotherapy. The exact mechanism by which TD occurs is unknown. Dopamine dysfunction is thought to be a related cause. Although it may be a necessary factor, it is not sufficient to explain this troublesome syndrome.

SIGNS AND SYMPTOMS　There is wide variation in the severity of the signs and symptoms of TD. These signs and symptoms generally include involuntary choreoathetoid; repetitive, purposeless hyperkinetic movements involving the face, jaw, lips, mouth, or tongue (e.g., puffing of the cheeks, chewing movements, puckering of the mouth, protrusion of the tongue), trunk, and extremities. The prevalence of TD varies. When the mildest signs and symptoms are included, prevalence can be as high as 70%. For severe signs and symptoms, the rates are generally 2.5%. The frequency and severity of TD increase with age, and TD is more common among women, particularly those who are elderly and require high-dosage phenothiazine pharmacotherapy.

TREATMENT　There is no known effective treatment for TD. For some patients, the syndrome may remit, partially or completely, when phenothiazine pharmacotherapy is discontinued. For other patients, the signs and symptoms of TD may occur upon the discontinuation of pharmacotherapy. Phenothiazine pharmacotherapy itself may suppress the signs and symptoms of this syndrome and, thus, mask its underlying effects.

PREVENTION　Prescribe phenothiazine and other antipsychotic pharmacotherapy with attention to minimizing the occurrence of TD. Prescribe the lowest dosage and the shortest duration of pharmacotherapy for patients who require long-term phenothiazine pharmacotherapy. Monitor patients regularly for early signs and symptoms of TD. Whenever clinically possible, immediately reduce the dosage of the phenothiazine at the first sign or symptom of TD. The immediate reduction in dosage may help to prevent the further development of the syndrome. Reevaluate at regular intervals the need for continued phenothiazine pharmacotherapy, and discontinue pharmacotherapy immediately if the signs and symptoms of TD are identified. Unfortunately, some patients may require continued phenothiazine pharmacotherapy despite the presence of TD.

Neuroleptic (Antipsychotic) Malignant Syndrome　The NMS is a potentially fatal condition associated with phenothiazine and other antipsychotic pharmacotherapy. It generally occurs after several weeks or months of pharmacotherapy. The signs and symptoms of NMS include drowsiness, hyperpyrexia, lethargy, muscle rigidity, uncharacteristic behavior, and signs and symptoms of autonomic nervous system instability (e.g., cardiac dysrhythmias, such as tachycardia or an irregular pulse; excessive sweating; irregular blood pressure).

The accurate diagnosis of NMS is difficult. Diagnosis requires (1) untreated, or inadequately treated, extrapyramidal signs and symptoms; and (2) a serious medical disorder (e.g., pneumonia, systemic infection). Other signs and symptoms may include anticholinergic toxicity with an elevated CPK enzyme level, drug fever, heat stroke, kidney failure (acute), leukocytosis, and liver dysfunction. A catatonic-like state has been associated with dosages of fluphenazine far exceeding the recommended dosage. Reactivation or aggravation of psychotic signs and symptoms also may occur.

Collaboration with the patient's family physician is required for the medical diagnosis of NMS. The therapeutic management of NMS requires immediate discontinuation of phenothiazine and other nonessential pharmacotherapy and intensive symptomatic medical management and monitoring. There is no general agreement about specific pharmacotherapy for uncomplicated NMS. If antipsychotic pharmacotherapy is required after recovery from NMS, frequent, regular monitoring of patient response is needed because of the possible recurrence of NMS.

Cutaneous

Angioneurotic edema, contact dermatitis (see Available Dosage Forms, Storage, and Compatibility, Notes), eczema, erythema, exfoliative dermatitis, itching, photosensitivity, systemic lupus erythematous-like syndrome, sweating (excessive), and seborrhea. Long-term phenothiazine pharmacotherapy, particularly chlorpromazine pharmacotherapy, has been associated with skin pigmentation and photosensitivity. To prevent photosensitivity reactions, advise patient to avoid direct sun exposure or to wear protective clothing (e.g., hat, long sleeve shirt) to minimize solar erythema.

Gastrointestinal

Constipation, diarrhea (rare), dry mouth, dyspepsia, fecal impaction, loss of appetite (anorexia), nausea, and paralytic ileus. An "oral syndrome" has occasionally been reported and may include cracking of the lips and corners of the mouth, denture stomatitis, diffuse redness of the mucous membranes of the mouth, dryness of the mouth, loosened teeth, pseudomembrane formation throughout the oral cavity, and tongue changes (i.e., bald, beefy, red tongue; black or white, hairy tongue).

Genitourinary

Bladder paralysis and increased urination (see also Metabolic/Endocrine)

Hematologic

Blood disorders, including agranulocytosis, eosinophilia, leukopenia, pancytopenia, and thrombocytopenic or nonthrombocytopenic purpura. Agranulocytosis is the most frequently reported blood disorder. It occurs most commonly among women between the fourth and tenth week of phenothiazine pharmacotherapy. Obtain blood counts at regular intervals, and monitor patients for signs and symptoms of blood disorders. These signs and symptoms include signs and symptoms of upper respiratory infections and soreness of the mouth, gums, and throat. If a decrease in blood counts or other signs and symptoms are noted, refer patients for medical evaluation and confirmation of blood disorders. A confirmatory leukocyte count indicates hematologic cellular depression. In the event of cellular depression, discontinue phenothiazine pharmacotherapy. Other appropriate medical treatment may be required.

Hepatic

Cholestatic jaundice may occur during the first months of phenothiazine pharmacotherapy and appears to be a hypersensitivity reaction. Cholestatic jaundice indicates liver damage and requires the immediate discontinuation of phenothiazine pharmacotherapy. Collaboration with the patient's family physician or a specialist (e.g., internist) is indicated to confirm a diagnosis of cholestatic jaundice. Appropriate medical management is required.

Metabolic/Endocrine

Absent menses (amenorrhea), abnormal lactation (galactorrhea), anorgasmia, breast enlargement among men (gynecomastia), breast pain (mastalgia), impotence, increased appetite, menstrual irregularities, peripheral edema, pregnancy test inaccuracy, and weight gain. Many of these ADRs are related to increased blood prolactin levels. Changes also may occur in glucose utilization characterized by sugar in the urine (glycosuria), high glucose tolerance, and increases or decreases in blood sugar concentration (e.g., hyperglycemia or hypoglycemia, respectively).

Ocular

Blurred vision and glaucoma. Long-term phenothiazine pharmacotherapy has been associated with corneal and lenticular opacities. Pigmentary retinopathy has been associated particularly with long-term thioridazine pharmacotherapy. Monitor patients regularly who are receiving long-term phenothiazine pharmacotherapy for corneal and lenticular opacities. Collaboration with the patient's ophthalmologist is indicated.

Respiratory

Asthma, laryngeal edema, and nasal congestion

Miscellaneous

Anaphylactic reactions, including angioedema, bronchospasm, and spasm of the larynx (laryngospasm) among susceptible patients, and high fever (hyperpyrexia)

OVERDOSAGE

The phenothiazines have a high therapeutic index. Although deaths have been associated with phenothiazine overdosages, particularly among children, they are relatively rare among adults unless alcohol or other drugs have been implicated. Signs and symptoms of phenothiazine overdosage include extensions of the common ADRs associated with phenothiazine pharmacotherapy, such as EPRs, hypotension, and sedation. Phenothiazine overdosage requires emergency symptomatic medical support of body systems with attention to increasing phenothiazine elimination. There is no known antidote.

PHENTERMINE

(fen'ter meen)

TRADE NAMES

Adipex-P®
Banobese®

Fastin®
Ionamin®
Obenix®

CLASSIFICATION

Anorexiant (CNS stimulant, amphetamine-related) (sympathomimetic) (C-IV)

APPROVED INDICATIONS FOR PSYCHOLOGICAL DISORDERS

Adjunctive pharmacotherapy for the short-term (maximum of 12 weeks) symptomatic management of:

Eating Disorders: Exogenous Obesity

USUAL DOSAGE AND ADMINISTRATION

Eating Disorders: Exogenous Obesity

Adults: 24 mg phentermine base regular tablets daily orally in three divided doses 30 minutes before meals. Avoid late evening dosing because of associated insomnia. If preferred, 15 to 30 mg phentermine base extended-release capsules daily orally in a single dose approximately two hours after breakfast. A dosage of 30 mg phentermine base extended-release capsule daily orally is usually adequate to suppress appetite for up to 14 hours.

MAXIMUM: 30 mg phentermine base daily orally or 37.5 mg phentermine hydrochloride daily orally

Women who are, or who may become, pregnant: FDA Pregnancy Category "not established." Safety and efficacy of phentermine pharmacotherapy for women who are pregnant have not been established. Avoid prescribing phentermine pharmacotherapy to women who are pregnant. If phentermine pharmacotherapy is required, advise patients of potential benefits and possible risks to themselves and the embryo, fetus, or neonate. Collaboration with the patient's obstetrician is indicated.

Women who are breast-feeding: Safety and efficacy of phentermine pharmacotherapy for women who are breast-feeding and their neonates and infants have not been established. Avoid prescribing phentermine pharmacotherapy to women who are breast-feeding. If phentermine pharmacotherapy is required, breast-feeding probably should be discontinued. If desired, lactation may be maintained and breast-feeding resumed following the discontinuation of short-term phentermine pharmacotherapy.

Elderly: Safety and efficacy of phentermine pharmacotherapy for elderly patients have not been established. Phentermine pharmacotherapy is *not* recommended for this age group.

Children younger than 12 years of age: Safety and efficacy of phentermine pharmacotherapy for children who are younger than 12 years of age have not been established. Phentermine pharmacotherapy is *not* recommended for this age group.

Notes, Eating Disorders: Exogenous Obesity

Prescribe phentermine pharmacotherapy as a component of a comprehensive weight reduction program that includes medically supervised dietary restrictions (e.g., restrictions in calories and fat), an individualized exercise program, and appropriate psychotherapy. Phentermine pharmacotherapy is only indicated for short-term (maximum of 12 weeks) adjunctive pharmacotherapy. Phentermine reportedly has limited therapeutic effectiveness for this indication. Thus, its use must be weighed against potential risks, including addiction and habituation (see also Adverse Drug Reactions).

Prescribe the lowest effective dosage adjusted to individual patient response for no longer than a few weeks. Abrupt discontinuation following regular long-term use has resulted in fatigue and mental depression. Discontinue phentermine pharmacotherapy gradually for these patients.

AVAILABLE DOSAGE FORMS, STORAGE, AND COMPATIBILITY

Capsules, oral extended-release: 15, 30 mg (phentermine base); 18.5, 37.5 mg (hydrochloride salt)
Tablets, oral: 8 mg (phentermine base), 37.5 mg (hydrochloride salt)

Notes

Note that 37.5 mg of phentermine hydrochloride is equivalent to 30 mg of phentermine base.

General Instructions for Patients   Instruct patients who are receiving phentermine pharmacotherapy to

- swallow whole each dose of the phentermine oral extended-release capsules without breaking, chewing, or crushing. Also instruct them to ingest each dose with an adequate amount of water or compatible liquid chaser (60 to 120 ml).
- safely store phentermine oral tablets or extended-release capsules out of the reach of children in tightly closed child-resistant containers at controlled room temperature (15° to 30°C; 59° to 86°F).
- obtain an available patient information sheet regarding phentermine pharmacotherapy from their pharmacist at the time that their prescription is dispensed. Encourage patients to clarify any questions that they may have concerning phentermine pharmacotherapy with their pharmacist or, if needed, to consult their prescribing psychologist.

PROPOSED MECHANISM OF ACTION

Phentermine is a CNS stimulant sympathomimetic amine pharmacologically similar to the amphetamines. Actions include CNS stimulation and the elevation of blood pressure. Phentermine has been associated with tachyphylaxis and tolerance. Drugs such as phentermine, which are used for the symptomatic management of exogenous obesity, commonly are referred to as anorexiants, anorectics, or anorexigenics. The exact mechanism of phentermine's anorexiant action, including appetite suppression, has not yet been fully determined. However, it appears to be related to direct CNS stimulation.

PHARMACOKINETICS/PHARMACODYNAMICS

Phentermine is well absorbed (~100%) following oral ingestion. Phentermine and its metabolites are excreted by the kidneys. Additional data are unavailable.

RELATIVE CONTRAINDICATIONS

Agitation
Arteriosclerosis, advanced
Cardiovascular disorders, severe, including valvular heart disease
Glaucoma
Hypersensitivity to phentermine or sympathomimetic amines
Hypertension, moderate to severe
Hyperthyroidism
MAOI pharmacotherapy, concurrent or within 14 days. Concurrent pharmacotherapy may result in hypertensive crisis.
Pregnancy
Problematic patterns of amphetamine or other CNS stimulant use, history of

CAUTIONS AND COMMENTS

Phentermine is addicting and habituating. It is chemically and pharmacologically related to the amphetamines, which have high abuse potential. Patients may attempt to increase their dosages to many times those recommended. Monitor patients for problematic patterns of use and for signs and symptoms of phentermine toxicity, including dermatoses (severe), hyperactivity, irritability, insomnia, and personality changes. One of the most serious signs and symptoms of phentermine toxicity is psychosis. Phentermine-induced psychosis is often clinically indistinguishable from schizophrenia. Prescribe short-term pharmacotherapy with the lowest effective dosage and the least amount of phentermine feasible for dispensing at one time. These measures will help to minimize the possible development of problematic patterns of use and prevent associated toxicity.

Phentermine was approved for the short-term symptomatic management of obesity during the 1970s, as was fenfluramine (Pondimin®). Commonly referred to as "phen-fen," the combined use of these two anorexiants became popular during the mid-1990s. Unfortunately, this combination of pharmacotherapy, which was not part of their approved labeling, became associated with serious ADRs among women, including valvular heart disease. In the summer of 1997, the FDA began to issue Public Health Advisory statements regarding the combined use of phentermine and fenfluramine and the associated risk for developing valvular heart disease. In response to a request from the FDA and increasing reports of the occurrence of valvular heart disease among women treated for obesity with this combination of pharmacotherapy, the manufacturer of fenfluramine voluntarily withdrew it from the U.S. market on September 15, 1997 (see Fenfluramine Monograph for additional details).

Prescribe phentermine pharmacotherapy cautiously to patients who

- have hypertension. Phentermine's stimulant action may exacerbate this condition. Collaboration with the patient's family physician or advanced practice nurse is indicated.
- have insulin-dependent diabetes mellitus. Phentermine pharmacotherapy, particularly with caloric restriction and an exercise program, may alter insulin requirements. Collaboration with the patient's family physician or advanced practice nurse is indicated when phentermine is prescribed for these patients.

Caution patients who are receiving phentermine pharmacotherapy against performing activities that require alertness, judgment, and physical coordination (e.g., driving an automobile, operating dangerous equipment, supervising children) until their response to phentermine pharmacotherapy is known.

In addition to this general precaution, caution patients to inform their prescribing psychologist if they begin or discontinue any other pharmacotherapy while receiving phentermine pharmacotherapy.

CLINICALLY SIGNIFICANT DRUG INTERACTIONS

Concurrent phentermine pharmacotherapy and the following may result in clinically significant drug interactions:

Guanethidine Pharmacotherapy

Phentermine may decrease the neuronal uptake of guanethidine (Ismelin®) and, thus, decrease its antihypertensive action. Collaboration with the prescriber of the guanethidine is indicated.

Monoamine Oxidase Inhibitor Pharmacotherapy

Phentermine may interact with MAOIs (e.g., phenelzine, tranylcypromine). This combination of pharmacotherapy, concurrent or within 14 days, may result in hypertensive crisis and, thus, is contraindicated.

See also Amphetamines General Monograph

ADVERSE DRUG REACTIONS

Phentermine pharmacotherapy commonly has been associated with constipation, dry mouth, and insomnia. Other ADRs include the following, listed according to body system:

Cardiovascular: high blood pressure (hypertension), rapid heart beat (tachycardia), or rapid throbbing or fluttering of the heart (palpitations)
CNS: dizziness, euphoria or dysphoria, headache, overstimulation, psychosis, restlessness, and tremor. Addiction and habituation may be associated with long-term pharmacotherapy or regular personal use.
Cutaneous: hives (urticaria)
Genitourinary: changes in sex drive and impotence

GI: diarrhea, nausea, unpleasant taste, and vomiting
Metabolic/Endocrine: see Genitourinary

See also Amphetamines General Monograph

OVERDOSAGE

Signs and symptoms of acute phentermine overdosage include abdominal cramps, assaultiveness, belligerence, circulatory collapse, confusion, diarrhea, dysrhythmias, hallucinations, hypertension or hypotension, hyporeflexia, hyperventilation, nausea, panic, restlessness, tremor, and vomiting. Depression and fatigue usually follow the CNS stimulation. Fatal phentermine overdosage usually terminates in coma and convulsions. Acute phentermine overdosage requires emergency symptomatic medical support of body systems with attention to increasing phentermine elimination. There is no known antidote.

PIMOZIDE

(pi'moe zide)

TRADE NAME

Orap®

CLASSIFICATION

Antipsychotic (diphenylbutylpiperidine derivative)

APPROVED INDICATIONS FOR PSYCHOLOGICAL DISORDERS

Adjunctive pharmacotherapy for the symptomatic management of:

- Tic Disorders: Tourette's Disorder (Gilles de la Tourette's Syndrome). Pimozide pharmacotherapy is indicated for the suppression of associated motor and phonic tics among patients who have failed to respond to standard pharmacotherapy (e.g., haloperidol pharmacotherapy). (Indication FDA but *not* HPB approved)
- Psychotic Disorders: Schizophrenia and Other Psychotic Disorders (Indication HPB but *not* FDA approved)

USUAL DOSAGE AND ADMINISTRATION

Gilles de la Tourette's Syndrome

Adults: Initially, 1 to 2 mg daily orally in two divided doses. Increase the dosage gradually according to individual patient response.

MAXIMUM: 10 mg daily orally

Women who are, or who may become, pregnant: FDA Pregnancy Category C. Safety and efficacy of pimozide pharmacotherapy for women who are pregnant have not been established. Avoid prescribing pimozide pharmacotherapy to women who are pregnant, particularly during the first trimester. If pimozide pharmacotherapy is required, advise patients (or their legal guardians in regard to the patient) of the potential benefits and possible risks to themselves and the embryo, fetus, or neonate. Collaboration with the patient's obstetrician is indicated.

Women who are breast-feeding: Safety and efficacy of pimozide pharmacotherapy for women who are breast-feeding and their neonates and infants have not been established. Avoid prescribing pimozide pharmacotherapy to women who are breast-feeding. If pimozide pharmacotherapy is required, breast-feeding probably should be discontinued. Collaboration with the patient's pediatrician is indicated.

Elderly, frail, or debilitated patients: Initially prescribe lower dosages for elderly, frail, or debilitated patients. Increase the dosage gradually, if needed, according to individual patient response. These patients may be more sensitive to the pharmacologic actions of pimozide than are younger or healthier adult patients. Monitor these patients particularly for hypotension. Pimozide pharmacotherapy has been associated with transient hypotension among elderly, frail, or debilitated patients.

Children younger than 2 years of age: Safety and efficacy of pimozide pharmacotherapy for children younger than 2 years of age have not been established. Pimozide pharmacotherapy is *not* recommended for this age group.

Children 2 years of age and older: Initially, 0.05 mg/kg daily orally, preferably in a single daily dose at bedtime. Increase the dosage gradually according to individual patient response.

MAXIMUM: 0.2 mg/kg daily orally *or* 10 mg daily orally, whichever dosage is the lower.

Notes, Gilles de la Tourette's Syndrome

See Notes, Schizophrenia and Other Psychotic Disorders

Schizophrenia and Other Psychotic Disorders

Adults: Initially, 2 to 4 mg daily orally each morning. Increase the daily dosage weekly by 2 to 4 mg increments until desired therapeutic response is achieved or signs and symptoms of toxicity are observed.

MAINTENANCE: 2 to 12 mg daily orally. Average maintenance dosage is 6 mg daily orally.

MAXIMUM: 20 mg daily orally. Dosages exceeding 20 mg daily are *not* recommended.

Women who are, or who may become, pregnant: FDA Pregnancy Category C. Safety and efficacy of pimozide pharmacotherapy for women who are pregnant have not been established. Avoid prescribing pimozide pharmacotherapy to women who are pregnant, particularly during the first trimester. If pimozide pharmacotherapy is required, advise patients (or their legal guardians in regard to the patient) of the potential benefits and possible risks to themselves and the embryo, fetus, or neonate. Collaboration with the patient's obstetrician is indicated.

Women who are breast-feeding: Safety and efficacy of pimozide pharmacotherapy for women who are breast-feeding and their neonates and infants have not been established. Avoid prescribing pimozide pharmacotherapy for women who are breast-feeding. If pimozide pharmacotherapy is required, breast-feeding should be discontinued. Collaboration with the patient's pediatrician is indicated.

Elderly, frail, or debilitated patients: Initially prescribe lower dosages of pimozide for elderly, frail, or debilitated patients (i.e., 1 to 2 mg daily orally). Increase the dosage gradually according to individual patient response. Monitor these patients for hypotension. Transient hypotension, which may last for several hours following the ingestion of pimozide, has been reported among these patients.

Children: Safety and efficacy of pimozide pharmacotherapy for the symptomatic management of schizophrenia and other psychotic disorders among children have not been established. Pimozide pharmacotherapy is *not* recommended for these indications for this age group.

Notes, Schizophrenia and Other Psychotic Disorders

Adjunctive pimozide pharmacotherapy has been found to be of benefit for the symptomatic management of chronic schizophrenia. Pimozide has little sedative action and can be dosed once daily. A single morning dose is generally recommended for adult patients. Discontinue pimozide pharmacotherapy gradually.

Sudden unexpected deaths have been associated with pimozide pharmacotherapy, particularly among patients who were receiving dosages exceeding 20 mg daily. Prolongation of the QT interval, which predisposes patients to ventricular dysrhythmias, may be a related factor in these deaths. Obtain an ECG before initiating pimozide pharmacotherapy and periodically during pharmacotherapy, especially when the dosage is adjusted upward toward 20 mg daily. Collaboration with the patient's family physician or a cardiologist is indicated. Monitor patients for any repolarization changes, such as prolongation of the QT interval beyond 0.52 seconds among adults, or more than 25% above the patient's baseline, and T-wave or U-wave changes. If repolarization changes are noted, do not increase the dosage further. If possible, decrease the dosage and reevaluate the patient's need for continued pimozide pharmacotherapy.

AVAILABLE DOSAGE FORMS, STORAGE, AND COMPATIBILITY

Tablets, oral: 2, 4, 10 mg

Notes

Some pimozide oral tablets contain tartrazine (FD&C Yellow No. 5). Tartrazine has been associated with hypersensitivity reactions, including bronchial asthma, among susceptible patients, particularly those who are hypersensitive to aspirin. The 2 mg Orap® tablets do *not* contain tartrazine.

General Instructions for Patients   Instruct patients who are receiving pimozide pharmacotherapy to

- safely store pimozide tablets out of the reach of children in tightly closed light- and child-resistant containers at controlled room temperature (15° to 30°C; 59° to 86°F).
- obtain an available patient information sheet regarding pimozide pharmacotherapy from their pharmacist at the time that their prescription is dispensed. Encourage patients to clarify any questions that they may have concerning pimozide pharmacotherapy with their pharmacist or, if needed, to consult their prescribing psychologist.

PROPOSED MECHANISM OF ACTION

The exact mechanism of pimozide's action is complex and has not yet been fully determined. Its antipsychotic activity appears to be related to its interaction with dopamine-containing neurons, specifically the blockade of dopamine receptors both pre- and post-synaptically. Higher dosages of pimozide affect the intracellular metabolism of norepinephrine. Although not a butyrophenone, pimozide is chemically and pharmacologically similar to haloperidol.

PHARMACOKINETICS/PHARMACODYNAMICS

Pimozide is slowly and variably absorbed (~50%) following oral ingestion and undergoes significant first-pass hepatic metabolism. Peak blood levels occur between 3 and 8 hours and decrease slowly to about 50% within 48 to 72 hours. Pimozide is highly plasma protein-bound (~99%). It has a mean apparent volume of distribution of approximately 25 L/kg. Pimozide is metabolized extensively in the liver. Approximately 50% is excreted in the urine and 20% in the feces, primarily as metabolites. Less than 1% is excreted in the urine in unchanged form. The mean half-life of elimination is approximately 55 hours. There is wide inter-patient variability in regard to pimozide's pharmacokinetic parameters.

RELATIVE CONTRAINDICATIONS

Blood disorders
Cardiac dysrhythmias
CNS depression, severe
Coma
Congenital long QT syndrome or concurrent pharmacotherapy with drugs that may prolong
     the QT interval. Pimozide prolongs the QT interval.
Depression, moderate to severe
Hypersensitivity to pimozide or related compounds
Hypersensitivity to tartrazine (some oral tablets contain tartrazine)
Kidney dysfunction

Liver dysfunction

Macrolide antibiotic pharmacotherapy, concurrent (see Clinically Significant Drug Interactions)

Phenothiazine pharmacotherapy, concurrent (see Clinically Significant Drug Interactions)

Parkinsonism

Schizophrenia, chronic *and associated with agitation, anxiety, and excitement.* Pimozide pharmacotherapy has been found to be ineffective for this clinical situation and should not be prescribed for these patients.

TCA pharmacotherapy, concurrent (see Clinically Significant Drug Interactions)

Tics, simple or drug (e.g., amphetamine, methylphenidate, pemoline) induced. Pimozide pharmacotherapy is only indicated for the symptomatic management of tics specifically associated with Tourette's Disorder (Gilles de la Tourette's syndrome).

CAUTIONS AND COMMENTS

Prescribe pimozide pharmacotherapy cautiously to patients who

- are elderly, frail, or debilitated, or those who have cardiovascular disorders. Pimozide may cause among these patients hypotension, tachycardia, and a prolongation of the QT interval on the ECG. Electrolyte imbalances, particularly hypokalemia, should be considered a risk factor.
- have seizure disorders. Pimozide may decrease the seizure threshold and, thus, increase the risk for seizures among these patients.

Caution patients who are receiving pimozide pharmacotherapy against performing activities that require alertness, judgment, and physical coordination (e.g., driving an automobile, operating dangerous equipment, supervising children) until their response to pimozide is known. Pimozide may affect these mental and physical functions adversely.

In addition to this general precaution, caution patients to obtain an available patient information sheet regarding pimozide pharmacotherapy from their pharmacist at the time that their prescription is dispensed. Encourage patients to clarify any questions that they may have concerning pimozide pharmacotherapy with their pharmacist or, if needed, to consult their prescribing psychologist.

CLINICALLY SIGNIFICANT DRUG INTERACTIONS

Concurrent pimozide pharmacotherapy and the following may result in clinically significant drug interactions:

Macrolide Antibiotic Pharmacotherapy

Concurrent pimozide (Orap®) and macrolide antibiotic pharmacotherapy (e.g., azithromycin [Zithromax®], clarithromycin [Biaxin®], dirithromycin [Dynabac®], erythromycin [E-Mycin®], and troleandomycin [TAO®]) can result in severe cardiac dysrhythmias. Concurrent pimozide and clarithromycin pharmacotherapy has resulted in death. Concurrent pimozide and macrolide antibiotic pharmacotherapy is *contraindicated.*

Phenothiazine Pharmacotherapy

Pimozide (Orap®) prolongs the QT interval of the ECG. The phenothiazines (e.g., chlorpromazine [Largactil®, Thorazine®]) can also prolong the QT interval. Thus, concurrent pharmacotherapy may result in serious risk for significant prolongation of the QT interval (i.e., a cardiac dysrhythmia). Concurrent pimozide and phenothiazine pharmacotherapy is *contraindicated*.

Tricyclic Antidepressant Pharmacotherapy

Pimozide (Orap®) prolongs the QT interval of the electrocardiogram. The TCAs (e.g., desipramine [Norpramin®], imipramine [Tofranil®]) can also prolong the QT interval. Thus, concurrent pharmacotherapy may result in serious risk for significant prolongation of the QT interval (i.e., a cardiac dysrhythmia). Concurrent pimozide and TCA pharmacotherapy is *contraindicated*.

ADVERSE DRUG REACTIONS

A number of ADRs have been associated with phenothiazine antipsychotic pharmacotherapy (see Phenothiazines General Monograph). Although pimozide is a dopaminergic blocker, these ADRs also may occur with pimozide pharmacotherapy because of its chemical and pharmacological similarity to the phenothiazines. The following ADRs, listed according to body system, have been specifically associated with pimozide pharmacotherapy:

Cardiovascular

Rarely, hypotension and, occasionally, hypertension, tachycardia, and fluctuations in blood pressure. Changes in ECG may include prolongation of the QT interval, lowering and inversion of the T-wave, and ST changes. Sudden, unexpected deaths have been associated with pimozide pharmacotherapy at dosages exceeding 20 mg daily. Sudden, unexpected deaths may also be associated with prolongation of the QT interval, which predisposes patients to ventricular dysrhythmias.

Central Nervous System

Commonly causes EPRs, including akathisia, dystonia (particularly torticollis), and Parkinsonism. Long-term pimozide pharmacotherapy has been associated with the development of TD, particularly among elderly patients. The NMS also has been associated with pimozide pharmacotherapy.

Neuroleptic Malignant Syndrome   Monitor for altered mental status, including catatonia, hyperpyrexia, muscle rigidity, and signs and symptoms of ANS instability (e.g., cardiac dysrhythmias, excessive sweating, irregular pulse or blood pressure, and tachycardia). Elevated CPK, myoglobin in the urine (myoglobinuria), which may be associated with rhabdomyolysis (an acute, sometimes fatal medical disorder characterized by destruction of skeletal muscle), and acute renal failure may occur.

Collaboration with the patient's family physician is required to assist with the diagnosis of NMS, which can be difficult. A diagnosis of NMS requires a serious medical disorder (e.g., pneumonia, systemic infection) and untreated (or inadequately treated) EPRs. Anticholinergic toxicity characterized by heat stroke, drug fever, and primary CNS pathology also may substantiate a diagnosis. In the event of NMS, discontinue pimozide pharmacotherapy immediately. Emergency symptomatic medical support of body systems and appropriate medical treatment of related medical disorders are required. If antipsychotic pharmacotherapy is needed after recovery from NMS, reintroduce antipsychotic pharmacotherapy cautiously and monitor patients closely for the reoccurrence of NMS.

Cutaneous

Erythematous rash, hives (urticaria), and, rarely, facial edema

Gastrointestinal

Abdominal cramps or pain, altered taste, constipation, diarrhea, loss of appetite (anorexia), nausea, salivation (excessive), and vomiting

Genitourinary

Urinary incontinence and urinary retention. See also Metabolic/Endocrine.

Metabolic/Endocrine

Abnormal lactation (galactorrhea, mild); impotence; loss of sex drive; menstrual irregularities, including absent or painful menses (amenorrhea, dysmenorrhea, respectively); and weight loss or weight gain (weight loss rather than weight gain has been more commonly observed among patients receiving pimozide pharmacotherapy).

Ocular

Accommodation difficulty, blurred vision, cataracts, and sensitivity to light

OVERDOSAGE

The signs and symptoms of pimozide overdosage generally are exaggerations of its known pharmacologic actions. The most prominent of these signs and symptoms are ECG abnormalities, severe EPRs, hypotension, and coma with respiratory depression. Pimozide overdosage requires emergency symptomatic medical support of body systems with attention to increasing pimozide elimination. There is no known antidote. Patients should be medically monitored closely for at least four days following pimozide overdosage because of its long half-life of elimination.

PIPOTIAZINE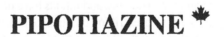

(pip oh tye'a zeen)

TRADE NAME

Piportil L4®

CLASSIFICATION

Antipsychotic (phenothiazine)

See also Phenothiazines General Monograph

APPROVED INDICATIONS FOR PSYCHOLOGICAL DISORDERS

Adjunctive pharmacotherapy for the symptomatic management of:

Psychotic Disorders: Schizophrenia and Other Psychotic Disorders. Pipotiazine, a long-acting depot phenothiazine formulation, has been found to be of particular benefit for patients who have chronic, non-agitated schizophrenia and require long-term maintenance pharmacotherapy.

USUAL DOSAGE AND ADMINISTRATION

Schizophrenia and Other Psychotic Disorders

Adults: Initially, 50 to 100 mg intramuscularly. Increase the dosage by 25 mg every two or three weeks, if needed, to achieve a monthly dosage of 75 to 150 mg.

MAXIMUM: 250 mg monthly intramuscularly

Women who are, or who may become, pregnant: FDA Pregnancy Category "not established." Safety and efficacy of pipotiazine pharmacotherapy for women who are pregnant have not been established (see Phenothiazines General Monograph). Avoid prescribing pipotiazine pharmacotherapy to women who are pregnant. If pipotiazine pharmacotherapy is required, advise patients (or their legal guardians in regard to the patient) of potential benefits and possible risks to themselves and the embryo, fetus, or neonate. Collaboration with the patient's obstetrician is indicated.

Women who are breast-feeding: Safety and efficacy of pipotiazine pharmacotherapy for women who are breast-feeding and their neonates and infants have not been established (see Phenothiazines General Monograph). Avoid prescribing pipotiazine pharmacotherapy to women who are breast-feeding. If pipotiazine pharmacotherapy is required, breast-feeding probably should be discontinued. Collaboration with the patient's pediatrician is indicated.

Elderly, frail, or debilitated patients: Generally prescribe lower dosages of pipotiazine for elderly, frail, or debilitated patients. Increase the dosage gradually, if needed, according to individual patient response. These patients may be more sensitive to the pharmacologic actions of pipotiazine than are younger or healthier adult patients.

Children and adolescents younger than 18 years of age: Safety and efficacy of pipotiazine pharmacotherapy for children and adolescents have not been established. Pipotiazine pharmacotherapy is *not* recommended for this age group.

Notes, Schizophrenia and Other Psychotic Disorders

Pipotiazine, a long-acting depot phenothiazine formulation is indicated for patients who are stabilized on short-acting antipsychotic pharmacotherapy (preferably, phenothiazine pharmacotherapy) and who may benefit from long-acting antipsychotic pharmacotherapy (e.g., patients for whom daily dosing is unsatisfactory). Discontinue the short-acting antipsychotic pharmacotherapy prior to initiating pipotiazine pharmacotherapy.

A single intramuscular injection of pipotiazine generally manages the signs and symptoms of schizophrenia for three to six weeks. Most patients can be satisfactorily dosed once monthly (i.e., every four weeks). Some patients may require lower dosages more frequently (i.e., every three weeks). Pipotiazine intramuscular injections are usually well tolerated and have been associated with few local reactions at the injection site.

A dry, sterile syringe and needle (at least 21-gauge) should be used for intramuscular pharmacotherapy. The use of a wet needle or syringe may cause the solution to become cloudy.

AVAILABLE DOSAGE FORMS, STORAGE, AND COMPATIBILITY

Injectables, intramuscular: 25, 50 mg/ml (in sesame oil)

Notes

The injectable is formulated with sesame oil. Assure that patients do not have a history of hypersensitivity to sesame oil or sesame seeds prior to use.

Store the injectables safely protected from light at room temperature.

PROPOSED MECHANISM OF ACTION

Pipotiazine is a potent phenothiazine antipsychotic with weak sedative activity and a prolonged duration of action. It has a relatively weak propensity for causing hypotension or for potentiating the actions of CNS depressants. The exact mechanism of antipsychotic action for pipotiazine has not been clearly determined. However, its action appears to be similar to that of the other phenothiazines.

See Phenothiazines General Monograph

PHARMACOKINETICS/PHARMACODYNAMICS

Data are unavailable.

RELATIVE CONTRAINDICATIONS

Blood disorders
Circulatory collapse
Coma
Depression, severe
Hypersensitivity to pipotiazine or other phenothiazines
Hypersensitivity to sesame oil or sesame seeds. The injectable is formulated with sesame oil.
Kidney dysfunction, severe
Liver dysfunction, severe
Pheochromocytoma
Subcortical brain damage. A hyperthermic reaction with body temperatures exceeding 40°C (104°F) has been associated with pipotiazine pharmacotherapy among patients who have this medical disorder.

CAUTIONS AND COMMENTS

Caution patients who require pipotiazine pharmacotherapy against performing activities that require alertness, judgment, or physical coordination (e.g., driving an automobile, operating dangerous equipment, supervising children) until their response to pipotiazine is known. Pipotiazine's pharmacologic actions may adversely affect these mental and physical functions.

See also Phenothiazines General Monograph

CLINICALLY SIGNIFICANT DRUG INTERACTIONS

Concurrent pipotiazine pharmacotherapy and the following may result in clinically significant drug interactions:

Alcohol Use

Concurrent alcohol use may increase the CNS depressant action of pipotiazine. Advise patients to avoid, or limit, their use of alcohol while receiving pipotiazine pharmacotherapy.

Pharmacotherapy With Anticholinergics or Other Drugs That Produce Anticholinergic Actions

Concurrent pipotiazine pharmacotherapy with anticholinergics (e.g., atropine) and other drugs that produce anticholinergic actions (e.g., TCAs) may result in additive anticholinergic actions, including paralytic ileus. Paralytic ileus can be fatal, particularly among elderly, frail, or debilitated patients. Avoid, whenever possible, concurrent pharmacotherapy. Collaboration with other prescribers may be indicated.

See also Phenothiazines General Monograph

ADVERSE DRUG REACTIONS

Pipotiazine pharmacotherapy commonly has been associated with EPRs, including akathisia, dyskinesia, dystonia, excessive salivation (sialorrhea), hyperreflexia, oculogyric crisis, opisthotonos, rigidity, and tremor. The EPRs generally occur during the first few days following an injection of pipotiazine. These reactions are often dose-related and tend to resolve with continued pipotiazine pharmacotherapy or with a decrease in dosage. Serious EPRs may be managed with anti-parkinsonian pharmacotherapy. If unresponsive to anti-parkinsonian pharmacotherapy, these EPRs may require the discontinuation of pipotiazine pharmacotherapy. In addition to EPRs, pipotiazine pharmacotherapy has been associated with the following ADRs, listed according to body system:

Cardiovascular: fainting (syncope), hypotension, and tachycardia
CNS: depression, dizziness, drowsiness, fatigue, and insomnia
Cutaneous: hives (urticaria), itching (severe), redness of the skin (erythema), and sweating (excessive)
Genitourinary: excessive urination and urinary incontinence
GI: constipation, dry mouth, loss of appetite, nausea, thirst (excessive), and vomiting
Hepatic: cholestatic jaundice. Cholestatic jaundice may occur during the first few months of pipotiazine pharmacotherapy. The occurrence of cholestatic jaundice requires immediate discontinuation of pipotiazine pharmacotherapy. Collaboration with the patient's family physician or specialist (e.g., internist) is indicated for the confirmation of the diagnosis and its medical management.
Metabolic/Endocrine: breast enlargement among males (gynecomastia), impotence, and menstrual irregularities (see also Genitourinary)
Ocular: nasal congestion
Respiratory: blurred vision

See also Phenothiazines General Monograph

OVERDOSAGE

Signs and symptoms of pipotiazine overdosage resemble those associated with other phenothiazine overdosage. Severe EPRs, hypotension, lethargy, and sedation are most commonly observed. Pipotiazine overdosage requires emergency symptomatic medical support of body systems with attention to increasing pipotiazine elimination. There is no known antidote.

PROCHLORPERAZINE

(proe klor per'a zeen)

TRADE NAMES

Compazine®
Stemetil®

CLASSIFICATION

Antipsychotic (phenothiazine, piperazine derivative)

See also Phenothiazines General Monograph

APPROVED INDICATIONS FOR PSYCHOLOGICAL DISORDERS

Adjunctive pharmacotherapy for the symptomatic management of:

Psychotic Disorders: Schizophrenia and Other Psychotic Disorders. *Note:* Prochlorperazine is rarely prescribed for this indication. It is more commonly prescribed for the medical management of severe nausea and vomiting.

USUAL DOSAGE AND ADMINISTRATION

Schizophrenia and Other Psychotic Disorders

Adults, hospitalized: Initially, 30 to 40 mg daily orally in three or four divided doses. Increase the dosage gradually until the signs and symptoms of psychosis are managed or ADRs occur. The occurrence of ADRs may be minimized by gradually increasing the dosage every two to three days. Although therapeutic benefit generally may be achieved with dosages of 50 to 75 mg daily, some patients may require 100 to 150 mg daily.

Adults, non-hospitalized: Initially, 15 to 20 mg daily orally or rectally in three or four divided doses

Adults, immediate management of severe signs and symptoms of psychoses: Initially, 10 to 20 mg intramuscularly. Repeat the initial dose every one to four hours until the severe signs and symptoms of psychosis have been managed. Inject prochlorperazine deeply into large healthy muscle sites (e.g., dorsogluteal site). Do *not* inject subcutaneously because of associated irritation and pain at the injection site. More than three or four doses rarely are required. Once severe signs and symptoms are managed, replace intramuscular pharmacotherapy with oral pharmacotherapy. Generally prescribe the same or a higher dosage.

Adults, long-term pharmacotherapy: Inject 10 to 20 mg intramuscularly every four to six hours, as needed. Rotate injection sites for each injection. Monitor for pain and irritation at injection sites. For intravenous injection, dilute the injectable formulation with normal saline or dextrose and water for injection to a concentration of 1 mg/ml. Infuse intravenously at a rate of 1 ml/minute. Long-term injectable pharmacotherapy rarely is required for the symptomatic management of psychotic disorders.

Women who are, or who may become, pregnant: FDA Pregnancy Category C. Safety and efficacy of prochlorperazine pharmacotherapy for women who are pregnant have not been established. Numerous studies and case reports tend to indicate that prochlorperazine is not a human teratogen, and, if it is a teratogen, the associated incidence of teratogenesis is extremely low. However, animal studies have demonstrated prochlorperazine to be teratogenic. For this reason, the manufacturer recommends that prochlorperazine *not* be prescribed to women during pregnancy.

Women who are breast-feeding: Safety and efficacy of prochlorperazine pharmacotherapy for women who are breast-feeding and their neonates and infants have not been established. Prochlorperazine pharmacotherapy is not recommended for women who are breast-feeding because there is evidence that phenothiazines are excreted into breast milk. Avoid prescribing prochlorperazine pharmacotherapy to women who are breast-feeding. If prochlorperazine pharmacotherapy is required, breast-feeding probably should be discontinued. Collaboration with the patient's pediatrician is indicated.

Elderly, frail, and debilitated patients: Generally prescribe lower dosages of prochlorperazine for elderly, frail, and debilitated patients. Increase the dosage gradually according to individual patient response. These patients may be more sensitive to the pharmacologic actions of prochlorperazine, including hypotension and neuromuscular reactions, than are younger or healthier adult patients. Closely monitor these patients for these ADRs.

Children, 2 to 12 years of age: Initially, 5 to 7.5 mg daily orally or rectally in two or three divided doses. Do not prescribe more than 10 mg during the first day of pharmacotherapy. Increase the dosage gradually according to individual patient response. If intramuscular prochlorperazine pharmacotherapy is required, calculate each dose on the basis of 0.132 mg/kg body weight. Inject deeply into healthy muscle sites. The signs and symptoms of psychosis generally are managed with one dose. Once the signs and symptoms of psychosis are managed, replace injectable prochlorperazine pharmacotherapy with oral pharmacotherapy. Prescribe the same, or a higher, dosage according to individual patient response.

MAXIMUM: 20 mg daily orally or rectally for children 2 to 5 years of age; 25 mg daily orally or rectally for children 6 to 12 years of age

Notes, Schizophrenia and Other Psychotic Disorders

Prescribe prochlorperazine pharmacotherapy either orally or by deep intramuscular injection for the symptomatic management of schizophrenia and other psychotic disorders. Intravenous and rectal administration generally are reserved for the medical management of nausea and vomiting.

Initiate prochlorperazine pharmacotherapy with the lowest recommended dosage. Note that 5 mg of prochlorperazine base is approximately equivalent to 7.5 mg of prochlorperazine edisylate or 8 mg of prochlorperazine maleate. Adjust dosage to the severity of signs and symptoms and individual patient response. Although therapeutic response may be observed within a few days, long-term pharmacotherapy is usually required before maximal therapeutic benefit is achieved.

AVAILABLE DOSAGE FORMS, STORAGE, AND COMPATIBILITY

Capsules, oral: 10, 15, 30, 75 mg
Capsules, oral extended-release (e.g., Compazine® Spansule): 10, 15, 30 mg
Concentrate, oral: 10 mg/ml
Injectable, intramuscular, intravenous: 5 mg/ml (contains 0.75% alcohol)
Injectable, intramuscular disposable syringe: 5 mg/ml (contains 0.75% alcohol)
Suppositories, rectal: 2.5, 5, 10, 25 mg
Syrup, oral: 1 mg/ml (fruit flavored, Compazine®)
Tablets, oral: 5, 10, 25 mg

Notes

Injectable Formulations   Inspect prochlorperazine injectable formulations before use. Do not use darkly discolored injectable solutions. Return these solutions to the dispensing pharmacy or manufacturer for safe and appropriate disposal.

Do not mix the prochlorperazine injectable with other drugs in the same syringe. Do not dilute contents of Compazine® ampules with any diluent that contains parabens as a preservative because of physical incompatibility.

Compazine® injectable contains sodium bisulfite and sodium sulfite. Sulfites have been associated with hypersensitivity reactions among susceptible patients, particularly those who have a history of asthma. These reactions include life-threatening anaphylaxis or less severe asthmatic episodes.

Store prochlorperazine injectable formulations safely below 30°C (86°F); do not freeze.

Oral Formulations   The prochlorperazine extended-release capsule (Compazine® Spansule) is formulated to release an initial dose promptly and to release the remaining dose over a prolonged period.

General Instructions for Patients   Instruct patients who are receiving prochlorperazine pharmacotherapy, or those involved with their pharmacotherapy, to

- dilute each dose of the prochlorperazine oral concentrate with 60 ml (2 ounces) of compatible beverage just prior to ingestion to increase palatability. If preferred, the oral concentrate may be gently mixed in a small amount of compatible soft food just prior to ingestion.
- avoid getting the oral concentrate in the eyes, on the skin, or on the clothes because it is irritating to the skin and contact dermatitis may result.
- safely store prochlorperazine oral dosage forms out of the reach of children in tightly closed child- and light-resistant containers.
- safely store prochlorperazine rectal suppositories below 30°C (86°F) and out of the reach of children.
- obtain an available patient information sheet regarding prochlorperazine pharmacotherapy from their pharmacist at the time that their prescription is dispensed. Encourage patients to clarify any questions that they may have concerning prochlorperazine pharmacotherapy with their pharmacist or, if needed, to consult their prescribing psychologist.

PROPOSED MECHANISM OF ACTION

The exact mechanism of action of prochlorperazine is complex and has not yet been fully determined. Its antipsychotic activity appears to be related primarily to its interaction with dopamine-containing neurons, specifically the blockade of dopamine receptors both pre- and post-synaptically. It has greater antiemetic and extrapyramidal actions than most phenothiazines. The antiemetic action appears to be related to the blockade of dopamine receptors in the CTZ of the medulla.

See also Phenothiazines General Monograph

PHARMACOKINETICS/PHARMACODYNAMICS

Prochlorperazine appears to be well absorbed following oral ingestion. However, it has limited bioavailability (~15%), probably because of significant first-pass hepatic metabolism. The onset of action of prochlorperazine following oral ingestion generally is within 30 to 40 minutes. The onset of action is more rapid following intramuscular injection (i.e., within 10 to 20 minutes). The duration of action following oral or intramuscular administration is approximately 3 to 4 hours. The extended-release oral capsules have a prolonged duration of action of 10 to 12 hours. The mean apparent volume of distribution is 13 L/kg. Prochlorperazine and its metabolites undergo enterohepatic recirculation and are excreted primarily in the feces. The mean half-life of elimination is approximately 8 hours. The mean total body clearance is ~70 L/hour.

RELATIVE CONTRAINDICATIONS

Blood disorders
Cardiovascular dysfunction, severe
CNS depression, including that associated with CNS depressant pharmacotherapy (e.g., barbiturates, benzodiazepines, opiate analgesics) or the regular personal use of these drugs or alcohol
Circulatory collapse
Coma
Liver dysfunction, severe
Hypersensitivity to prochlorperazine or other phenothiazines
Parkinson's disease
Pregnancy

CAUTIONS AND COMMENTS

Prescribe prochlorperazine pharmacotherapy cautiously to patients who are children and/or are hospitalized for the treatment of psychological disorders. The incidence of EPRs appears to be significantly higher among these patients.

Caution patients who are receiving prochlorperazine pharmacotherapy against performing activities that require alertness, judgment, or physical coordination (e.g., driving an automobile, operating dangerous equipment, supervising children). Prochlorperazine may adversely affect these mental and physical functions, particularly during the first few days of pharmacotherapy.

In addition to this general precaution, caution patients to inform their prescribing psychologist if they begin or discontinue any other pharmacotherapy while receiving prochlorperazine pharmacotherapy.

See also Phenothiazines General Monograph

CLINICALLY SIGNIFICANT DRUG INTERACTIONS

Concurrent prochlorperazine pharmacotherapy and the following may result in clinically significant drug interactions:

Guanethidine Pharmacotherapy

Prochlorperazine may decrease the neuronal uptake of guanethidine (Ismelin®) and, thus, decrease its antihypertensive action. An adjustment in the dosage of the guanethidine may be required. Collaboration with the prescriber of the guanethidine is indicated.

Pharmacotherapy With Anticholinergics or Other Drugs That Produce Anticholinergic Actions

Concurrent prochlorperazine pharmacotherapy with anticholinergics (e.g., atropine) and other drugs that produce anticholinergic actions (e.g., TCAs) may result in additive anticholinergic actions, including paralytic ileus.

ADVERSE DRUG REACTIONS

Prochlorperazine pharmacotherapy has been associated with the following ADRs, listed according to body system:

Cardiovascular: hypotension
CNS: dizziness, drowsiness, and EPRs
Cutaneous: skin reactions
Hematologic: blood disorders, including a reduction in circulating white blood cells (i.e., leukopenia) and a reduction in neutrophils (i.e., agranulocytosis, granulocytopenia, neutropenia), which may result in an increased susceptibility to bacterial and fungal infections. Severe neutropenia may be life-threatening.
Hepatic: cholestatic jaundice
Ocular: blurred vision

See also Phenothiazines General Monograph

OVERDOSAGE

Signs and symptoms of prochlorperazine overdosage are primarily extensions of its pharmacologic actions and include, particularly, EPRs with dystonic reactions. Other signs and symptoms of prochlorperazine overdosage include agitation, anticholinergic actions (e.g., dry mouth, hypotension, paralytic ileus), cardiac dysrhythmias, convulsions, depression with somnolence, fever, and restlessness. Prochlorperazine overdosage requires emergency symptomatic medical support of body systems with attention to increasing prochlorperazine elimination. Emergency medical treatment should be continued for as long as the signs and symptoms of overdosage remain. Signs and symptoms of prochlorperazine overdosage may be prolonged when overdosages involve the ingestion of extended-release formulations (e.g., Compazine® Spansules). There is no known antidote.

PROMAZINE *

(proe'ma zeen)

TRADE NAME

Sparine®

CLASSIFICATION

Antipsychotic (phenothiazine, propylamino derivative)

See also Phenothiazines General Monograph

APPROVED INDICATIONS FOR PSYCHOLOGICAL DISORDERS

Adjunctive pharmacotherapy for the symptomatic management of psychotic disorders:

Schizophrenia and Other Psychotic Disorders

USUAL DOSAGE AND ADMINISTRATION

Schizophrenia and Other Psychotic Disorders

Adults: 40 to 1000 mg daily orally, intramuscularly, or intravenously in four to six divided doses

MAXIMUM: 1000 mg daily

Women who are, or who may become, pregnant: FDA Pregnancy Category C. Safety and efficacy of promazine pharmacotherapy for women who are pregnant have not been established (see Phenothiazines General Monograph). Avoid prescribing promazine pharmacotherapy to women who are pregnant. If promazine pharmacotherapy is required, advise patients (or their legal guardians in regard to the patient) of potential benefits and possible risks to themselves and the embryo, fetus, or neonate. Collaboration with the patient's obstetrician is indicated.

Women who are breast-feeding: Safety and efficacy of promazine pharmacotherapy for women who are breast-feeding and their neonates and infants have not been established (see Phenothiazines General Monograph). Avoid prescribing promazine pharmacotherapy to women who are breast-feeding. If promazine pharmacotherapy is required, breast-feeding probably should be discontinued. Collaboration with the patient's pediatrician is indicated.

Children younger than 12 years of age: Safety and efficacy of promazine pharmacotherapy for children younger than 12 years of age have not been established. Promazine pharmacotherapy is *not* recommended for this age group.

Children and adolescents 12 years of age and older: 40 to 150 mg daily orally in four to six divided doses

Notes, Schizophrenia and Other Psychotic Disorders

The antipsychotic activity of promazine is relatively weak when compared to the other phenothiazines. Therefore, although generally efficacious, promazine is *not* recommended as a drug of first choice for the symptomatic management of psychotic disorders.

Injectable Promazine Pharmacotherapy

INTRAMUSCULAR PHARMACOTHERAPY   Inject intramuscularly deeply into large healthy muscle sites (e.g., dorsogluteal site). Rotate injection sites carefully.

INTRAVENOUS PHARMACOTHERAPY   Intravenous injection should not exceed a concentration of 25 mg/ml. Inject intravenously slowly into the lumen of a large vein. Carefully aspirate before injecting. Avoid intra-arterial injection, which has been associated with arterial spasm. Monitor intravenous injection sites for cellulitis or thrombophlebitis.

AVAILABLE DOSAGE FORMS, STORAGE, AND COMPATIBILITY

Concentrates, oral: 30, 100 mg/ml
Injectables, intramuscular, intravenous: 25, 50 mg/ml
Syrup, oral: 2 mg/ml
Tablets, oral: 10, 25, 50, 100, 200 mg

Notes

Injectable Formulations   Some injectable formulations of promazine contain sodium bisulfite. Sulfites have been associated with hypersensitivity reactions, including anaphylactic reactions, among susceptible patients. Although relatively uncommon, these reactions appear to occur with a higher incidence among patients who have asthma.

Oral Formulations   The promazine oral tablets (e.g., 25 mg Sparine®) may contain tartrazine (FD&C Yellow No. 5). Tartrazine has been associated with hypersensitivity reactions (e.g., bronchial asthma) among susceptible patients, particularly those who have a hypersensitivity to aspirin.

General Instructions for Patients   Instruct patients who are receiving promazine pharmacotherapy to

- dilute each dose of the promazine oral concentrate in a small amount (i.e., 60 to 120 ml) of flavored drink, fruit juice, or milk before ingestion to increase palatability.
- safely store promazine oral dosage forms out of the reach of children in tightly closed child- and light-resistant containers at controlled room temperature (15° to 30°C; 59° to 86°F).
- obtain an available patient information sheet regarding promazine pharmacotherapy from their pharmacist at the time that their prescription is dispensed. Encourage patients to clarify any questions that they may have concerning promazine pharmacotherapy with their pharmacist or, if needed, to consult their prescribing psychologist.

PROPOSED MECHANISM OF ACTION

The exact mechanism of action of promazine is complex and has not yet been fully determined. Its antipsychotic activity appears to be primarily related to its interaction with dopamine-containing neurons, specifically the blockade of dopamine receptors both pre- and post-synaptically. Promazine possesses relatively weak antipsychotic activity and moderate antiemetic activity. It has relatively strong anticholinergic actions.

See also Phenothiazines General Monograph

PHARMACOKINETICS/PHARMACODYNAMICS

Following oral ingestion, the bioavailability of promazine is limited and varies (range 8% to 25%). Additional data are unavailable.

RELATIVE CONTRAINDICATIONS

Blood disorders
Cardiovascular dysfunction, severe
Coma
Liver dysfunction, severe
Hypersensitivity to promazine or other phenothiazines
Parkinson's disease

CAUTIONS AND COMMENTS

Prescribe promazine pharmacotherapy cautiously to patients who have histories of seizure disorders. Promazine may lower the seizure threshold.

Caution patients who are receiving promazine pharmacotherapy against performing activities that require alertness, judgment, and physical coordination (e.g., driving an automobile, operating dangerous equipment, supervising children) until their response to promazine pharmacotherapy is known. Promazine may adversely affect these mental and physical functions.

In addition to this general precaution, caution patients to inform their prescribing psychologist if they begin or discontinue any other pharmacotherapy while receiving promazine pharmacotherapy.

See also Phenothiazines General Monograph

CLINICALLY SIGNIFICANT DRUG INTERACTIONS

Concurrent promazine pharmacotherapy and the following may result in clinically significant drug interactions:

Guanethidine Pharmacotherapy

Promazine may decrease the neuronal uptake of guanethidine (Ismelin®) and, thus, decrease its pharmacologic action. An adjustment in the guanethidine dosage may be required. Collaboration with the prescriber of the guanethidine is indicated.

Pharmacotherapy With Anticholinergics or Other Drugs That Produce Anticholinergic Actions

Concurrent promazine pharmacotherapy and pharmacotherapy with anticholinergics (e.g., atropine) and other drugs that have anticholinergic actions (e.g., TCAs) may result in additive anticholinergic actions, including paralytic ileus.

See also Phenothiazines General Monograph

ADVERSE DRUG REACTIONS

Promazine pharmacotherapy commonly is associated with ADRs due to its anticholinergic actions (e.g., decreased gastrointestinal secretions, drowsiness, dry mouth, and urinary retention). Hypotension is prominent with higher dosages.

See also Phenothiazines General Monograph

OVERDOSAGE

Signs and symptoms of promazine overdosage generally are extensions of its pharmacologic actions. Promazine overdosage requires emergency symptomatic medical support of body systems with attention to increasing promazine elimination. There is no known antidote.

PROPOXYPHENE

(proe pox'i feen)

TRADE NAMES

Darvon®
Darvon-N®
Novo-Propoxyn®

CLASSIFICATION

Opiate analgesic (C-IV)

See also Opiate Analgesics General Monograph

APPROVED INDICATIONS FOR PSYCHOLOGICAL DISORDERS

Adjunctive pharmacotherapy for the symptomatic management of:

- Pain Disorders: Acute Pain, Mild to Moderate
- Pain Disorders: Chronic Cancer Pain, Mild to Moderate

USUAL DOSAGE AND ADMINISTRATION

Acute Pain or Chronic Cancer Pain, Mild to Moderate

Adults: 65 mg (chloride salt) *or* 100 mg (napsylate salt) orally every four hours, as needed

MAXIMUM: 390 mg (chloride salt) daily orally *or* 600 mg (napsylate salt) daily orally

Women who are, or who may become, pregnant: FDA Pregnancy Category C. Safety and efficacy of propoxyphene pharmacotherapy for women who are pregnant have not been established. Various physical malformations (e.g., beaked nose, congenital hip dislocation, micrognathia) and the signs and symptoms of the neonatal opiate analgesic withdrawal syndrome (e.g., irritability, seizures, tremors) have been reported. However, the data are inconclusive (see also the Opiate Analgesics General Monograph). Avoid prescribing propoxyphene pharmacotherapy to women who are pregnant. If propoxyphene pharmacotherapy is required, advise patients of potential benefits and possible risks to themselves and the embryo, fetus, or neonate. Collaboration with the patient's obstetrician is indicated.

Women who are breast-feeding: Safety and efficacy of propoxyphene pharmacotherapy for women who are breast-feeding and their neonates and infants have not been established. Low concentrations of propoxyphene are excreted in breast milk and would appear to be unlikely to affect breast-fed neonates or infants. However, adverse reactions have been noted among breast-fed neonates of mothers who were prescribed propoxyphene during the postpartum period (see also the Opiate Analgesics General Monograph). Avoid prescribing propoxyphene pharmacotherapy to women who are breast-feeding. If propoxyphene pharmacotherapy is required, breast-feeding probably should be discontinued. If desired, lactation may be maintained and breast-feeding resumed following the discontinuation of short-term propoxyphene pharmacotherapy. Collaboration with the patient's pediatrician is indicated.

Children: Safety and efficacy of propoxyphene pharmacotherapy for children have not been established. Propoxyphene pharmacotherapy is *not* recommended for this age group.

AVAILABLE DOSAGE FORMS, STORAGE, AND COMPATIBILITY

Capsules, oral (chloride salt): 32, 65 mg
Suspension, oral (napsylate salt): 10 mg/ml
Tablets, oral (napsylate salt): 50, 100 mg

Notes

General Instructions for Patients   Instruct patients who are receiving propoxyphene pharmacotherapy to

- shake well the propoxyphene oral suspension prior to measuring each dose to assure that an accurate dose is measured.

- safely store propoxyphene oral dosage forms out of the reach of children in tightly closed child-resistant containers.
- obtain an available patient information sheet regarding propoxyphene pharmacotherapy from their pharmacist at the time that their prescription is dispensed. Encourage patients to clarify any questions that they may have concerning propoxyphene pharmacotherapy with their pharmacist or, if needed, to consult their prescribing psychologist.

PROPOSED MECHANISM OF ACTION

Propoxyphene elicits its analgesic, CNS depressant, and respiratory depressant actions primarily by binding to the endorphin receptors in the CNS. The exact mechanism of action has not yet been fully determined.

See also Opiate Analgesics General Monograph

PHARMACOKINETICS/PHARMACODYNAMICS

Propoxyphene is well absorbed following oral ingestion. Peak blood concentrations are achieved within 3 hours. Propoxyphene is metabolized extensively in the liver and excreted almost entirely as metabolites in the urine. The half-life of elimination ranges from 6 to 12 hours. The duration of action generally is 4 to 6 hours. Additional data are unavailable.

RELATIVE CONTRAINDICATIONS TO USE

Addiction and habituation to propoxyphene or other abusable psychotropics, history of
Hypersensitivity to propoxyphene
Ritonavir (Norvir®) pharmacotherapy, concurrent (see Clinically Significant Drug Interactions)
Suicide ideation

CAUTIONS AND COMMENTS

Long-term propoxyphene pharmacotherapy, or regular personal use, has been associated with the development of addiction and, particularly, habituation. Propoxyphene will only partially suppress the opiate analgesic withdrawal syndrome among people who are addicted to opiate analgesics. Therefore, the sudden substitution of propoxyphene pharmacotherapy for other opiate analgesic pharmacotherapy among patients who are addicted to opiate analgesics may result in the opiate analgesic withdrawal syndrome. To avoid precipitating the opiate analgesic withdrawal syndrome, reduce the dosage of the other opiate analgesic gradually prior to initiating propoxyphene pharmacotherapy.

Despite its reputation as being much less addictive than other opiate analgesics (i.e., the abuse liability of propoxyphene is qualitatively similar to that of codeine, although quantitatively less), propoxyphene is an abusable psychotropic. Frequent requests for repeat prescriptions require careful investigation. Propoxyphene has no real advantage over aspirin or acetaminophen for the symptomatic management of mild to moderate pain. Avoid prescribing propoxyphene when pain disorders can be managed by non-opiate analgesics.

Prescribe propoxyphene pharmacotherapy cautiously to patients who

- are receiving pharmacotherapy with other CNS depressants (e.g., opiate analgesics, sedative-hypnotics) or other drugs that produce CNS depression (e.g., antihistamines, phenothiazines, TCAs). Concurrent pharmacotherapy may result in additive CNS depression.
- exhibit depression, suicidal ideation or have attempted suicide, or have histories of problematic patterns of abusable psychotropic use. Avoid, whenever possible, prescribing opiate analgesics to these patients. While some overdosage deaths have been associated with accidental ingestion, many deaths associated with propoxyphene overdosage reportedly involved patients who had previous histories of mental disorders, suicidal ideation or attempted suicide, and problematic patterns of abusable psychotropic use. Prescribe only for dispensing small quantities of propoxyphene, and monitor patient response closely. Reevaluate the need for continued propoxyphene pharmacotherapy carefully.

Caution patients who are receiving propoxyphene pharmacotherapy against

- drinking alcohol while receiving propoxyphene pharmacotherapy. Alcohol can potentiate the CNS depressant actions of propoxyphene and may result in serious CNS depression.
- performing activities that require alertness, judgment, and physical coordination (e.g., driving an automobile, operating dangerous equipment, supervising children). Propoxyphene pharmacotherapy may adversely affect these mental and physical functions.

In addition to these general precautions, caution patients to inform their prescribing psychologist if they begin or discontinue any other pharmacotherapy while receiving propoxyphene pharmacotherapy.

CLINICALLY SIGNIFICANT DRUG INTERACTIONS

Concurrent propoxyphene pharmacotherapy and the following may result in clinically significant drug interactions:

Alcohol Use

Concurrent alcohol use may increase the CNS depressant action of propoxyphene. In addition, alcohol reportedly enhances the bioavailability of propoxyphene by 25%, probably by reducing its first-pass hepatic metabolism. Advise patients to avoid, or limit, their use of alcohol while receiving propoxyphene pharmacotherapy.

Pharmacotherapy With Central Nervous System Depressants and Other Drugs That Produce Central Nervous System Depression

Concurrent propoxyphene pharmacotherapy with other opiate analgesics, sedative-hypnotics, or other drugs that produce CNS depression (e.g., antihistamines, phenothiazines, TCAs) may result in additive CNS depression.

Ritonavir Pharmacotherapy

Ritonavir (Norvir®), an antiretroviral drug indicated for the pharmacologic management of HIV infection, can significantly inhibit the hepatic microsomal enzyme metabolism of propoxyphene. This interaction may result in severe toxicity, including cardiotoxicity and respiratory depression. Concurrent propoxyphene and ritonavir pharmacotherapy is *contraindicated*.

Tobacco Smoking

Concurrent tobacco smoking may increase the metabolism of propoxyphene. Thus, smokers may experience less pain relief than non-smokers when equal dosages of propoxyphene are prescribed. Higher dosages of propoxyphene may be required for patients who smoke tobacco.
See also Opiate Analgesics General Monograph

ADVERSE DRUG REACTIONS

Propoxyphene pharmacotherapy has been associated with dizziness; drowsiness; dysphoria or euphoria; gastrointestinal complaints, including abdominal pain, constipation, nausea, and vomiting; headache; insomnia; light-headedness; paradoxical excitement; sedation; skin rash; and visual disturbances (minor). Long-term pharmacotherapy with dosages exceeding 800 mg daily has been associated with convulsions and toxic psychosis.
See also Opiate Analgesics General Monograph

OVERDOSAGE

Signs and symptoms of propoxyphene overdosage resemble those associated with other opiate analgesic overdosage and include respiratory depression (e.g., decrease in respiratory rate and tidal volume; Cheyne-Stokes respirations), extreme somnolence progressing to stupor or coma, initial contraction of the pupils followed by dilation of the pupils as hypoxia increases, and circulatory collapse (see also Opiate Analgesics General Monograph). In addition to the signs and symptoms of general opiate analgesic overdosage, local and generalized seizures occur in most cases of severe propoxyphene overdosage. Propoxyphene overdosage, alone or in combination with alcohol or other CNS depressants, has resulted in a significant number of overdosage deaths. Fatalities within the first hour of overdosage are common.
Propoxyphene overdosage requires emergency symptomatic medical support of body systems with attention to increasing propoxyphene elimination. The opiate antagonist naloxone (Narcan®) is a specific antidote against the respiratory depression produced by propoxyphene.

PROTRIPTYLINE

(proe trip'ti leen)

TRADE NAMES

Triptil®
Vivactil®

CLASSIFICATION

Antidepressant, tricyclic

See also Tricyclic Antidepressants General Monograph

APPROVED INDICATIONS FOR PSYCHOLOGICAL DISORDERS

Adjunctive pharmacotherapy for the symptomatic management of:

Mood Disorders, Depressive Disorders: Major Depressive Disorder

USUAL DOSAGE AND ADMINISTRATION

Major Depressive Disorder

Adults, hospitalized: Initially, 30 to 60 mg daily orally in three or four divided doses. To avoid associated insomnia, prescribe the afternoon dose for the mid-afternoon, and prescribe any increases in the daily dosage, if needed, for the morning dose.

Adults, non-hospitalized: Initially, 15 to 40 mg daily orally in three or four divided doses. When a satisfactory response is achieved, reduce the dosage to the lowest effective dosage, according to individual patient response.

MAINTENANCE: May prescribe the maintenance dosage as a single daily dose

MAXIMUM: 60 mg daily orally

Women who are, or who may become, pregnant: FDA Pregnancy Category "not established." Safety and efficacy of protriptyline pharmacotherapy for women who are pregnant have not been established (see Tricyclic Antidepressants General Monograph). Avoid prescribing protriptyline pharmacotherapy to women who are pregnant. If protriptyline pharmacotherapy is required, advise patients of potential benefits and possible risks to themselves and the embryo, fetus, or neonate. Collaboration with the patient's obstetrician is indicated.

Women who are breast-feeding: Safety and efficacy of protriptyline pharmacotherapy for women who are breast-feeding and their neonates and infants have not been established (see Tricyclic Antidepressants General Monograph). Avoid prescribing protriptyline pharmacotherapy to women who are breast-feeding. If protriptyline pharmacotherapy is required, breast-feeding probably should be discontinued. Collaboration with the patient's pediatrician is indicated.

Elderly, frail, or debilitated patients: Initially, 15 mg daily orally in three divided doses. Increase the dosage gradually, if needed, according to individual patient response. Generally prescribe lower dosages for elderly, frail, or debilitated patients. These patients may be more sensitive to the pharmacologic actions of protriptyline than are younger or healthier adult patients.

MAXIMUM: 20 mg daily

Children: Safety and efficacy of protriptyline pharmacotherapy for children have not been established. Protriptyline pharmacotherapy is *not* recommended for this age group.

Notes, Major Depressive Disorder

Initiating Protriptyline Pharmacotherapy Prescribe the initial dosage according to the severity of the signs and symptoms of the major depressive disorder and individual patient response. Adjust the dosage as needed according to individual patient response. Therapeutic benefit is usually achieved by the fifth day of protriptyline pharmacotherapy. However, for some patients, it may be delayed for up to two weeks or longer. Maximal therapeutic benefit generally occurs within two to three weeks following the initiation of pharmacotherapy. Some elderly patients may require dosages exceeding 20 mg daily. Overstimulation and cardiovascular reactions may occur among these patients. Observe these patients for overstimulation, and monitor cardiovascular function carefully. Collaboration with the patient's family physician or specialist (e.g., cardiologist) is required.

The rapid onset of action associated with protriptyline pharmacotherapy is clinically useful for patients who are suicidal. It also is useful for patients who require ECT, which can be initiated concurrently with protriptyline pharmacotherapy. Concurrent protriptyline pharmacotherapy may reduce the number of ECT treatments required for these patients. Protriptyline pharmacotherapy and effective psychotherapy may be a satisfactory substitute for ECT for patients who are not at acute risk for suicide. Spontaneous remission may occur among some of these patients following treatment.

Maintaining Protriptyline Pharmacotherapy Maintenance protriptyline pharmacotherapy should be continued for at least three months following improvement in the signs and symptoms of depression. Maintenance pharmacotherapy for this length of time has been associated with decreased risk for relapse. Relapse following the discontinuation of protriptyline pharmacotherapy may require reinstitution of pharmacotherapy.

AVAILABLE DOSAGE FORMS, STORAGE, AND COMPATIBILITY

Tablets, oral: 5, 10 mg

Notes

General Instructions for Patients Instruct patients who are receiving protriptyline pharmacotherapy to

- safely store protriptyline oral tablets out of the reach of children in tightly closed child-resistant containers at controlled room temperature (15° to 30°C; 59° to 86°F).

- obtain an available patient information sheet regarding protriptyline pharmacotherapy from their pharmacist at the time that their prescription is dispensed. Encourage patients to clarify any questions that they may have concerning protriptyline pharmacotherapy with their pharmacist or, if needed, to consult their prescribing psychologist.

PROPOSED MECHANISM OF ACTION

Protriptyline is a potent, rapidly acting antidepressant. It appears to produce its antidepressant action primarily by blocking the re-uptake of CNS biogenic amines, specifically norepinephrine and serotonin at the pre-synaptic nerve terminals. This inhibition of re-uptake increases the amount of norepinephrine and serotonin in the synapses and, consequently, results in increased activity at the post-synaptic neuron receptor sites. The anticholinergic activity of protriptyline appears to be primarily centrally mediated.

See also Tricyclic Antidepressants General Monograph

PHARMACOKINETICS/PHARMACODYNAMICS

Protriptyline is well absorbed (77% to 93%) following oral ingestion. Peak blood concentrations are generally obtained within 12 hours. Protriptyline is highly bound to plasma protein ($\sim$92%). It has an apparent volume of distribution of $\sim$22 L/kg. Protriptyline is extensively metabolized primarily in the liver. Total body clearance ranges from 210 to 294 ml/minute. The mean half-life of elimination is approximately 3 days. The therapeutic blood concentrations associated with protriptyline's antidepressant action are generally between 70 and 250 ng/ml.

RELATIVE CONTRAINDICATIONS

Congestive heart failure
Glaucoma, narrow-angle. Protriptyline's anticholinergic action may exacerbate this condition.
Hypersensitivity to protriptyline or other TCAs
MAOI pharmacotherapy, concurrent or within 14 days
Myocardial infarction, acute recovery phase
Pregnancy
Urinary retention. Protriptyline's anticholinergic action may exacerbate this condition.

CAUTIONS AND COMMENTS

Prescribe protriptyline pharmacotherapy cautiously to patients who

- have cardiovascular disorders. Protriptyline can produce tachycardia. Collaboration with the patient's family physician or a specialist (e.g., cardiologist) may be required.
- have histories of seizure disorders. Protriptyline can lower the seizure threshold. Seizure precautions may be needed for these patients. Collaboration with the patient's family physician or a specialist (e.g., neurologist) may be required.
- have hyperthyroidism
- require elective surgery. Discontinue protriptyline pharmacotherapy several days prior to elective surgery. Collaboration with the patient's surgeon or anesthesiologist may be required.

Caution patients who are receiving protriptyline pharmacotherapy against performing activities that require alertness, judgment, and physical coordination (e.g., driving an automobile, operating dangerous equipment, supervising children) until their individual response to protriptyline pharmacotherapy is known. Protriptyline may adversely affect these mental and physical functions.

In addition to this general precaution, caution patients to inform their prescribing psychologist if they begin or discontinue any other pharmacotherapy while receiving protriptyline pharmacotherapy.

CLINICALLY SIGNIFICANT DRUG INTERACTIONS

Concurrent protriptyline pharmacotherapy and the following may result in clinically significant drug interactions:

Alcohol Use

Concurrent alcohol use may increase the CNS depressant action of protriptyline. It may also increase clinical depression. Advise patients to avoid, or limit, their use of alcohol while receiving protriptyline pharmacotherapy.

Clonidine Pharmacotherapy

Protriptyline may decrease the antihypertensive action of clonidine (Catapres®). An adjustment in the clonidine dosage may be required. Collaboration with the prescriber of the clonidine is indicated.

Guanethidine Pharmacotherapy

Protriptyline may decrease the neuronal uptake of guanethidine (Ismelin®) and, thus, decrease its antihypertensive action. An adjustment in the dosage of the guanethidine may be required. Collaboration with the prescriber of the guanethidine is indicated.

Monoamine Oxidase Inhibitor Pharmacotherapy

Protriptyline may interact with MAOIs to increase the therapeutic actions and toxic effects of both drugs. Protriptyline and MAOI pharmacotherapy, concurrent or within 14 days, is *contraindicated*.

Pharmacotherapy With Central Nervous System Depressants and Other Drugs That Produce Central Nervous System Depression

Concurrent protriptyline pharmacotherapy with opiate analgesics, sedative-hypnotics, or other drugs that produce CNS depression (e.g., antihistamines, phenothiazines) may result in additive CNS depression.

See also Tricyclic Antidepressants General Monograph

ADVERSE DRUG REACTIONS

Protriptyline pharmacotherapy commonly is associated with dizziness, feelings of restlessness and jitteriness, insomnia, rapid pulse, sweating (excessive), tiredness, and weakness. It also has been associated with the following ADRs, listed according to body system. Anticholinergic reactions (e.g., blurred vision, dry mouth) generally may be managed by reducing the dosage.

Cardiovascular: heart block, tachycardia, and, rarely, postural hypotension
CNS: rarely, drowsiness and incoordination (ataxia)
Cutaneous: rarely, hives, petechiae, and skin rash
Genitourinary: urinary retention
GI: constipation, dry mouth, GI upset, and, rarely, unpleasant taste in the mouth
Hematologic: rarely, bone marrow depression
Musculoskeletal: rarely, tremor
Ocular: blurred vision

See also Tricyclic Antidepressants General Monograph

OVERDOSAGE

Signs and symptoms of protriptyline overdosage include the signs and symptoms associated with other TCA overdosage (see Tricyclic Antidepressants General Monograph). Protriptyline overdosage requires emergency symptomatic medical support of body systems with attention to increasing protriptyline elimination. There is no known antidote.

QUAZEPAM *

(kway'ze pam)

TRADE NAME

Doral®

CLASSIFICATION

Sedative-hypnotic (benzodiazepine) (C-IV)

See also Benzodiazepines General Monograph

APPROVED INDICATIONS FOR PSYCHOLOGICAL DISORDERS

Adjunctive pharmacotherapy for the short-term symptomatic management of:

Sleep Disorders: Insomnia (difficulty falling asleep, frequent nocturnal awakenings, and/or early morning awakenings)

USUAL DOSAGE AND ADMINISTRATION

Insomnia

Adults: Initially, 15 mg daily orally 30 minutes before retiring for bed in the evening

Women who are, or who may become, pregnant: FDA Pregnancy Category X. Safety and efficacy of quazepam pharmacotherapy for women who are pregnant have not been established. However, quazepam pharmacotherapy is contraindicated during pregnancy because it has been associated with teratogenic effects in animal studies. Its chemical and pharmacological similarity to other benzodiazepines that have been associated with teratogenic effects in humans also supports its contraindication during pregnancy.
See Benzodiazepines General Monograph

Women who are breast-feeding: Safety and efficacy of quazepam pharmacotherapy for women who are breast-feeding and their neonates and infants have not been established. Quazepam is excreted in breast milk. Breast-fed neonates and infants may display expected pharmacologic actions (e.g., drowsiness or lethargy). They also may become addicted. Avoid prescribing quazepam pharmacotherapy to women who are breast-feeding. If quazepam pharmacotherapy is required, breast-feeding probably should be discontinued. If desired, lactation may be maintained and breast-feeding resumed following the discontinuation of short-term quazepam pharmacotherapy. Collaboration with the patient's pediatrician is indicated.

Elderly, frail, or debilitated patients: Initially, 7.5 mg daily orally 30 minutes before retiring for bed in the evening. Initiate quazepam pharmacotherapy with the lowest dosage to avoid associated incoordination (ataxia) or over-sedation. Increase the dosage gradually, if needed, according to individual patient response. Do *not* exceed 15 mg per dose for elderly, frail, or debilitated patients. These patients may be more sensitive to quazepam's pharmacologic actions than are younger or healthier adult patients.

Children and adolescents younger than 18 years of age: Safety and efficacy of quazepam pharmacotherapy for children and adolescents have not been established. Quazepam pharmacotherapy is *not* indicated for this age group.

Notes, Insomnia

Adjust dosage according to individual patient response for optimal therapeutic benefit. Although usual recommended dosages will meet the needs of most patients, some patients may require higher dosages. Increase the dosage gradually for these patients to avoid associated ADRs.

The safety and efficacy of quazepam pharmacotherapy for longer than 30 days have not been established. Reevaluate patients who appear to require quazepam pharmacotherapy for longer than 30 days. A benzodiazepine withdrawal syndrome similar to the alcohol withdrawal syndrome may occur upon abrupt discontinuation of long-term quazepam pharmacotherapy, or regular personal use. Discontinue quazepam pharmacotherapy gradually for these patients.

AVAILABLE DOSAGE FORMS, STORAGE, AND COMPATIBILITY

Tablets, oral: 7.5, 15 mg

Notes

General Instructions for Patients Instruct patients who are receiving quazepam pharmacotherapy to

- safely store quazepam tablets in tightly closed child-resistant containers at controlled temperature (2° to 30°C; 36° to 86°F) out of the reach of children.
- obtain an available patient information sheet regarding quazepam pharmacotherapy from their pharmacist at the time that their prescription is dispensed. Encourage patients to clarify any questions that they may have concerning quazepam pharmacotherapy with their pharmacist or, if needed, to consult their prescribing psychologist.

PROPOSED MECHANISM OF ACTION

Quazepam is a benzodiazepine with hypnotic action. The exact mechanism of action of quazepam has not yet been fully determined. It appears to be mediated or act in concert with the inhibitory neurotransmitter GABA.

See also Benzodiazepines General Monograph

PHARMACOKINETICS/PHARMACODYNAMICS

Quazepam is rapidly and well absorbed following oral ingestion. Peak blood concentrations generally are achieved within 2 hours. Quazepam is ~95% plasma protein-bound. It is extensively metabolized in the liver. Quazepam and its metabolites are excreted primarily in the urine, with less than 5% of quazepam excreted in unchanged form. The mean half-life of elimination is ~39 hours. Additional data are unavailable.

RELATIVE CONTRAINDICATIONS

Hypersensitivity to quazepam or other benzodiazepines
Pregnancy
Sleep apnea syndrome

CAUTIONS AND COMMENTS

Long-term quazepam pharmacotherapy, or regular personal use, may result in addiction and habituation. Abrupt discontinuation of long-term high dosage pharmacotherapy, or regular personal use, has been associated with a benzodiazepine withdrawal syndrome similar to the alcohol withdrawal syndrome. Signs and symptoms of the benzodiazepine withdrawal syndrome include abdominal and muscle cramps, convulsions, sweating, tremor, and vomiting. The abrupt discontinuation of benzodiazepine pharmacotherapy among patients who were receiving recommended dosages over several months also has been associated with signs and symptoms of withdrawal. However, these signs and symptoms generally are milder and include such signs and symptoms as dysphoria and insomnia. Avoid abrupt discontinuation of quazepam pharmacotherapy, particularly when pharmacotherapy has been extended over several months. Reduce the dosage gradually before completely discontinuing quazepam pharmacotherapy.

Prescribe quazepam pharmacotherapy cautiously to patients who

- are severely depressed or have evidence of latent depression. Similar to other benzodiazepines, quazepam may exacerbate the depression. Monitor these patients for increased suicide risk. Suicide precautions may be indicated.
- histories of problematic patterns of alcohol or other abusable psychotropic use. These patients may be at risk for developing problematic patterns of quazepam use. Monitor these patients closely for signs and symptoms of problematic patterns of use.
- have kidney or liver dysfunction. The half-life of elimination may be significantly increased among these patients.

Caution patients who are receiving quazepam pharmacotherapy against

- concurrent use of alcohol or other drugs that produce CNS depression because of the potential for additive CNS depression.
- increasing their prescribed dosage, using their quazepam more often than prescribed, or abruptly discontinuing their quazepam pharmacotherapy without first consulting with their prescribing psychologist. Quazepam is addicting and habituating.
- performing activities that require alertness, judgment, and physical coordination (e.g., driving an automobile, operating dangerous equipment, or supervising children) until their response to quazepam is known. The CNS depressant action of quazepam may affect these mental and physical functions.

In addition to these general precautions, caution patients to inform their prescribing psychologist if they begin or discontinue any other pharmacotherapy while receiving quazepam pharmacotherapy.

CLINICALLY SIGNIFICANT DRUG INTERACTIONS

Concurrent quazepam pharmacotherapy and the following may result in clinically significant drug interactions:

Alcohol Use

Concurrent alcohol use may increase the CNS depressant action of quazepam. Advise patients to avoid, or limit, their use of alcohol while receiving quazepam pharmacotherapy.

Pharmacotherapy With Central Nervous System Depressants and Other Drugs That Produce Central Nervous System Depression

Concurrent quazepam pharmacotherapy with opiate analgesics, other sedative-hypnotics, or other drugs that produce CNS depression (e.g., antihistamines, phenothiazines, TCAs) may result in additive CNS depression.

See also Benzodiazepines General Monograph

ADVERSE DRUG REACTIONS

Quazepam pharmacotherapy commonly has been associated with drowsiness and headache. Other ADRs, listed according to body system, include the following:

Cardiovascular: rarely, palpitations
CNS: dizziness; fatigue; and paradoxical reactions, including acute anxiety. If these ADRs are observed, discontinue quazepam pharmacotherapy.
Cutaneous: severe itching (pruritus) and skin rash
Genitourinary: rarely, involuntary urination (incontinence)

See also Benzodiazepines General Monograph

OVERDOSAGE

Signs and symptoms of quazepam overdosage include confusion, somnolence, coma, and diminished reflexes. Quazepam overdosage requires emergency symptomatic medical support of body systems with attention to increasing quazepam elimination. Flumazenil (Anexate®, Romazicon®), the benzodiazepine antagonist, may be required.

QUETIAPINE

(kwoo tye'a peen)

TRADE NAME

Seroquel®

CLASSIFICATION

Antipsychotic (atypical, dibenzothiazepine derivative)

APPROVED INDICATIONS FOR PSYCHOLOGICAL DISORDERS

Adjunctive pharmacotherapy for the short-term symptomatic management of:

Psychotic Disorders: Schizophrenia and Other Psychotic Disorders

USUAL DOSAGE AND ADMINISTRATION

Schizophrenia and Other Psychotic Disorders

Adults: Initially, 50 mg daily orally in two divided doses. On the second and third days of pharmacotherapy, increase the dosage to 150 to 300 mg daily orally in two or three divided doses, as tolerated. By the fourth day, achieve an optimal dosage of 300 to 400 mg daily orally in two or three divided doses. Adjust the dosage according to individual patient response.

MAXIMUM: 750 mg daily orally

Women who are, or who may become, pregnant: FDA Pregnancy Category C. Safety and efficacy of quetiapine pharmacotherapy for women who are pregnant have not been established. Avoid prescribing quetiapine pharmacotherapy to women who are pregnant. If quetiapine pharmacotherapy is required, advise patients of potential benefits and possible risks to themselves and the embryo, fetus, or neonate. Collaboration with the patient's obstetrician is indicated.

Women who are breast-feeding: Safety and efficacy of quetiapine pharmacotherapy for women who are breast-feeding and their neonates and infants have not been established. Avoid prescribing quetiapine pharmacotherapy to women who are breast-feeding. If quetiapine pharmacotherapy is required, breast-feeding probably should be discontinued. Collaboration with the patient's pediatrician is indicated.

Elderly, frail, or debilitated patients: Generally prescribe lower dosages for elderly, frail, or debilitated patients. These patients may be more sensitive to quetiapine's pharmacologic actions than are younger or healthier adult patients. The total body clearance of quetiapine reportedly is reduced by up to 40% among elderly patients.

Children and adolescents younger than 18 years of age: Safety and efficacy of quetiapine pharmacotherapy for children and adolescents have not been established. Quetiapine pharmacotherapy is *not* recommended for this age group.

Notes, Schizophrenia and Other Psychotic Disorders

Adjust dosage according to individual patient response for optimal therapeutic benefit.

AVAILABLE DOSAGE FORMS, STORAGE, AND COMPATIBILITY

Tablets, oral: 25, 100, 200 mg

Notes

General Instructions for Patients Instruct patients who are receiving quetiapine pharmacotherapy to

- safely store quetiapine tablets in tightly closed child-resistant containers at controlled room temperature (~25°C; ~77°F) out of the reach of children.
- obtain an available patient information sheet regarding quetiapine pharmacotherapy from their pharmacist at the time that their prescription is dispensed. Encourage patients to clarify any questions that they may have concerning quetiapine pharmacotherapy with their pharmacist or, if needed, to consult their prescribing psychologist.

PROPOSED MECHANISM OF ACTION

Quetiapine is a multiple receptor antagonist. The exact mechanism of action of quetiapine's action is complex and has not been fully determined. However, it appears to be primarily related to antagonism of dopamine (D2) and serotonin (5HT2) receptors within the CNS. The higher selectivity for 5HT2 relative to D2 receptors is believed to contribute to the reportedly low liability of quetiapine for inducing EPRs.

PHARMACOKINETICS/PHARMACODYNAMICS

Quetiapine is rapidly and well absorbed following oral ingestion. Peak blood concentrations generally are achieved in approximately 1.5 hours. Quetiapine is widely distributed throughout the body with an apparent volume of distribution of 10 ± 4 L/kg. At therapeutic concentrations, quetiapine is moderately bound (i.e., 83%) to plasma proteins. It is metabolized extensively in the liver, primarily by the cytochrome P450 3A4 isoenzyme (i.e., CYP3A4), to pharmacologically inactive metabolites. Total body clearance is reduced by approximately 40%, on average, among elderly patients.

RELATIVE CONTRAINDICATIONS

Hypersensitivity to quetiapine

CAUTIONS AND COMMENTS

Prescribe quetiapine pharmacotherapy cautiously to patients who

- are receiving antihypertensive pharmacotherapy, have cardiovascular dysfunction (e.g., congestive heart failure, history of myocardial infarction), have conditions that predispose them to hypotension (e.g., dehydration, loss of blood volume [hypovolemia]), or require elective surgery. Quetiapine pharmacotherapy may produce postural hypotension with associated dizziness, fainting (syncope), and tachycardia. Thus, quetiapine pharmacotherapy may exacerbate the hypotension associated with these conditions. Advise patients to inform their family physician and other health care providers (e.g., advanced practice nurse, cardiologist, surgeon) that they are receiving quetiapine pharmacotherapy. Collaboration with the patient's family physician or other health care providers is indicated.
- have histories of breast cancer. Quetiapine elevates serum prolactin levels. Tissue culture experiments provide evidence that approximately one-third of human breast cancers are prolactin dependent. Collaboration with the patient's oncologist is indicated.
- have histories of hypercholesterolemia. Quetiapine pharmacotherapy is associated with increases from baseline cholesterol and triglyceride blood concentrations of 11% and 17%, respectively. These increases in blood lipids appear to be relatively independent of quetiapine-related weight gain.
- have histories of seizure disorders. Quetiapine pharmacotherapy has been associated with seizures in less than 1% of patients. However, caution is indicated when quetiapine pharmacotherapy is prescribed to patients who have histories of seizure disorders or conditions that potentially lower the seizure threshold (e.g., Alzheimer's dementia). Collaboration with the patient's family physician or neurologist may be indicated.
- have Parkinson's disease. Quetiapine is a dopamine receptor antagonist. Thus, quetiapine pharmacotherapy may cause a deterioration in the clinical condition of these patients.

Caution patients who are receiving quetiapine pharmacotherapy against performing activities that require alertness, judgment, and physical coordination (e.g., driving an automobile, operating dangerous equipment, or supervising children) until their response to quetiapine pharmacotherapy is known. Quetiapine may adversely affect these mental and physical functions.

In addition to this general precaution, caution patients to

- understand that quetiapine pharmacotherapy may be associated with the development of TD. Advise all patients for whom long-term quetiapine pharmacotherapy is required of this potential risk. The decision to inform patients, or their legal guardians, must take into account the clinical circumstances and the competency of the patient to understand the information provided.
- inform their prescribing psychologist if they begin or discontinue any other pharmacotherapy while receiving quetiapine pharmacotherapy.

CLINICALLY SIGNIFICANT DRUG INTERACTIONS

Concurrent quetiapine pharmacotherapy and the following may result in clinically significant drug interactions:

Alcohol Use

Concurrent alcohol use may increase the CNS depressant action of quetiapine. Advise patients to avoid, or limit, their use of alcohol while receiving quetiapine pharmacotherapy.

Pharmacotherapy with Levodopa and Other Dopamine Agonists

Quetiapine directly antagonizes the action of levodopa (Dopar®) and other dopamine agonists.

Phenytoin Pharmacotherapy

Concurrent quetiapine and phenytoin pharmacotherapy may result in significant increases in quetiapine clearance (by up to 5-fold). Avoid concurrent quetiapine and phenytoin pharmacotherapy. If concurrent pharmacotherapy cannot be avoided, monitor patients carefully, and increase the quetiapine dosage as indicated by patient response.

Thioridazine Pharmacotherapy

Concurrent quetiapine and thioridazine pharmacotherapy may result in a significant increase in quetiapine clearance (by ~65%). Monitor patients carefully who require concurrent pharmacotherapy, and increase the quetiapine dosage according to individual patient response.

ADVERSE DRUG REACTIONS

Quetiapine pharmacotherapy commonly has been associated with constipation, dizziness, dry mouth, dyspepsia, headache, postural hypotension, somnolence, tachycardia, and weight gain. Other ADRs, listed according to body system, include the following:

Cardiovascular: peripheral edema, and rapid, throbbing or fluttering of the heart (palpitations) (see also Musculoskeletal)

CNS: *Note:* Available data do *not* support an association between quetiapine pharmacotherapy and EPRs.

Cutaneous: rash and sweating

GI: abdominal pain and loss of appetite (anorexia)

Hematologic: white blood cell count below 5,000/mm^3 (leukopenia [i.e., granulocytopenia or leukocytopenia])

Metabolic/Endocrine: hypothyroidism

Musculoskeletal: back pain, difficult or defective speech due to the impairment of the tongue or other muscles essential to speech (dysarthria), lack of strength and weakness (asthenia), and tension of muscles (hypertonia) (see also CNS)

Ocular: cataracts (see Cautions and Comments)

Otic: ear pain
Respiratory: cough (increased), difficult or labored breathing (dyspnea), inflammation of the pharynx (pharyngitis), and runny nose (rhinitis)
Miscellaneous: fever

OVERDOSAGE

Signs and symptoms of acute quetiapine overdosage generally are extensions of its pharmacologic actions. These signs and symptoms include drowsiness, hypotension, sedation, and tachycardia. No deaths have been associated with quetiapine overdosage. Regardless, quetiapine overdosage requires emergency symptomatic medical support of body systems with attention to increasing quetiapine elimination. There is no known antidote.

RISPERIDONE

(ris per'i done)

TRADE NAME

Risperdal®

CLASSIFICATION

Antipsychotic (atypical, benzisoxazole)

APPROVED INDICATIONS FOR PSYCHOLOGICAL DISORDERS

Adjunctive pharmacotherapy for the symptomatic management of:

Psychotic Disorders: Schizophrenia and Other Psychotic Disorders

USUAL DOSAGE AND ADMINISTRATION

Schizophrenia and Other Psychotic Disorders

Adults: Initially, 2 mg daily orally in two divided doses. Increase the dosage by 2 mg daily to achieve an optimal dosage of 6 mg daily orally in two divided doses. Adjust the dosage according to individual patient response. Some patients may require a more gradual increase in dosage. Alternatively, risperidone may be prescribed as a single daily dose. This dosing schedule may be of benefit to patients who have difficulty managing twice daily dosing. Patients who experience excessive drowsiness associated with their risperidone pharmacotherapy also may benefit from single daily dosing. For these patients, prescribe their daily dose for ingestion 30 minutes before retiring for bed in the evening.

MAXIMUM: 16 mg daily orally

Women who are, or who may become, pregnant: FDA Pregnancy Category C. Safety and efficacy of risperidone pharmacotherapy for women who are pregnant have not been established. Avoid prescribing risperidone pharmacotherapy to women who are pregnant. If risperidone pharmacotherapy is required, advise patients of potential benefits and possible risks to themselves and the embryo, fetus, or neonate. Collaboration with the patient's obstetrician is indicated.

Women who are breast-feeding: Safety and efficacy of risperidone pharmacotherapy for women who are breast-feeding and their neonates and infants have not been established. Avoid prescribing risperidone pharmacotherapy to women who are breast-feeding. If risperidone pharmacotherapy is required, breast-feeding probably should be discontinued. Collaboration with the patient's pediatrician may be indicated.

Elderly, frail, or debilitated patients: Initially, 1 mg daily orally in two divided doses. Increase the dosage gradually, if needed, by 1 mg daily according to individual patient response. Alternatively, risperidone may be prescribed as a single daily dose. This dosing schedule may be of benefit to elderly patients who have difficulty managing twice daily dosing. Elderly patients who experience excessive drowsiness associated with their risperidone pharmacotherapy also may benefit from single daily dosing. For these patients, prescribe the daily dose for ingestion 30 minutes before retiring for bed in the evening. Generally prescribe lower dosages for elderly, frail, or debilitated patients. These patients may be more sensitive to the pharmacologic actions of risperidone than are younger or healthier adult patients.

MAXIMUM: 3 mg daily orally

Children and adolescents younger than 18 years of age: Safety and efficacy of risperidone pharmacotherapy for children and adolescents have not been established. Risperidone pharmacotherapy is *not* recommended for this age group.

Notes, Schizophrenia and Other Psychotic Disorders

Some patients may require dosages of up to 16 mg daily for the symptomatic management of psychotic disorders. However, dosages exceeding 6 mg daily generally do not increase therapeutic benefit and may increase the incidence and severity of ADRs, particularly EPRs. The safety and efficacy of risperidone pharmacotherapy for longer than several months have not been established.

AVAILABLE DOSAGE FORMS, STORAGE, AND COMPATIBILITY

Solution, oral: 1 mg/ml
Tablets, oral: 1, 2, 3, 4 mg

Notes

General Instructions for Patients   Instruct patients who are receiving risperidone pharmacotherapy to

- dilute each dose of the risperidone oral solution with coffee, low-fat milk, orange juice, or water. Advise them *not* to dilute their doses with cola beverages or tea because of incompatibility.
- safely store risperidone oral dosage forms in tightly closed child- and light-resistant containers at room temperature (15° to 30°C; 59° to 86°F) out of the reach of children.

- obtain an available patient information sheet regarding risperidone pharmacotherapy from their pharmacist at the time that their prescription is dispensed. Encourage patients to clarify any questions that they may have concerning risperidone pharmacotherapy with their pharmacist or, if needed, to consult their prescribing psychologist.

PROPOSED MECHANISM OF ACTION

The exact mechanism of risperidone's antipsychotic action is complex and has not yet been fully determined. However, it appears to be primarily related to antagonism of dopamine (D2) and serotonin (5HT2) receptors within the CNS.

PHARMACOKINETICS/PHARMACODYNAMICS

Risperidone is relatively well absorbed following oral ingestion (F = 0.7). Peak blood concentrations are achieved within 1 to 2 hours. The ingestion of food does not appear to affect the bioavailability of risperidone. Risperidone is highly plasma protein-bound ($\sim$90%) and has an apparent volume of distribution of $\sim$1.5 L/kg. Risperidone is metabolized extensively in the liver to an active metabolite, 9-hydroxyrisperidone. The metabolism of risperidone is subject to genetic polymorphism. Approximately 8% of Caucasians and a small percentage of Asians have little of the major metabolizing enzyme (i.e., cytochrome P450 2D6 or debrisoquin hydroxylase). These patients are referred to as "poor metabolizers." Poor metabolizers excrete 20% of risperidone in unchanged form in the urine, while "extensive metabolizers" (i.e., the majority of the population) excrete 3% of risperidone in unchanged form in the urine. The mean half-life of elimination of risperidone for extensive metabolizers is $\sim$3 hours, while for poor metabolizers it is $\sim$20 hours.

RELATIVE CONTRAINDICATIONS

Hypersensitivity to risperidone

CAUTIONS AND COMMENTS

Prescribe risperidone pharmacotherapy cautiously to patients who

- are receiving antihypertensive pharmacotherapy, have cardiovascular dysfunction (e.g., congestive heart failure, history of myocardial infarction), have conditions that predispose them to hypotension (e.g., dehydration, loss of blood volume [hypovolemia]), or require elective surgery. Risperidone can produce postural hypotension with associated dizziness, fainting (syncope), and tachycardia. Thus, risperidone pharmacotherapy may exacerbate the hypotension associated with these conditions. Advise patients to inform their family physician and other health care providers (e.g., cardiologist, surgeon) that they are receiving risperidone pharmacotherapy. Collaboration with the patient's family physician or other health care providers is indicated.
- have histories of breast cancer. Risperidone elevates serum prolactin levels. Tissue culture experiments provide evidence that approximately one-third of human breast cancers are prolactin dependent. Collaboration with the patient's oncologist is indicated.

- have histories of seizure disorders. Risperidone pharmacotherapy has been associated with seizures in less than 1% of patients. However, caution is indicated when risperidone pharmacotherapy is prescribed to patients who have histories of seizure disorders. Collaboration with the patient's physician or neurologist may be indicated.
- have Parkinson's disease. Risperidone is a dopamine receptor antagonist. Thus, risperidone pharmacotherapy may cause a deterioration in the clinical condition of these patients.

Caution patients who are receiving risperidone pharmacotherapy against performing activities that require alertness, judgment, and physical coordination (e.g., driving an automobile, operating dangerous equipment, supervising children) until their response to risperidone pharmacotherapy is known. The sedative action of risperidone may adversely affect these mental and physical functions.

In addition to this general precaution, caution patients to

- understand that risperidone pharmacotherapy may be associated with the development of TD. Advise all patients requiring long-term high-dosage risperidone pharmacotherapy of this risk. The decision to inform patients, or their legal guardians, must take into account the clinical circumstances and the competency of the patient to understand the information provided.
- inform their prescribing psychologist if they begin or discontinue any other pharmacotherapy while receiving risperidone pharmacotherapy.

CLINICALLY SIGNIFICANT DRUG INTERACTIONS

Concurrent risperidone pharmacotherapy and the following may result in clinically significant drug interactions:

Alcohol Use

Concurrent alcohol use may increase the CNS depressant action of risperidone. Advise patients to avoid, or limit, their use of alcohol while receiving risperidone pharmacotherapy.

Carbamazepine Pharmacotherapy

Concurrent carbamazepine pharmacotherapy may result in significant decreases in the plasma concentration of the active metabolite of risperidone (i.e., 9-hydroxyrisperidone).

Pharmacotherapy With Central Nervous System Depressants and Other Drugs That Produce Central Nervous System Depression

Concurrent risperidone pharmacotherapy with opiate analgesics, sedative-hypnotics, or other drugs that produce CNS depression (e.g., antihistamines, phenothiazines, or TCAs) may result in additive CNS depression.

Pharmacotherapy With Levodopa and Other Dopamine Agonists

Risperidone directly antagonizes the action of levodopa (Dopar®) and other dopamine agonists.

ADVERSE DRUG REACTIONS

Risperidone pharmacotherapy commonly has been associated with agitation, anxiety, constipation, dyspepsia, EPRs, headache, insomnia, rash, runny nose (rhinitis), tachycardia, and weight gain. Other ADRs, listed according to body system, include:

Cardiovascular: AV block, myocardial infarction, postural (orthostatic) hypotension, prolonged QT interval, and rapid throbbing or fluttering of the heart (palpitations)

CNS: attempted suicide, confusion, depression, dizziness, excessive drowsiness (somnolence), fatigue, increased dreaming, increased sleep duration, nervousness, and seizures

Cutaneous: dry skin, hair loss (alopecia, rare), increased pigmentation, and sensitivity to light (photosensitivity)

Genitourinary: excessive urination (polyuria), and involuntary urination (urinary incontinence) (see also Metabolic/Endocrine)

GI: bitter taste (rare), dry mouth, excessive gas in the stomach and intestines (flatulence), excessive thirst (polydipsia), loss of appetite (anorexia), and nausea

Hematologic: anemia; hemorrhages into the skin, mucous membranes, internal organs, and other tissues (hemorrhages into the skin discolor the skin red to dark purple, then brownish yellow, and finally disappear in two to three weeks, purpura); and nose bleeds (epistaxis)

Hepatic: rarely, hepatitis and liver failure

Metabolic/Endocrine: breast enlargement among men (gynecomastia), breast pain, decreased sex drive, and excessive menstrual bleeding or duration of menses (menorrhagia)

Musculoskeletal: joint pain (arthralgia) and muscle pain (myalgia)

Ocular: abnormal accommodation, double vision (diplopia, rare), and dryness of the mucous membrane lining the eyelids and reflected onto the eyeball (conjunctiva, xerophthalmia)

Otic: rarely, decreased hearing and ringing in the ears (tinnitus)

Respiratory: increased minute volume ventilation that results in a lowered carbon dioxide level (hyperventilation), inflammation of the pharynx (pharyngitis), narrowing with obstruction of the lumen of the bronchi due to spasm of the peribronchial smooth muscle that is characterized by coughing and wheezing (bronchospasm), and pneumonia

OVERDOSAGE

Signs and symptoms of acute risperidone overdosage generally are extensions of its pharmacologic actions and include drowsiness, EPRs, hypotension, sedation, and tachycardia. No deaths have been associated with risperidone overdosage. Regardless, risperidone overdosage requires emergency symptomatic medical support of body systems with attention to increasing risperidone elimination. There is no known antidote.

SECOBARBITAL [Quinalbarbitone]

(see koe bar'bi tal)

TRADE NAMES

Novo-Secobarb®
Seconal®

CLASSIFICATION

Sedative-hypnotic (barbiturate) (C-II)

See Barbiturates General Monograph

APPROVED INDICATIONS FOR PSYCHOLOGICAL DISORDERS

Adjunctive pharmacotherapy for the short-term symptomatic management of:

Sleep Disorders: Insomnia

USUAL DOSAGE AND ADMINISTRATION

Insomnia

Adults: 100 mg daily orally 30 minutes before retiring for bed in the evening; *or* 120 to 200 mg daily rectally upon retiring for bed in the evening; *or* 100 to 200 mg daily intramuscularly upon retiring for bed in the evening

Women who are, or who may become, pregnant: FDA Pregnancy Category D. Safety and efficacy of secobarbital pharmacotherapy for women who are pregnant have not been established. Secobarbital pharmacotherapy during pregnancy appears unlikely to result in physical birth defects. However, use near term or during labor may result in neonatal respiratory depression and the neonatal barbiturate withdrawal syndrome, which can be delayed in onset for up to 14 days. Avoid prescribing secobarbital pharmacotherapy to women who are pregnant, particularly near term. If secobarbital pharmacotherapy is required, advise patients of potential benefits and possible risks to themselves and the embryo, fetus, or neonate. Collaboration with the patient's obstetrician is indicated.

Women who are breast-feeding: Safety and efficacy of secobarbital pharmacotherapy for women who are breast-feeding and their neonates and infants have not been established. Secobarbital is generally excreted in low concentrations in breast milk. Breast-fed neonates and infants may display expected pharmacologic actions (e.g., drowsiness, lethargy). They also may become addicted (see also Barbiturates General Monograph). Avoid prescribing secobarbital pharmacotherapy to women who are breast-feeding. If secobarbital pharmacotherapy is required, breast-feeding probably should be discontinued. If desired, lactation may be maintained and breast-feeding resumed following the discontinuation of short-term secobarbital pharmacotherapy. Collaboration with the patient's pediatrician is indicated.

Elderly, frail, or debilitated patients: Generally prescribe lower dosages of secobarbital for elderly, frail, or debilitated patients. Increase the dosage gradually, if needed, according to individual patient response. These patients may be more sensitive to the pharmacologic actions of secobarbital than are younger or healthier adult patients.

Infants up to 6 months of age: 15 to 60 mg daily rectally at bedtime

Infants and children 6 months to 3 years of age: 60 mg daily rectally at bedtime

Children 3 years of age and older: 60 to 100 mg daily orally at bedtime, *or* 60 to 100 mg daily rectally at bedtime, *or* 3 to 5 mg/kg daily intramuscularly (maximum 100 mg) at bedtime

Notes, Insomnia

Tolerance to the hypnotic action of secobarbital generally occurs after two weeks of pharmacotherapy. Secobarbital pharmacotherapy exceeding two weeks for the symptomatic management of insomnia is *not* recommended. Reevaluate patients who appear to require longer secobarbital pharmacotherapy.

Injectable Secobarbital Pharmacotherapy

INTRAMUSCULAR PHARMACOTHERAPY   The injectable formulation of secobarbital is highly alkaline. Inject intramuscularly deeply into healthy muscle sites to minimize possible tissue necrosis. For adults, do not inject more than 5 ml at any one intramuscular injection site.

INTRAVENOUS PHARMACOTHERAPY   Use extreme care to avoid extravasation during intravenous injection. Intravenous pharmacotherapy is *not* recommended because of the danger of respiratory depression. Intravenous secobarbital pharmacotherapy is generally reserved for hospitalized patients.

AVAILABLE DOSAGE FORMS, STORAGE, AND COMPATIBILITY

Capsules, oral: 50, 100 mg
Injectable, intramuscular, intravenous: 50 mg/ml
Suppositories, rectal: 30, 60, 100, 120 mg
Tablets, oral: 100 mg

Notes

Inspect the secobarbital injectable formulations prior to use. Do not use injectable formulations that are discolored or contain a precipitate. Return these injectable products to the dispensing pharmacy or manufacturer for safe and appropriate disposal.

Store the secobarbital injectable and rectal suppositories safely in light-resistant containers under refrigeration (2° to 8°C; 36° to 46°F).

General Instructions for Patients   Instruct patients who are receiving secobarbital to

- safely store secobarbital capsules and tablets out of the reach of children in tightly closed child-resistant containers at controlled room temperature (15° to 30°C; 59° to 86°F).
- obtain an available patient information sheet regarding secobarbital pharmacotherapy from their pharmacist at the time that their prescription is dispensed. Encourage patients to clarify any questions that they may have concerning secobarbital pharmacotherapy with their pharmacist or, if needed, to consult their prescribing psychologist.

PROPOSED MECHANISM OF ACTION

The exact mechanism of secobarbital's hypnotic action has not yet been fully determined. It appears to act primarily at the level of the thalamus, where it interferes with impulse transmission to the cortex.

See also Barbiturates General Monograph

PHARMACOKINETICS/PHARMACODYNAMICS

Absorption generally is rapid and complete (~90%) following oral ingestion. Once absorbed, distribution is rapid. Of the barbiturates, secobarbital has the highest degree of lipid solubility and, thus, the fastest distribution. Approximately 45% of secobarbital is bound to plasma proteins. The onset of action depends on the method of administration but generally is within 10 to 15 minutes. The onset of action following rectal insertion is similar to that following oral ingestion. The onset of action following intramuscular injection is slightly faster than that following either oral ingestion or rectal insertion. The duration of action is three to four hours. Secobarbital is almost completely metabolized, with less than 5% excreted in the urine in unchanged form. The mean half-life of elimination for adults is approximately 30 hours (range 15 to 40 hours). Alterations in urinary volume or pH do not significantly affect the elimination of secobarbital.

See also Barbiturates General Monograph

RELATIVE CONTRAINDICATIONS

Hypersensitivity to secobarbital or other barbiturates
Liver dysfunction, severe
Pain, uncontrolled
Porphyria, active or latent
Respiratory depression, moderate to severe

CAUTIONS AND COMMENTS

Secobarbital is a popular illicit street drug, the capsules of which are commonly known as "reds" or "red devils." Long-term secobarbital pharmacotherapy, or regular personal use, may result in addiction and habituation. Sudden discontinuation of long-term secobarbital pharmacotherapy, or regular personal use, may result in the barbiturate withdrawal syndrome. The barbiturate withdrawal syndrome is considered to be a medical emergency that can result in death if not treated appropriately.

Prescribe secobarbital pharmacotherapy cautiously to patients who

- are receiving oral anticoagulant pharmacotherapy because of the difficulty in stabilizing prothrombin times.
- have CNS depression. Secobarbital pharmacotherapy may result in severe CNS depression among these patients.
- have liver dysfunction. The half-life of elimination may be prolonged among these patients.
- have respiratory depression. Secobarbital may increase respiratory depression among these patients.

Caution patients who are receiving secobarbital pharmacotherapy against performing activities that require alertness, judgment, and physical coordination (e.g., driving an automobile, operating dangerous equipment, supervising children) until their response to secobarbital is known. Secobarbital may adversely affect these mental and physical functions.

In addition to this general precaution, caution patients who are receiving secobarbital pharmacotherapy to inform their prescribing psychologist if they begin or discontinue any other pharmacotherapy while receiving secobarbital pharmacotherapy.

See also Barbiturates General Monograph

CLINICALLY SIGNIFICANT DRUG INTERACTIONS

Concurrent secobarbital pharmacotherapy and the following may result in clinically significant drug interactions:

Alcohol Use

Concurrent alcohol use may increase the CNS depressant action of secobarbital to dangerous and, possibly, fatal levels. Caution patients to refrain from alcohol use while receiving secobarbital pharmacotherapy.

Pharmacotherapy With Central Nervous System Depressants and Other Drugs That Produce Central Nervous System Depression

Concurrent secobarbital pharmacotherapy with opiate analgesics, other sedative-hypnotics, or other drugs that produce CNS depression (e.g., antihistamines, phenothiazines, TCAs) may result in additive CNS depression.

Pharmacotherapy With Drugs That Are Primarily Metabolized in the Liver

Secobarbital may stimulate the production of the hepatic microsomal enzymes responsible for the metabolism of many different drugs (e.g., corticosteroids, oral anticoagulants, oral contraceptives, quinidine [Biquin®]). Whenever secobarbital is added to or removed from a patient's pharmacotherapy, attention must be given to the effect on other pharmacotherapy that the patient may be receiving. Collaboration with other prescribers may be needed, so that dosages can be appropriately adjusted (i.e., increased or decreased) if necessary.

See also Barbiturates General Monograph

ADVERSE DRUG REACTIONS

Secobarbital pharmacotherapy commonly has been associated with respiratory depression, particularly following intramuscular or intravenous injection. Other ADRs, listed according to body system, include:

Cardiovascular: bradycardia and hypotension
CNS: headache, lethargy, and, rarely, excitement. Secobarbital suppresses REM sleep and, thus, may be associated with "hangover" effects.
Cutaneous: skin rash
GI: GI complaints
Miscellaneous: hypersensitivity reactions

See also Barbiturates General Monograph

OVERDOSAGE

See Barbiturates General Monograph

SELECTIVE SEROTONIN RE-UPTAKE INHIBITORS
General Monograph

GENERIC NAMES

(for trade names, see individual SSRI monographs)

Fluoxetine
Fluvoxamine
Paroxetine
Sertraline
Venlafaxine

CLASSIFICATION

Antidepressant (SSRI)

See also individual SSRI monographs

APPROVED INDICATIONS FOR PSYCHOLOGICAL DISORDERS

Adjunctive pharmacotherapy for the symptomatic management of:

- Anxiety Disorders: Obsessive-Compulsive Disorder
- Mood Disorders, Depressive Disorders: Major Depressive Disorder

USUAL DOSAGE AND ADMINISTRATION

Major Depressive Disorder and Obsessive-Compulsive Disorder

Adults: See individual SSRI monographs

Women who are, or who may become, pregnant: FDA Pregnancy Category B. Safety and efficacy of SSRI pharmacotherapy for women who are pregnant have not been established. Available data suggest that the risk for congenital malformations (birth defects) associated with SSRIs is low. However, the effects of in utero exposure on behavior, cognition, learning, or memory during infancy and childhood have not been adequately studied. Avoid prescribing SSRI pharmacotherapy to women who are pregnant. If SSRI pharmacotherapy is required, advise patients of potential benefits and possible risks to themselves and the embryo, fetus, or neonate. Collaboration with the patient's obstetrician is indicated.

Women who are breast-feeding: Safety and efficacy of SSRI pharmacotherapy for women who are breast-feeding and their neonates and infants have not been established. SSRIs are excreted in breast milk. Avoid prescribing SSRI pharmacotherapy to women who are breast-feeding. If SSRI pharmacotherapy is required, breast-feeding probably should be discontinued. Collaboration with the patient's pediatrician may be required.

Elderly, frail, or debilitated patients and those who have liver dysfunction: Generally prescribe lower dosages of the SSRIs for elderly, frail, or debilitated patients and those who have liver dysfunction. Increase the dosage gradually, if needed, according to individual patient response. These patients may be more sensitive to the pharmacologic actions of the SSRIs than are younger or healthier adult patients.

Children and adolescents younger than 18 years of age: Safety and efficacy of SSRI pharmacotherapy for children and adolescents have not been established. SSRI pharmacotherapy is *not* recommended for this age group.

Notes, Major Depressive Disorder and Obsessive-Compulsive Disorder

Initiating SSRI Pharmacotherapy *Before* initiating SSRI pharmacotherapy, ensure that an accurate diagnosis of major depressive disorder or obsessive-compulsive disorder has been properly made and documented. Depending upon the clinical situation, also assure for patients and their legal guardians, as appropriate, that the following are completed as soon as possible:

- assess the patient's perception of his or her condition and need for adjunctive SSRI pharmacotherapy. Include as part of the psychological assessment a family history of mental disorders. Ascertain the presence of any current or active medical disorders, or a history of such disorders, and identify any related pharmacotherapy for their medical management. Note particularly any pharmacotherapy that has been associated with mimicking, exacerbating, or inducing the signs and symptoms of major depressive disorder or obsessive-compulsive disorder. Also identify any problematic patterns of abusable psychotropic use, including any heavy alcohol, barbiturate, benzodiazepine, or other sedative-hypnotic use that may induce or exacerbate depression.
- depending on the indication for use, note any previous antidepressant pharmacotherapy or pharmacotherapy for obsessive-compulsive disorder and the patient's general response.
- identify possible hypersensitivity to the SSRIs and other potential contraindications and cautions that may require consideration when prescribing SSRI pharmacotherapy.
- assess the patient's abilities to manage his or her SSRI pharmacotherapy.
- ensure civil liberties in relation to the following:

  - obtain the patient's (or legal guardian's) informed consent for SSRI pharmacotherapy. Patients (or their legal guardians) require, commensurate with their intelligence and mental status, information regarding the potential benefits (i.e., management of the mental disorder) and risks (e.g., serotonin syndrome) associated with SSRI pharmacotherapy.
  - the implementation of suicide precautions. Severely depressed patients may require the implementation of suicide precautions. Some patients may require supervised administration of their SSRI pharmacotherapy in order to help to ensure that oral doses are swallowed. Such patients may require alternative approaches to drug administration (e.g., contracting) or the direct observation of ingestion of oral dosage forms that will prevent them from "cheeking" or "hoarding" their doses for potential later overdosage associated with attempted suicide.

- ensure that patients (or their legal guardians) have an understanding of the planned pharmacotherapy and any adjunctive psychotherapy or other related therapy (e.g., ECT). For example, they should know that, generally, a low dosage of the SSRI will be prescribed initially and increased gradually until therapeutic benefit is achieved. They should know that it may take several days, weeks, or months before optimal therapeutic benefit is fully achieved. They also should understand that during this period of time, they will be monitored for common ADRs, such as weight loss, and that they will be helped to manage these ADRs. Any questions that patients or their legal guardians may have regarding SSRI pharmacotherapy should be answered honestly.
- ensure that the patient knows the exact name of the required SSRI. They also should know its general action, dosage and administration, and storage requirements. They should know how to monitor for therapeutic benefit and identify and manage common ADRs. They should know the signs and symptoms of toxicity and know when it may be necessary to contact the prescribing psychologist immediately or to access emergency medical facilities for evaluation and treatment.

- individualize the dosage according to the severity of signs and symptoms and patient response. Most patients (~80%) respond to lower dosages as steady state is achieved. The achievement of steady state usually requires a period of time equivalent to five times the half-life of elimination of the SSRI. Avoid increasing the dosage prior to achieving steady state. Increasing the dosage before achieving steady state may significantly and unnecessarily increase the incidence and severity of associated ADRs. Many of the SSRIs have a long half-life of elimination and, thus, a long duration of action. Once steady state has been achieved, most patients may be dosed once daily with these SSRIs. See individual SSRI monographs.
- advise patients and their legal guardians, as appropriate, that many of the ADRs associated with SSRI pharmacotherapy usually diminish over the first few weeks of pharmacotherapy and that these ADRs do not necessarily mean that the patient has a more serious mental disorder or has relapsed. They should be encouraged to continue SSRI pharmacotherapy despite mild ADRs and be assisted with the management of these ADRs. More troublesome ADRs may require a reduction of the dosage or changes in dosage schedule (e.g., ingesting each dose of an oral dosage form in the morning rather than the evening if insomnia proves to be a troublesome ADR). Explore these and other possible countermeasures (see following discussion) with patients, as needed.
- ensure that patients understand that if ADRs occur, they can, for the most part, be treated quickly. It is important to acknowledge how annoying and uncomfortable ADRs can be. Patients should be encouraged to discuss their feelings about ADRs and to assist with their management. Special attention should be given to the management of common mild ADRs because the inability to manage or tolerate ADRs is often a major reason for patients to discontinue SSRI pharmacotherapy. For patients who want to discontinue their SSRI pharmacotherapy because of associated ADRs, it is often helpful to weigh with them and their legal guardians, as appropriate, the discontinuation of pharmacotherapy with expected or actual benefits and the risk for the return of the signs and symptoms of the mental disorder being treated.
- assist patients to manage common or troublesome ADRs, such as loss of appetite (anorexia) and weight loss, by suggesting that patients do the following:

  - follow a balanced diet and exercise program to maintain their normal weight
  - monitor their daily caloric intake
  - eat nutritious snack foods. Collaboration with the patient's advanced practice nurse or a nutritional consultant may be required.

- provide realistic information regarding SSRI pharmacotherapy and other recommended therapy. Patients and their legal guardians, as appropriate, should have a realistic view of what to expect in relation to SSRI pharmacotherapy and other recommended therapy. They should understand that SSRI pharmacotherapy will not solve all of the patient's problems but will help him or her to be better able to work on the problems. They should understand that SSRI pharmacotherapy will not improve judgment, improve poor socialization or interpersonal skills, or change their personality. However, they can expect that adjunctive SSRI pharmacotherapy will help the patient to better manage the mental disorder being treated.
- clarify misconceptions. Patients and their legal guardians, as appropriate, should be aware that SSRIs are not addicting or habituating. They should also be aware that high dosages do not necessarily indicate a more serious mental disorder. Dosage selection depends on several factors, such as age, gender, weight, metabolism, and response to previous antidepressant pharmacotherapy. Patients and their legal guardians, as appropriate, should recognize that concurrent participation in other recommended therapy and the maintenance of regular appointments with the clinical psychologist are important adjuncts for the symptomatic management of major depressive disorder or obsessive-compulsive disorder.

Patients and their legal guardians, as appropriate, should be encouraged to ask questions about the individualized therapeutic plan as active consumers of comprehensive psychologic services. They also should be directed to available support groups for additional help.
- involve patients and their legal guardians, as appropriate, in treatment planning, whenever possible. Provide them with frequent evaluations of the patient's progress.

Maintaining SSRI Pharmacotherapy   Most patients will require long-term SSRI pharmacotherapy for the symptomatic management of depression or obsessive-compulsive disorder. Monitor initial and continued therapeutic response to SSRI pharmacotherapy characterized by:

- improvement in mood and activity level, if being treated for major depressive disorder.
- decreased compulsive behavior, if being treated for obsessive-compulsive disorder.

Continue to monitor patients for ADRs, particularly those associated with long-term SSRI pharmacotherapy (see also Adverse Drug Reactions and individual SSRI monographs)

Discontinuing SSRI Pharmacotherapy   See individual SSRI monographs
See also Cautions and Comments

AVAILABLE DOSAGE FORMS, STORAGE, AND COMPATIBILITY

See individual SSRI monographs

Notes

SSRIs are available in oral dosage forms only.

General Instructions for Patients   Instruct patients who are receiving SSRI pharmacotherapy to

- safely store their SSRI oral dosage forms out of the reach of children in tightly closed child-resistant containers below 30°C (86°F).
- obtain an available patient information sheet regarding SSRI pharmacotherapy from their pharmacist at the time that their prescription is dispensed. Encourage patients to clarify any questions that they may have concerning SSRI pharmacotherapy with their pharmacist or, if needed, to consult their prescribing psychologist.

PROPOSED MECHANISM OF ACTION

The exact mechanism of antidepressant, anti-obsessional, and other related actions of the SSRIs has not yet been fully determined. The SSRIs appear to act at both pre- and post-synaptic neuronal sites by selectively inhibiting the re-uptake of serotonin. The blockage of serotonin re-uptake results in an acute increase in synaptic serotonin. This increase in serotonin allows it to act for an extended period of time at the synaptic binding sites.

The SSRIs also inhibit the uptake of serotonin into human platelets. However, the clinical significance of this action is unknown. In addition, they bind, although with much lower affinity, to other CNS neurotransmitter receptors (e.g., adrenergic [α_1, α_2, β], dopaminergic, and opiate analgesic receptors). The lower affinity of the SSRIs for these receptors may help to explain the lower incidence of ADRs associated with this group of antidepressants.

PHARMACOKINETICS/PHARMACODYNAMICS

The SSRIs are slowly, but well absorbed following oral ingestion. However, some SSRIs (e.g., sertraline) undergo significant first-pass hepatic metabolism. Peak blood concentrations are reached within 2 to 8 hours. The SSRIs are highly plasma protein-bound (i.e., greater than 95% protein-bound, except for fluvoxamine, which is 77% protein-bound). Thus, the SSRIs may displace other drugs from plasma protein binding sites. The SSRIs are metabolized by the liver and also have the potential to inhibit, to varying degrees, the hepatic cytochrome P450 metabolizing enzymes (see Clinically Significant Drug Interactions).

See also individual SSRI monographs

RELATIVE CONTRAINDICATIONS

Hypersensitivity to the SSRIs

MAOI pharmacotherapy, concurrent or within 14 days. *Note:* It is recommended that MAOI pharmacotherapy not be initiated for five weeks following the discontinuation of fluoxetine pharmacotherapy because of the long half-life of elimination of fluoxetine and its active metabolite (see Fluoxetine Monograph). Concurrent MAOI and fluoxetine pharmacotherapy has resulted in the serotonin syndrome. The signs and symptoms of this syndrome include hypertension, hyperthermia, myoclonus, rigidity, and tachycardia. Mental, cardiovascular, and respiratory function are subject to rapid changes and marked fluctuations. The serotonin syndrome can progress, if untreated, to cardiovascular collapse and death.

CAUTIONS AND COMMENTS

Abrupt discontinuation of the SSRIs may result in a withdrawal syndrome. The signs and symptoms of this syndrome include agitation, anxiety, dizziness, fatigue, headache, insomnia, lightheadedness, and sensory disturbances. The etiology of the withdrawal syndrome is unknown but probably includes both biological (e.g., serotonin deficiency related to receptor down-regulation) and psychological (e.g., personality) factors. The signs and symptoms of the withdrawal syndrome may be eliminated or minimized by gradually tapering-off the dosage over a period of one to two weeks, prescribing a SSRI that has a longer half-life of elimination (e.g., fluoxetine), or reinstituting SSRI pharmacotherapy if the signs and symptoms of withdrawal occur upon discontinuation of SSRI pharmacotherapy and become troublesome for the patient.

Prescribe SSRI pharmacotherapy cautiously to patients who

- have anorexia nervosa, are cachectic, or are underweight. SSRI pharmacotherapy has been associated with loss of appetite (anorexia) and loss of body weight and may exacerbate these conditions.
- have anxiety, insomnia, or nervousness. Up to 20% of patients receiving SSRI pharmacotherapy may experience anxiety, insomnia, or nervousness. These ADRs may be

significant enough to warrant discontinuation of pharmacotherapy for approximately one-quarter of these patients.

- are receiving ECT. Although data are limited, an increase in the incidence and duration of seizures among these patients has been reported.
- have histories of bipolar disorder. SSRI pharmacotherapy may induce mania in 20% of patients who have bipolar disorder. It also may induce mania in a much smaller percentage of patients who have unipolar disorders.
- have histories of seizure disorders. Although the risk is reportedly low, the SSRIs may increase seizure activity among these patients.

Caution patients who are receiving SSRI pharmacotherapy against

- giving, selling, or trading their prescribed SSRI to any friends, relatives, or others.
- performing activities that require alertness, judgment, and physical coordination (e.g., driving an automobile, operating dangerous equipment, supervising children) until their response to SSRI pharmacotherapy is known. The SSRIs may adversely affect these mental and physical functions.

In addition to these general precautions, caution patients to

- inform their prescribing psychologist if they begin or discontinue any other pharmacotherapy while receiving SSRI pharmacotherapy.
- carry a card, to use in the event of an emergency, indicating that they are receiving SSRI pharmacotherapy and other relevant information (e.g., the name and telephone numbers of their prescribing psychologist, a family member).
- inform their advanced practice nurse, dentist, family physician, and other health care providers that they are receiving SSRI pharmacotherapy.

CLINICALLY SIGNIFICANT DRUG INTERACTIONS

The SSRIs can interact with other drugs by a variety of mechanisms. However, one of the most important mechanisms involves the inhibition of the cytochrome P450 isoenzyme systems. This interaction varies among the SSRIs, as noted in the following table.

Inhibitory potential	Cytochrome P450 isoenzyme system				
	CYP1A2	CYP3A3/4	CYP2C9	CYP2C19	CYP2D6
None	fluoxetine paroxetine sertraline venlafaxine	venlafaxine	paroxetine venlafaxine		fluvoxamine venlafaxine
Low		paroxetine	fluvoxamine	fluoxetine	
Moderate		fluoxetine sertraline	fluoxetine		sertraline
High	fluvoxamine	fluvoxamine	sertraline	fluvoxamine	fluoxetine paroxetine

Concurrent SSRI pharmacotherapy and the following may result in clinically significant drug interactions:

Cimetidine Pharmacotherapy

Cimetidine (Tagamet®) pharmacotherapy, and to a lesser extent other histamine receptor-2 antagonist pharmacotherapy (e.g., ranitidine [Zantac®]), may significantly inhibit the first-pass hepatic metabolism of the SSRIs. This interaction may result in increased SSRI blood concentrations and toxicity.

Pharmacotherapy With Drugs That Are Highly Bound to Plasma Proteins

The SSRIs may displace from their binding sites other drugs that are highly bound to plasma proteins (e.g., digitoxin [Digitaline®], warfarin [Coumadin®]). This interaction may result in significantly higher concentrations of free drug and associated pharmacologic actions, including ADRs. Conversely, depending upon their affinity for the plasma protein binding sites, other drugs may displace the SSRIs.

Monoamine Oxidase Inhibitor Pharmacotherapy

See Relative Contraindications

Pharmacotherapy With Drugs That Are Primarily Metabolized by the Hepatic Cytochrome P450 Enzyme System

The SSRIs inhibit, to varying degrees, these hepatic enzymes (see previous table). Thus, they may reduce the rate and extent of metabolism of a number of drugs, as noted in the following table. Note that some drugs are metabolized by more than one isoenzyme.

Drugs metabolized by the various cytochrome P450 isoenzymes.[1]

CYP1A2	CYP3A3/4	CYP2C9	CYP2C19	CYP2D6
caffeine	**alprazolam**	**amitriptyline**	**diazepam**	**amitriptyline**
clozapine	astemizole	nonsteroidal	**imipramine**	**clomipramine**
imipramine	calcium channel	anti-inflammatory	omeprazole	**clozapine**
propranolol	blockers	drugs (NSAIDs)	propranolol	**codeine**
theophylline	**carbamazepine**	**phenytoin**		**desipramine**
warfarin	cisapride	warfarin		flecainide
	clozapine			**haloperidol**
	corticosteroids			**imipramine**
	diazepam			**nortriptyline**
	imipramine			**paroxetine**
	midazolam			**perphenazine**
	quinidine			propafenone
	terfenadine			propranolol
	triazolam			**risperidone**
	verapamil			**sertraline**
				thioridazine
				venlafaxine

[1]Psychotropics are indicated in bold.

Pharmacotherapy With Tryptophan and Other Serotonergics

Tryptophan is an essential amino acid and a serotonin precursor (i.e., tryptophan can be metabolized to serotonin). It is found in some foods (e.g., milk) and in significant amounts in some vitamin and dietary supplements. Concurrent SSRI pharmacotherapy with tryptophan may result in the potentially fatal serotonin syndrome. The serotonin syndrome also may occur with concurrent SSRI and other serotonergic pharmacotherapy (e.g., fenfluramine pharmacotherapy) (see Fenfluramine Monograph).

ADVERSE DRUG REACTIONS

The SSRIs are associated with the fewest and lowest incidence of ADRs when compared to the other available antidepressants. Thus, they have the best ADR profile. For example, the SSRIs cause minimal sedation or weight gain and virtually no anticholinergic, cardiovascular (i.e., dysrhythmias), or CNS (i.e., seizures) ADRs. However, the ADRs associated with SSRI pharmacotherapy have resulted in discontinuation of treatment in up to 15% of patients. SSRI pharmacotherapy commonly has been associated with anorgasmia, anxiety, asthenia, decreased sex drive, dizziness, drowsiness, dry mouth, headache, and insomnia. Other ADRs associated with SSRI pharmacotherapy, listed according to body system, include:

Cardiovascular: hypotension (relatively infrequent with most SSRIs but may occur with fluoxetine)
CNS: light-headedness and nervousness
Cutaneous: hair loss (alopecia), rare; itching, severe (pruritus); rash; and sweating (excessive)
Genitourinary: painful menstruation (dysmenorrhea)
GI: constipation, diarrhea, loss of appetite (anorexia), and nausea
Hematologic: anemia (rare)
Metabolic/Endocrine: see Genitourinary
Musculoskeletal: arthritis, back pain, joint pain, and muscle pain
Ocular: blurred vision, conjunctivitis, and reduction or dimness of vision (amblyopia)
Respiratory: asthma, bronchitis, and runny nose (rhinitis)
Miscellaneous: chills, malaise, and weight loss

See also individual SSRI monographs

OVERDOSAGE

Signs and symptoms of SSRI overdosage include agitation, hypomania, irritability, nausea, restlessness, seizures, tachycardia, tremor, and vomiting. Overdosages involving the SSRIs are generally less severe than those involving MAOIs or TCAs and have been associated with fewer deaths. Regardless, SSRI overdosage requires emergency symptomatic medical support of body systems with attention to increasing SSRI elimination. There is no known antidote.

SERTRALINE

(ser'tra leen)

TRADE NAME

Zoloft®

CLASSIFICATION

Antidepressant (SSRI)

See also Selective Serotonin Re-Uptake Inhibitors General Monograph

APPROVED INDICATIONS FOR PSYCHOLOGICAL DISORDERS

Adjunctive pharmacotherapy for the symptomatic management of:

- Mood Disorders, Depressive Disorders: Major Depressive Disorder
- Anxiety Disorders: Obsessive-Compulsive Disorder
- Anxiety Disorders: Panic Disorder

USUAL DOSAGE AND ADMINISTRATION

Depressive Disorders: Major Depressive Disorder

Adults: Initially, 50 mg daily orally in a single morning or evening dose. Increase the daily dosage weekly by 25 to 50 mg increments according to individual patient response.

MAXIMUM: 200 mg daily orally

Women who are, or who may become, pregnant: FDA Pregnancy Category C. Safety and efficacy of sertraline pharmacotherapy for women who are pregnant have not been established (see Selective Serotonin Re-Uptake Inhibitors General Monograph). Avoid prescribing sertraline pharmacotherapy to women who are pregnant. If sertraline pharmacotherapy is required, advise patients of potential benefits and possible risks to themselves and the embryo, fetus, or neonate. Collaboration with the patient's obstetrician is indicated.

Women who are breast-feeding: Safety and efficacy of sertraline pharmacotherapy for women who are breast-feeding and their neonates and infants have not been established (see Serotonin Re-Uptake Inhibitors General Monograph). Avoid prescribing sertraline pharmacotherapy to women who are breast-feeding. If sertraline pharmacotherapy is required, breast-feeding probably should be discontinued. Collaboration with the patient's pediatrician may be indicated.

Elderly, frail, or debilitated patients and those who have liver dysfunction: Generally prescribe lower dosages of sertraline for elderly, frail, or debilitated patients and those who have liver dysfunction. Increase the dosage gradually, if needed, according to individual patient response. These patients may be more sensitive to the pharmacologic actions of sertraline than are younger or healthier adult patients. Total body clearance of sertraline is reportedly reduced by up to 40% among elderly patients.

Children and adolescents younger than 18 years of age: Safety and efficacy of sertraline pharmacotherapy for children and adolescents have not been established. Sertraline pharmacotherapy is *not* recommended for this age group.

Notes, Depressive Disorders: Major Depressive Disorder

Each daily dose of sertraline should be ingested with food, preferably with the evening meal. If preferred, the daily dose may be ingested in the morning with breakfast (see also Available Dosage Forms, Storage, and Compatibility, Notes; and Pharmacokinetics/Pharmacodynamics).

Safety and efficacy of long-term sertraline pharmacotherapy (i.e., longer than 16 weeks) have not been established. Patients who require pharmacotherapy for longer than 16 weeks require regular periodic re-evaluation for the need for continued sertraline pharmacotherapy.

Anxiety Disorders: Obsessive-Compulsive Disorder

Adults: Initially, 50 mg daily orally in a single morning or evening dose. Increase the daily dosage weekly by 25 to 50 mg increments according to individual patient response.

MAXIMUM: 200 mg daily orally

Women who are, or who may become, pregnant: See Major Depressive Disorder

Women who are breast-feeding: See Major Depressive Disorder

Elderly, frail, or debilitated patients and those who have liver dysfunction: See Major Depressive Disorder

Children and adolescents younger than 18 years of age: See Major Depressive Disorder

Notes, Anxiety Disorders: Obsessive-Compulsive Disorder

See Notes, Major Depressive Disorder

Anxiety Disorders: Panic Disorder

Adults: Initially, 25 mg daily orally in a single morning or evening dose. Increase the daily dosage weekly by 25 to 50 mg increments according to individual patient response.

MAXIMUM: 200 mg daily orally

Women who are, or who may become, pregnant: See Major Depressive Disorder

Women who are breast-feeding: See Major Depressive Disorder

Elderly, frail, or debilitated patients and those who have liver dysfunction: See Major Depressive Disorder

Children and adolescents younger than 18 years of age: See Major Depressive Disorder

Notes, Anxiety Disorders: Panic Disorder

See Notes, Major Depressive Disorder

AVAILABLE DOSAGE FORMS, STORAGE, AND COMPATIBILITY

Capsules, oral: 25, 50, 100 mg
Tablets, oral: 25, 50, 100 mg

Notes

General Instructions for Patients   Instruct patients who are receiving sertraline pharmacotherapy to

- always ingest each dose of their sertraline capsules or tablets with their breakfast or evening meal in order to maximize absorption (i.e., oral availability) and to help maintain constant sertraline blood levels (i.e., to ensure consistent bioavailability) (see Pharmacokinetics/Pharmacodynamics).
- safely store sertraline capsules and tablets out of the reach of children in tightly closed child-resistant containers at controlled room temperature (15° to 30°C; 59° to 86°F).
- obtain an available patient information sheet regarding sertraline pharmacotherapy from their pharmacist at the time that their prescription is dispensed. Encourage patients to clarify any questions that they may have concerning sertraline pharmacotherapy with their pharmacist or, if needed, to consult their prescribing psychologist.

PROPOSED MECHANISM OF ACTION

The exact mechanism of sertraline's antidepressant and other related actions has not yet been fully determined. These actions appear to be directly related to sertraline's ability to selectively inhibit the neuronal re-uptake of serotonin. It also appears to down-regulate CNS norepinephrine and serotonin receptors.

See also the Selective Serotonin Re-Uptake Inhibitors General Monograph

PHARMACOKINETICS/PHARMACODYNAMICS

Sertraline is relatively well absorbed following oral ingestion. However, it is subject to extensive first-pass hepatic metabolism. Peak blood concentrations are achieved within 6 to 8 hours. The ingestion of food increases the bioavailability of sertraline by ~40%. Sertraline is highly plasma protein-bound (~98%). Its mean apparent volume of distribution is 76 L/kg. Sertraline is metabolized extensively in the liver. Virtually no sertraline (i.e., less than 1%) is excreted in unchanged form in the urine. However, ~14% is excreted in unchanged form in the feces. The mean half-life of elimination is ~26 hours, and the mean total body clearance is ~2.8 L/minute.

RELATIVE CONTRAINDICATIONS

Hypersensitivity to sertraline

MAOI pharmacotherapy, concurrent or within 14 days. This combination of pharmacotherapy, concurrent or within 14 days, may result in the serotonin syndrome (see Selective Serotonin Re-Uptake Inhibitors General Monograph).

CAUTIONS AND COMMENTS

Prescribe sertraline pharmacotherapy cautiously to patients who

- have anorexia nervosa, are cachectic, or are underweight. Sertraline pharmacotherapy has been associated with anorexia and weight loss and, thus, may exacerbate these conditions.
- are receiving concurrent pharmacotherapy with astemizole (an antihistamine removed in 1998 from the U.S. market at the request of the FDA), cisapride (a GI motility regulator), or terfenadine (an antihistamine). These drugs are metabolized by the cytochrome P450 isoenzyme CYP3A4. Potent inhibitors of this enzyme, such as fluvoxamine and ketoconazole (an antifungal), can significantly increase the blood concentrations of these drugs. This interaction may result in a potentially fatal torsades de pointes-type ventricular tachycardia. Although this interaction has not yet been directly associated with sertraline, extreme caution is required because sertraline is a moderate inhibitor of CYP3A4 (see Selective Serotonin Re-Uptake Inhibitors General Monograph).
- have histories of bipolar disorder. Mania may occur more frequently among these patients. Monitor these patients carefully.

Caution patients who are receiving sertraline pharmacotherapy against performing activities that require alertness, judgment, and physical coordination (e.g., driving an automobile, operating dangerous equipment, supervising children) until their response to sertraline pharmacotherapy is known. Sertraline may adversely affect these mental and physical functions.

In addition to this general precaution, caution patients to inform their prescribing psychologist if they begin or discontinue any other pharmacotherapy while receiving sertraline pharmacotherapy.

CLINICALLY SIGNIFICANT DRUG INTERACTIONS

Concurrent sertraline pharmacotherapy and the following may result in clinically significant drug interactions:

Pharmacotherapy With Drugs That Are Highly Bound to Plasma Proteins

Sertraline may displace from their binding sites other drugs that are highly bound to plasma proteins (e.g., digitoxin [Digitaline®], warfarin [Coumadin®]). This interaction results in significantly higher concentrations of free drug and associated actions, including ADRs. Conversely, other drugs, depending upon their affinity for plasma proteins, may displace sertraline from its binding sites.

Pharmacotherapy With Drugs That Are Metabolized by the Hepatic Cytochrome P450 Enzyme System, Particularly Isoenzyme CYP2C9

Sertraline inhibits this particular hepatic isoenzyme. Consequently, sertraline reduces the rate and extent of metabolism of a number of drugs. These drugs include amitriptyline (Elavil®), clozapine (Clozaril®), NSAIDS (e.g., ibuprofen [Motrin®]), phenytoin (Dilantin®), and warfarin (Coumadin®). Concurrent sertraline pharmacotherapy with these drugs may result in their toxicity.

See also Selective Serotonin Re-Uptake Inhibitors General Monograph

ADVERSE DRUG REACTIONS

Sertraline pharmacotherapy commonly has been associated with delayed ejaculation, diarrhea, dizziness, dry mouth, dyspepsia, headache, insomnia, nausea, somnolence, sweating (excessive), and tremor. Other ADRs associated with sertraline pharmacotherapy, listed according to body system, include:

Cardiovascular: hypertension, hypotension, palpitations, fainting (syncope), and tachycardia

CNS: abnormal dreams, agitation, anxiety, emotional lability, mania (rare), and migraine

Cutaneous: acne, cold and clammy or dry skin, edema, flushing, hair loss (alopecia), itching (severe), and rash

Genitourinary: decreased sex drive, excessive urination (polyuria), excessive urination during the night (nocturia), painful menstruation (dysmenorrhea), painful or difficult urination (dysuria), and urinary incontinence

GI: abdominal pain, abnormal taste, belching (eructation), constipation, difficulty swallowing (dysphagia), loss of appetite (anorexia), and vomiting

Hematologic: rarely, anemia

Metabolic/Endocrine: breast enlargement among males (gynecomastia, rare), and hot flushes (see also Genitourinary and Ocular)

Musculoskeletal: incoordination (ataxia), joint pain (arthralgia), muscle cramps, muscle pain (myalgia), muscle weakness (asthenia), and prolonged muscle contractions associated with twisting and repetitive movements or abnormal posture (dystonia)

Ocular: abnormal accommodation, abnormal dilation of the pupils (mydriasis), abnormal protrusion of the eyeball (exophthalmos), conjunctivitis, double vision (diplopia), and eye pain

Otic: ear ache and ringing in the ears (tinnitus)

Respiratory: bronchospasm, coughing, difficult breathing (dyspnea), pharyngitis, and runny nose (rhinitis)

Miscellaneous: fatigue and malaise

See also Selective Serotonin Re-Uptake Inhibitors General Monograph

OVERDOSAGE

Signs and symptoms of sertraline overdosage include anxiety, dilated pupils, nausea, somnolence, tachycardia, and vomiting. Sertraline overdosage requires emergency symptomatic medical support of body systems with attention to increasing sertraline elimination. There is no known antidote.

TEMAZEPAM

(te maz'e pam)

TRADE NAME

Restoril®

CLASSIFICATION

Sedative-hypnotic (benzodiazepine) (C-IV)

See also Benzodiazepines General Monograph

APPROVED INDICATIONS FOR PSYCHOLOGICAL DISORDERS

Adjunctive pharmacotherapy for the short-term symptomatic management of:

Sleep Disorders: Insomnia (difficulty falling asleep, frequent nocturnal awakenings, and/or early morning awakenings)

USUAL DOSAGE AND ADMINISTRATION

Insomnia

Adults: 15 to 30 mg daily orally 30 minutes before retiring for bed in the evening

Women who are, or who may become, pregnant: FDA Pregnancy Category X. Safety and efficacy of temazepam pharmacotherapy for women who are pregnant have not been established. However, temazepam pharmacotherapy is contraindicated during pregnancy because it has been associated with teratogenic effects in animal studies. Its similarity to other benzodiazepines that have been associated with teratogenic effects in humans also supports its contraindication during pregnancy. In addition, maternal use of therapeutic dosages of a benzodiazepine during the last weeks of pregnancy may place neonates at risk for CNS depression and flaccidity due to transplacental distribution. Long-term benzodiazepine pharmacotherapy during pregnancy also may place neonates at risk for the neonatal benzodiazepine withdrawal syndrome (see also Benzodiazepines General Monograph). Do *not* prescribe temazepam pharmacotherapy to women who are pregnant.

Women who are breast-feeding: Safety and efficacy of temazepam pharmacotherapy for women who are breast-feeding and their neonates and infants have not been established. Temazepam is excreted into breast milk. Breast-fed neonates and infants may display expected pharmacologic actions (e.g., drowsiness, lethargy). They also may become addicted (see Benzo-diazepines General Monograph). Avoid prescribing temazepam pharmacotherapy to women who are breast-feeding. If temazepam pharmacotherapy is required, breast-feeding probably should be discontinued. If desired, lactation may be maintained and breast-feeding resumed following the discontinuation of short-term temazepam pharmacotherapy. Collaboration with the patient's pediatrician may be indicated.

Elderly, frail, or debilitated patients and those who have organic brain syndrome (OBS) or kidney dysfunction: Initially, 7.5 mg daily orally 30 minutes before retiring for bed in the evening. Generally prescribe lower dosages for elderly, frail, or debilitated patients. These patients may be more sensitive to the pharmacologic actions of temazepam, particularly its dose-related ADRs (e.g., dizziness, drowsiness, impaired coordination) than are younger or healthier adult patients. Debilitated patients and those who have OBS are prone to CNS depression even when lower dosages of temazepam or other benzodiazepines are prescribed. These patients may experience paradoxical reactions. Prescribe the lowest effective dosage of temazepam cautiously for these patients. Adjust the dosage, as needed, according to individual patient response. Inappropriate over-sedation among elderly and other sensitive patients has been associated with accidental falls and other adverse events. Lower dosages also may be required for patients who have kidney dysfunction.

MAXIMUM: 15 mg daily orally

Children and adolescents younger than 18 years of age: Safety and efficacy of temazepam pharmacotherapy for children and adolescents have not been established. Temazepam pharmacotherapy is *not* recommended for this age group.

Notes, Insomnia

Initiating Temazepam Pharmacotherapy   Prescribe temazepam pharmacotherapy only for the short-term symptomatic management of insomnia associated with disturbed sleep that results in impaired daytime functioning. An appropriate hypnotic dose should produce desired sleep while avoiding over-sedation and impaired performance the following day (i.e., "hang-over" effect). In this regard, do *not* prescribe for longer than seven to ten consecutive days. Do not prescribe quantities exceeding those required for short-term pharmacotherapy, and do not renew prescriptions without reevaluating the patient's need for continued temazepam pharmacotherapy.

The failure of insomnia to remit after seven to ten days of temazepam pharmacotherapy may indicate the presence of a primary mental disorder, medical disorder, or sleep state misperception. Pharmacotherapy that appears to be required for longer than two to three consecutive weeks requires reevaluation of the patient. Collaboration with a psychologist specializing in sleep disorders or another specialist (e.g., neurologist) may be indicated. Worsening of insomnia, or the emergence of new signs and symptoms, including abnormal thinking or behavior, may or may not be ADRs associated with temazepam pharmacotherapy and also require careful evaluation.

Discontinuing Temazepam Pharmacotherapy   A benzodiazepine withdrawal syndrome similar to that observed with alcohol has occurred following the abrupt discontinuation of benzodiazepine pharmacotherapy, including temazepam pharmacotherapy. Signs and symptoms of this syndrome include abdominal and muscle cramps, convulsions, dysphoria, insomnia, perceptual disturbances, sweating, tremor, and vomiting. Severe signs and symptoms are generally associated with higher dosages and long-term regular use. Patients who have received pharmacotherapy with recommended dosages for as few as one to two weeks also may display signs and symptoms of withdrawal upon discontinuation of pharmacotherapy. These signs and symptoms include daytime anxiety between evening doses. Avoid the abrupt discontinuation of temazepam pharmacotherapy. Discontinue temazepam pharmacotherapy gradually, particularly for patients who have histories of seizure disorders and those who have received more than the lowest dosage for longer than a few weeks.

AVAILABLE DOSAGE FORMS, STORAGE, AND COMPATIBILITY

Capsules, oral: 7.5, 15, 30 mg

Notes

General Instructions for Patients Instruct patients who are receiving temazepam pharmacotherapy to

- safely store temazepam capsules out of the reach of children and protected from moisture or excessive heat in tightly closed child-resistant containers at controlled room temperature (15° to 30°C; 59° to 86°F).
- obtain an available patient information sheet regarding temazepam pharmacotherapy from their pharmacist at the time that their prescription is dispensed. Encourage patients to clarify any questions that they may have concerning temazepam pharmacotherapy with their pharmacist or, if needed, to consult their prescribing psychologist.

PROPOSED MECHANISM OF ACTION

Temazepam is a benzodiazepine with hypnotic action. Its exact mechanism of action has not yet been fully determined. However, it appears to be mediated by or to work in concert with the inhibitory neurotransmitter GABA. Temazepam appears to produce hypnosis by binding to benzodiazepine receptors within the GABA complex.

See also Benzodiazepines General Monograph

PHARMACOKINETICS/PHARMACODYNAMICS

Temazepam is well absorbed after oral ingestion and has a mean bioavailability of ~90%. Therapeutic blood concentrations are achieved within 30 minutes, with peak blood concentrations occurring in two to three hours. Temazepam displays minimal first-pass hepatic metabolism (~8%) and has no active metabolites. Temazepam is approximately 96% bound to plasma protein. The mean apparent volume of distribution is 1 L/kg. Temazepam blood concentration levels decline bi-phasically with a mean half-life of elimination of 10 hours (range 3.5 to 18 hours). The mean total body clearance is ~4.2 L/hour.

RELATIVE CONTRAINDICATIONS

Glaucoma, acute narrow-angle
Hypersensitivity to temazepam or other benzodiazepines
Myasthenia gravis
Paradoxical reactions to alcohol use or sedative-hypnotic pharmacotherapy, history of
Pregnancy
Sleep apnea syndrome

CAUTIONS AND COMMENTS

Temazepam pharmacotherapy has been associated with addiction and habituation. The risk for addiction and habituation is increased among patients who have histories of alcoholism or other problematic patterns of abusable psychotropic use. It also may be increased among patients who have marked personality disorders. Inter-dose daytime anxiety and rebound anxiety also have been associated with increased risk for addiction and habituation among patients who are receiving temazepam pharmacotherapy. Limit repeat prescriptions, and reevaluate patient need for continued pharmacotherapy. Discontinue temazepam pharmacotherapy gradually for all patients to avoid the benzodiazepine withdrawal syndrome.

Prescribe temazepam pharmacotherapy cautiously to patients who

- have depression, severe or latent. Temazepam may potentiate CNS depression and exacerbate suicidal tendencies. Monitor patients for depression, and evaluate suicidal risk. Implement appropriate suicide precautions, as needed.
- have histories of problematic patterns of alcohol or other abusable psychotropic use. These patients may be at greater risk for developing problematic patterns of temazepam use.
- have kidney dysfunction. Temazepam is primarily excreted by the kidneys. These patients may be at risk for prolonged action or toxicity.
- have liver dysfunction. Temazepam is metabolized in the liver. These patients may be at risk for prolonged action or toxicity.
- have pulmonary dysfunction. Temazepam-related respiratory depression has been reported among these patients.

Caution patients who are receiving temazepam pharmacotherapy against

- drinking alcohol or using other drugs that depress the CNS. Concurrent use may result in severe CNS depression.
- performing activities that require alertness, judgment, or physical coordination (e.g., driving an automobile, operating dangerous equipment, supervising children) until their response to temazepam is known. Temazepam's CNS depressant action may adversely affect these mental and physical functions.

In addition to these general precautions, caution patients to inform their prescribing psychologist if they begin or discontinue any other pharmacotherapy while receiving temazepam pharmacotherapy.

CLINICALLY SIGNIFICANT DRUG INTERACTIONS

Concurrent temazepam pharmacotherapy and the following may result in clinically significant drug interactions:

Alcohol Use

Concurrent alcohol use may increase the CNS depressant action of temazepam. Advise patients to avoid, or limit, their use of alcohol while receiving temazepam pharmacotherapy.

Pharmacotherapy With Central Nervous System Depressants and Other Drugs That Produce Central Nervous System Depression

Concurrent temazepam pharmacotherapy with opiate analgesics, other sedative-hypnotics, or other drugs that produce CNS depression (e.g., antihistamines, phenothiazines, TCAs) may result in additive CNS depression.

See also Benzodiazepines General Monograph

ADVERSE DRUG REACTIONS

Temazepam pharmacotherapy commonly has been associated with dizziness, drowsiness, fatigue, headache, lethargy, and nervousness. Other ADRs, listed according to body system, include:

Cardiovascular: fainting (syncope) and rapid throbbing or fluttering of the heart (palpitations)

CNS: confusion; dreaming, increased; disequilibrium; euphoria; and hallucinations. Temazepam pharmacotherapy also has been rarely associated with amnesia, anxiety, confusion, depression, psychoses, and rebound insomnia.

Cutaneous: sweating (excessive)

GI: vomiting

Musculoskeletal: backache, incoordination (ataxia), and tremor

Ocular: burning of the eyes and constant, involuntary, cyclical, horizontal movement of the eyeball (horizontal nystagmus)

See also Benzodiazepines General Monograph

OVERDOSAGE

Signs and symptoms of acute temazepam overdosage are related to its CNS depressant action and include confusion and somnolence. Overdosage involving large amounts of temazepam may result in respiratory depression, hypotension, and coma with reduced or absent reflexes. Temazepam overdosage requires emergency symptomatic medical support of body systems with attention to increasing temazepam elimination. The benzodiazepine antagonist flumazenil (Anexate®, Romazicon®) is a specific antidote for known or suspected benzodiazepine overdosage.

THIOPROPERAZINE ♣

(thye oh proe per′a zeen)

TRADE NAME

Majeptil®

CLASSIFICATION

Antipsychotic (phenothiazine)

See also Phenothiazines General Monograph

APPROVED INDICATIONS FOR PSYCHOLOGICAL DISORDERS

Adjunctive pharmacotherapy for the symptomatic management of:

Psychotic Disorders: Schizophrenia and Other Psychotic Disorders

USUAL DOSAGE AND ADMINISTRATION

Schizophrenia and Other Psychotic Disorders

Adults: Initially, 5 mg daily orally in a single or divided doses. Increase the daily dosage gradually by 5 mg increments every two or three days until the usual effective dosage of 30 to 40 mg daily is achieved.

MAXIMUM: 90 mg daily orally

Women who are, or who may become, pregnant: FDA Pregnancy Category "not established." Safety and efficacy of thioproperazine pharmacotherapy for women who are pregnant have not been established. Avoid prescribing thioproperazine pharmacotherapy to women who are pregnant, particularly during the first trimester of pregnancy. If thioproperazine pharmacotherapy is required, advise patients of potential benefits and possible risks to themselves and the embryo, fetus, or neonate. Collaboration with the patient's obstetrician is indicated.

Women who are breast-feeding: Safety and efficacy of thioproperazine pharmacotherapy for women who are breast-feeding and their neonates and infants have not been established. Avoid prescribing thioproperazine pharmacotherapy to women who are breast-feeding. If thioproperazine pharmacotherapy is required, breast-feeding probably should be discontinued. Collaboration with the patient's pediatrician is required.

Elderly, frail, or debilitated patients: Generally prescribe lower dosages of thioproperazine for elderly, frail, or debilitated patients. Increase the dosage gradually, if needed, according to individual patient response. These patients may be more sensitive to the pharmacologic actions of thioproperazine than are younger or healthier adult patients.

Children younger than 3 years of age: Thioproperazine pharmacotherapy is *contraindicated* for children who are younger than 3 years of age.

Children younger than 10 years of age: Safety and efficacy of thioproperazine pharmacotherapy for children younger than 10 years of age have not been established. Thioproperazine pharmacotherapy is *not* recommended for this age group.

Children 10 years of age and older: Initially, 1 to 3 mg daily orally in a single or divided dose. Increase the daily dosage gradually by the same amount every two or three days until optimal therapeutic benefit is achieved. Do *not* exceed the recommended adult dosage.

Notes, Schizophrenia and Other Psychotic Disorders

Prescribe *general* or *discontinuous* thioproperazine pharmacotherapy according to the patient's signs and symptoms of psychosis and previous response to antipsychotic pharmacotherapy.

Initiating, Maintaining, and Discontinuing *General* Thioproperazine Pharmacotherapy Prior to initiating thioproperazine pharmacotherapy, establish that patients have satisfactory cardiovascular, kidney, and liver function. Referral to the patient's family physician or a specialist (e.g., cardiologist) for medical evaluation may be indicated. Initially prescribe a lower oral dosage. Increase the dosage gradually according to individual patient response.

For children and adults, reduce the dosage gradually to the lowest effective dosage. This dosage may be as low as a few milligrams daily. Maintain the dosage for as long as needed. However, discontinue thioproperazine pharmacotherapy if patients display signs and symptoms of a severe neurologic syndrome, including abnormal tension of muscles (hypertonia) accompanied by an inability to swallow or difficulty swallowing (dysphagia) and marked autonomic nervous system disturbances.

Initiating, Maintaining, and Discontinuing *Discontinuous* Thioproperazine Pharmacotherapy   Patients who are resistant to antipsychotic pharmacotherapy may occasionally benefit from discontinuous pharmacotherapy. Prescribe 5 to 10 mg of thioproperazine three times daily until the onset of severe EPRs. Once severe EPRs occur, withhold pharmacotherapy until the patient fully and spontaneously recovers from these EPRs. Following recovery from the EPRs, reinstitute thioproperazine pharmacotherapy. A total of three consecutive treatments is recommended. *Discontinuous pharmacotherapy requires hospitalization and close monitoring.* Collaboration with a clinical psychologist or a specialist (e.g., neurologist) who is experienced with initiating, maintaining, and discontinuing *discontinuous* thioproperazine pharmacotherapy may be indicated.

AVAILABLE DOSAGE FORMS, STORAGE, AND COMPATIBILITY

Tablets, oral: 10 mg

Notes

General Instructions for Patients   Instruct patients who are receiving thioproperazine pharmacotherapy to

- safely store thioproperazine oral tablets out of the reach of children in child-resistant containers at controlled room temperature (15° to 30°C; 59° to 86°F).
- obtain an available patient information sheet regarding thioproperazine pharmacotherapy from their pharmacist at the time that their prescription is dispensed. Encourage patients to clarify any questions that they may have concerning thioproperazine pharmacotherapy with their pharmacist or, if needed, to consult their prescribing psychologist.

PROPOSED MECHANISM OF ACTION

Thioproperazine is a potent antipsychotic that has cataleptic and antiemetic actions. It also has mild sedative, hypothermic, and spasmolytic actions. However, unlike other phenothiazines, thioproperazine does not have antiserotonin, antihistamine, or hypotensive actions. The exact mechanism of its antipsychotic action has not yet been fully determined. It appears to be similar to that of the other phenothiazines.

See also Phenothiazines General Monograph

PHARMACOKINETICS/PHARMACODYNAMICS

Data are unavailable.

RELATIVE CONTRAINDICATIONS

Blood disorders
Cardiovascular dysfunction, severe
Children younger than 3 years of age
Coma
Depression, including that associated with CNS depressant pharmacotherapy, or regular personal use
Hypersensitivity to thioproperazine or other phenothiazines
Liver dysfunction, severe
Parkinson's disease

CAUTIONS AND COMMENTS

Prescribe thioproperazine pharmacotherapy cautiously to patients who

- have histories of seizure disorders. The phenothiazines lower the seizure threshold and may induce seizures among these patients.
- regularly drink alcohol or are receiving concurrent pharmacotherapy with drugs that produce CNS depression (e.g., antihistamines, opiate analgesics, sedative-hypnotics, TCAs). Concurrent pharmacotherapy may result in possible additive CNS depression.

- have suspected or actual brain tumors or GI obstruction. The antiemetic action of thioproperazine may obscure nausea, vomiting, and other symptomatology important for the monitoring of the clinical course of these medical disorders.

Caution patients who are receiving thioproperazine pharmacotherapy against performing activities that require alertness, judgment, and physical coordination (e.g., driving an automobile, operating dangerous equipment, supervising children) until their response to thioproperazine is known. Thioproperazine may adversely affect these mental and physical functions.

In addition to this general precaution, caution patients to inform their prescribing psychologist if they begin or discontinue any other pharmacotherapy while receiving thioproperazine pharmacotherapy.

See also Phenothiazines General Monograph

CLINICALLY SIGNIFICANT DRUG INTERACTIONS

Concurrent thioproperazine pharmacotherapy and the following may result in clinically significant drug interactions:

Alcohol Use

Concurrent alcohol use may increase the CNS depressant action of thioproperazine. Advise patients to avoid, or limit, their use of alcohol while receiving thioproperazine pharmacotherapy.

Grapefruit Juice

Grapefruit juice inhibits the cytochrome P450 isoenzyme 3A4 (CYP3A4). This enzyme is responsible for the metabolism of many different drugs, including triazolam. The oral ingestion of triazolam with grapefruit juice (as compared with its ingestion with water) may result in a 1.5-fold higher AUC (i.e., the amount of drug available to the systemic circulation) and a corresponding increase in sedation. Instruct patients to refrain from ingesting their triazolam doses with grapefruit juice.

Guanethidine Pharmacotherapy

Thioproperazine may decrease the neuronal uptake of guanethidine (Ismelin®) and, thus, decrease its antihypertensive action. An adjustment in the guanethidine dosage may be required. Collaboration with the prescriber of the guanethidine is indicated.

Pharmacotherapy With Anticholinergics or Other Drugs That Produce Anticholinergic Actions

Concurrent thioproperazine pharmacotherapy with anticholinergics (e.g., atropine) and other drugs that produce anticholinergic actions (e.g., TCAs) may result in additive anticholinergic actions, including paralytic ileus among susceptible patients (e.g., elderly or bedridden patients).

Pharmacotherapy With Central Nervous System Depressants and Other Drugs That Produce Central Nervous System Depression

Concurrent thioproperazine pharmacotherapy with opiate analgesics, sedative-hypnotics, or other drugs that produce CNS depression (e.g., antihistamines, TCAs) may result in additive CNS depression.

See also Phenothiazines General Monograph

ADVERSE DRUG REACTIONS

Thioproperazine pharmacotherapy commonly has been associated with EPRs. These reactions are dose-related. Thus, they generally subside with a reduction in dosage or with the temporary discontinuation of thioproperazine pharmacotherapy. Some patients may require anti-parkinsonian pharmacotherapy for the reversal of EPRs. In addition to EPRs, thioproperazine pharmacotherapy has been associated with the following ADRs, listed according to body system:

CNS: anxiety, apathy, changes in mood (depression or elation), drowsiness, insomnia and, rarely, headache, and nausea
Cutaneous: sweating (excessive)
Genitourinary: rarely, diminished production of urine (oliguria)
GI: rarely, diarrhea, excessive salivation, and vomiting
Ocular: blurred vision, and, rarely, accommodation disturbances

See also Phenothiazines General Monograph

OVERDOSAGE

Signs and symptoms of thioproperazine overdosage include severe EPRs with an inability to swallow (dysphagia), unusually high persistent and rapidly increasing fever (hyperthermia), excessive salivation, respiratory depression, shock with pallor, and profuse sweating. These signs and symptoms may be followed by collapse and coma. Although mild signs and symptoms may be managed by discontinuing thioproperazine pharmacotherapy, more severe signs and symptoms require emergency symptomatic medical support of body systems with attention to increasing thioproperazine elimination. There is no known antidote.

THIORIDAZINE

(thye oh rid'a zeen)

TRADE NAMES

Mellaril®
Novo-Ridazine®

CLASSIFICATION

Antipsychotic (phenothiazine)

See also Phenothiazines General Monograph

APPROVED INDICATIONS FOR PSYCHOLOGICAL DISORDERS

Adjunctive pharmacotherapy for the symptomatic management of:

Psychotic Disorders: Schizophrenia and Other Psychotic Disorders

USUAL DOSAGE AND ADMINISTRATION

Schizophrenia and Other Psychotic Disorders

Adults: 150 to 300 mg daily orally in two to four divided doses

MAXIMUM: 800 mg daily orally. Dosages above 300 mg daily generally are reserved for hospitalized patients.

Women who are, or who may become, pregnant: FDA Pregnancy Category "not established." Safety and efficacy of thioridazine pharmacotherapy for women who are pregnant have not been established. Thioridazine crosses the placenta. However, both reproductive studies involving animals and reported clinical experience have failed to demonstrate teratogenic effects associated with thioridazine pharmacotherapy (see also Phenothiazines General Monograph). Until safety and efficacy are established, avoid prescribing thioridazine pharmacotherapy to women who are pregnant. If thioridazine pharmacotherapy is required, advise patients (or their legal guardians in regard to the patient) of potential benefits and possible risks to themselves and the embryo, fetus, or neonate. Collaboration with the patient's obstetrician is indicated.

Women who are breast-feeding: Safety and efficacy of thioridazine pharmacotherapy for women who are breast-feeding and their neonates and infants have not been established. Thioridazine is excreted in breast milk (see also Phenothiazines General Monograph). Avoid prescribing thioridazine pharmacotherapy to women who are breast-feeding. If thioridazine pharmacotherapy is required, breast-feeding probably should be discontinued. Collaboration with the patient's advanced practice nurse or pediatrician is indicated.

Elderly, frail, or debilitated patients: Initially, 75 mg daily orally in three divided doses. Increase the dosage gradually, if needed, according to individual patient response. Generally prescribe lower dosages for elderly, frail, or debilitated patients. These patients may be more sensitive to the pharmacologic actions of thioridazine than are younger or healthier adult patients.

Children 2 years of age and older: 0.5 to 3 mg/kg daily orally in two or three divided doses

MAXIMUM: 3 mg/kg daily orally

Notes, Schizophrenia and Other Psychotic Disorders

Adjust all thioridazine dosages to the severity of signs and symptoms and individual patient response. Initially prescribe lower dosages, and increase the dosage gradually until optimal therapeutic benefit is achieved.

AVAILABLE DOSAGE FORMS, STORAGE, AND COMPATIBILITY

Concentrate, oral: 30 mg/ml (cherry-like odor, contains 3% alcohol); 100 mg/ml (strawberry-like odor, contains 4.2% alcohol)
Solution, oral (with calibrated dropper): 30 mg/ml (contains 2.5% alcohol)
Suspension, oral (Mellaril-S®): 2 mg/ml (fruit flavored, contains 0.5% alcohol); 5, 20 mg/ml (buttermint flavored with a peppermint odor)
Tablets, oral: 10, 15, 25, 50, 100, 150, 200 mg

Notes

General Instructions for Patients   Instruct patients who are receiving thioridazine pharmacotherapy to

- dilute each dose of the thioridazine oral concentrate with distilled or acidified water or juice prior to ingestion.
- shake the thioridazine oral suspension well before measuring each dose, to ensure an accurate dose is measured.
- safely store thioridazine oral dosage formulations out of the reach of children in tightly closed child- and light-resistant containers at temperatures below 30°C (86°F). Discard darkly discolored oral solutions appropriately.
- obtain an available patient information sheet regarding thioridazine pharmacotherapy from their pharmacist at the time that their prescription is dispensed. Encourage patients to clarify any questions that they may have concerning thioridazine pharmacotherapy with their pharmacist or, if needed, to consult their prescribing psychologist.

PROPOSED MECHANISM OF ACTION

Thioridazine is similar to other phenothiazines in regard to its antipsychotic action. However, it differs in regard to its antiemetic action and low propensity to cause EPRs. It also does not affect temperature regulation.

The exact mechanism of action of thioridazine is complex and has not yet been fully determined. Its antipsychotic activity appears to be primarily related to its interaction with dopamine-containing neurons, specifically the blockade of dopamine receptors both pre- and post-synaptically.

See also Phenothiazines General Monograph

PHARMACOKINETICS/PHARMACODYNAMICS

Thioridazine is rapidly and completely absorbed following oral ingestion. However, its total bioavailability is ~60%, probably because of significant first-pass hepatic metabolism. Peak blood concentrations are achieved within two to four hours. Thioridazine is highly plasma protein-bound (>95%). The volume of distribution is ~10 L/kg. It is metabolized in the liver to the active metabolites mesoridazine and sulforidazine. Excretion is mainly through the feces (~50%) and urine (~35%). Less than 5% of thioridazine is excreted in the urine as unchanged drug. The mean half-life of elimination is approximately 10 hours.

RELATIVE CONTRAINDICATIONS

Blood disorders
Bone marrow depression
Cardiovascular dysfunction
Children younger than 1 year of age
CNS depression, severe
Coma
Hypersensitivity to thioridazine or other phenothiazines
Hypertension, severe
Liver dysfunction, severe

CAUTIONS AND COMMENTS

Prescribe thioridazine pharmacotherapy cautiously to patients who

- have histories of seizure disorders. Seizures rarely have been associated with thioridazine pharmacotherapy.
- have liver dysfunction. Monitor liver function regularly among these patients. Collaboration with the patient's family physician or a specialist (e.g., internist) may be required.
- have narrow-angle glaucoma or prostatic hypertrophy. Thioridazine produces anticholinergic actions, which can exacerbate these conditions.

Caution patients who are receiving thioridazine pharmacotherapy against performing activities that require alertness, judgment, and physical coordination (e.g., driving an automobile, operating dangerous equipment, supervising children) until their response to thioridazine is known. Thioridazine may adversely affect these mental and physical functions.

In addition to this general precaution, caution patients to inform their prescribing psychologist if they begin or discontinue any other pharmacotherapy while receiving thioridazine pharmacotherapy.

See also Phenothiazines General Monograph

CLINICALLY SIGNIFICANT DRUG INTERACTIONS

Concurrent thioridazine pharmacotherapy and the following may result in clinically significant drug interactions:

Guanethidine Pharmacotherapy

Thioridazine may decrease the neuronal uptake of guanethidine (Ismelin®) and, thus, decrease its antihypertensive action. An adjustment in the dosage of the guanethidine may be required. Collaboration with the prescriber of the guanethidine is indicated.

Pharmacotherapy With Anticholinergics or Other Drugs That Produce Anticholinergic Actions

Concurrent thioridazine pharmacotherapy with anticholinergics (e.g., atropine) and other drugs that produce anticholinergic actions (e.g., TCAs) may result in additive actions, including paralytic ileus among susceptible patients (e.g., elderly or bedridden patients).

See also Phenothiazines General Monograph

ADVERSE DRUG REACTIONS

Thioridazine pharmacotherapy commonly has been associated with ADRs related to its anticholinergic actions. These ADRs include confusion, drowsiness, dry mouth, inhibition of ejaculation, tachycardia, urinary retention, and rarely, parotid gland swelling. Thioridazine pharmacotherapy also has been associated with pigmentary retinopathy and postural hypotension, especially among women and elderly patients. Patients who have histories of problematic patterns of alcohol use also may be prone to hypotension.

The severity of the ADRs associated with thioridazine pharmacotherapy appears to be directly related to the dosage and duration of thioridazine pharmacotherapy. For example, pigmentary retinopathy, a serious ADR, generally has been associated with long-term thioridazine pharmacotherapy among patients who are receiving dosages exceeding the recommended maximum of 800 mg daily. Monitor patients regularly for ADRs. Patients who require high-dosage long-term thioridazine pharmacotherapy require additional monitoring for ocular changes. Collaboration with the patient's ophthalmologist is required for the completion of regular eye examinations, which are recommended for these patients.

See also Phenothiazines General Monograph

OVERDOSAGE

Signs and symptoms of thioridazine overdosage resemble those associated with other phenothiazine overdosage. However, acute thioridazine overdosage generally has not been associated with the occurrence of EPRs (e.g., prolonged muscle contractions with twisting, repetitive movements, or abnormal posture [dystonia]; oculogyric crisis), although they may occur. The signs and symptoms of thioridazine overdosage generally include an abnormally low body temperature (hypothermia); cardiac abnormalities, such as tachycardia or other dysrhythmias; confusion; convulsions; disorientation; drowsiness; increased action of the reflexes (hyperreflexia); and motor restlessness, which may be followed by coma and absent reflexes (areflexia). Anticholinergic signs and symptoms (e.g., blurred vision, dry mouth, nasal congestion, postural hypotension) may occur early after thioridazine overdosage and generally are severe and persistent. Respiratory depression may occur later and generally is a sign of severe phenothiazine overdosage. Thioridazine overdosage requires emergency symptomatic medical support of body systems with attention to increasing thioridazine elimination. There is no known antidote.

THIOTHIXENE

(thye oh thix'een)

TRADE NAME

Navane®

CLASSIFICATION

Antipsychotic (thioxanthene)

APPROVED INDICATIONS FOR PSYCHOLOGICAL DISORDERS

Adjunctive pharmacotherapy for the symptomatic management of:

Psychotic Disorders: Schizophrenia and Other Psychotic Disorders. Thiothixene pharmacotherapy has been found to be of benefit to patients who have had unsatisfactory response to other antipsychotic pharmacotherapy. It also may be of therapeutic benefit to patients who have schizophrenia and who are also apathetic or withdrawn.

USUAL DOSAGE AND ADMINISTRATION

Schizophrenia and Other Psychotic Disorders

Adults: Initially, 5 to 15 mg daily intramuscularly or orally in two to four divided doses. Increase the dosage gradually according to individual patient response. Once optimal therapeutic response has been achieved, reduce the dosage as soon as possible to the lowest effective maintenance dosage.

MAINTENANCE: 15 to 30 mg daily intramuscularly; *or* 15 to 60 mg daily orally as a single dose. Adjust the dosage according to individual patient response. Higher daily dosages may be equally divided into two or three doses.

MAXIMUM: 30 mg daily intramuscularly; *or* 60 mg daily orally

Women who are, or who may become, pregnant: FDA Pregnancy Category "not established." Safety and efficacy of thiothixene pharmacotherapy for women who are pregnant have not been established. Avoid prescribing thiothixene pharmacotherapy to women who are pregnant. If thiothixene pharmacotherapy is required, advise patients of potential benefits and possible risks to themselves and the embryo, fetus, or neonate. Collaboration with the patient's obstetrician is indicated.

Women who are breast-feeding: Safety and efficacy of thiothixene pharmacotherapy for women who are breast-feeding and their neonates and infants have not been established. Avoid prescribing thiothixene pharmacotherapy to women who are breast-feeding. If thiothixene pharmacotherapy is required, breast-feeding probably should be discontinued. Collaboration with the patient's pediatrician is indicated.

Elderly, frail, or debilitated patients: Generally prescribe lower dosages of thiothixene for elderly, frail, or debilitated patients. Increase the dosage gradually, if needed, according to individual patient response. These patients may be more sensitive to the pharmacologic actions of thiothixene than are younger or healthier adult patients.

Children younger than 12 years of age: Safety and efficacy of thiothixene pharmacotherapy for children younger than 12 years of age have not been established. Thiothixene pharmacotherapy is *not* recommended for this age group.

Notes, Schizophrenia and Other Psychotic Disorders

The thiothixene injectable is *only* for intramuscular injection. Inject intramuscularly into large healthy muscle sites (e.g., dorsogluteal, ventrogluteal, or vastus lateralis sites). Do *not* inject intravenously.

Monitor blood counts and liver function regularly for patients who require long-term thiothixene pharmacotherapy, particularly high-dosage pharmacotherapy. Monitor also for sudden onset of severe CNS or vasomotor signs and symptoms. Patients who have changes in blood counts or liver function, or have severe CNS or vasomotor signs and symptoms, may require a decrease in dosage or discontinuation of thiothixene pharmacotherapy. Collaboration with the patient's family physician or a specialist (e.g., hematologist, internist, neurologist) may be required.

AVAILABLE DOSAGE FORMS, STORAGE, AND COMPATIBILITY

> Capsules, oral: 1, 2, 5, 10, 20 mg
> Injectables, intramuscular: 2, 5 mg/ml
> Concentrate, oral (with calibrated dropper): 5 mg/ml (cherry and passion fruit flavored; contains 7% alcohol)

Notes

Injectable Formulation   The thiothixene injectable formulation must be reconstituted according to the manufacturer's directions with sterile water for injection prior to intramuscular use. The reconstituted solution is stable at room temperature for up to 48 hours. Discard any unused portion appropriately after 48 hours. If not used immediately, the reconstituted injectable solution should be clearly labeled as per hospital or other institutional policy (e.g., time, date, and initials of the person who reconstituted the solution). It should then be safely stored until used or discarded appropriately.

Oral Formulations

General Instructions for Patients   Instruct patients who are receiving thiothixene pharmacotherapy to

- safely store thiothixene oral capsules out of the reach of children in child-resistant containers at controlled room temperature (15° to 30°C; 59° to 86°F).
- obtain an available patient information sheet regarding thiothixene pharmacotherapy from their pharmacist at the time that their prescription is dispensed. Encourage patients to clarify any questions that they may have concerning thiothixene pharmacotherapy with their pharmacist or, if needed, to consult their prescribing psychologist.

PROPOSED MECHANISM OF ACTION

Thiothixene, a thioxanthene derivative, shares similar pharmacologic actions with the piperazine phenothiazines. Its exact mechanism of action is complex and has not yet been fully determined. Its antipsychotic activity appears to be primarily related to its interaction with dopamine-containing neurons, specifically the blockade of dopamine receptors (D1 and D2) both pre- and post-synaptically within the CNS.

PHARMACOKINETICS/PHARMACODYNAMICS

Thiothixene is well absorbed following oral ingestion and intramuscular injection. It is widely distributed in body tissues. Thiothixene is metabolized extensively in the liver. It is primarily eliminated by biliary excretion in the feces as unchanged drug and inactive metabolites. Additional data are unavailable.

RELATIVE CONTRAINDICATIONS

Blood disorders
Cardiac dysfunction, severe
Children younger than 12 years of age
Circulatory collapse
CNS depression, associated with any cause
Coma
Hypersensitivity to thiothixene
Liver dysfunction, severe

CAUTIONS AND COMMENTS

Prescribe thiothixene pharmacotherapy cautiously to patients who

- have histories of seizure disorders, including those associated with the alcohol withdrawal syndrome. Thiothixene can lower the seizure threshold.
- have known or suspected glaucoma, may be exposed to extreme heat, or are receiving concurrent pharmacotherapy with drugs that have anticholinergic actions (e.g., phenothiazines, TCAs). Thiothixene displays weak anticholinergic action that can exacerbate these conditions or potentiate the action of anticholinergic drugs.

- regularly drink alcohol or are receiving concurrent pharmacotherapy with drugs that depress the CNS (e.g., antihistamines, barbiturates, benzodiazepines, opiate analgesics). These patients may be at risk for excessive CNS depression.

CLINICALLY SIGNIFICANT DRUG INTERACTIONS

Concurrent thiothixene pharmacotherapy and the following may result in clinically significant drug interactions:

Alcohol Use

Concurrent alcohol use may increase the CNS depressant action of thiothixene. Advise patients to avoid, or limit, their use of alcohol while receiving thiothixene pharmacotherapy.

ADVERSE DRUG REACTIONS

Thiothixene pharmacotherapy commonly has been associated with agitation, drowsiness (initial and transient), EPRs, feelings of restlessness and an inability to sit down (akathisia), and insomnia. Nonspecific reversible ECG changes have been reported. These changes generally remit with the discontinuation of thiothixene pharmacotherapy. Thiothixene also has been associated with the following ADRs, listed according to body system:

Cardiovascular: fainting (syncope), hypotension, and tachycardia
CNS: depression; fatigue; headache; and tardive dyskinesia, particularly with long-term thiothixene pharmacotherapy and upon discontinuation of pharmacotherapy
Cutaneous: hives, itching (severe), and rash
Genitourinary: abnormal absence of menses (amenorrhea) and impotence
GI: constipation, dry mouth, loss of appetite (anorexia), nausea, salivation (excessive), and sweating (excessive)
Hematologic: a usually transient increase in the number of leukocytes (leukocytosis) and a reduction in the number of circulating white blood cells, including basophils, eosinophils, monocytes, and, in particular, lymphocytes (leukopenia)
Metabolic/Endocrine: abnormal breast enlargement among men (gynecomastia) and abnormal secretion of milk (galactorrhea)
Musculoskeletal: prolonged muscle contractions with twisting, repetitive movements, or abnormal posture (dystonia) (see also CNS)
Ocular: blurred vision and fine lenticular pigmentation (with long-term high-dosage pharmacotherapy)
Respiratory: nasal congestion

OVERDOSAGE

Signs and symptoms of mild thiothixene overdosage include dizziness, drowsiness, and muscular twitching. Severe overdosage may include such signs and symptoms as CNS depression and coma, difficulty swallowing, gait disturbances, hypotension, rigidity, salivation (excessive), tilting of the head associated with a deformity of the neck muscles to the affected side with the chin pointing to the other side (torticollis), tremor, and weakness. Thiothixene overdosage requires emergency symptomatic medical support of body systems with attention to increasing thiothixene elimination. There is no known antidote.

TRANYLCYPROMINE

(tran il sip'roe meen)

TRADE NAME

Parnate®

CLASSIFICATION

Antidepressant (MAOI)

APPROVED INDICATIONS FOR PSYCHOLOGICAL DISORDERS

Adjunctive pharmacotherapy for the symptomatic management of:

Mood Disorders, Depressive Disorders: Moderate to Severe Depression

USUAL DOSAGE AND ADMINISTRATION

Moderate to Severe Depression

Adults: Initially, 20 mg daily orally in two divided doses, morning and afternoon. Increase the dosage after two to three weeks to 30 mg daily in two divided doses, 20 mg upon arising and 10 mg in the afternoon. Continue for at least one week. When desired therapeutic response is achieved, gradually reduce the dosage to a maintenance dosage, according individual patient response. Discontinue tranylcypromine pharmacotherapy for patients who do not achieve therapeutic benefit by the end of one week. Continued tranylcypromine pharmacotherapy for these patients is unlikely to be of therapeutic benefit. Allow a "drug-free" interval of at least one week before replacing tranylcypromine pharmacotherapy with other antidepressant pharmacotherapy. When replacing tranylcypromine pharmacotherapy with other antidepressant pharmacotherapy, generally prescribe half of the usual recommended dosage (see Clinically Significant Drug Interactions).

MAXIMUM: 60 mg daily orally

Women who are, or who may become, pregnant: FDA Pregnancy Category "not established." Safety and efficacy of tranylcypromine pharmacotherapy for women who are pregnant have not been established. Avoid prescribing tranylcypromine pharmacotherapy to women who are pregnant. If tranylcypromine pharmacotherapy is required, advise patients of potential benefits and possible risks to themselves and the embryo, fetus, or neonate. Collaboration with the patient's obstetrician is indicated.

Women who are breast-feeding: Safety and efficacy of tranylcypromine pharmacotherapy for women who are breast-feeding and their neonates and infants have not been established. Tranylcypromine is excreted into breast milk. Avoid prescribing tranylcypromine pharmacotherapy to women who are breast-feeding. If tranylcypromine pharmacotherapy is required, breast-feeding probably should be discontinued. Collaboration with the patient's pediatrician is indicated.

Elderly, frail, or debilitated patients: Generally prescribe lower dosages of tranylcypromine for elderly, frail, or debilitated patients. Increase the dosage gradually, if needed, according to individual patient response. These patients may be more sensitive to the pharmacologic actions of tranylcypromine than are younger or healthier adult patients. Tranylcypromine pharmacotherapy is *contraindicated* for patients who are 60 years of age and older.

Children and adolescents younger than 18 years of age: Safety and efficacy of tranylcypromine pharmacotherapy for children and adolescents have not been established. Tranylcypromine pharmacotherapy is *not* recommended for this age group.

Notes, Moderate to Severe Depression

Tranylcypromine pharmacotherapy may be prescribed for patients who also require ECT. For these patients, prescribe tranylcypromine 20 mg daily orally in two divided doses. Reduce the dosage to 10 mg daily orally for maintenance pharmacotherapy.

AVAILABLE DOSAGE FORMS, STORAGE, AND COMPATIBILITY

Tablets, oral: 10 mg

Notes

General Instructions for Patients Instruct patients who are receiving tranylcypromine pharmacotherapy to

- safely store tranylcypromine oral tablets out of the reach of children in child-resistant containers protected from light at controlled room temperature (15° to 30°C; 59° to 86°F).
- obtain an available patient information sheet regarding tranylcypromine pharmacotherapy from their pharmacist at the time that their prescription is dispensed. Encourage patients to clarify any questions that they may have concerning tranylcypromine pharmacotherapy with their pharmacist or, if needed, to consult their prescribing psychologist.

PROPOSED MECHANISM OF ACTION

Tranylcypromine appears to produce its antidepressant action primarily by potentiating the actions of various biogenic amines (specifically, dopamine, epinephrine, norepinephrine, and serotonin) by inhibiting the enzyme (monoamine oxidase) that catalyses their oxidative de-amination. This inhibition of metabolism increases the amounts of these amines throughout the body, including the synapses, and, consequently, results in increased activity at the post-synaptic neuron receptor sites.

PHARMACOKINETICS/PHARMACODYNAMICS

Tranylcypromine is well and rapidly absorbed following oral ingestion. Peak blood concentrations generally are achieved within 1.5 hours. The mean apparent volume of distribution is 3 L/kg (range 1.1 to 5.7 L/kg). Tranylcypromine is metabolized extensively in the liver. The mean half-life of elimination is 2.5 hours (range 1.5 to 3.5 hours). Additional data are unavailable.

RELATIVE CONTRAINDICATIONS TO USE

Blood disorders

Cardiovascular dysfunction

Cerebrovascular dysfunction

Dopaminergic pharmacotherapy (e.g., dopamine [Intropin®], levodopa [Dopar®], methyldopa [Aldomet®]), concurrent or within 14 days. Concurrent tranylcypromine and dopaminergic pharmacotherapy has been associated with severe ADRs, including headache (severe), fever (hyperpyrexia), hypertension, and, rarely, cerebral (subarachnoid) hemorrhage.

Fluoxetine pharmacotherapy, concurrent or within five weeks. Concurrent tranylcypromine and fluoxetine pharmacotherapy has resulted in death. Allow five weeks between the discontinuation of fluoxetine pharmacotherapy and the initiation of tranylcypromine pharmacotherapy.

Headaches, frequent or recurring. Headaches commonly are the first symptom of a tranylcypromine-induced hypertensive reaction. This reaction may be masked among these patients.

Hypersensitivity to tranylcypromine

Hypertension

Liver dysfunction. Hepatitis rarely has been associated with tranylcypromine pharmacotherapy. Patients who have liver dysfunction may be at increased risk for hepatitis.

MAOI (i.e., phenelzine) pharmacotherapy, concurrent or within 14 days

Patients who are 60 years of age and older. Elderly patients are more likely to experience the ADRs associated with tranylcypromine pharmacotherapy. These ADRs are also associated with increased morbidity and mortality among the elderly.

Pheochromocytoma, known or suspected. Tumors associated with this condition secrete catecholamines (e.g., epinephrine, norepinephrine). Tranylcypromine may increase blood pressure and cause other related undesirable actions among patients who have this medical disorder.

Sympathomimetic pharmacotherapy (e.g., amphetamine, ephedrine, non-prescription cough and cold products containing phenylephrine and phenylpropanolamine), concurrent or within 14 days. Concurrent tranylcypromine and sympathomimetic pharmacotherapy may result in fever (hyperpyrexia), headache (severe), hypertension, and, rarely, cerebral (subarachnoid) hemorrhage.

Tryptophan pharmacotherapy, concurrent or within 14 days. Concurrent tranylcypromine and tryptophan pharmacotherapy has been associated with severe ADRs, including agitation; amnesia; Babinski signs; confusion; delirium; incoordination (ataxia); and syndromes involving disorientation, hyperreflexia, hypomania, ocular oscillations, shivering, and twitching or clonic spasm of a muscle or group of muscles (myoclonus).

CAUTIONS AND COMMENTS

Prescribe tranylcypromine pharmacotherapy cautiously to patients who

- have histories of seizure disorders. Tranylcypromine may lower the seizure threshold.
- have histories of Parkinsonism. Tranylcypromine pharmacotherapy may increase the incidence and severity of the signs and symptoms associated with Parkinsonism.
- regularly drink alcohol or are using or concurrently receiving pharmacotherapy with other drugs that produce CNS depression (e.g., barbiturates, benzodiazepines, opiate analgesics).
- require elective surgery. Discontinue tranylcypromine pharmacotherapy at least seven days prior to elective surgery in order to avoid possible interactions with general anesthetics. Collaboration with the patient's surgeon or anesthesiologist may be indicated.

Caution patients who are receiving tranylcypromine pharmacotherapy against

- ingesting beverages and foods that contain high levels of tyramine, which can precipitate the hypertensive crisis. Generally, these beverages and foods include those for which aging protein breakdown is used to increase flavor:

  > Alcoholic beverages, especially beer (including non-alcoholic beer), red wines (Chianti), and sherry
  > Avocados (particularly when over-ripe)
  > Banana peel
  > Bovril
  > Caviar
  > Cheese, other than cottage cheese or cream cheese
  > Chocolate
  > Figs (canned)
  > Liver
  > Meat prepared with tenderizers
  > Pickled herring
  > Pods of broad beans (e.g., fava beans)
  > Raisins
  > Sour cream
  > Soy sauce
  > Yeast extracts (e.g., marmite)

- ingesting excessive amounts of caffeine in any form (e.g., coffee, cola drinks, tea). The ingestion of excessive amounts of caffeine may increase tranylcypromine's CNS stimulant actions.
- performing activities that require alertness, judgment, and physical coordination (e.g., driving an automobile, operating dangerous equipment, supervising children) until their response to tranylcypromine is known. Tranylcypromine pharmacotherapy may adversely affect these mental and physical functions.

In addition to these general precautions, caution patients to

- carry, for emergency identification, a card stating that they are receiving MAOI pharmacotherapy and other pertinent information (e.g., the telephone numbers of their prescribing psychologist and the person to call in case of an emergency).
- immediately report to their prescribing psychologist the occurrence of headaches or other unusual signs and symptoms.

- inform their prescribing psychologist if they begin or discontinue any other pharmacotherapy while receiving tranylcypromine pharmacotherapy.

CLINICALLY SIGNIFICANT DRUG INTERACTIONS

Concurrent tranylcypromine pharmacotherapy and the following may result in clinically significant drug interactions:

Bupropion Pharmacotherapy

Concurrent bupropion (Wellbutrin®) and MAOI pharmacotherapy (e.g., phenelzine [Nardil®], tranylcypromine [Parnate®]) may result in bupropion toxicity. Concurrent bupropion and MAOI pharmacotherapy is contraindicated. At least 14 days should elapse between the discontinuation of MAOI pharmacotherapy and the initiation of bupropion pharmacotherapy.

Buspirone Pharmacotherapy

Concurrent buspirone (BuSpar®) and MAOI pharmacotherapy (e.g., phenelzine [Nardil®], tranylcypromine [Parnate®]) has resulted in severe hypertension. Avoid, if possible, concurrent buspirone and MAOI pharmacotherapy. If concurrent pharmacotherapy is unavoidable, carefully monitor the patient's blood pressure. Collaboration with the patient's advanced practice nurse or family physician may be indicated.

Dopaminergic Pharmacotherapy Including Dopamine (Intropin®), Levodopa (Dopar®), and Methyldopa (Aldomet®) Pharmacotherapy

See Relative Contraindications

Tyramine-containing Beverages and Foods

Concurrent ingestion of beverages and foods that contain high concentrations of tyramine (e.g., aged cheese, beer, caffeine (in excess), canned figs, chocolate, pickled herring, red wine, sherry, sour cream) (see Cautions and Comments) may result in hypertensive crisis. Tyramine is normally metabolized by monoamine oxidase in the intestines and liver. When monoamine oxidase is inhibited by tranylcypromine, or other MAOI pharmacotherapy, tyramine absorbed from the GI tract passes freely into the general circulation. This change in tyramine metabolism results in the release of norepinephrine from adrenergic neurons, which produces exaggerated hypertension and other adverse reactions.

Sympathomimetic Pharmacotherapy

See Relative Contraindications

Tricyclic Antidepressant Pharmacotherapy

Concurrent tranylcypromine and TCA (e.g., amitriptyline, imipramine) pharmacotherapy may increase the actions of both drugs.

ADVERSE DRUG REACTIONS

Tranylcypromine pharmacotherapy commonly has been associated with insomnia and the more serious hypertensive crisis. The insomnia may be managed by reducing the daily dosage or by prescribing the last dose of the day no later than 3 pm (1500 hr) in the afternoon. The hypertensive crisis, the occurrence of which appears to be independent of dosage, is characterized by a paradoxical increase in blood pressure and bradycardia or tachycardia with constricting chest pain and palpitations. Other signs and symptoms include dilated pupils; a headache (occipital) that may radiate frontally; nausea or vomiting; neck stiffness or soreness; sensitivity to light (photophobia); and sweating, accompanied by fever or cold, clammy skin. These signs and symptoms may culminate with intracranial bleeding and death. The hypertensive crisis requires immediate discontinuation of tranylcypromine pharmacotherapy. Emergency symptomatic medical support of body systems and the appropriate management of related medical disorders are required. Phentolamine (Regitine®) generally is considered the antihypertensive of choice in this clinical situation. With appropriate medical management, acute signs and symptoms generally subside within 24 hours.

In addition to insomnia and the more serious hypertensive crisis, tranylcypromine pharmacotherapy has been associated with the following ADRs, listed according to body system:

Cardiovascular: postural hypotension and, rarely, tachycardia
CNS: dizziness, drowsiness, and headache
Cutaneous: rarely, chills, skin rash, and sweating
Genitourinary: rarely, impotence and urinary retention
GI: abdominal pain, constipation, dry mouth, diarrhea, GI complaints, loss of appetite (anorexia, rare), and nausea
Hepatic: rarely, jaundice (mild)
Musculoskeletal: rarely, muscle spasms and paresthesias
Ocular: rarely, blurred vision
Otic: rarely, ringing in the ears (tinnitus)

OVERDOSAGE

Signs and symptoms of tranylcypromine overdosage generally are intensified ADRs. The severity of the signs and symptoms of overdosage depend on the degree of overdosage and include anxiety, insomnia, restlessness progressing to agitation, confusion, dizziness, drowsiness, hypotension, incoherence, and weakness progressing to extreme dizziness and shock. Hypertension with a severe headache and other signs and symptoms may occur. Hypertension also may be rarely associated with myoclonic fibrillation of the skeletal muscles or twitching and hyperpyrexia progressing to generalized rigidity and coma. Emergency symptomatic medical support of body symptoms is required with attention to increasing tranylcypromine elimination. Although tranylcypromine is rapidly excreted, its MAOI action may continue for up to one week. There is no known antidote.

TRAZODONE

(traz'oh done)

TRADE NAME

Desyrel®

CLASSIFICATION

Antidepressant (triazolopyridine derivative)

APPROVED INDICATIONS FOR PSYCHOLOGICAL DISORDERS

Adjunctive pharmacotherapy for the symptomatic management of:

Mood Disorders: Major Depressive Disorder, including that accompanied by anxiety or agitation

USUAL DOSAGE AND ADMINISTRATION

Major Depressive Disorder, including that accompanied by anxiety or agitation

Adults: Initially, 150 mg daily orally in three divided doses. Increase the dosage by 50 mg increments every three or four days according to individual patient response.

MAXIMUM: 600 mg daily orally (hospitalized adult patients); 400 mg daily orally (non-hospitalized adult patients)

Women who are, or who may become, pregnant: FDA Pregnancy Category C. Safety and efficacy of trazodone pharmacotherapy for women who are pregnant have not been established. Avoid prescribing trazodone pharmacotherapy to women who are pregnant. If trazodone pharmacotherapy is required, advise patients of potential benefits and possible risks to themselves and the embryo, fetus, or neonate. Collaboration with the patient's obstetrician is indicated.

Women who are breast-feeding: Safety and efficacy of trazodone pharmacotherapy for women who are breast-feeding and their neonates and infants have not been established. Trazodone is excreted in breast milk. Avoid prescribing trazodone pharmacotherapy to women who are breast-feeding. If trazodone pharmacotherapy is required, breast-feeding probably should be discontinued. Collaboration with the patient's advanced practice nurse or pediatrician is required.

Elderly, frail, or debilitated patients: Generally prescribe lower dosages of trazodone for elderly, frail, or debilitated patients. Increase the dosage gradually, if needed, according to individual patient response. These patients may be more sensitive to the pharmacologic actions of trazodone than are younger or healthier adult patients.

Children and adolescents younger than 18 years of age: Safety and efficacy of trazodone pharmacotherapy for children and adolescents have not been established. Trazodone pharmacotherapy is *not* recommended for this age group.

Notes, Major Depressive Disorder, including that accompanied by anxiety or agitation

The potential for suicide among patients receiving trazodone pharmacotherapy for the symptomatic management of depression remains until significant remission occurs. Prescribe the smallest quantity of tablets feasible for dispensing. Other suicide precautions may be indicated.

Trazodone pharmacotherapy has been associated with the development of severe blood disorders. Monitor patients for signs and symptoms of blood disorders, including fever, sore throat, and other signs of infection. Obtain white blood cell and differential counts for these patients. Collaboration with the patient's advanced practice nurse, family physician, or a specialist (e.g., hematologist) may be required. Discontinue trazodone pharmacotherapy if white blood cell or absolute neutrophil counts fall below the normal ranges. Refer patients for medical confirmation of suspected blood disorders and, if needed, related medical management.

AVAILABLE DOSAGE FORMS, STORAGE, AND COMPATIBILITY

Tablets, oral: 50, 100, 150, 300 mg

Tablets, oral (Desyrel Dividose®): 150 mg. Each bisected and trisected tablet can be accurately broken to provide any of the following dosages: 50 mg (1/3 tablet), 75 mg (1/2 tablet), 100 mg (2/3 tablet), 150 mg (entire tablet). To break a Dividose® tablet accurately and easily, hold the tablet between the thumbs and index fingers close to the appropriate score mark or groove in the tablet. Then, facing the tablet score mark, apply pressure and snap the tablet segments apart.

Notes

General Instructions for Patients Instruct patients who are receiving trazodone pharmacotherapy to

- ingest each dose of the trazodone oral tablets with meals. Ingesting each dose with meals may increase absorption by as much as 20%.
- safely store trazodone oral tablets out of the reach of children in tightly closed child- and light-resistant containers at temperatures below 40°C (104°F).
- obtain an available patient information sheet regarding trazodone pharmacotherapy from their pharmacist at the time that their prescription is dispensed. Encourage patients to clarify any questions that they may have concerning trazodone pharmacotherapy with their pharmacist or, if needed, to consult their prescribing psychologist.

PROPOSED MECHANISM OF ACTION

Trazodone has antidepressant and sedative actions. The exact mechanism of trazodone's antidepressant action has not yet been fully determined. It appears to be primarily related to its ability to block the re-uptake of serotonin at the pre-synaptic neuronal membrane. This inhibition of re-uptake increases the amount of serotonin at the synapses and, consequently, results in increased activity at the post-synaptic neuron receptor sites.

PHARMACOKINETICS/PHARMACODYNAMICS

Trazodone is well absorbed following oral ingestion (mean bioavailability of 80%). Peak blood concentration levels are achieved within one hour. Absorption may be significantly enhanced by ingesting each dose with meals. However, absorption is delayed (i.e., absorption may be increased by up to 20%, but the achievement of peak blood concentrations is delayed for two hours). Trazodone is highly plasma protein-bound (~93%) and has an apparent volume of distribution of approximately 1 L/kg. Trazodone is metabolized extensively to at least three major metabolites. It is eliminated mainly by urinary excretion with less than 1% excreted as unchanged drug. The mean half-life of elimination is 6 hours (range is from 4 to 9 hours). The mean total body clearance is ~8 L/hour.

RELATIVE CONTRAINDICATIONS

Hypersensitivity to trazodone

CAUTIONS AND COMMENTS

Prescribe trazodone pharmacotherapy cautiously to patients who

- are receiving ECT. The safety and efficacy of concurrent trazodone pharmacotherapy and ECT have not been established. Avoid prescribing trazodone pharmacotherapy to patients who are receiving ECT.
- have histories of breast cancer. Long-term trazodone pharmacotherapy may increase prolactin secretion. Prolactin has been tentatively associated with approximately one-third of breast cancers. Avoid prescribing trazodone pharmacotherapy to patients who have histories of breast cancer. Collaboration with the patient's oncologist may be indicated.
- have histories of seizure disorders. Episodes of grand mal seizures have been reported among patients who were concurrently receiving trazodone pharmacotherapy and anticonvulsant pharmacotherapy for a previously diagnosed seizure disorder.
- have pre-existing heart disease. Trazodone may produce dysrhythmias among these patients, including isolated premature ventricular contractions, ventricular couplets, and, rarely, ventricular tachycardia. Monitor patients carefully for cardiac dysrhythmias. Collaboration with the patient's family physician or a specialist (e.g., cardiologist) is required. Avoid prescribing trazodone pharmacotherapy to patients during the initial recovery phase of myocardial infarction. Trazodone pharmacotherapy is *not* recommended for these patients.

Caution patients who are receiving trazodone pharmacotherapy against

performing activities that require alertness, judgment, and physical coordination (e.g., driving an automobile, operating dangerous equipment, supervising children) until their response to trazodone pharmacotherapy is known. Trazodone may adversely affect these mental and physical functions.

In addition to this general precaution, caution patients to inform their prescribing psychologist if they begin or discontinue any other pharmacotherapy while receiving trazodone pharmacotherapy.

CLINICALLY SIGNIFICANT DRUG INTERACTIONS

Concurrent trazodone pharmacotherapy and the following may result in clinically significant drug interactions:

Alcohol Use

Concurrent alcohol use may increase the CNS depressant action of trazodone. Advise patients to avoid, or limit, their use of alcohol while receiving trazodone pharmacotherapy.

Clonidine Pharmacotherapy

Trazodone may decrease the antihypertensive action of clonidine (Catapres®). Collaboration with the prescriber of the clonidine is indicated.

Pharmacotherapy With Central Nervous System Depressants and Other Drugs That Produce Central Nervous System Depression

Concurrent trazodone pharmacotherapy with opiate analgesics, sedative-hypnotics, or other drugs that produce CNS depression (e.g., antihistamines, phenothiazines, TCAs) may result in additive CNS depression.

ADVERSE DRUG REACTIONS

Trazodone pharmacotherapy commonly has been associated with dizziness, drowsiness, headache, dry mouth, and nausea or vomiting. It also has been associated with the following ADRs, listed according to body system:

Cardiovascular: cardiac arrest, chest pain, dysrhythmias (e.g., atrial fibrillation, bradycardia or tachycardia, and ventricular ectopic activity, including ventricular tachycardia), hypertension, myocardial infarction, postural hypotension, and rapid throbbing or fluttering of the heart (palpitations)

CNS: agitation, anger, confusion, difficulty concentrating, disorientation, excitement, fatigue, hostility, insomnia, lethargy, light-headedness, memory impairment, nervousness, nightmares, restlessness (akathisia), seizures (grand mal), slurred speech, and tremor; rarely, delusions, hallucinations, hypomania, and paranoia

Cutaneous: edema, itching, photosensitivity, purpura, maculopapular eruptions, rash, and sweating (excessive)

Genitourinary: blood in the urine (hematuria), urinary frequency, urinary incontinence, and urinary retention. Rarely, menstrual irregularities, inhibition of ejaculation, and retrograde ejaculation. Trazodone pharmacotherapy also has been associated with priapism, which has required surgery for some patients with resultant permanently impaired erectile function or impotence. Discontinue trazodone pharmacotherapy for men who have prolonged or inappropriate erections. Refer these patients for immediate medical evaluation.

GI: constipation, diarrhea, GI discomfort, increased or loss of appetite, peculiar taste, and salivation (excessive)

Hematologic: rarely, hemolytic anemia, leukocytoblastic vasculitis, and methemoglobinemia

Hepatic: liver enzyme alterations and obstructive jaundice

Metabolic/Endocrine: weight gain or loss

Musculoskeletal: aching joints and muscles; muscular incoordination, especially when voluntary muscle movement is attempted (ataxia); motor restlessness; and muscle stiffness. Rarely, dystonia and involuntary movements; muscle twitching, prickling, or tingling of the extremities (paresthesia); and sensation of numbness.

Ocular: abnormal contraction of the pupils (miosis); blurred vision; double vision (diplopia); red, tired, and itchy eyes; and visual distortions

Otic: ringing in the ears (tinnitus)

Respiratory: apnea, nasal congestion, and shortness of breath

Miscellaneous: fever

OVERDOSAGE

Signs and symptoms of trazodone overdosage are similar to the ADRs associated with trazodone pharmacotherapy. However, there is an increase in their incidence or severity. Trazodone overdosage requires emergency symptomatic medical support of body systems with attention to trazodone elimination. There is no known antidote.

TRIAZOLAM

(trye ay'zoe lam)

TRADE NAMES

Apo-Triazo®
Halcion®
Novo-Triolam®

CLASSIFICATION

Sedative-hypnotic (benzodiazepine) (C-IV)

See also Benzodiazepines General Monograph

APPROVED INDICATIONS FOR PSYCHOLOGICAL DISORDERS

Adjunctive pharmacotherapy for the short-term symptomatic management of:

Sleep Disorders: Insomnia

USUAL DOSAGE AND ADMINISTRATION

Insomnia

Adults: Initially, 0.125 mg daily orally 30 minutes before retiring for bed in the evening. If required, the dosage may be increased to 0.25 mg daily orally 30 minutes before retiring for bed in the evening.

MAXIMUM: 0.5 mg daily orally. Dosages exceeding 0.5 mg daily may produce an altered sense of taste or smell and non-specific personality changes, such as depersonalization, paranoia, severe anxiety, or suicidal ideation.

Women who are, or who may become, pregnant: FDA Pregnancy Category X. Safety and efficacy of triazolam pharmacotherapy for women who are pregnant have not been established. Based upon animal studies and the association of other benzodiazepines with congenital malformations (birth defects), particularly when used during the first trimester of pregnancy, triazolam pharmacotherapy is contraindicated during pregnancy. Maternal use of therapeutic dosages of benzodiazepines during the last weeks of pregnancy also has resulted in neonatal CNS depression and the neonatal benzodiazepine withdrawal syndrome as a result of transplacental distribution (see Benzodiazepines General Monograph). Do *not* prescribe triazolam pharmacotherapy to women who are, or who may become, pregnant. Caution women who are not yet pregnant to avoid pregnancy while receiving triazolam pharmacotherapy.

Women who are breast-feeding: Safety and efficacy of triazolam pharmacotherapy for women who are breast-feeding and their neonates and infants have not been established. Triazolam is excreted in breast milk. Breast-fed neonates and infants may display expected pharmacologic actions (e.g., drowsiness, lethargy). They also may become addicted (see Benzodiazepines General Monograph). Avoid prescribing triazolam pharmacotherapy to women who are breast-feeding. If triazolam pharmacotherapy is required, breast-feeding probably should be discontinued. If desired, lactation may be maintained and breast-feeding resumed following the discontinuation of short-term triazolam pharmacotherapy. Collaboration with the patient's pediatrician is indicated.

Elderly, frail, or debilitated patients and those who have kidney or liver dysfunction: Initially, 0.125 mg daily orally 30 minutes before retiring for bed in the evening. If required, the dosage may be cautiously increased to 0.25 mg daily orally 30 minutes before retiring for bed in the evening. Elderly, frail, or debilitated patients, and those who have kidney or liver dysfunction, may be overly sensitive to usual adult dosages of triazolam. They also may be overly sensitive to dose-related ADRs, including dizziness, drowsiness, and incoordination (ataxia). Prescribe the lowest effective dosage for these patients. Safety precautions may be indicated (e.g., supervised ambulation, supervised tobacco smoking).

MAXIMUM: 0.25 mg daily orally

Children and adolescents younger than 18 years of age: Safety and efficacy of triazolam pharmacotherapy for children and adolescents have not been established. Triazolam pharmacotherapy is *not* recommended for this age group.

Notes, Insomnia

Triazolam pharmacotherapy is restricted for the short-term symptomatic management of insomnia that impairs daytime functioning. It is not recommended for the symptomatic relief of early morning awakenings. Prescribe the lowest effective dosage for a period not exceeding seven to ten consecutive days. Patients who require triazolam pharmacotherapy for longer than this period of time require re-evaluation. Failure of insomnia to remit after seven to ten days of adjunctive triazolam pharmacotherapy may indicate the presence of another mental or medical disorder that may require further evaluation or referral for appropriate treatment. Worsening of insomnia, or the emergence of new signs and symptoms, may be the consequence of an unrecognized mental or medical disorder. In no case should triazolam pharmacotherapy be prescribed for longer than two to three consecutive weeks.

AVAILABLE DOSAGE FORMS, STORAGE, AND COMPATIBILITY

Tablets, oral: 0.125, 0.25, 0.5, 1 mg

Notes

General Instructions for Patients Instruct patients who are receiving triazolam pharmacotherapy to

- safely store triazolam oral tablets out of the reach of children in child-resistant containers at controlled room temperature (15° to 30°C; 59° to 86°F).
- obtain an available patient information sheet regarding triazolam pharmacotherapy from their pharmacist at the time that their prescription is dispensed. Encourage patients to clarify any questions that they may have concerning triazolam pharmacotherapy with their pharmacist or, if needed, to consult their prescribing psychologist.

PROPOSED MECHANISM OF ACTION

The exact mechanism of action of triazolam has not been fully determined. However, it appears to be mediated by, or to work in concert with, the inhibitory neurotransmitter GABA. Thus, its action appears to be accomplished by binding to benzodiazepine receptors within the GABA complex.

See also Benzodiazepines General Monograph

PHARMACOKINETICS/PHARMACODYNAMICS

Triazolam is rapidly, but only moderately, absorbed (mean bioavailability of 45%) following oral ingestion. Peak blood concentrations are achieved within two hours. Bioavailability is increased (mean of 55%) with sublingual administration. Triazolam is moderately plasma protein-bound (~90%) and has an apparent volume of distribution of approximately 1 L/kg. It is metabolized extensively in the liver to inactive metabolites. These metabolites are excreted in the urine as conjugated glucuronides (~2% are excreted in unchanged form). Triazolam has a short half-life of elimination of ~3 hours (range 1.5 to 5.5 hours). Its mean total body clearance is ~25 L/hour.

The pharmacokinetics of triazolam display significant age effects. Although peak blood concentrations and AUC may be significantly higher and clearance significantly lower among elderly patients, the time to peak blood concentration and differences in elimination half-life generally are insignificant.

RELATIVE CONTRAINDICATIONS

Addiction or habituation to benzodiazepines or other abusable psychotropics, history of
Glaucoma, acute narrow-angle (untreated)
Hypersensitivity to triazolam or other benzodiazepines
Myasthenia gravis
Paradoxical reactions to alcohol or other sedative-hypnotics, history of
Pregnancy

CAUTIONS AND COMMENTS

Triazolam, like other benzodiazepines, is addicting and habituating (see Benzodiazepines General Monograph).

Prescribe triazolam pharmacotherapy cautiously to patients who have respiratory dysfunction, including sleep apnea. Triazolam pharmacotherapy may adversely affect respiratory function among these patients.

Caution patients who are receiving triazolam pharmacotherapy against

- drinking alcohol. Concurrent use of alcohol is associated with additive CNS depression.
- performing activities that require alertness, judgment, or physical coordination (e.g., driving an automobile, operating dangerous equipment, supervising children). Triazolam produces CNS depression and may adversely affect these mental and physical functions.

In addition to these general precautions, caution patients to inform their prescribing psychologist if they begin or discontinue any other pharmacotherapy while receiving triazolam pharmacotherapy.

CLINICALLY SIGNIFICANT DRUG INTERACTIONS

Concurrent triazolam pharmacotherapy and the following may result in clinically significant drug interactions:

Alcohol Use

Concurrent alcohol use may increase the CNS depressant action of triazolam. Advise patients to avoid, or limit, their use of alcohol while receiving triazolam pharmacotherapy.

Pharmacotherapy With Central Nervous System Depressants and Other Drugs That Produce Central Nervous System Depression

Concurrent triazolam pharmacotherapy with opiate analgesics, other sedative-hypnotics, or other drugs that produce CNS depression (e.g., antihistamines, phenothiazines, TCAs) may result in additive CNS depression.

See also Benzodiazepines General Monograph

ADVERSE DRUG REACTIONS

The most common ADRs associated with triazolam pharmacotherapy are extensions of its pharmacologic actions and include dizziness, drowsiness (morning), somnolence (extreme drowsiness), incoordination (ataxia), irritability, and nervousness. Triazolam pharmacotherapy also has been associated with abnormal thinking or behavior, anxiety, confusion, and depression. Other ADRs, listed according to body system, include:

Cardiovascular: chest pain, fainting (syncope), and hypertension
CNS: dream abnormalities and hallucinations
Cutaneous: abnormal sensations, such as a feeling of burning or cutting pain; heightened sensitivity, numbness, prickling, or tingling (dysesthesia/paresthesia); edema; and sweating
Genitourinary: difficulty urinating and sexual dysfunction
GI: constipation, flatulence, and oral irritation
Metabolic/Endocrine: hot and cold flashes
Musculoskeletal: muscular cramps, muscle tone disorders, muscular weakness, and tremor
Ocular: eye irritation and redness
Otic: ear ringing (tinnitus) and hearing impairment
Respiratory: labored or difficult breathing (dyspnea)
Miscellaneous: malaise

See also Benzodiazepines General Monograph

OVERDOSAGE

Signs and symptoms of triazolam overdosage generally are extensions of its pharmacological actions and include confusion, excessive drowsiness, incoordination, slurred speech, and, ultimately, coma. Respiratory depression, apnea, and death have been associated with triazolam overdosage, alone, or in combination with the use of alcohol. In the latter cases, blood concentrations of triazolam and alcohol were lower than those usually associated with overdosage death for each drug alone. Triazolam overdosage requires emergency symptomatic medical support of body systems with attention to increasing triazolam elimination. The benzodiazepine antagonist flumazenil (Anexate®, Romazicon®) is the specific antidote for benzodiazepine overdosage.

TRICYCLIC ANTIDEPRESSANTS
General Monograph

GENERIC NAMES

(for trade names, see individual TCA monographs)

Amitriptyline (dibenzocycloheptene derivative)
Amoxapine (dibenzoxazepine derivative)
Clomipramine (dibenzazepine derivative)
Desipramine (dibenzazepine derivative)
Doxepin (dibenzoxepin derivative)
Imipramine (dibenzazepine derivative)
Nortriptyline (dibenzocycloheptene derivative)
Protriptyline (dibenzocycloheptene derivative)
Trimipramine (dibenzazepine derivative)

CLASSIFICATION

Tricyclic antidepressant (TCA)

APPROVED INDICATIONS FOR PSYCHOLOGICAL DISORDERS

Adjunctive pharmacotherapy for the symptomatic management of:

Mood Disorders, Depressive Disorders: Major Depressive Disorder

See also individual TCA monographs

USUAL DOSAGE AND ADMINISTRATION

Major Depressive Disorder

Adults: The TCAs generally are prescribed as a single daily oral dose. An evening dose may be prescribed for patients who would benefit from their sedative actions or for whom daytime sedation is troublesome. A morning dose may be prescribed for patients for whom insomnia is troublesome when their TCA is dosed in the evening. Dosages are subject to wide interpatient variation in regard to clinical response. See individual TCA monographs for recommended dosages and administration.

Women who are, or who may become, pregnant: FDA Pregnancy Category C. Safety and efficacy of TCA pharmacotherapy for women who are pregnant have not been generally established. Avoid prescribing TCA pharmacotherapy to women who are pregnant. If TCA pharmacotherapy is required, advise patients of potential benefits and possible risks to themselves and the embryo, fetus, or neonate. Collaboration with the patient's obstetrician is indicated. See also individual TCA monographs.

Women who are breast-feeding: Safety and efficacy of TCA pharmacotherapy for women who are breast-feeding and their neonates and infants have not been generally established. Amitriptyline, desipramine, doxepin, imipramine, nortriptyline, and, likely, other TCAs are excreted in breast milk. Avoid prescribing TCA pharmacotherapy to women who are breast-feeding unless their safety has been demonstrated. If TCA pharmacotherapy is required, breast-feeding probably should be discontinued. Collaboration with the patient's pediatrician is required. See also individual TCA monographs.

Elderly, frail, or debilitated patients: Generally prescribe lower dosages of TCAs for elderly, frail, or debilitated patients. Increase the dosage gradually, if needed, according to individual patient response. These patients may be more sensitive to the pharmacologic actions of TCAs than are younger or healthier adult patients. See also individual TCA monographs.

Children younger than 12 years of age: Safety and efficacy of TCA pharmacotherapy for the symptomatic management of depressive disorders among children younger than 12 years of age have not been established. TCA pharmacotherapy for this indication is generally *not* recommended for this age group.

Adolescents: See individual TCA monographs

Notes, Major Depressive Disorder

Precise daily dosages for the TCAs that will be therapeutically beneficial for all patients have not been established. Initiate TCA pharmacotherapy with lower dosages, and increase the dosage gradually according to individual patient response. Lower dosages are particularly recommended for adolescents and elderly, frail, or debilitated patients. Lower dosages also are recommended for non-hospitalized patients as compared to hospitalized patients who may be more closely monitored.

The etiology of depressive disorders is complex and multifactorial. Spontaneous remission or exacerbations commonly occur among patients regardless if they are, or are not, receiving antidepressant pharmacotherapy. Thus, recommended dosages are only a guide and require adjustment in relation to such patient factors as age, signs and symptoms of depression, body system function, concurrent medical and psychological disorders, and individual response to psychotherapy or other therapy (e.g., ECT).

Most antidepressants have a latency period of approximately two to four weeks before maximal therapeutic benefit is achieved. Increasing the recommended dosage will not shorten this latency period and may increase the incidence or severity of ADRs and, thus, is not recommended. The possibility of suicide is always present among severely depressed patients and persists following clinical improvement of the signs and symptoms of depression. For non-hospitalized patients, evaluate their abilities to manage their TCA pharmacotherapy. Prescribe the smallest quantity (i.e., a two-week supply) of TCAs feasible for dispensing to these patients in order to decrease the possibility of intentional TCA overdosage. Other suicide precautions also may be indicated. Patients who are unable to manage their TCA pharmacotherapy, or are at high risk for suicide, may require hospitalization and alternative therapies, such as ECT.

Initiating and Maintaining TCA Pharmacotherapy *Before* initiating TCA pharmacotherapy, ensure that an accurate diagnosis of major depressive disorder has been properly made and documented. Depending upon the clinical situation, also assure for patients and their family members or legal guardians, as appropriate, that the following are completed as soon as possible:

- assess the patient's perception of his or her condition and the need for adjunctive TCA pharmacotherapy. Include as part of the psychological assessment a family history of depression or other mental disorders. Ascertain the presence of any current or active medical disorders (e.g., alcoholism, Cushing's syndrome, premenstrual syndrome), or a history of such disorders, and identify any related pharmacotherapy prescribed for their medical management. Note particularly any pharmacotherapy (e.g., prescription sedative-hypnotic pharmacotherapy) that may cause or exacerbate the signs and symptoms of major depressive disorder. Also identify any problematic patterns of abusable psychotropic use, including any heavy alcohol, barbiturate, benzodiazepine, or other sedative-hypnotic use that my induce or exacerbate depression. Initial psychological assessment also should include the identification of other psychological or medical disorders and the use of any additional drugs (e.g., cimetidine [Tagamet®], corticosteroids, reserpine [Serpasil®]) that may cause or exacerbate depression.
- note any previous antidepressant pharmacotherapy or other therapy for the symptomatic management of major depressive disorder and the patient's general response. Question patients or their family members or legal guardians, as appropriate, regarding the history of the present depressive disorder. Note any previous episodes and their duration and any suicide attempts. Carefully explore the presence of suicidal thoughts or plans, including the presence of recent behaviors, such as giving away valued possessions, making out a will, obtaining additional life insurance, or recording a final message on videotape. Identify the recent occurrence or anniversary of significant losses or separations. Seriously depressed patients require appropriate assessment for the need for suicide precautions.
- ensure civil liberties in relation to the following:

  - obtain the patient's or legal guardian's informed consent for TCA pharmacotherapy. Patients (or their legal guardians) require, commensurate with their intelligence and mental status, information regarding the potential benefits (e.g., management of the mental disorder) and risks (e.g., headache, seizures) associated with TCA pharmacotherapy (see Adverse Drug Reactions).
  - the implementation of suicide precautions. Severely depressed patients may require the implementation of suicide precautions. Some patients may require supervised administration of their TCA pharmacotherapy to help to ensure that oral doses are swallowed. Such patients may require alternative approaches to drug administration (e.g., contracting) or the prescription of dosage forms (e.g., liquid oral dosage forms) that will prevent them from "cheeking" or "hoarding" their doses for potential later overdosage associated with attempted suicide.

- ensure that patients (or their legal guardians) have an understanding of the planned pharmacotherapy and any adjunctive psychotherapy or other related therapy (e.g., ECT). For example, they should know that a low dosage of the TCA will be initially prescribed and gradually increased until therapeutic benefit is achieved. They should know that it may take several days, weeks, or months before optimal therapeutic benefit is fully achieved. They also should understand that during this time, they will be monitored for common

ADRs, such as weight gain or loss, and that they will be helped to manage these ADRs. Any questions that patients or their legal guardians may have regarding TCA pharmacotherapy should be answered honestly.

- ensure that patients know the exact name of the required TCA. They also should know its general action, dosage and administration, and storage requirements. They should know how to monitor for therapeutic benefit and identify and manage common ADRs. They also should know the signs and symptoms of toxicity and know when it may be necessary to contact immediately the prescribing psychologist or access emergency medical facilities for evaluation and treatment.

- individualize the dosage according to the severity of signs and symptoms and patient response. Most patients respond to lower dosages as steady state is achieved. The achievement of steady state usually requires a period of time equivalent to five times the half-life of elimination of the TCA. Avoid increasing the dosage prior to achieving steady state. Increasing the dosage before achieving steady state may significantly and unnecessarily increase the incidence and severity of associated ADRs. Many of the TCAs have long half-lives of elimination and, therefore, long durations of action. Once steady state has been achieved, most patients may be dosed once daily with these TCAs. See individual TCA monographs.

- advise patients, and their family members or legal guardians as appropriate, that many of the ADRs associated with TCA pharmacotherapy usually diminish over the first few weeks of pharmacotherapy and that these ADRs do not necessarily mean that the patient has a more serious mental disorder or has relapsed. They should be encouraged to continue TCA pharmacotherapy despite mild ADRs and be assisted with the management of these ADRS. More troublesome ADRs may require a reduction of the dosage or changes in the dosage schedule (e.g., ingesting each dose of an oral dosage form in the evening before retiring for bed in order to minimize associated daytime drowsiness). Explore these and other possible countermeasures (see following discussion) with patients, as needed.

- ensure that patients understand that if ADRs occur, they can, for the most part, be treated quickly. It is important to acknowledge how annoying and uncomfortable ADRs can be. Patients should be encouraged to discuss their feelings about ADRs and to assist with their management. Special attention should be given to the management of common mild ADRs because the inability to manage or tolerate ADRs is often a major reason for patients to discontinue TCA pharmacotherapy. For patients who want to discontinue their TCA pharmacotherapy because of associated ADRs, it is often helpful to weigh with them the discontinuation of pharmacotherapy with expected or actual benefits and the risk for the return of the signs and symptoms of major depression.

- assist patients to manage common or troublesome ADRs, such as dry mouth, constipation, and weight gain or loss (see Adverse Drug Reactions).

- provide realistic information regarding TCA pharmacotherapy and other recommended therapy. Patients and their family members or legal guardians, as appropriate, should have a realistic view of what to expect in relation to TCA pharmacotherapy and other recommended therapy. They should understand that TCA pharmacotherapy will not solve all of the patient's problems, but will help him or her to be better able to work on the problems. They should understand that TCA pharmacotherapy will not improve judgment, improve poor socialization or interpersonal skills, or change their personality. However, they can expect that adjunctive TCA pharmacotherapy will help the patient to manage better the major depressive disorder.

- clarify misconceptions. Patients and their legal guardians, as appropriate, should be aware that TCAs are not addicting or habituating. They should also be aware that high dosages do not necessarily indicate a more serious mental disorder. Dosage selection depends on several factors, such as age, gender, weight, metabolism, and response to previous antidepressant pharmacotherapy. Patients and their family members or legal guardians, as appropriate, should recognize that concurrent participation in other recommended therapy and the maintenance of regular appointments with the clinical psychologist are important adjuncts for the symptomatic management of major depressive disorder. Patients and their family members or legal guardians, as appropriate, should be encouraged to ask questions about the individualized therapeutic plan as active consumers of comprehensive psychologic services. They also should be directed to available support groups for additional help.

- involve patients and their legal guardians, as appropriate, in treatment planning, whenever possible. Provide them with frequent evaluations of the patient's progress.

Maintaining TCA Pharmacotherapy Monitor the patient's attitude and behavior during the early weeks of TCA pharmacotherapy. A greater interest in the environment (i.e., resolution of anhedonia) and improvement in affect, appetite, mood, personal appearance, and sleep pattern may not be observed for two or more weeks following the initiation of TCA pharmacotherapy.

As therapeutic benefit is achieved, observe patients for mood changes and increased suicidal tendencies, which generally occur at this time. Implement suicide precautions, as needed. Although risk may be greatest when patients begin to respond to their TCA pharmacotherapy, monitor for suicidal ideation throughout the course of therapy. In this regard, express a genuine concern for patients and a sincere desire to protect them from self-destructive impulses. Other therapy (e.g., ECT) or precautions (e.g., hospitalization with suicide monitoring) also may be required, particularly for patients who have severe refractory depression and for whom the risk for suicide is clinically ascertained to be high (see also Clinically Significant Drug Interactions and Cautions and Comments).

Assess the patient's abilities to manage TCA pharmacotherapy in the home setting, and plan to promote these abilities. Provide psychological support for patients and their families while awaiting initial therapeutic response, which may require up to several weeks of pharmacotherapy before becoming apparent. Encourage patients not to become discouraged while awaiting therapeutic benefit. In addition, as previously noted, assist patients with the management of common ADRs that can occur readily upon the initiation of TCA pharmacotherapy. Involve patients and families in treatment planning whenever possible, and provide frequent evaluation of patient progress. Direct patients and their families to appropriate support groups and other services, as needed.

As early as possible, involve patients and their families in treatment planning and provide frequent evaluations of the patient's progress. Ensure that patients understand that they may experience common ADRs that may affect their daily living. Provide instruction regarding the general management of these common ADRs. When providing antidepressant pharmacotherapy to patients, it is important for clinical psychologists to recognize that most common ADRs can be minimized or avoided by gradually adjusting the dosage of the prescribed TCA according to individual patient response.

Discontinuing TCA Pharmacotherapy Discontinue TCA pharmacotherapy gradually. Although TCAs are classified as nonabusable psychotropics, abrupt discontinuation of long-term pharmacotherapy may result in a withdrawal-like syndrome with anxiety, chills, diarrhea, dizziness, feelings of restlessness and an inability to sit (akathisia), headache, insomnia, malaise, muscle pain (myalgia), nausea, profuse nasal discharge associated with acute inflammation of the nasal mucous membrane (coryza), restlessness, and vomiting. To discontinue long-term TCA pharmacotherapy, reduce the dosage gradually over two weeks. During this time, monitor for dream and sleep disturbances, irritability, restlessness, and other transient signs and symptoms.

Also monitor patients for hypomania and mania, which rarely may occur between two and seven days following the discontinuation of long-term TCA pharmacotherapy.

If a gradual reduction in dosage is not effective for the symptomatic management of troublesome signs and symptoms of withdrawal, then TCA pharmacotherapy may need to be reinstituted. Alternatively, anticholinergic (e.g., benztropine [Cogentin®]) pharmacotherapy may need to be prescribed for some patients to treat troublesome signs and symptoms of withdrawal.

AVAILABLE DOSAGE FORMS, STORAGE, AND COMPATIBILITY

See individual TCA monographs for available dosage forms, storage, and compatibility.

Notes

General Instructions for Patients Instruct patients who are receiving TCA pharmacotherapy to

- safely store TCA oral dosage forms safely out of the reach of children in child-resistant containers.
- obtain an available patient information sheet regarding TCA pharmacotherapy from their pharmacist at the time that their prescription is dispensed. Encourage patients to clarify any questions that they may have concerning TCA pharmacotherapy with their pharmacist or, if needed, to consult their prescribing psychologist.

See individual TCA monographs for additional notes.

PROPOSED MECHANISM OF ACTION

Many depressive disorders are thought to have a biochemical basis in the form of a relative deficiency of neurotransmitters, such as norepinephrine and serotonin. While the precise mechanism of action of the TCAs is unknown, one theory suggests that they restore normal levels of neurotransmitters (predominantly norepinephrine, although, also serotonin) by blocking their re-uptake at the neuronal membrane from synapses into pre-synaptic neurons within the CNS. The actions of norepinephrine and serotonin are, thus, augmented.

Available data suggest that the secondary amine TCAs (e.g., desipramine) may have a greater blocking activity than the other TCAs in regard to norepinephrine re-uptake. Tertiary amine TCAs (e.g., amitriptyline) may have a greater blocking activity on serotonin re-uptake. In addition to these actions, the TCAs generally possess strong anticholinergic actions. These actions may contribute to the efficacy of adjunctive TCA pharmacotherapy for the symptomatic management of childhood enuresis (see Imipramine Monograph). The ADRs affecting the cardiovascular system (e.g., ECG changes, postural hypotension, tachycardia) are a result of direct quinidine-like cardiotoxicity, indirect anticholinergic activity, and potentiation of norepinephrine action.

PHARMACOKINETICS/PHARMACODYNAMICS

The TCAs are well and rapidly absorbed following oral ingestion. Some TCAs, such as imipramine and nortriptyline, undergo significant first-pass hepatic metabolism. TCAs are highly bound to plasma proteins and are widely distributed in body tissues. Most TCAs appear to cross the placenta readily and are likely excreted in breast milk. The TCAs are metabolized extensively in the liver. Their rates of metabolism, which may be genetically determined and also display age effects, vary widely among patients. Generally, elderly adults metabolize TCAs more slowly than do younger adults. Consequently, the half-life of elimination for the various TCAs demonstrates wide inter-patient variation. Only relatively small amounts of TCAs are excreted in unchanged form in the urine.

Therapeutic Drug Monitoring

Routine monitoring of TCA blood concentrations is not warranted but may be useful to evaluate the patient's ability to manage his or her TCA pharmacotherapy or confirm suspected toxicity. Therapeutic drug monitoring may be particularly helpful for monitoring desipramine, imipramine, and nortriptyline pharmacotherapy (see individual TCA monographs).

RELATIVE CONTRAINDICATIONS

Clomipramine pharmacotherapy, concurrent or within 14 days (see Clinically Significant Drug Interactions)
Congestive heart failure, severe
Glaucoma, narrow angle
Hypersensitivity to any of the TCAs
Liver failure
Myocardial infarction, acute recovery phase

CAUTIONS AND COMMENTS

Prescribe TCA pharmacotherapy cautiously to patients who

- have benign prostatic hypertrophy. The anticholinergic actions of the TCAs can exacerbate this condition.
- have histories of cardiovascular disorders. Some TCAs (e.g., trimipramine) have been associated with the occurrence of conduction defects; dysrhythmias, including tachycardia; myocardial infarction; and strokes among these patients.
- have histories of hiatal hernia. The anticholinergic actions of the TCAs may result in reduced tone of the esophago-gastric sphincter. This action may induce or exacerbate a hiatal hernia. If symptoms of esophageal reflux occur, the TCA should be discontinued. Collaboration with the patient's family physician or a specialist (e.g., gastroenterologist) is indicated.
- have histories of hyperthyroidism or are receiving thyroid pharmacotherapy. Some TCAs (e.g., trimipramine) have been associated with cardiovascular toxicity among these patients.
- have histories of increased intraocular pressure, including narrow-angle glaucoma. The anticholinergic actions of the TCAs may exacerbate this condition.
- have histories of seizure disorders. Some TCAs (e.g., trimipramine) may lower the seizure threshold.
- have histories of urinary retention. The anticholinergic actions of the TCAs may exacerbate this condition.
- require concurrent ECT. Concurrent TCA pharmacotherapy may increase the risks associated with ECT (e.g., seizures). Prescribe concurrent TCA (e.g., trimipramine) pharmacotherapy and ECT only for patients for whom it is essential.

Caution patients who are receiving TCA pharmacotherapy against

• drinking alcohol or using other drugs that produce CNS depression. The concurrent use of these drugs may increase the CNS depression associated with the anticholinergic actions of several of the TCAs (e.g., trimipramine).
• giving, selling, or trading their TCA to any friends, relatives, or others.
• performing activities that require alertness, judgment, and physical coordination (e.g., driving an automobile, operating dangerous equipment, supervising children). The CNS depressant action of some TCAs (e.g., trimipramine) may adversely affect these mental and physical functions.

In addition to these general precautions, caution patients to inform their prescribing psychologist if they begin or discontinue any other pharmacotherapy while receiving TCA pharmacotherapy.

See also individual TCA monographs

CLINICALLY SIGNIFICANT DRUG INTERACTIONS

Concurrent TCA pharmacotherapy and the following may result in clinically significant drug interactions:

Alcohol Use

Concurrent alcohol use may increase the CNS depressant action of the TCAs. Advise patients to avoid, or limit, their use of alcohol while receiving TCA pharmacotherapy.

Barbiturate Pharmacotherapy

Barbiturates induce liver enzyme activity. Thus, they increase the metabolism of the TCAs and other drugs that are metabolized by the liver. As a result of this action, barbiturates may reduce TCA blood concentrations. However, the clinical significance of this interaction is difficult to evaluate. The relationship between TCA blood concentrations and therapeutic response for the various TCAs is unclear. In addition, this interaction has not been established for some TCAs (e.g., desipramine). See also Pharmacotherapy With CNS Depressants and Other Drugs That Produce CNS Depression.

Cimetidine Pharmacotherapy

Cimetidine (Tagamet®) inhibits liver enzyme activity. Thus, concurrent TCA and cimetidine pharmacotherapy may result in a significant increase in the blood concentration of the TCA. This interaction may result in TCA toxicity. Conversely, the discontinuation of concurrent cimetidine pharmacotherapy may decrease the blood concentration of the TCA. This interaction may result in the loss of the therapeutic efficacy of the TCA. Ranitidine (Zantac®) and other histamine-2 receptor antagonists appear less likely to interact with the TCAs than does cimetidine.

Clomipramine Pharmacotherapy

Concurrent TCA and clomipramine (Anafranil®) pharmacotherapy may result in the potentially fatal serotonin syndrome. Associated signs and symptoms of this syndrome include cardiovascular disturbances, coma, confusion, excessive sweating (diaphoresis), fever (hyperpyrexia), myoclonus, rigidity, and seizures. See Relative Contraindications.

Fluoxetine Pharmacotherapy

Fluoxetine (Prozac®) inhibits liver enzyme activity. Thus, concurrent TCA and fluoxetine pharmacotherapy may result in a greater than 2-fold increase in a previously stable blood concentration of the TCA. This interaction may result in TCA toxicity.

Monoamine Oxidase Inhibitor Pharmacotherapy

Concurrent TCA and MAOI pharmacotherapy has resulted in a severe increase in body temperature (hyperpyretic crisis), seizures, and death. However, this interaction usually has occurred in the context of either overdosage (often deliberate suicide attempts) or injectable pharmacotherapy. Concurrent oral TCA and MAOI pharmacotherapy with recommended dosages has resulted in confusion, fever, hypertension, seizures, and tachycardia. This combination of pharmacotherapy is occasionally prescribed for the management of severe refractory depression among selected patients. However, this combination of pharmacotherapy is recommended *only* for patients who are hospitalized and can receive close monitoring and immediate symptomatic medical management should any serious ADRs (e.g., seizures) occur. See also Clinically Significant Drug Interactions, Clomipramine Pharmacotherapy.

Pharmacotherapy With Anticholinergics and Other Drugs That Produce Anticholinergic Actions

Concurrent TCA and anticholinergic (e.g., atropine) pharmacotherapy or pharmacotherapy with other drugs that produce anticholinergic actions (e.g., phenothiazines) may result in significant exacerbation of anticholinergic activity (e.g., blurred vision; constipation and paralytic ileus; hyperthermia, particularly when patients are exposed to high environmental temperatures; and urinary retention).

Pharmacotherapy With Central Nervous System Depressants and Other Drugs That Produce Central Nervous System Depression

Concurrent TCA pharmacotherapy with opiate analgesics, sedative-hypnotics, or other drugs that produce CNS depression (e.g., antihistamines, phenothiazines) may result in additive CNS depression.

Pharmacotherapy With Central Nervous System Stimulants

Concurrent TCA and CNS stimulant (e.g., amphetamine, methylphenidate) pharmacotherapy may increase the blood concentration of the TCA. The CNS stimulants compete for the same metabolic enzyme systems. In addition, the TCAs can potentiate the actions of amphetamines and other CNS stimulants by the same mechanism. See also Clinically Significant Drug Interactions, Sympathomimetic Pharmacotherapy.

Pharmacotherapy With Clonidine and Similarly Acting Antihypertensives

Concurrent TCA pharmacotherapy, particularly desipramine or imipramine pharmacotherapy, may inhibit the hypotensive action of clonidine (Catapres®) and similarly acting antihypertensives (e.g., guanabenz [Wytensin®], guanfacine [Tenex®]). Initiating or discontinuing TCA pharmacotherapy for patients who are stabilized on clonidine, or a similarly acting hypertensive, may have significant impact upon its antihypertensive actions. An adjustment of the clonidine, or similarly acting hypertensive, dosage may be required. Collaboration with the prescriber of the clonidine, or similar antihypertensive, is indicated. See also Clinically Significant Drug Interactions, Pharmacotherapy With Guanethidine and Similarly Acting Antihypertensives.

Pharmacotherapy With Guanethidine and Similarly Acting Antihypertensives

Concurrent TCA pharmacotherapy may decrease the neuronal uptake of guanethidine (Ismelin®) and similar antihypertensives. This interaction may result in a decrease in their antihypertensive actions. Collaboration with the prescriber of the guanethidine is indicated. See also Clinically Significant Drug Interactions, Pharmacotherapy With Clonidine and Similarly Acting Antihypertensives.

Phenothiazine Pharmacotherapy

Concurrent TCA and phenothiazine pharmacotherapy may increase the blood concentration level of the TCA. Phenothiazines compete for the same metabolic enzyme systems.

Pimozide Pharmacotherapy

Pimozide (Orap®) prolongs the QT interval of the ECG. The TCAs (e.g., desipramine [Norpramin®], imipramine [Tofranil®]) can also prolong the QT interval. Thus, concurrent pharmacotherapy may result in serious risk for significant prolongation of the QT interval (i.e., a cardiac dysrhythmia). Concurrent pimozide and TCA pharmacotherapy is *contraindicated*.

Sympathomimetic Pharmacotherapy

Concurrent TCA and sympathomimetic (e.g., amphetamines, epinephrine, isoproterenol, norepinephrine, phenylephrine) pharmacotherapy may result in increased cardiac (e.g., increased heart rate) and pressor (e.g., increased blood pressure) actions of the sympathomimetic. This interaction may be fatal among susceptible patients (e.g., those who have serious cardiovascular disorders or cerebral aneurysms). See also Clinically Significant Drug Interactions, Pharmacotherapy With CNS Stimulants.

Tobacco Smoking

Concurrent tobacco smoking may increase the CNS depressant action of the TCAs. Advise patients to avoid, or limit, their tobacco smoking while receiving TCA pharmacotherapy.

See also individual TCA monographs

ADVERSE DRUG REACTIONS

Although some ADRs may not be directly associated with all TCA pharmacotherapy, the pharmacological similarities among the TCAs require that these ADRs be considered whenever a TCA is prescribed (see also individual TCA monographs). *Note:* Tolerance to the postural hypotensive and sedative actions of the TCAs usually develops with continued TCA pharmacotherapy. However, the following anticholinergic ADRs, including dry mouth, constipation, and weight gain, occur more commonly and usually can be managed by instructing patients to do the following:

Dry mouth

 • relieve by sucking on a sugarless hard candy.

Constipation

 • prevent or manage by eating a balanced diet including bran, fresh fruits, vegetables, and stewed prunes.
 • drink at least 8 glasses of water each day. If persistent or troublesome, advise patients to notify their prescribing psychologist. Collaboration with the patient's advanced practice nurse or pharmacist may be indicated.

Weight gain

 • weight gain is usually caused by an increase in appetite. Instruct patients to monitor their weight and eat a well-balanced diet. Encourage them to exercise regularly and avoid sweets.
 • if assistance with diet planning or developing an exercise program is needed, instruct patients to consult their prescribing psychologist. Referral to an advanced practice nurse or dietician also may be indicated.

Tricyclic antidepressant pharmacotherapy also has been associated with the following ADRs, listed according to body system.

Cardiovascular: asystole; AV conduction changes; congestive heart failure; fainting (syncope); heart block; dysrhythmias (e.g., bradycardia, tachycardia); hypertension; hypotension, particularly postural hypotension; myocardial infarction; nonspecific ECG changes, including flattening or inversion of T waves; palpitations; peripheral vasospasm; premature ventricular fibrillation; and stroke. "Acute collapse" and "sudden death" have been reported involving an 8-year old boy who received TCA pharmacotherapy over two years for the symptomatic management of hyperactivity. There have been additional reports of sudden death among children.

CNS: agitation; alteration in EEG patterns; anxiety; coma; confusion with hallucinations, particularly among elderly patients; delusions; disorientation; disturbed concentration; dizziness; drowsiness; euphoria; exacerbation of psychosis; excitement; EPRs (e.g., abnormal involuntary movements and TD); fatigue; hallucinations; headache; hypomania;

incoordination (ataxia); insomnia; lethargy; nervousness; nightmares; panic; restlessness; and seizures. The TCAs reportedly produce varying degrees of sedation among patients who have, or do not have, depressive disorders. They also may lower the seizure threshold.

Cutaneous: edema of the face and tongue, flushing, hives (urticaria), itching (pruritus), loss of hair (alopecia), petechiae, sensitivity to light (photosensitivity, advise patients to avoid excessive exposure to sunlight), skin rash, and sweating (excessive). Most of these reactions may be hypersensitivity reactions.

Genitourinary: excessive urination during the night (nocturia), impotence, increased or decreased sex drive, painful ejaculation, urinary frequency, urinary hesitancy (delayed urination), urinary retention, and urinary tract dilation

GI: absence, partial loss, or impairment of the sense of taste (ageusia); black tongue; constipation; diarrhea; dry mouth; epigastric distress; hiatal hernia (induce or exacerbate); increased pancreatic enzymes; inflammation of the mouth (stomatitis); loss of appetite (anorexia); nausea; paralytic ileus; parotid swelling; peculiar taste (bitter); salivation (excessive); sublingual adenitis; and vomiting

Hematologic: a reduction in circulating white blood cells, including basophils, eosinophils, monocytes, and, particularly, lymphocytes (leukopenia); bone marrow depression (rare), including a reduction in blood neutrophils often resulting in an increased susceptibility to bacterial and fungal infections (neutropenia); hemorrhages into the skin (purpura); and reduction in circulating blood platelets (thrombocytopenia). These reactions may be due to a hypersensitivity reaction.

Hepatic: elevated liver function tests and obstructive jaundice. Rarely, hepatitis, with or without, jaundice, and hepatic failure. The development of hepatitis or jaundice generally is reversible but requires immediate discontinuation of TCA pharmacotherapy. Continued TCA pharmacotherapy may be fatal.

Metabolic/Endocrine: abnormal breast enlargement among males (gynecomastia), breast enlargement and abnormal lactation among females (galactorrhea), edema, elevation and lowering of blood sugar concentrations, syndrome of inappropriate antidiuretic hormone secretion (SIADH), testicular swelling, and weight gain or loss

Musculoskeletal: difficult or defective speech due to impairment of the tongue or other muscles essential to speech (mental function is intact, dysarthria); numbness, tingling, and other paresthesias of the extremities; peripheral neuropathy; tremors; and weakness. In addition, a lupus-like syndrome (migratory arthritis; positive ANA and rheumatoid factor) has been associated with TCA pharmacotherapy.

Ocular: abnormal dilation of the pupils (mydriasis), accommodation disturbances, blurred vision, and increased intraocular pressure (glaucoma)

Otic: ringing in the ears (tinnitus)

Respiratory: nasal congestion

Miscellaneous: cross-hypersensitivity to other TCAs, drug fever (hyperpyrexia), and weakness

See also individual TCA monographs

OVERDOSAGE

Signs and symptoms of TCA overdosage most often involve the CNS and cardiovascular system. Accidental or intentional overdosage may be fatal. Within a few hours of ingestion, patients may become agitated, restless, confused, delirious, stuporous, and comatose. They may complain of blurred vision, constipation, dizziness, and drowsiness. Overdosages involving large amounts of TCAs may cause temporary confusion, disturbed concentration, or transient visual hallucinations. Other signs and symptoms include abnormal dilation of the pupils (mydriasis), diminished bowel sounds, dry mouth, fever, hyperactive reflexes, hypothermia, muscle rigidity, ocular motility disorders, polyradiculoneuropathy (i.e., Guillain-Barre syndrome), renal failure, respiratory depression, vomiting, and urinary retention. Generalized seizures, both early and late after the ingestion of an overdosage, have been reported.

Cardiovascular signs and symptoms may include severe dysrhythmias, such as tachycardia and bundle-branch block. Other cardiovascular signs and symptoms may include hypotension (severe) and shock. The ECG evidence of impaired conduction, congestive heart failure, and serious disturbances of cardiac rate, rhythm, and output may occur. The duration of the QRS complex on the ECG may be a helpful guide to the severity of TCA overdosage.

TCA overdosage requires emergency symptomatic medical support of body systems with attention to increasing TCA elimination. There is no known antidote. A fatal dysrhythmia occurring as late as 56 hours after amitriptyline overdosage has been reported. Cardiac function should be monitored for no less than five days following the stabilization of body systems. Physostigmine (Antilirium®) may be required for the medical management of amitriptyline overdosage. Close medical monitoring is essential after apparent recovery because of the possible recurrence of signs and symptoms.

TRIFLUOPERAZINE

(trye floo oh per'a zeen)

TRADE NAMES

Novo-Flurazine®
Stelazine®
Terfluzine®

CLASSIFICATION

Antipsychotic (phenothiazine)

See also Phenothiazines General Monograph

APPROVED INDICATIONS FOR PSYCHOLOGICAL DISORDERS

Adjunctive pharmacotherapy for the symptomatic management of:

Psychotic Disorders: Schizophrenia and Other Psychotic Disorders

USUAL DOSAGE AND ADMINISTRATION

Schizophrenia and Other Psychotic Disorders

Adults, hospitalized: Initially, 10 to 20 mg daily orally in two or three divided doses. Increase the dosage gradually until the signs and symptoms of the psychotic disorder are managed.

Rarely, some patients may require 40 to 80 mg daily. The optimal dosage is usually achieved within two to three weeks. Maintain the optimal dosage for a sufficient time to achieve maximal improvement. For most hospitalized patients, two to three weeks of trifluoperazine pharmacotherapy at the optimal dosage will be adequate before initiating a gradual reduction of the dosage to a maintenance dosage. Some patients who are refractory to trifluoperazine or other antipsychotic pharmacotherapy may require several months to a year before a reduction in their optimal dosage can be initiated.

MAXIMUM: 20 mg daily intramuscularly; 80 mg daily orally

Adults, non-hospitalized: Initially, 4 to 10 mg daily orally in two divided doses; *or* 1 to 2 mg intramuscularly every 4 to 6 hours, as needed. Increase the dosage gradually until the signs and symptoms of the psychotic disorder are managed. The optimal dosage is generally achieved within two to three weeks.

MAINTENANCE: 4 to 12 mg daily orally in two to four divided doses or as a single dose 30 minutes before retiring for bed in the evening

MAXIMUM: 10 mg daily intramuscularly; 40 mg daily orally

Women who are, or who may become, pregnant: FDA Pregnancy Category C. Safety and efficacy of trifluoperazine pharmacotherapy for women who are pregnant have not been established. Although congenital malformations (i.e., birth defects) have occasionally been associated with trifluoperazine pharmacotherapy, multiple studies of trifluoperazine use during pregnancy have failed to demonstrate an associated increase in the rate of congenital malformations (see also Phenothiazines General Monograph). Avoid prescribing trifluoperazine pharmacotherapy to women who are pregnant. If trifluoperazine pharmacotherapy is required, advise patients (or their legal guardians in regard to the patient) of potential benefits and possible risks to themselves and the embryo, fetus, or neonate. Collaboration with the patient's obstetrician is indicated.

Women who are breast-feeding: Safety and efficacy of trifluoperazine pharmacotherapy for women who are breast-feeding and their neonates and infants have not been established. There is evidence that trifluoperazine is excreted in breast milk (see Phenothiazines General Monograph). Avoid prescribing trifluoperazine pharmacotherapy to women who are breast-feeding. If trifluoperazine pharmacotherapy is required, breast-feeding probably should be discontinued. Collaboration with the patient's pediatrician is indicated.

Elderly, frail, or debilitated patients, hospitalized: Initially, 4 to 6 mg daily orally in two or three divided doses. Increase the dosage gradually until the signs and symptoms of the psychotic disorder are managed. The optimal dosage generally is achieved within two to three weeks.

Elderly, frail, or debilitated patients, non-hospitalized: Initially, 2 to 4 mg daily orally in a single or two divided doses. Increase the dosage gradually, if needed, according to individual patient response. Generally prescribe lower dosages for elderly, frail, or debilitated patients. These patients may be more sensitive to the pharmacologic actions of trifluoperazine than are younger or healthier adult patients.

Children younger than 6 years of age: Safety and efficacy of trifluoperazine pharmacotherapy for children younger than 6 years of age have not been established. Trifluoperazine pharmacotherapy is *not* recommended for this age group.

Children 6 to 12 years of age: Initially, 1 to 2 mg daily orally or intramuscularly in a single or two divided doses. Increase the dosage gradually until the signs and symptoms of the psychotic disorder are managed. *Note:* Trifluoperazine pharmacotherapy is *not* recommended for children who are 6 to 12 years of age or those who weigh less than 36.4 kg *unless* they are hospitalized or otherwise closely monitored.

MAXIMUM: 2 mg daily intramuscularly; 15 mg daily orally

Notes, Schizophrenia and Other Psychotic Disorders

Two to three weeks of trifluoperazine pharmacotherapy are usually required for optimal therapeutic benefit. For maintenance trifluoperazine pharmacotherapy, adjust the dosage to the lowest effective dosage according to individual patient response. The ADRs that become troublesome during dosage adjustment can usually be promptly managed with concurrent anti-parkinsonian pharmacotherapy. Patients who require more than 10 mg daily of trifluoperazine may benefit from prophylactic anti-parkinsonian pharmacotherapy. Collaboration with the patient's family physician or a specialist (e.g., neurologist) may be required.

The injectable formulation of trifluoperazine is for intramuscular injection only. Do *not* inject intravenously. Intramuscular injections of trifluoperazine generally are well-tolerated, with little, if any, pain or irritation at the injection site. However, oral pharmacotherapy is preferred over intramuscular pharmacotherapy. Prescribe intramuscular pharmacotherapy *only* when necessary for the prompt control of severe signs and symptoms. Replace intramuscular pharmacotherapy with oral pharmacotherapy as soon as feasible.

AVAILABLE DOSAGE FORMS, STORAGE, AND COMPATIBILITY

Concentrate, oral: 10 mg/ml (banana-vanilla flavored)
Injectable, intramuscular: 2 mg/ml
Tablets, oral: 1, 2, 5, 10 mg

Notes

Injectable Formulations   Inspect the trifluoperazine injectable formulations prior to use. Do not use darkly discolored injectable solutions. Return these products to the dispensing pharmacy or manufacturer for safe and appropriate disposal. Protect the injectable from light, and store at controlled room temperature (15° to 30°C; 59° to 86°F).

Oral Formulations   The trifluoperazine oral concentrate contains sodium bisulfite. Sulfites have been associated with hypersensitivity reactions, including anaphylactic reactions, among susceptible patients. Although relatively uncommon, these reactions appear to occur with a higher incidence among patients who have asthma.

General Instructions for Patients Instruct patients who are receiving trifluoperazine pharmacotherapy to

- dilute each dose of the trifluoperazine oral concentrate immediately before ingestion with 60 ml (2 ounces) of a compatible beverage (e.g., carbonated soft drinks, coffee, fruit or tomato juice, milk, tea, water) or gently mix in 60 ml (2 ounces) of soft food (e.g., applesauce, pudding) to increase palatability.
- avoid getting the trifluoperazine oral concentrate on the skin or clothing because it is irritating and has been associated with contact dermatitis.
- safely store trifluoperazine oral concentrate and tablets out of the reach of children in tightly closed child- and light-resistant containers at controlled room temperature (15° to 30°C; 59° to 86°F).
- obtain an available patient information sheet regarding trifluoperazine pharmacotherapy from their pharmacist at the time that their prescription is dispensed. Encourage patients to clarify any questions that they may have concerning trifluoperazine pharmacotherapy with their pharmacist or, if needed, to consult their prescribing psychologist.

PROPOSED MECHANISM OF ACTION

The exact mechanism of action of trifluoperazine is complex and has not been fully determined. Its antipsychotic activity appears to be primarily related to its interaction with dopamine-containing neurons, specifically the blockade of dopamine receptors both pre- and post-synaptically.

See also Phenothiazines General Monograph

PHARMACOKINETICS/PHARMACODYNAMICS

Data are unavailable.

RELATIVE CONTRAINDICATIONS

Blood disorders
Bone marrow depression
Cardiovascular dysfunction, severe
CNS depression, severe, including that associated with the ingestion of alcohol or CNS
    depressant (e.g., sedative-hypnotic, opiate analgesic) pharmacotherapy
Coma
Hypersensitivity to trifluoperazine or other phenothiazines
Liver dysfunction, severe
Parkinson's disease

CAUTIONS AND COMMENTS

Prescribe trifluoperazine pharmacotherapy cautiously to patients who have cardiovascular dysfunction. Trifluoperazine pharmacotherapy has been associated with CNS and cardiovascular stimulation. For some patients, such as those who have angina pectoris, this action may be undesirable. Collaboration with the patient's cardiologist is indicated. If any undesired response is noted among these patients, discontinue trifluoperazine pharmacotherapy. Trifluoperazine pharmacotherapy is *contraindicated* for patients who have severe cardiovascular dysfunction.

Caution patients who are receiving trifluoperazine pharmacotherapy against performing activities that require alertness, judgment, and physical coordination (e.g., driving an automobile, operating dangerous equipment, supervising children), especially during the first few days of pharmacotherapy. Trifluoperazine may depress the CNS and adversely affect these mental and physical functions.

See also Phenothiazines General Monograph

CLINICALLY SIGNIFICANT DRUG INTERACTIONS

Concurrent trifluoperazine pharmacotherapy and the following may result in clinically significant drug interactions:

Guanethidine Pharmacotherapy

Trifluoperazine may decrease the neuronal uptake of guanethidine (Ismelin®) and, thus, decrease its antihypertensive action. An adjustment to the guanethidine dosage may be required. Collaboration with the prescriber of the guanethidine is indicated.

Pharmacotherapy With Anticholinergics and Other Drugs That Produce Anticholinergic Actions

Concurrent trifluoperazine pharmacotherapy with anticholinergics (e.g., atropine) or other drugs that produce anticholinergic actions (e.g., TCAs) may result in additive anticholinergic actions.

See also Phenothiazines General Monograph

ADVERSE DRUG REACTIONS

Adverse drug reactions have been infrequently associated with trifluoperazine pharmacotherapy. When ADRs do occur, they are usually mild and transient. These ADRs, listed according to body system, include the following:

CNS: dizziness, drowsiness, fatigue, insomnia, and over-stimulation. Elderly, frail, or debilitated patients may be more sensitive to ADRs affecting the CNS. EPRs and TD have been reported rarely, particularly among patients who were receiving high daily dosages (20 to 40 mg).

The EPRs may include motor restlessness (dystonic type) or Parkinsonism. Depending on the severity of the EPRs, reduce the daily dosage or, if necessary, discontinue trifluoperazine pharmacotherapy. If trifluoperazine pharmacotherapy requires reinstitution, prescribe lower dosages. If EPRs are observed among children or pregnant women, trifluoperazine pharmacotherapy should be discontinued, and it should *not* be reinstituted.

Anti-parkinsonian pharmacotherapy usually rapidly reverses EPRs. Some EPRs may require symptomatic medical management. Collaboration with the patient's family physician is indicated.

See also Phenothiazines General Monograph

Cutaneous: skin rashes

GI: dry mouth and loss of appetite (anorexia)

Genitourinary: abnormal absence of menses (amenorrhea)

Hematologic: rarely, blood disorders such as anemia; a reduction in the circulating white blood cells, including basophils, eosinophils, monocytes, and, in particular, lymphocytes (leukopenia); a reduction in blood neutrophils, often resulting in an increased susceptibility to bacterial and fungal infections, which, if severe, may be fatal (neutropenia [agranulocytosis, granulocytopenia]); abnormal decrease in the number of blood platelets (thrombocytopenia); and a reduction in all cellular elements of the blood (pancytopenia). Patients who are receiving high dosages (20 to 40 mg) of trifluoperazine may be at particular risk for these ADRs affecting the hematologic system.

Hepatic: rarely, cholestatic jaundice. Patients who require high dosages (i.e., 20 to 40 mg) of trifluroperazine may be at particular risk for this ADR.

Metabolic/Endocrine: abnormal lactation

Musculoskeletal: EPRs (see CNS)

Ocular: blurred vision

See also Phenothiazines General Monograph

OVERDOSAGE

Signs and symptoms of trifluoperazine overdosage can range from mild to severe. Mild signs and symptoms include dizziness, drowsiness, and muscle twitching. More severe signs and symptoms include marked dystonic reactions and other EPRs. Other signs and symptoms of trifluoperazine overdosage include agitation, CNS depression (severe), difficulty swallowing, gait disturbances, restlessness, salivation (excessive), torticollis, tremor, and weakness. Trifluoperazine overdosage requires emergency symptomatic medical support of body systems with attention to increasing trifluoperazine elimination. There is no known antidote.

TRIMIPRAMINE

(trye mi′pra meen)

TRADE NAMES

Apo-Trimip®
Novo-Tripramine®
Rhotrimine®
Surmontil®

CLASSIFICATION

Antidepressant, tricyclic (dibenzazepine)

APPROVED INDICATIONS FOR PSYCHOLOGICAL DISORDERS

Adjunctive pharmacotherapy for the symptomatic management of:

Mood Disorders, Depressive Disorders: Major Depressive Disorder, particularly when associated with signs and symptoms of anxiety

USUAL DOSAGE AND ADMINISTRATION

Major Depressive Disorder, particularly when associated with anxiety

Adults, hospitalized: Initially, 100 mg daily orally in divided doses. Increase the dosage gradually to 200 mg daily, according to individual patient response. If therapeutic benefit is not achieved by three weeks, increase the dosage to the maximum recommended daily dosage for hospitalized adults of 250 to 300 mg.

MAXIMUM: 300 mg daily orally

Adults, non-hospitalized: Initially, 75 mg daily orally in divided doses. Increase the dosage gradually to 150 mg daily, according to individual patient response. Prescribe dosage increases for late afternoon or evening doses to avoid associated daytime drowsiness. Dosages exceeding 200 mg daily are *not* recommended.

MAXIMUM: 200 mg daily orally

MAINTENANCE: Prescribe the lowest effective dosage as a single daily dose 30 minutes before retiring for bed in the evening.

Women who are, or who may become, pregnant: FDA Pregnancy Category C. Safety and efficacy of trimipramine pharmacotherapy for women who are pregnant have not been established (see Tricyclic Antidepressants General Monograph). Avoid prescribing trimipramine pharmacotherapy to women who are pregnant. If trimipramine pharmacotherapy is required, advise patients of potential benefits and possible risks to themselves and the embryo, fetus, or neonate. Collaboration with the patient's obstetrician is indicated.

Women who are breast-feeding: Safety and efficacy of trimipramine pharmacotherapy for women who are breast-feeding and their neonates and infants have not been established (see Tricyclic Antidepressants General Monograph). Avoid prescribing trimipramine pharmacotherapy to women who are breast-feeding. If trimipramine pharmacotherapy is required, breast-feeding probably should be discontinued. Collaboration with the patient's pediatrician is required.

Elderly, frail, or debilitated patients: Initially, 12.5 to 25 mg orally with monitoring in 45 minutes for postural hypotension. If postural hypotension is not observed, then 50 mg daily orally beginning the following day. Increase the daily dosage weekly by 25 mg increments to a maximal dosage of 100 mg daily, if needed, according to individual patient response.

MAXIMUM: 100 mg daily orally

MAINTENANCE: Maintenance trimipramine pharmacotherapy may be required for up to three months following the clinical improvement of the signs and symptoms of depression. Prescribe the lowest effective dosage as a single daily dose 30 minutes before retiring for bed in the evening.

Adolescents: Initially, 50 mg daily orally in divided doses. Increase the dosage gradually to 100 mg daily, if needed, according to individual patient response.

MAXIMUM: 150 mg daily orally

Children: Safety and efficacy of trimipramine pharmacotherapy for children have not been established. Trimipramine pharmacotherapy is *not* recommended for this age group.

Notes, Major Depressive Disorder, particularly when associated with anxiety

Initiating and Maintaining Trimipramine Pharmacotherapy Precise daily dosages of therapeutic benefit for all patients have not been established. Initiate trimipramine pharmacotherapy with a lower dosage, and increase the dosage gradually according to individual patient response. Lower dosages are particularly recommended for adolescents and elderly, frail, or debilitated patients. Lower dosages also are recommended for non-hospitalized patients as compared to hospitalized patients, who may be more closely monitored.

The etiology of depressive disorders is complex and multifactored. Spontaneous remission or exacerbations commonly occur among patients who are, or who are not, receiving antidepressant pharmacotherapy. Thus, recommended dosages are only a guide and require adjustments in regard to age, symptomatology, body system function, concurrent psychological and medical disorders, individual response to psychotherapy, and other appropriate therapy (e.g., ECT).

Most antidepressants have a latency period of approximately two to four weeks before therapeutic benefit is achieved. Increasing the recommended dosage will *not* shorten this latency period and may increase the incidence or severity of ADRs and, thus, is *not* recommended.

The possibility of suicide is always present among severely depressed patients and persists following the initial clinical improvement of the signs and symptoms of depression. Prescribe for dispensing the smallest quantity (i.e., two-week supply) of trimipramine as feasible for non-hospitalized patients in order to decrease the possibility of intentional overdosage. Other suicide precautions also may be indicated.

Discontinuing Trimipramine Pharmacotherapy Discontinue trimipramine pharmacotherapy gradually. Although trimipramine is classified as a nonabusable psychotropic, abrupt discontinuation of long-term pharmacotherapy may result in a withdrawal-like syndrome with headache, malaise, and nausea.

AVAILABLE DOSAGE FORMS, STORAGE, AND COMPATIBILITY

Capsules, oral: 25, 50, 75, 100 mg
Tablets, oral: 12.5, 25, 50, 100 mg

Notes

General Instructions for Patients   Instruct patients who are receiving trimipramine pharmacotherapy to

- safely store trimipramine oral capsules and tablets out of the reach of children in tightly closed child-resistant containers at controlled room temperature (15° to 30°C; 59° to 86°F). Protect capsules and tablets packaged in blister strips from moisture.
- obtain an available patient information sheet regarding trimipramine pharmacotherapy from their pharmacist at the time that their prescription is dispensed. Encourage patients to clarify any questions that they may have concerning trimipramine pharmacotherapy with their pharmacist or, if needed, to consult their prescribing psychologist.

PROPOSED MECHANISM OF ACTION

Trimipramine appears to produce its antidepressant action primarily by potentiating the CNS biogenic amines, specifically norepinephrine and serotonin, by blocking their re-uptake at the presynaptic nerve terminals. This inhibition of re-uptake increases the amount of norepinephrine and serotonin in the synapses and, consequently, results in increased activity at the post-synaptic neuron receptor sites. The anticholinergic activity of trimipramine appears to be primarily centrally mediated. The anxiety-reducing sedative component of trimipramine's action may be related to its anticholinergic activity.

See also Tricyclic Antidepressants General Monograph

PHARMACOKINETICS/PHARMACODYNAMICS

Trimipramine is absorbed from the GI tract following oral ingestion and generally achieves peak blood concentrations within 2 hours. Trimipramine is metabolized extensively, primarily in the liver, to over 15 different metabolites. The mean half-life of elimination is 10 hours. Additional data are unavailable.

RELATIVE CONTRAINDICATIONS TO USE

Dibenzazepine pharmacotherapy, concurrent
Hypersensitivity to trimipramine or other TCAs

MAOI pharmacotherapy, concurrent or within 14 days
Myocardial infarction, acute recovery phase

CAUTIONS AND COMMENTS

Prescribe trimipramine pharmacotherapy cautiously to patients who

- have histories of cardiovascular dysfunction. Trimipramine pharmacotherapy has been associated with the possible occurrence of conduction defects; dysrhythmias, including tachycardia; myocardial infarction; and strokes among these patients.
- have histories of hyperthyroidism or are receiving thyroid pharmacotherapy. Trimipramine pharmacotherapy has been associated with cardiovascular toxicity among these patients.
- have histories of increased intraocular pressure, including narrow-angle glaucoma. Trimipramine's anticholinergic action may exacerbate this condition.
- have histories of liver dysfunction. Trimipramine is metabolized extensively in the liver. Its half-life of elimination may be prolonged among these patients, resulting in toxicity.
- have histories of seizure disorders. Trimipramine pharmacotherapy may lower the seizure threshold.
- have histories of urinary retention. Trimipramine's anticholinergic action may exacerbate this condition.

Caution patients who are receiving trimipramine pharmacotherapy against

- drinking alcohol or using other drugs that produce CNS depression. These drugs may increase the sedation associated with trimipramine's anticholinergic action. See also Clinically Significant Drug Interactions.
- performing activities that require alertness, judgment, and physical coordination (e.g., driving an automobile, operating dangerous equipment, supervising children) until their response to trimipramine pharmacotherapy is known. Trimipramine's CNS action may adversely affect these mental and physical functions.

In addition to these general precautions, caution patients to inform their prescribing psychologist if they begin or discontinue any other pharmacotherapy while receiving trimipramine pharmacotherapy.

See also Phenothiazines General Monograph

CLINICALLY SIGNIFICANT DRUG INTERACTIONS

Concurrent trimipramine pharmacotherapy and the following may result in clinically significant drug interactions:

Alcohol Use

Concurrent alcohol use may increase the CNS depressant action of trimipramine. Advise patients to avoid, or limit, their use of alcohol while receiving trimipramine pharmacotherapy.

Clonidine Pharmacotherapy

Concurrent trimipramine pharmacotherapy may decrease the antihypertensive action of clonidine (Catapres®). Collaboration with the prescriber of the clonidine is indicated.

Guanethidine Pharmacotherapy

Concurrent trimipramine pharmacotherapy may block or decrease the antihypertensive action of guanethidine (Ismelin®) and related drugs. Collaboration with the prescriber of the guanethidine, or related drugs, is indicated.

Monoamine Oxidase Inhibitor Pharmacotherapy

Trimipramine may interact with MAOIs to increase the therapeutic action and toxic effects of both drugs.

Pharmacotherapy With Central Nervous System Depressants and Other Drugs That Produce Central Nervous System Depression

Concurrent trimipramine pharmacotherapy with opiate analgesics, sedative-hypnotics, or other drugs that produce CNS depression (e.g., antihistamines, phenothiazines) may result in additive CNS depression.

See also Tricyclic Antidepressants General Monograph

ADVERSE DRUG REACTIONS

Trimipramine pharmacotherapy has been associated with bone marrow depression, cardiac dysrhythmias, confusion, dry mouth, GI complaints, postural hypotension, and skin rash. Although the ADRs generally associated with the TCAs may not be directly associated with trimipramine pharmacotherapy, the chemical and pharmacological similarities among the TCAs require that these ADRs also be considered when any of the TCAs are prescribed.

See Tricyclic Antidepressants General Monograph

OVERDOSAGE

Signs and symptoms of trimipramine overdosage include abnormal dilation of the pupils (mydriasis), agitation, athetoid and choreiform movements, cardiac dysrhythmias, coma, convulsions, cyanosis, hyperactive reflexes, hyperpyrexia, hypotension, incoordination (ataxia), muscle rigidity, respiratory depression, restlessness, shock, signs and symptoms of congestive heart failure (e.g., impaired conduction as displayed by ECG, tachycardia), sweating (excessive), and vomiting. Signs and symptoms of trimipramine overdosage vary in relation to such factors as the patient's age, amount ingested and absorbed, and interval between ingestion and initiation of emergency treatment. Trimipramine overdosage should be regarded as serious and potentially fatal, particularly accidental overdosage among infants and young children. Trimipramine overdosage requires emergency symptomatic medical support of body systems with attention to increasing trimipramine elimination. There is no known antidote.

VALPROIC ACID
[Divalproex sodium, Sodium valproate]

(val proe'ik)

TRADE NAMES

Depakene®(valproic acid)
Depakote®(divalproex sodium)
Deproic®(valproic acid)
Epival®(divalproex sodium)

CLASSIFICATION

Antimanic (anticonvulsant, valproic acid derivative)

APPROVED INDICATIONS FOR PSYCHOLOGICAL DISORDERS

Adjunctive pharmacotherapy for the symptomatic management of:

Mood Disorders: Mania Associated With Bipolar Disorder (Indication is *not* HPB or FDA approved)

USUAL DOSAGE AND ADMINISTRATION

Mania Associated With Bipolar Disorder

Adults: Initially, 750 mg daily orally in two or three equally divided doses. Increase the dosage gradually by 250 mg increments every two or three days according to individual patient response.

MAXIMUM: 60 mg/kg daily orally

Women who are, or who may become, pregnant: FDA Pregnancy Category D. Valproic acid crosses the placenta and achieves higher blood concentrations in the embryo and fetus than in the mother. Valproic acid pharmacotherapy during pregnancy has been associated with congenital malformations (i.e., birth defects). These birth defects include cardiovascular malformations and anomalies involving various other body systems, cranial defects, and spina bifida. The incidence of neural tube defects among neonates born to women who received valproic acid pharmacotherapy during the first trimester of pregnancy is significantly increased (e.g., risk of spina bifida is approximately 1% to 2%). Liver failure resulting in the death of a neonate and an infant have been reported following the maternal use of valproic acid during pregnancy. Do *not* prescribe valproic acid pharmacotherapy to women who are pregnant. Caution women who may become pregnant to avoid pregnancy while receiving valproic acid pharmacotherapy.

Women who are breast-feeding:　Safety and efficacy of valproic acid pharmacotherapy for women who are breast-feeding and their neonates and infants have not been established. Valproic acid in the form of valproate is excreted in breast milk in concentrations reportedly up to 10% of maternal blood concentrations. Although this concentration of valproic acid generally poses little significant risk to neonates and infants who are breast-feeding, rare, apparently idiosyncratic cases of hepatic failure have been reported. Avoid prescribing valproic acid pharmacotherapy to women who are breast-feeding. If valproic acid pharmacotherapy is required, breast-feeding should be discontinued. Collaboration with the patient's pediatrician may be indicated.

Elderly, frail, or debilitated patients:　Generally prescribe lower dosages of valproic acid for elderly, frail, or debilitated patients. Increase the dosage gradually, if needed, according to individual patient response. These patients may be more sensitive to the pharmacologic actions of valproic acid than are younger or healthier adult patients.

Children and adolescents younger than 18 years of age:　Safety and efficacy of valproic acid pharmacotherapy for the symptomatic management of acute mania associated with bipolar disorder among children and adolescents have not been established. Valproic acid pharmacotherapy for this indication is *not* recommended for this age group.

Notes, Mania Associated With Bipolar Disorder

Initiating and Maintaining Valproic Acid Pharmacotherapy　Evaluate liver function (e.g., obtain liver function tests) prior to initiating valproic acid pharmacotherapy. Also monitor liver function at regular intervals, especially during the first six months of valproic acid pharmacotherapy. Collaboration with the patient's family physician or a specialist (e.g., internist) may be required. Discontinue valproic acid pharmacotherapy immediately if liver dysfunction is suspected or medically confirmed. Unfortunately, liver dysfunction rarely has progressed among some patients following the discontinuation of valproic acid pharmacotherapy. The frequency of ADRs, particularly elevated liver enzymes, may be dose-related. The benefit of higher dosages must be weighed against the potential for the increased frequency or severity of ADRs, including possible liver toxicity. See also Cautions and Comments.

AVAILABLE DOSAGE FORMS, STORAGE, AND COMPATIBILITY

Capsules, oral (soft): 250, 500 mg (Depakene®)
Capsules, oral sprinkle: 125 mg (Depakote®Sprinkle)
Syrup, oral: 250 mg/5 ml (Depakene®)
Tablets, oral enteric-coated: 125, 250, 500 mg (Epival®)
Tablets, oral enteric-coated extended-release: 125, 250, 500 mg (Depakote®)

Notes

All oral dosage formulations are listed in terms of valproic acid equivalents, even though some (e.g., Depakote®, Epival®) contain the valproic acid prodrug, divalproex sodium.

Depakene® 50 mg capsules contain tartrazine (FD&C Yellow No. 5). Tartrazine has been associated with hypersensitivity reactions (e.g., bronchial asthma) among susceptible patients, particularly those who are hypersensitive to aspirin.

General Instructions for Patients   Instruct patients who are receiving valproic acid pharmacotherapy to

- ingest each oral dose of valproic acid with food to decrease associated GI complaints.
- swallow each dose of the valproic acid oral capsules whole without breaking, chewing, or crushing in order to avoid associated local irritation of the mouth and throat.
- swallow each dose of the valproic acid oral enteric-coated tablets whole without breaking, chewing, or crushing.
- avoid ingesting valproic acid oral enteric-coated tablets within 1 hour of ingesting antacids or milk, which may, theoretically, destroy the enteric coating.
- safely store valproic acid oral dosage forms out of the reach of children in child-resistant containers at controlled room temperature (15° to 30°C; 59° to 86°F).
- obtain an available patient information sheet regarding valproic acid pharmacotherapy from their pharmacist at the time that their prescription is dispensed. Encourage patients to clarify any questions that they may have concerning valproic acid pharmacotherapy with their pharmacist or, if needed, to consult their prescribing psychologist.

PROPOSED MECHANISM OF ACTION

Valproic acid appears to elicit its anticonvulsant action by means of increasing the availability of GABA, an inhibitory neurotransmitter, within the CNS. However, the exact mechanism of its antimanic action has not yet been determined.

PHARMACOKINETICS/PHARMACODYNAMICS

Divalproex sodium dissociates in the GI tract into valproic acid, which, in turn, becomes valproate ion. Valproic acid is rapidly and virtually completely absorbed (approximately 100%) following oral ingestion. Absorption may be slightly delayed if divalproex sodium is ingested with meals. However, this does not affect total absorption, and the ingestion of various oral formulations of valproic acid with food, or their substitution with each other, should not be clinically problematic. However, any change in dosage or formulation, or change in other concurrent pharmacotherapy, should be accompanied with close monitoring of valproate blood concentrations and individual patient response.

The valproate ion is moderately to highly plasma protein-bound (80% to 95%, concentration dependent) and has an apparent volume of distribution of approximately 0.2 L/kg. Valproic acid is metabolized extensively by the liver, with less than 4% excreted in unchanged form in the urine. The mean total plasma clearance is ∼0.5 L/hour. The mean half-life of elimination is ∼12 hours.

Therapeutic Drug Monitoring

Blood concentrations of 50 to 125 μg/ml (350 to 875 μmol/L) generally are achieved following oral ingestion of valproic acid. Oral formulations of valproic acid generally are well tolerated by 80% of patients receiving valproic acid pharmacotherapy for the symptomatic management of acute mania. These blood concentrations may be used as a *general* guide when prescribing and managing valproic acid pharmacotherapy. However, a direct relationship between valproic acid blood concentrations and clinical antimanic response has not been clearly established. The optimal dosage must be ultimately determined by individual patient response. Blood concentrations also may be helpful for monitoring the patient's ability to manage his or her valproic acid pharmacotherapy or to confirm suspected overdosage. For the former, it generally is recommended that blood samples be obtained from trough concentrations just prior to the next dose. In regard to the latter, samples may be obtained at anytime.

RELATIVE CONTRAINDICATIONS

Hypersensitivity to divalproex sodium or valproic acid
Liver dysfunction, severe
Pregnancy, first trimester

CAUTIONS AND COMMENTS

Prescribe valproic acid pharmacotherapy cautiously to patients who

- are receiving pharmacotherapy with several different drugs for the management of seizure disorders (see Clinically Significant Drug Interactions).
- have histories of liver dysfunction. Fatal liver failure has been reported during the first six months of valproic acid pharmacotherapy. These deaths generally have occurred among infants and children younger than 2 years of age. In addition to valproic acid pharmacotherapy, these infants and children were receiving anticonvulsant pharmacotherapy with several different drugs, and also had congenital metabolic disorders, severe seizure disorders and mental retardation, or other organic brain disease. Thus, valproic acid pharmacotherapy was not conclusively implicated. Although the incidence of fatal hepatotoxicity decreases significantly among progressively older patient groups, monitor liver function carefully and observe all patients for non-specific signs and symptoms of liver dysfunction. These signs and symptoms include facial edema, lethargy, loss of appetite (anorexia), malaise, and vomiting.

Caution patients who are receiving valproic acid pharmacotherapy against performing activities that require alertness, judgment, and physical coordination (e.g., driving an automobile, operating dangerous equipment, supervising children) until their response to valproic acid is known. Valproic acid may adversely affect these mental and physical functions.

In addition to this general precaution, caution patients to inform their prescribing psychologist if they begin or discontinue any other pharmacotherapy while receiving valproic acid pharmacotherapy.

In addition to these general precautions, caution women to inform their prescribing psychologist if they become, or intend to become, pregnant while receiving valproic acid pharmacotherapy, so that their pharmacotherapy can be safely discontinued and appropriately replaced, if needed.

CLINICALLY SIGNIFICANT DRUG INTERACTIONS

Concurrent valproic acid pharmacotherapy and the following may result in clinically significant drug interactions:

Alcohol Use

Concurrent alcohol use may increase the CNS depressant action of valproic acid. Advise patients to avoid, or limit, their use of alcohol while receiving valproic acid pharmacotherapy.

Amitriptyline Pharmacotherapy

Valproic acid may decrease the first-pass hepatic metabolism of amitriptyline and inhibit its systemic metabolism. This interaction may result in a significant increase in amitriptyline's bioavailability. Amitriptyline blood concentrations may be increased by approximately one-third.

Anticonvulsant Pharmacotherapy

Concurrent valproic acid pharmacotherapy may displace diazepam (Valium®) or phenytoin (Dilantin®) from plasma protein binding sites. Thus, this interaction may result in an increase in diazepam's or phenytoin's anticonvulsant and other actions.

Pharmacotherapy With Central Nervous System Depressants and Other Drugs That Produce Central Nervous System Depression

Concurrent valproic acid pharmacotherapy with opiate analgesics, sedative-hypnotics, or other drugs that produce CNS depression (e.g., antihistamines, phenothiazines) may result in additive CNS depression.

Pharmacotherapy With Drugs That Induce Hepatic Enzyme Metabolism

Hepatic enzyme inducers (e.g., carbamazepine, phenobarbital, phenytoin, primidone) may decrease valproic acid blood concentrations. This interaction may result in a lowered therapeutic response to valproic acid pharmacotherapy (see also Clinically Significant Drug Interactions, Phenobarbital Pharmacotherapy).

Phenobarbital Pharmacotherapy

Concurrent valproic acid pharmacotherapy may increase phenobarbital blood concentrations by decreasing its hepatic metabolism. This interaction may result in phenobarbital toxicity (see also Clinically Significant Drug Interactions, Pharmacotherapy With Drugs That Induce Hepatic Enzyme Metabolism and Pharmacotherapy with CNS Depressants And Other Drugs That Produce CNS Depression).

ADVERSE DRUG REACTIONS

There are limited data regarding the ADRs associated with valproic acid pharmacotherapy when prescribed for the symptomatic management of mania associated with bipolar disorder. Valproic acid pharmacotherapy traditionally has been indicated for the management of seizure disorders.

Thus, the following ADRs, listed according to body system, have been ascribed in the available literature to valproic acid alone, or in combination with other psychotropics that are indicated for the symptomatic management of seizure disorders. More data are needed. Several ADRs (e.g., anemia, hepatotoxicity, irregular menses) may require appropriate collaboration with the patient's family physician or a specialist (e.g., gynecologist, internist) for appropriate medical evaluation and management.

Cardiovascular: edema of the extremities

CNS: sedation, particularly with concurrent CNS depressant pharmacotherapy. This ADR may usually be managed with a reduction in dosage. Other ADRs affecting the CNS include aggression, behavioral deterioration, depression, dizziness, emotional upset, hyperactivity, incoordination (ataxia), and psychosis, which may be dose-related. Coma rarely has been reported with valproic acid pharmacotherapy alone, or in combination with phenobarbital pharmacotherapy. Encephalopathy with fever rarely occurs following the initiation of valproic acid pharmacotherapy. This ADR may occur among patients who have no evidence of liver dysfunction or inappropriate valproic acid blood concentrations. Recovery usually occurs upon discontinuation of valproic acid pharmacotherapy.

Cutaneous: erythema multiform, generalized itching (pruritus), hair loss (transient), lupus erythematosus, sensitivity to light (photosensitivity), and Stevens-Johnson syndrome. Fatal epidermal necrolysis has been reported involving a 6 month old infant who was receiving multiple combination pharmacotherapy, including valproic acid.

Genitourinary: abnormal absence of menses (amenorrhea) and involuntary urination (enuresis)

GI: indigestion, nausea, and vomiting commonly have been associated with the initiation of valproic acid pharmacotherapy. These ADRs are usually transient and generally do not require discontinuation of valproic acid pharmacotherapy. Other ADRs affecting the GI system include abdominal cramps, constipation, and diarrhea. An increased appetite with some associated weight gain or a loss of appetite with some associated weight loss also has been associated with valproic acid pharmacotherapy. Replacing valproic acid pharmacotherapy with divalproex sodium pharmacotherapy may be of benefit for patients who experience troublesome ADRs affecting the GI system.

Hematologic: anemia, including macrocytic anemia with or without folate deficiency; bone marrow depression; eosinophilia; hypofibrinogenemia; inhibition of the secondary phase of platelet aggregation reflected by an altered bleeding time, bruising, hemorrhage, hematoma, and petechiae; leukopenia; lymphocytosis; macrocytosis; and thrombocytopenia

Hepatic: minor elevations of liver enzyme tests, which may be dose-related, and abnormal changes in other liver function tests, including increases in serum bilirubin. These changes in liver function tests may occasionally indicate potentially serious hepatotoxicity.

Metabolic/Endocrine: abnormal breast enlargement, abnormal lactation (galactorrhea), abnormal thyroid function tests, acute intermittent porphyria, hyperammonemia, hyponatremia, inappropriate ADH secretion, irregular menses, and parotid gland swelling. Fatal hyperglycemia has been reported among patients who had pre-existing non-ketonic hyperglycemia. Valproic acid pharmacotherapy also has been associated with fatal pancreatitis.

Musculoskeletal: abnormal muscle tremor, which may be dose-related, or involuntary jerking movements of the hands, feet, or tongue (asterixis); difficulty speaking due to tongue and other muscular dysfunction (dysarthria); and weakness

Ocular: double vision (diplopia) and "spots before the eyes"

Otic: hearing loss, which may be irreversible

Miscellaneous: fever

OVERDOSAGE

Signs and symptoms of valproic acid overdosage include somnolence, heart block, and deep coma. Deaths have been associated with valproic acid overdosage. Valproic acid overdosage requires emergency symptomatic medical support of body systems with attention to increasing valproic acid elimination. The opiate analgesic antagonist naloxone (Narcan®) reportedly reverses the CNS depression associated with valproic acid overdosage. Caution is required when used for patients who have histories of seizure disorders because it may also reverse, theoretically, valproic acid's anticonvulsant actions. There is no known antidote.

VENLAFAXINE

(ven'la fax een)

TRADE NAME

Effexor®

CLASSIFICATION

Antidepressant (SSRI)

See also Selective Serotonin Re-Uptake Inhibitors General Monograph

APPROVED INDICATIONS FOR PSYCHOLOGICAL DISORDERS

Adjunctive pharmacotherapy for the symptomatic management of:

Mood Disorders, Depressive Disorders: Major Depressive Disorder

USUAL DOSAGE AND ADMINISTRATION

Major Depressive Disorder

Adults, hospitalized and severely depressed: Severely depressed patients who are hospitalized may require 350 to 375 mg daily orally in two or three divided doses with meals. It generally is recommended that these higher dosages be reserved for patients who are hospitalized and can be closely monitored.

MAXIMUM: 375 mg daily orally (see also Notes, Major Depressive Disorder)

Adults, non-hospitalized: Initially, 75 mg daily orally in two or three divided doses with meals. Increase the daily dosage by 37.5 to 75 mg increments every four to seven days, according to individual patient response. Most non-hospitalized patients benefit from dosages of 225 mg daily (or less). Note that the entire daily dosage may be prescribed for once daily dosing with the venlafaxine oral extended-release capsules (see Available Dosage Forms, Storage, and Compatibility).

Women who are, or who may become, pregnant: FDA Pregnancy Category C. Safety and efficacy of venlafaxine pharmacotherapy for women who are pregnant have not been established (see Serotonin Re-Uptake Inhibitors General Monograph). Avoid prescribing venlafaxine pharmacotherapy to women who are pregnant. If venlafaxine pharmacotherapy is required, advise patients of potential benefits and possible risks to themselves and the embryo, fetus, or neonate. Collaboration with the patient's obstetrician is indicated.

Women who are breast-feeding: Safety and efficacy of venlafaxine pharmacotherapy for women who are breast-feeding and their neonates and infants have not been established (see Serotonin Re-Uptake Inhibitors General Monograph). Avoid prescribing venlafaxine pharmacotherapy to women who are breast-feeding. If venlafaxine pharmacotherapy is required, breast-feeding probably should be discontinued. Collaboration with the patient's pediatrician is indicated.

Elderly, frail, or debilitated patients and those who have kidney or liver dysfunction: Initially, 25 to 37.5 mg daily orally in two or three divided doses. Generally prescribe lower dosages for elderly, frail, or debilitated patients and those who have kidney or liver dysfunction. Increase the daily dosage by 25 to 37.5 mg increments every four to seven days, if needed, according to individual patient response. These patients may be more sensitive to the pharmacologic actions of venlafaxine than are younger or healthier adult patients.

Children and adolescents younger than 18 years of age: Safety and efficacy of venlafaxine pharmacotherapy for children and adolescents have not been established. Venlafaxine pharmacotherapy is *not* recommended for this age group.

Notes, Major Depressive Disorder

Discontinue venlafaxine pharmacotherapy gradually over one to two weeks. Abrupt discontinuation of venlafaxine pharmacotherapy has been associated with dizziness, dry mouth, dysphoria, headache, insomnia, irritability, light-headedness, loss of strength or weakness (asthenia), nausea, nervousness, and sweating (excessive).

AVAILABLE DOSAGE FORMS, STORAGE, AND COMPATIBILITY

Capsules, oral extended-release: 37.5, 75, 150, 225 mg
Tablets, oral: 25, 37.5, 50, 75, 100 mg

Notes

General Instructions for Patients   Instruct patients who are receiving venlafaxine pharmacotherapy to

- safely store venlafaxine oral capsules and tablets out of the reach of children in tightly closed child-resistant containers at controlled room temperature (20° to 25°C; 68° to 77°F).
- obtain an available patient information sheet regarding venlafaxine pharmacotherapy from their pharmacist at the time that their prescription is dispensed. Encourage patients to clarify any questions that they may have concerning venlafaxine pharmacotherapy with their pharmacist or, if needed, to consult their prescribing psychologist.

PROPOSED MECHANISM OF ACTION

The exact mechanism of venlafaxine's antidepressant and other related actions has not been fully determined. These actions appear to be directly related to venlafaxine's ability to selectively inhibit the neuronal re-uptake of serotonin. Venlafaxine and its active metabolite O-desmethylvenlafaxine also are potent inhibitors of norepinephrine re-uptake (see also the Selective Serotonin Re-Uptake Inhibitors General Monograph).

PHARMACOKINETICS/PHARMACODYNAMICS

Venlafaxine is well absorbed (~92%) following oral ingestion. However, it is subject to extensive first-pass hepatic metabolism. The ingestion of food does not significantly affect the bioavailability of venlafaxine. Peak blood concentration levels occur within 2 hours. Venlafaxine is only 30% plasma protein-bound, and its mean apparent volume of distribution is ~8 L/kg. Venlafaxine is metabolized extensively in the liver to several metabolites, including its principal active metabolite, O-desmethylvenlafaxine. Approximately 5% of venlafaxine is excreted in unchanged form in the urine. The mean half-life of elimination is 5 hours, and the mean total body clearance is ~1.5 L/minute. The mean half-life of elimination of the principal active metabolite, O-desmethylvenlafaxine, is ~10 hours.

RELATIVE CONTRAINDICATIONS

Hypersensitivity to venlafaxine

MAOI pharmacotherapy, concurrent or within 14 days. This combination of pharmacotherapy, concurrent or within 14 days, may result in the serotonin syndrome (see Selective Serotonin Re-Uptake Inhibitors General Monograph).

CAUTIONS AND COMMENTS

Venlafaxine pharmacotherapy has been associated with a lower incidence of seizures (~0.3%) and mania (~0.5%) than most of the other SSRIs. In addition, venlafaxine does not appear to cause significant sedation or to interfere with cognitive or psychomotor performance.

Prescribe venlafaxine pharmacotherapy cautiously to patients who

- have anorexia nervosa, are cachectic, or are underweight. Venlafaxine pharmacotherapy has been associated with a loss of appetite (anorexia) and associated weight loss among ~11% of patients. Thus, venlafaxine pharmacotherapy may exacerbate these disorders.
- have hypertension. Venlafaxine pharmacotherapy has been associated with sustained increases in blood pressure. The increases in blood pressure appear to be dose-dependent and generally are within the 10 to 15 mm Hg range (mean increase in lying [supine] diastolic blood pressure of ~7 mm Hg). A reduction in the venlafaxine dosage or discontinuation of venlafaxine pharmacotherapy is indicated for patients who experience a sustained increase in blood pressure. The discontinuation of venlafaxine pharmacotherapy was required for ~1% of patients. It generally is recommended that patients who are receiving venlafaxine pharmacotherapy have their blood pressure monitored regularly. Collaboration with the patient's advanced practice nurse, cardiologist, or family physician may be indicated.

Caution patients who are receiving venlafaxine pharmacotherapy against performing activities that require alertness, judgment, and physical coordination (e.g., driving an automobile, operating dangerous equipment, supervising children) until their response to venlafaxine is known. The psychotropic action of venlafaxine may adversely affect these mental and physical functions.

In addition to this general precaution, caution patients to inform their prescribing psychologist if they begin or discontinue any other pharmacotherapy while receiving venlafaxine pharmacotherapy.

See also Selective Serotonin Re-Uptake Inhibitors General Monograph

CLINICALLY SIGNIFICANT DRUG INTERACTIONS

Concurrent venlafaxine pharmacotherapy and the following may result in clinically significant drug interactions:

Cimetidine Pharmacotherapy

Concurrent cimetidine (Tagamet®) pharmacotherapy may inhibit the hepatic metabolism and elimination of venlafaxine. However, the effect upon venlafaxine's principal active metabolite is not significant. Therefore, dosage adjustment generally is not required unless patients have pre-existing hypertension or hepatic dysfunction.

Haloperidol Pharmacotherapy

Concurrent venlafaxine pharmacotherapy may significantly increase haloperidol (Haldol®) blood concentrations by an as yet undetermined mechanism. This interaction may require a reduction in the haloperidol dosage by 50%.

See also Selective Serotonin Re-Uptake Inhibitors General Monograph

ADVERSE DRUG REACTIONS

Venlafaxine pharmacotherapy commonly has been associated with abnormal dreams, anxiety, blurred vision, constipation, delayed ejaculation, dizziness, dry mouth, impotence, lack of strength (asthenia), loss of appetite (anorexia), nausea, nervousness, somnolence, sweating (excessive), tremor, and vomiting. Other ADRs associated with venlafaxine pharmacotherapy, listed according to body system, include:

Cardiovascular: angina pectoris, fainting (syncope), hypertension, postural hypotension, tachycardia, and vasodilation

CNS: agitation, decreased sex drive, headache, insomnia, migraine, and vertigo

Cutaneous: acne, brittle nails, dry skin, edema, itching (severe), loss of hair (alopecia), rash, and sweating (excessive)

Genitourinary: abnormal absence of menses (amenorrhea), abnormal bleeding from the uterus (metrorrhagia), albumin in the urine (albuminuria), anorgasmia, blood in the urine (hematuria), difficult or painful urination (dysuria), prostatitis, urinary frequency, uterine spasm (rare), and vaginal hemorrhage

GI: abdominal pain, belching (eructation), diarrhea, difficulty swallowing (dysphagia), dyspepsia, excessive gas in the stomach and intestines (flatulence), inflammation of the stomach (gastritis), inflammation of the tongue (glossitis), and swelling of the tongue

Hematologic: abnormal decrease in the number of blood platelets (thrombocytopenia), anemia, bruising (ecchymosis), disease of the lymph nodes (lymphadenopathy), and increase in the number of leukocytes (leukocytosis)

Metabolic/Endocrine: abnormal breast enlargement among males (gynecomastia) (rare), breast pain, and goiter (rare) (see also Genitourinary)

Musculoskeletal: arthritis, bone pain, incoordination (ataxia), muscle weakness and abnormal fatigue (myasthenia), neck pain, and tonic contraction of the muscles of mastication (trismus)

Ocular: abnormal vision, cataract formation, conjunctivitis, double vision (diplopia), dry eyes, eye pain, and photophobia

Otic: ear pain

Respiratory: asthma, bronchitis, labored breathing (dypsnea), and laryngitis

Miscellaneous: chills and malaise

See also Selective Serotonin Re-Uptake Inhibitors General Monograph

OVERDOSAGE

Signs and symptoms of venlafaxine overdosage include generalized convulsions, somnolence, and mild tachycardia. No overdosage deaths have been reported involving venlafaxine alone. Regardless, venlafaxine overdosage requires emergency symptomatic medical support of body systems with attention to increasing venlafaxine elimination. There is no known antidote.

ZOLPIDEM *

(zole pi'dem)

TRADE NAME

Ambien®

CLASSIFICATION

Sedative-hypnotic (imidazopyridine derivative) (C-IV)

APPROVED INDICATIONS FOR PSYCHOLOGICAL DISORDERS

Adjunctive pharmacotherapy for the short-term symptomatic management of:

Sleep Disorders: Insomnia (difficulty falling asleep, frequent nocturnal awakenings, and/or early morning awakenings)

USUAL DOSAGE AND ADMINISTRATION

Insomnia

Adults: 10 mg daily orally 30 minutes before retiring for bed in the evening

MAXIMUM: 10 mg daily orally

Women who are, or who may become, pregnant: FDA Pregnancy Category B. Safety and efficacy of zolpidem pharmacotherapy for women who are pregnant have not been established. Avoid prescribing zolpidem pharmacotherapy to women who are pregnant. If zolpidem pharmacotherapy is required, advise patients of potential benefits and possible risks to themselves and the embryo, fetus, or neonate. Collaboration with the patient's obstetrician is indicated.

Women who are breast-feeding: Safety and efficacy of zolpidem pharmacotherapy for women who are breast-feeding and their neonates and infants have not been established. Avoid prescribing zolpidem pharmacotherapy to women who are breast-feeding. If zolpidem pharmacotherapy is required, breast-feeding probably should be discontinued. If desired, lactation may be maintained and breast-feeding resumed following the discontinuation of short-term zolpidem pharmacotherapy.

Elderly, frail, or debilitated patients, and those who have liver dysfunction: Initially, 5 mg daily orally 30 minutes before retiring for bed in the evening. Increase the dosage gradually, if needed, according to individual patient response. Generally prescribe lower dosages for elderly, frail, or debilitated patients and those who have liver dysfunction. These patients may be more sensitive to the pharmacologic actions of zolpidem than are younger or healthier adult patients.

MAXIMUM: 10 mg daily orally

Children and adolescents younger than 18 years of age: Safety and efficacy of zolpidem pharmacotherapy for children and adolescents have not been established. Zolpidem pharmacotherapy is *not* recommended for this age group.

Notes, Insomnia

The safety and efficacy of zolpidem pharmacotherapy for longer than 21 days have not been established. Reevaluate patients who appear to require zolpidem pharmacotherapy for longer than 21 days.

AVAILABLE DOSAGE FORMS, STORAGE, AND COMPATIBILITY

Tablets, oral: 5, 10 mg

Notes

General Instructions for Patients Instruct patients who are receiving zolpidem pharmacotherapy to

- ingest each dose of zolpidem oral tablets on an empty stomach for optimal absorption.
- safely store zolpidem oral tablets out of the reach of children in child-resistant containers at room temperature below 30°C (86°F).
- obtain an available patient information sheet regarding zolpidem pharmacotherapy from their pharmacist at the time that their prescription is dispensed. Encourage patients to clarify any questions that they may have concerning zolpidem pharmacotherapy with their pharmacist or, if needed, to consult their prescribing psychologist.

PROPOSED MECHANISM OF ACTION

The exact mechanism of action of zolpidem has not yet been fully determined. It appears to be mediated or work in concert with the inhibitory neurotransmitter GABA. Although not a benzodiazepine, zolpidem appears to interact with the benzodiazepine receptor ($GABA_A$) and to share some of the pharmacological properties of the benzodiazepines.

PHARMACOKINETICS/PHARMACODYNAMICS

Zolpidem is rapidly absorbed following oral ingestion. Peak blood concentrations generally are obtained within 1.5 hours. However, ingesting zolpidem with food delays and decreases its absorption. Zolpidem is ~92% bound to plasma proteins. It is metabolized extensively in the liver, and its metabolites are primarily excreted in the urine. The mean half-life of elimination is 2.5 hours (range 1.5 to 4.5 hours). The half-life of zolpidem may be prolonged for patients who have liver dysfunction. However, the half-life is not significantly affected by kidney dysfunction. Additional data are unavailable.

RELATIVE CONTRAINDICATIONS

None currently identified

CAUTIONS AND COMMENTS

Zolpidem pharmacotherapy has been associated with the development of problematic patterns of use, including addiction and habituation. Prescribe zolpidem only for the short-term symptomatic management of insomnia associated with disturbed sleep that results in impaired daytime functioning. The risk for addiction and habituation is increased among patients who have histories of alcoholism or other problematic patterns of abusable psychotropic use. It also may be increased among patients who have marked personality disorders. Limit repeat prescriptions for the symptomatic management of insomnia, and reevaluate patients who appear to require continued zolpidem pharmacotherapy.

Prescribe zolpidem pharmacotherapy cautiously to patients who

- have depression, severe or latent. Zolpidem may potentiate CNS depression and exacerbate suicidal tendencies among these patients. Assess patients for suicide risk, and implement appropriate precautions.
- have liver dysfunction. Zolpidem is metabolized in the liver, and its elimination may be significantly prolonged among these patients.
- have sleep apnea. Zolpidem may cause respiratory insufficiency and exacerbate the signs and symptoms of sleep apnea.

Caution patients who are receiving zolpidem pharmacotherapy against

- drinking alcohol or using other drugs that produce CNS depression. Concurrent use of these drugs may result in severe CNS depression.
- performing activities that require alertness, judgment, and physical coordination (e.g., driving an automobile, operating dangerous equipment, supervising children). The CNS depressant action of zolpidem may adversely affect these mental and physical functions.

CLINICALLY SIGNIFICANT DRUG INTERACTIONS

Concurrent zolpidem pharmacotherapy and the following may result in clinically significant drug interactions:

Ritonavir Pharmacotherapy

Ritonavir (Norvir®), an antiretroviral drug indicated for the pharmacologic management of HIV infection, can significantly inhibit the hepatic microsomal enzyme metabolism of zolpidem (Ambien®). This interaction may result in severe zolpidem toxicity, including cardiotoxicity and respiratory depression. Concurrent zolpidem and ritonavir pharmacotherapy is *contraindicated*.

ADVERSE DRUG REACTIONS

Zolpidem pharmacotherapy commonly has been associated with dizziness, drowsiness, incoordination, and light-headedness. Other ADRs, listed according to body system, include the following:

Cardiovascular: hypertension, postural hypotension, and tachycardia
CNS: confusion, euphoria, and insomnia
Cutaneous: edema, itching, pallor, and sweating (excessive)
Genitourinary: impotence (rare), painful menses (dysmenorrhea), urinary bladder infections (infrequent), and urinary incontinence (infrequent)
GI: constipation, difficulty swallowing (dysphagia), and hiccups
Hematologic: rarely, anemia
Musculoskeletal: arthritis (infrequent), incoordination (ataxia), and weakness (asthenia)
Ocular: blurred vision, double vision (diplopia), eye irritation, and eye pain (infrequent)
Miscellaneous: fever, high blood sugar concentrations (hyperglycemia), and malaise

OVERDOSAGE

Signs and symptoms of zolpidem overdosage primarily involve impairment of consciousness ranging from drowsiness to light coma. Zolpidem overdosage requires emergency symptomatic medical support of body systems with attention to increasing zolpidem elimination. There is no known antidote. However, the benzodiazepine antagonist flumazenil (Anexate®, Romazicon®) reportedly has been of some benefit (see Proposed Mechanism of Action).

ZUCLOPENTHIXOL ✤

(zoo kloe′pen thix ole)

TRADE NAME

Clopixol®

CLASSIFICATION

Antipsychotic (thioxanthene derivative)

APPROVED INDICATIONS FOR PSYCHOLOGICAL DISORDERS

Adjunctive pharmacotherapy for the symptomatic management of:

Psychotic Disorders: Schizophrenia and Other Psychotic Disorders

USUAL DOSAGE AND ADMINISTRATION

Schizophrenia and Other Psychotic Disorders

Adults: Initially, 10 to 50 mg daily orally in two or three divided doses. Increase the daily dosage by 10 to 20 mg increments every two or three days according to individual patient response. Once optimal therapeutic benefit has been achieved, reduce the dosage as soon as possible to the lowest effective maintenance dosage (see also Notes, Schizophrenia and Other Psychotic Disorders).

MAINTENANCE: 20 to 40 mg daily orally as a single evening dose

MAXIMUM: 100 mg daily orally (see also Notes, Schizophrenia and Other Psychotic Disorders)

Women who are, or who may become, pregnant: FDA Pregnancy Category "not established." Safety and efficacy of zuclopenthixol pharmacotherapy for women who are pregnant have not been established. Avoid prescribing zuclopenthixol pharmacotherapy to women who are pregnant. If zuclopenthixol pharmacotherapy is required, advise patients (or their legal guardians in regard to the patient) of potential benefits and possible risks to themselves and the embryo, fetus, or neonate. Collaboration with the patient's obstetrician is indicated.

Women who are breast-feeding: Safety and efficacy of zuclopenthixol pharmacotherapy for women who are breast-feeding and their neonates and infants have not been established. Zuclopenthixol is excreted into breast milk in concentrations that are approximately one-third of the maternal blood concentration. Avoid prescribing zuclopenthixol pharmacotherapy to women who are breast-feeding. If zuclopenthixol pharmacotherapy is required, breast-feeding probably should be discontinued. Collaboration with the patient's pediatrician is indicated.

Elderly, frail, or debilitated patients and those who have kidney or liver dysfunction: Generally prescribe lower dosages of zuclopenthixol for elderly, frail, or debilitated patients and those who have kidney or liver dysfunction. Increase the dosage gradually, if needed, according to individual patient response. These patients may be more sensitive to the pharmacologic actions of zuclopenthixol than are younger or healthier adult patients.

Children and adolescents younger than 18 years of age: Safety and efficacy of zuclopenthixol pharmacotherapy for children and adolescents have not been established. Zuclopenthixol pharmacotherapy is *not* recommended for this age group.

Notes, Schizophrenia and Other Psychotic Disorders

Generally initiate zuclopenthixol pharmacotherapy with lower dosages, and increase the dosage gradually until optimal therapeutic benefit is achieved. Individualize dosage according to the severity of the signs and symptoms of the psychotic disorder and individual patient response. Some patients who have acute or chronic psychosis may require either short-term or long-term maintenance intramuscular zuclopenthixol pharmacotherapy.

Short-Term Intramuscular Zuclopenthixol Pharmacotherapy for the Symptomatic Management of Acute Psychosis, Adults Initially, 50 to 150 mg zuclopenthixol acetate (Clopixol-Acuphase®) intramuscularly. Repeat initial dosage at two- or three-day intervals according to individual patient response. Zuclopenthixol acetate is only intended for short-term pharmacotherapy. Zuclopenthixol pharmacotherapy should *not* exceed two weeks. The total number of injections should *not* exceed four injections, and the maximal cumulative dosage should *not* exceed 400 mg.

Long-Term Maintenance Intramuscular Zuclopenthixol Pharmacotherapy for the Symptomatic Management of Chronic Psychosis, Adults Zuclopenthixol decanoate (Clopixol Depot®) intramuscular pharmacotherapy may be required by some patients who have chronic psychosis. This formulation provides long-acting maintenance pharmacotherapy for patients who would benefit from once monthly or twice monthly dosing. The usual maintenance dosage is 150 to 300 mg intramuscularly every two to four weeks according to individual patient response.

The following table provides approximate dosage equivalents for the three available zuclopenthixol dosage formulations and should be used as an initial guideline for replacing one dosage formulation with another.

Zuclopenthixol dihydrochloride (tablet, oral)	Zuclopenthixol acetate (injectable, intramuscular)	Zuclopenthixol decanoate (injectable, intramuscular)
20 mg daily	50 mg every 2 or 3 days	100 mg every 2 weeks
40 mg daily	100 mg every 2 or 3 days	200 mg every 2 weeks
60 mg daily	150 mg every 2 or 3 days	300 mg every 2 weeks

AVAILABLE DOSAGE FORMS, STORAGE, AND COMPATIBILITY

Injectable, intramuscular (acetate salt): 50 mg/ml (equivalent to zuclopenthixol base 45.25 mg/ml)

Injectable, intramuscular (decanoate salt): 200, 500 mg/ml (equivalent to zuclopenthixol base 144.4, 361.1 mg/ml)

Tablets, oral: 10, 25, 40 mg

Notes

Injectable Formulations All zuclopenthixol injectable formulations contain coconut oil. Note the difference in duration of action for the acetate versus the decanoate formulations. Zuclopenthixol acetate and zuclopenthixol decanoate may be mixed in a single syringe and administered as a single injection for the symptomatic management of psychosis among patients who have exacerbation of chronic psychosis. Do *not* mix with other injectable drugs. Safely store injectables protected from light at controlled room temperature (15° to 25°C; 59° to 77°F).

Oral Formulations See General Instructions for Patients

General Instructions for Patients Instruct patients who are receiving zuclopenthixol pharmacotherapy to

- safely store zuclopenthixol oral tablets out of the reach of children in tightly closed child- and light-resistant containers at controlled room temperature (15° to 25°C; 59° to 77°F).
- obtain an available patient information sheet regarding zuclopenthixol pharmacotherapy from their pharmacist at the time that their prescription is dispensed. Encourage patients to clarify any questions that they may have concerning zuclopenthixol pharmacotherapy with their pharmacist or, if needed, to consult their prescribing psychologist.

PROPOSED MECHANISM OF ACTION

Zuclopenthixol, a thioxanthene derivative, shares some pharmacologic actions with the piperazine phenothiazines. Its exact mechanism of action is complex and has not yet been fully determined. Its antipsychotic activity appears to be primarily related to its interaction with dopamine-containing neurons, specifically the blockade of dopamine receptors (i.e., D1 and D2) both pre- and post-synaptically. Zuclopenthixol also has a high affinity for adrenergic (α-1) and serotonin ($5HT_2$) receptors.

PHARMACOKINETICS/PHARMACODYNAMICS

Zuclopenthixol is highly plasma protein-bound ($\sim$98%) and has a mean apparent volume of distribution of 20 L/kg. It is metabolized extensively in the liver and is excreted mainly in the feces. Approximately 10% is excreted in the urine, with less than 0.1% in unchanged form. The mean half-life of elimination is 20 hours (range 12 to 28 hours). The mean total body clearance is $\sim$1 L/minute.

RELATIVE CONTRAINDICATIONS

Alcohol, barbiturate, or opiate intoxication (acute)
Blood disorders
Circulatory collapse
CNS depression

Hypersensitivity to zuclopenthixol (or any of its constituents [i.e., the injectables are formulated with coconut oil and, thus, are contraindicated for patients who are hypersensitive to coconut]) or other thioxanthenes
Pheochromocytoma
Subcortical brain damage

CAUTIONS AND COMMENTS

Prescribe zuclopenthixol pharmacotherapy cautiously to patients who

- have histories of breast cancer. Zuclopenthixol elevates prolactin levels. Some breast cancers (approximately one-third) are prolactin dependent. Collaboration with the patient's oncologist is indicated.
- have histories of seizure disorders. Zuclopenthixol can lower the seizure threshold.
- have Parkinson's disease. Zuclopenthixol is a dopamine antagonist and, thus, can exacerbate the signs and symptoms of this medical disorder.

Caution patients who are receiving zuclopenthixol pharmacotherapy against performing activities that require alertness, judgment, and physical coordination (e.g., driving an automobile, operating dangerous equipment, or supervising children) until their response to zuclopenthixol is known. The CNS sedation caused by zuclopenthixol may adversely affect these mental and physical functions.

In addition to this general precaution, caution patients to inform their prescribing psychologist if they begin or discontinue any other pharmacotherapy while receiving zuclopenthixol pharmacotherapy.

CLINICALLY SIGNIFICANT DRUG INTERACTIONS

Concurrent zuclopenthixol pharmacotherapy and the following may result in clinically significant drug interactions:

Alcohol Use

Concurrent alcohol use may increase the CNS depressant action of zuclopenthixol. Advise patients to avoid, or limit, their use of alcohol while receiving zuclopenthixol pharmacotherapy.

Guanethidine Pharmacotherapy

Concurrent zuclopenthixol pharmacotherapy may decrease the neuronal uptake of guanethidine (Ismelin®) and, thus, decrease its antihypertensive action. An adjustment in the guanethidine dosage may be required. Collaboration with the prescriber of the guanethidine is indicated.

ADVERSE DRUG REACTIONS

Zuclopenthixol pharmacotherapy commonly has been associated with dizziness; drowsiness; EPRs, including TD; and fatigue. Zuclopenthixol also has been associated with the following ADRs, listed according to body system:

Cardiovascular: postural (orthostatic) hypotension, rapid throbbing or fluttering of the heart (palpitations), and tachycardia

CNS: agitation, amnesia, anxiety, apathy, decreased motor reaction to stimulus (hypokinesia), depression, fatigue, a feeling of restlessness and an inability to sit (akathisia), hallucinations, headache, insomnia, nervousness, and prolonged muscle contractions with twisting, repetitive movements, or abnormal posture (dystonia)

Cutaneous: itching, seborrhea, and sweating (excessive)

Genitourinary: decreased sex drive, impotence, urinary incontinence, and urinary retention

GI: constipation, dry mouth, loss of appetite, nausea, salivation (excessive), and thirst (increased)

Metabolic/Endocrine: abnormal breast enlargement (gynecomastia) and abnormal lactation (galactorrhea)

Musculoskeletal: abnormal tension of the muscles (hypertonia); muscle pain (myalgia); prolonged muscle contractions, or rhythmic jerks, that may cause twisting and repetitive movements or abnormal posture; and tremor

Ocular: abnormal accommodation

Miscellaneous: malaise and the neuroleptic (antipsychotic) malignant syndrome

OVERDOSAGE

Cases of zuclopenthixol overdosage have not been reported. On the basis of its pharmacologic actions, and those of similar antipsychotics, the signs and symptoms of zuclopenthixol overdosage would probably include coma, convulsions EPRs, hypotension, hyper- or hypothermia, shock, and somnolence. Zuclopenthixol overdosage would require emergency symptomatic medical support of body systems with attention to increasing zuclopenthixol elimination. There is no known antidote.

References[1,2]

Airaudo, C. B., Gayte-Sorbier, A., Bianchi, C., & Verdier, M. (1993). Interactions between six psychotherapeutic drugs and plastic containers. *International Journal of Clinical Pharmacology, Therapy and Toxicology, 31*, 261–266.

Alcohol-medication interactions. (1995, January). *National Institute on Alcohol Abuse and Alcoholism, 237*, 1–4.

Alcohol-medication interactions. (1995, January). *Alcohol Alert, 27*, 1–3.

American Psychiatric Association. (1994). *Diagnostic and statistical manual of mental disorders* (4th ed.). Washington, DC.

Andrews, J. M., & Nemeroff, C. B. (1994). Contemporary management of depression. *American Journal of Medicine, 97*(6A), 24S–32S.

Ascher, J. A., Cole, C. O., Colin, J. N., Feighner, J. P., Ferris, R. M., Ribiger, H. C., Goldern, R. N., Martin, P., Potter, W. Z., & Richelson, E. (1995). Bupropion: A review of its mechanism of antidepressant activity. *Journal of Clinical Psychiatry, 56*, 395–401.

Ashton, H. (1994). Guidelines for the rational use of benzodiazepines. When and what to use. *Drugs, 48*, 25–40.

Ashton, H. (1994). The treatment of benzodiazepine dependence. *Addiction, 89*, 1535–1541.

Azorin, J. M. (1995). Long-term treatment of mood disorders in schizophrenia. *Acta Psychiatrica Scandinavica, 388*, 20–23.

Bailey, R. T., Jr., Bonavina, L., Nwakama, P. E., DeMeester, T. R., & Cheng, S. C. (1990). Influence of dissolution rate and pH of oral medications on drug-induced esophageal injury. *DICP, The Annals of Pharmacotherapy, 24*, 571–573.

Baldassano, C. F., Truman, C. J., Nierenberg, A., Ghaemi, S. N., & Sachs, G. S. (1996). Akathisia: A review and case report following paroxetine treatment. *Comprehensive Psychiatry, 37*, 122–124.

Bapna, J. S. (1989). Education on the concept of essential drugs and rationalized drug use. *Clinical Pharmacology & Therapeutics, 45*, 217–219.

Barden, N., Reul, J. M., & Holsboer, F. (1995). Do antidepressants stabilize mood through actions on the hypothalamic-pituitary-adrenocortical system? *Trends in Neurosciences, 18*, 6–11.

Beasley, C. M., Jr., Masica, D. N., Heiligenstein, J. H., Wheadon, D. E., & Zerbe, R. L. (1993). Possible monoamine oxidase inhibitor-serotonin uptake inhibitor interaction: Fluoxetine clinical data and preclinical findings. *Journal of Clinical Psychopharmacology, 13*, 312–320.

---

[1] The references cited in this appendix were used in the writing of this text. They were integrated with over 30 years of clinical experience and academic knowledge of each of the coauthors. As noted in the Preface, this text and the others in this series were based on the "Hierarchical Series of Graduate and Postgraduate Courses in Pharmacopsychology." This series was developed by the coauthors in 1989 and continues to be taught by the coauthors. Thus, the references are not meant to provide an exhaustive review of the related literature, but may be better interpreted as a starting point. Additional comprehensive referencing, particularly to earlier classical and initial foundational works in the field can be found in previous textbooks by the coauthors.

[2] The references are meant to provide readers with examples that document ADRs and drug interactions cited in the body of this text. For this reason, secondary reviews have been cited where possible. Readers are encouraged to perform current CD-ROM searches of relevant computerized databases (e.g., Medline, PsychLIT) to obtain additional references. Although the Internet provides databases reporting ADRs and drug interactions, these reports generally have *not* been externally reviewed and, therefore, should be interpreted with caution.

Benet, L. Z., & Pagliaro, L. A. (1986). Pharmacokinetic considerations in drug response. In A. M. Pagliaro & L. A. Pagliaro (Eds.), *Pharmacologic aspects of nursing* (pp. 118–129). St. Louis, MO: C. V. Mosby.

Bhatara, V. S., & Bandettini, F. C. (1993). Possible interaction between sertraline and tranylcypromine. *Clinical Pharmacy, 12*, 222–225.

Bhatara, V. S., & Bandettini, F. (1993). Serotonin syndrome and drug interactions [Letter]. *Clinical Pharmacology & Therapeutics, 53*, 230.

Biegon, A., & Volkow, N. D. (Eds.) (1995). *Sites of drug action in the human brain.* Boca Raton, FL: CRC.

Blaisdell, G. D. (1994). Akathisia: A comprehensive review and treatment summary. *Pharmacopsychiatry, 27*, 139–146.

Block, L. H. (1983). Drug interactions in the geriatric client. In L. A. Pagliaro & A. M. Pagliaro (Eds.), *Pharmacologic aspects of aging* (pp. 140–191). St. Louis, MO: C. V. Mosby.

Bloomfield, S. S., Cissell, G. B., Mitchell, J., Barden, T. P., Kaiko, R. F., Fitzmartin, R. D., Grandy, R. P., Komorowski, J., & Goldenheim, P. D. (1993). Analgesic efficacy and potency of two oral controlled-release morphine preparations. *Clinical Pharmacology and Therapeutics, 53*, 469–478.

Borison, R. L. (1995). Clinical efficacy of serotonin-dopamine antagonists relative to classic neuroleptics. *Journal of Clinical Psychopharmacology, 15*(S1), 24S–29S.

Bostrom-Ezrati, J., Dibble, S., & Rizzuto, C. (1990). Intravenous therapy management: Who will develop insertion site symptoms? *Applied Nursing Research, 3*, 146–152.

Bowden, C. L. (1996). Role of newer medications for bipolar disorder. *Journal of Clinical Psychopharmacology, 16*(S1), 48S–55S.

Boyer, W. F., & Blumhardt, C. L. (1992). The safety profile of paroxetine. *Journal of Clinical Psychiatry, 53*, 61–66.

Bristow, M. R. (1993). Changes in myocardial and vascular receptors in heart failure. *Journal of the American College of Cardiology, 22*(4, Suppl. A), 61A–71A.

Brodde, O. E. (1993). Beta-adrenoceptors in cardiac disease. *Pharmacology & Therapeutics, 60*, 405–430.

Brosen, K. (1995). Drug interactions and the cytochrome P450 system. The role of cytochrome P450 1A2. *Clinical Pharmacokinetics, 29*(S1), 20–25.

Brosen, K. (1996). Are pharmacokinetic drug interactions with the SSRIs an issue? *International Clinical Psychopharmacology, 11*(S1), 23–27.

Bruera, E., Legris, M. A., & Kuehn, N. (1990). Hypodermoclysis for the administration of fluids and narcotic analgesics in patients with advanced cancer. *Journal of Pain and Symptom Management, 5*, 218–220.

Buchanan, R. W. (1995). Clozapine: Efficacy and safety. *Schizophrenia Bulletin, 21*, 579–591.

Buck, M. L., & Blumer, J. L. (1991). Phenothiazine associated apnea in two siblings. *The Annals of Pharmacotherapy, 25*, 244–247.

Butler, S. H. (1986). Analgesics and narcotic antagonists. In A. M. Pagliaro & L. A. Pagliaro (Eds.), *Pharmacologic aspects of nursing* (pp. 299–324). St. Louis, MO: C. V. Mosby.

Caccia, S., & Garattini, S. (1990). Formation of active metabolites of psychotropic drugs: An updated review of their significance. *Clinical Pharmacokinetics, 18*, 434–459.

Cardella, J. F., Fox, P. S., & Lawler, J. B. (1993). Interventional radiologic placement of peripherally inserted central catheters. *Journal of Vascular & Interventional Radiology, 4*, 653–660.

Cohen, M. R., & Davis, N. M. (1992). Free flow associated with electronic infusion devices: An underestimated danger. *Hospital Pharmacy, 27*, 384–390.

Connolly, M. J. (1993). Ageing, late-onset asthma and the beta-adrenoceptor. *Pharmacology & Therapeutics, 60*, 389–404.

Cooper, J. R., Bloom, F. E., & Roth, R. H. (1996). *The biochemical basis of neuropharmacology* (7th ed.). New York, NY: Oxford.

Corso, D. M., Pucino, F., DeLeo, J. M., Calis, K. A., & Gallelli, J. F. (1992). Development of a questionnaire for detecting potential adverse drug reactions. *The Annals of Pharmacotherapy, 26,* 890–892.

Costa, E., & Guidotti, A. (1996). Benzodiazepines on trial: A research strategy for their rehabilitation. *Trends in Pharmacological Sciences, 17,* 192–200.

Currier, G. W., & Simpson, G. M. (1998). Antipsychotic medications and fertility. *Psychiatric Services, 49,* 175–176.

Davis, J. M., Matalon, L., Watanabe, M. D., Blake, L., & Metalon, L. (1994). Depot antipsychotic drugs. Place in therapy. *Drugs, 47,* 741–773.

Denny, D. F. (1993). Placement and management of long-term central venous access catheter ports. *American Journal of Roentgenology, 161,* 385–393.

DeVane, C. L. (1994). Pharmacokinetics of the newer antidepressants: Clinical relevance. *American Journal of Medicine, 97*(6A), 13S–23S.

DeVane, C. L. (1995). Brief comparison of the pharmacokinetics and pharmacodynamics of the traditional and newer antipsychotic drugs. *American Journal of Health-System Pharmacy, 52*(S1), S15–S18.

Devinsky, O., & Pacia, S.V. (1994). Seizures during clozapine therapy. *Journal of Clinical Psychiatry, 55*(Suppl. B), 153–156.

Dewhurst, W. G. (1986). Drugs used to treat affective disorders. In A. M. Pagliaro & L. A. Pagliaro (Eds.), *Pharmacologic aspects of nursing* (pp. 352–381). St. Louis, MO: C. V. Mosby.

DiPadova, C., Roine, R., Frezza, M., Gentry, R. T., Baraona, E., & Lieber, C. S. (1992). Effects of ranitidine on blood alcohol levels after ethanol ingestion. *Journal of the American Medical Association, 267,* 83–86.

DiSalvo, T. G., & O'Gara, P. T. (1995). Torsade de pointes caused by high-dose intravenous haloperidol in cardiac patients. *Clinical Cardiology, 18,* 285–290.

Dockens, R. C., Greene, D. S., & Barbhaiya, R.H. (1996). Assessment of pharmacokinetic and pharmacodynamic drug interactions between nefazodone and digoxin in healthy male volunteers. *Journal of Clinical Pharmacology, 36,* 160–167.

Drug/drug interaction: Fluoxetine/Phenytoin. (1994). *Drug Evaluations Monitor, 2,* 7.

Drugs that cause psychiatric symptoms. (1993). *Medical Letter on Drugs and Therapeutics, 35,* 65–70.

Dubovsky, S. L., & Thomas, M. (1996). Tardive dyskinesia associated with fluoxetine. *Psychiatric Services, 47,* 991–993.

Ellingrod, V. L., & Perry, P. J. (1994). Venlafaxine: A heterocyclic antidepressant. *American Journal of Hospital Pharmacy, 51,* 3033–3046.

Ellingrod, V. L., & Perry, P. J. (1995). Nefazodone: A new antidepressant. *American Journal of Health-System Pharmacy, 52,* 2799–2812.

Ereshefsky, L., Riesenman, C., & Lan, Y. W. (1995). Antidepressant drug interactions and the cytochrome P450 system. The role of cytochrome P450 2D6. *Clinical Pharmacokinetics, 29*(Suppl. 1), 10–18.

Estes, J. W. (1995). The road to tranquillity: The search for selective anti-anxiety agents. *Synapse, 21*(1), 10–20.

Evans, R. J., Miranda, R. N., Jordan, J., & Krolikowski, F. J. (1995). Fatal acute pancreatitis caused by valproic acid. *American Journal of Forensic Medicine & Pathology, 16,* 62–65.

Fava, M., Mulroy, R., Alpert, J., Nierenberg, A., & Fosenbaum, J. (1997). Emergence of adverse events following discontinuation of treatment with extended-release venlafaxine. *American Journal of Psychiatry, 154,* 1760–1762.

Feighner, J. P. (1994). The role of venlafaxine in rational antidepressant therapy. *Journal of Clinical Psychiatry, 55*(Suppl. A), 62–68.

Fernstrom, M. H. (1995). Drugs that cause weight gain. *Obesity Research, 3*(Suppl. 4), 435S–439S.

Fleischhacker, W. W. (1995). New drugs for the treatment of schizophrenic patients. *Acta Psychiatrica Scandinavica, 388*(Suppl.), 24–30.

Friesen, A. J. D. (1983). Adverse drug reactions in the geriatric client. In L. A. Pagliaro & A. M. Pagliaro (Eds.), *Pharmacologic aspects of aging* (pp. 257–293). St. Louis, MO: C. V. Mosby.

Garcia, B., Zaborras, E., Areas, V., Obeso, G., Jimenez, I., de Juana, P., & Bermejo, T. (1992). Interaction between isoniazid and carbamazepine potentiated by cimetidine [Letter]. *The Annals of Pharmacotherapy, 26,* 841.

Geller, J. L., Gaulin, B. D., & Barreira, P. J. (1992). A practitioner's guide to use of psychotropic medication in liquid form. *Hospital and Community Psychiatry, 43,* 969–971.

Generali, J. A. (1996). Drug-nutrient interactions: New drug update. *Drug Newsletter, 15*(6), 42–44.

Generali, J. A. (1996). Serotonin syndrome. *Drug Newsletter, 15*(10), 76–77.

Generali, J. A. (1998). Unlabelled use of medications. *Drug Link,* 2(1), 2–4.

Gerlach, J. (1994). Oral versus depot administration in relapse prevention. *Acta Psychiatrica Scandinavica, 382*(Suppl.), 28–32.

Gerlach, J. (1995). Depot neuroleptics in relapse prevention: Advantages and disadvantages. *International Clinical Psychopharmacology, 9*(Suppl. 5), 17–20.

Gibaldi, M. (1992). Drug interactions: Part I. *The Annals of Pharmacotherapy, 26,* 709–713.

Gibaldi, M. (1992). Drug interactions: Part II. *The Annals of Pharmacotherapy, 26,* 829–834.

Gitlin, M. J. (1994). Psychotropic medications and their effects on sexual function: Diagnosis, biology, and treatment approaches. *Journal of Clinical Psychiatry, 55,* 406–413.

Gitlin, M. J. (1995). Effects of depression and antidepressants on sexual functioning. *Bulletin of the Menninger Clinic, 59,* 232–248.

Givens, B., Oberle, S., & Lander, J. (1993). Taking the jab out of needles. *The Canadian Nurse, 89*(10), 37–40.

Goff, D. C., Henderson, D. C., & Amico, E. (1992). Cigarette smoking in schizophrenia: Relationship to psychopathology and medication side effects. *American Journal of Psychiatry, 149,* 1189–1194.

Gold, P. W., Licinio, J., Wong, M. L., & Chrousos, G. P. (1995). Corticotropin releasing hormone in the pathophysiology of melancholic and atypical depression and in the mechanism of action of the antidepressant drugs. *Annals of the New York Academy of Sciences, 771,* 716–729.

Goodnick, P. J. (1994). Pharmacokinetic optimisation of therapy with newer antidepressants. *Clinical Pharmacokinetics, 27,* 307–330.

Graber, M. A., Hoehns, T. B., & Perry, P. J. (1994). Sertraline-phenelzine drug interaction: A serotonin syndrome reaction. *Annals of Pharmacotherapy, 28,* 732–735.

Graham, D. R., Keldermans, M. M., Klemm, L. W., Semenza, N. J., & Shafer, M. L. (1991). Infectious complications among patients receiving home intravenous therapy with peripheral, central, or peripherally placed central venous catheters. *American Journal of Medicine, 91*(3B), 95S–100S.

Haggett, R. R., & Gionet, P. J. (1992). Peripherally inserted central catheters—review and case reports. *Alaska Medicine, 34,* 140–141.

Hansten, P. D. (1986). Drug interactions. In A. M. Pagliaro & L. A. Pagliaro (Eds.), *Pharmacologic aspects of nursing* (pp. 170–179). St. Louis, MO: C. V. Mosby.

Hansten, P. D. (1995). Pediatric drug interactions. In L. A. Pagliaro & A. M. Pagliaro (Eds.), *Problems in pediatric drug therapy* (3rd ed.) (pp. 463–504). Hamilton, IL: Drug Intelligence.

Haria, M., Fitton, A., & McTavish, D. (1994). Trazodone: A review of its pharmacology, therapeutic use in depression and therapeutic potential in other disorders. *Drugs & Aging, 4,* 331–355.

Harth, Y., & Rapoport, M. (1996). Photosensitivity associated with antipsychotics, antidepressants and anxiolytics. *Drug Safety, 14,* 252–259.

Hedges, C., & Karas, B. S. (1993). Peripherally-inserted central catheters: Challenges for hospital management. *Medical Surgical Nursing, 2*, 443–450.

Hensley, J. R. (1991). Continuous SC morphine for cancer pain. *American Journal of Nursing*, 98–101.

Hirschfeld, R. M. (1994). Guidelines for the long-term treatment of depression. *Journal of Clinical Psychiatry, 55*(Suppl.), 61–69.

Hoener, B. (1986). Drug availability and distribution. In A. M. Pagliaro & L. A. Pagliaro (Eds.), *Pharmacologic aspects of nursing* (pp. 78–94). St. Louis, MO: C. V. Mosby.

Holsboer, F., Grasser, A., Friess, E., & Wiedemann, K. (1994). Steroid effects on central neurons and implications for psychiatric and neurological disorders. *Annals of the New York Academy of Sciences, 746*, 345–359.

Human, S. E., & Nestler, E. J. (1996). Initiation and adaptation: A paradigm for understanding psychotropic drug action. *American Journal of Psychiatry, 153*, 151–162.

Hunt, N., & Stern, T. A. (1995). The association between intravenous haloperidol and torsade de pointes. Three cases and a literature review. *Psychosomatics, 36*, 541–549.

James, L., Bledsoe, L., & Hadaway, L. C. (1993). A retrospective look at tip location and complications of peripherally inserted central catheter lines. *Journal of Intravenous Nursing, 16*, 104–109.

Janai, H. (1990). Adverse drug reactions: United States experience. Part I. *Pediatric Infectious Disease Journal, 9*, S115–S116.

Janicak, P. G. (1993). The relevance of clinical pharmacokinetics and therapeutic drug monitoring. Anticonvulsant mood stabilizers and antipsychotics. *Journal of Clinical Psychiatry, 54*(Suppl.), 35–41.

Johnson, M. S., Pesko, L. J., Wood, C. F., & Reinders, T. P. (1990). Cost and acceptability of three syringe-pump infusion systems. *American Journal of Hospital Pharmacy, 47*, 1794–1798.

Joyce, T. H. (1993). Topical anesthesia and pain management before venipuncture. *The Journal of Pediatrics, 22*(5, part 2), S24–S29.

Kalow, W. (1993). Pharmacogenetics: Its biologic roots and the medical challenge. *Clinical Pharmacology & Therapeutics, 54*, 235–241.

Kane, J. M., Jeste, D. V., & Barnes, T. R. E. (1992). *Tardive dyskinesia: A task force report of the American Psychiatric Association.* Washington, DC: American Psychiatric Association.

Kane, J. M., & Lieberman, J. A. (Eds.). (1992). *Adverse effects of psychotropic drugs.* New York, NY: Guilford.

Keck, P. E., Caroff, S. N., & McElroy, S. L. (1995). Neuroleptic malignant syndrome and malignant hyperthermia: End of a controversy? *Journal of Neuropsychiatry & Clinical Neurosciences, 7*, 135–144.

Ketter, T. A., Flockhart, D. A., Post, R. M., Denicoff, K., Pazzaglia, P. J., Marangell, L. B., George, M. S., & Callahan, A. M. (1995). The emerging role of cytochrome P450 3A in psychopharmacology. *Journal of Clinical Psychopharmacology, 15*, 387–398.

Kittel, J. F. (1986). Sedative-hypnotics. In A. M. Pagliaro & L. A. Pagliaro (Eds.), *Pharmacologic aspects of nursing* (pp. 252–283). St. Louis, MO: C. V. Mosby.

Koch, K. E. (1990). Use of standardized screening procedures to identify adverse drug reactions. *American Journal of Hospital Pharmacy, 47*, 1314–1320.

Kopala, L. C. (1996). Risperidone for child and adolescent schizophrenia. *Child & Adolescent Psychopharmacology News, 1*(2), 1–4.

Kostowski, W. (1995). Recent advances in the GABA-A-benzodiazepine receptor pharmacology. *Polish Journal of Pharmacology, 47*, 237–246.

Kulin, N. A., Pastuszak, A., Sage, S. R., Schick-Boschetto, R., Spivey, G., Feldkamp, M., Ormond, K., Matsui, D., Stein-Schechman, A. K., Cook, L., Brochu, J., Rieder, M., & Korne, G. (1998). Pregnancy outcome following maternal use of the new selective serotonin reuptake inhibitors: A prospective controlled multicenter study. *Journal of the American Medical Association, 279*, 609–610.

Kunovac, J. L., & Stahl, S. M. (1995). Future directions in anxiolytic pharmacotherapy. *Psychiatric Clinics of North America, 18*, 895–909.

Latimer, P. R. (1995). Tardive dyskinesia: A review. *Canadian Journal of Psychiatry, 40* (Suppl. 2), S49–S54.

Lean, M. E. (1997). Sibutramine: A review of clinical efficacy. *International Journal of Obesity, 21*(Suppl. 1), S30–S36.

Lejoyeux, M., Ades, J., Mourad, I., Solomon, J., & Dilsaver, S. (1996). Antidepressant withdrawal syndrome. *CNS Drugs, 5*, 278–292.

Levinson, M. L., Lipsy, R. J., & Fuller, D. K. (1991). Adverse effects and drug interactions associated with fluoxetine therapy. *Drug Intelligence and Clinical Pharmacy, 25*, 657–661.

Lindenmayer, J. P. (1995). New pharmacotherapeutic modalities for negative symptoms in psychosis. *Acta Psychiatrica Scandinavica, 388*(Suppl.), 15–19.

Logan, M., & Fothergill-Bourbonnais, F. (1990). Continuous subcutaneous infusion of narcotics (CSCI)—Preparing family caregivers for managing chronic pain in the home. *Canadian Nurse, 85*(4), 31–32.

Lumpkin, M. M. (1997). Reports of valvular heart disease in patients receiving concomitant fenfluramine and phentermine. *FDA Medical Bulletin, 27*(2), 1–2.

MacMorran, W. S., & Krahn, L. E. (1997). Adverse cutaneous reactions to psychotropic drugs. *Psychosomatics, 38*, 413–422.

Marder, S. R. (1994). The role of dosage and plasma levels in neuroleptic relapse prevention. *Acta Psychiatrica Scandinavica, 382*(Suppl.), 25–27.

Marti-Masso, J. F., Lopez de Munain, A., & Lopez de Dicastillo, G. (1992). Ataxia following gastric bleeding due to omeprazole-benzodiazepine interaction. *Annals of Pharmacotherapy, 26*, 429–430.

McLean, D. R. (1986). Antiparkinsonian medications and stimulants. In A. M. Pagliaro & L. A. Pagliaro (Eds.), *Pharmacologic aspects of nursing* (pp. 382–404). St. Louis: C. V. Mosby.

McLean, D. R. (1986). Drugs used to treat epilepsy. In A. M. Pagliaro & L. A. Pagliaro (Eds.), *Pharmacologic aspects of nursing* (pp. 405–432). St. Louis, MO: C. V. Mosby.

Medication errors. (1996). *Prescriber's Letter, 3*(12), 72.

Megens, A. A., Awouters, F. H., Schotte, A., Meert, T. F., Dugovic, C., Niemegeers, C. J., & Leysen, J. E. (1994). Survey on the pharmacodynamics of the new antipsychotic risperidone. *Psychopharmacology, 114*, 9–23.

Merrell, S. W., Peatross, B. G., Grossman, M. D., Sullivan, J. J., & Harker, W. G. (1994). Peripherally inserted central venous catheters: Low-risk alternatives for ongoing venous access. *Western Journal of Medicine, 160*(1), 25–30.

Meyer, F. P., Tröger, U., & Röhl, F.-W. (1996). Pharmacoepidemiology and drug utilization. *Clinical Pharmacology & Therapeutics, 60*, 347–352.

Mitchell, J. F., & Pawlicki, K. S. (1994). Oral dosage forms that should not be crushed: 1994 revision. *Hospital Pharmacy, 29*, 666–668, 670–675.

Morton, W. A., Sonne, S. C., & Verga, M. A. (1995). Venlafaxine: A structurally unique and novel antidepressant. *Annals of Pharmacotherapy, 29*, 387–395.

Moulin, D. E., Kreeft, J. H., Murray-Parsons, N., & Bouquillon, A. I. (1991). Comparison of continuous subcutaneous and intravenous hydromorphone infusions for management of cancer pain. *The Lancet, 337*, 465–468.

Mulligan, S. C., Masterson, J. G., Devane, J. G., & Kelly, J. G. (1990). Clinical and pharmacokinetic properties of a transdermal nicotine patch. *Clinical Pharmacology and Therapeutics, 47*, 331–337.

Murray, M. (1992). P450 enzymes: Inhibition mechanisms, genetic regulation and effects of liver disease. *Clinical Pharmacokinetics, 23*, 132–146.

Naganuma, H., & Fujii, I. (1994). Incidence and risk factors in neuroleptic malignant syndrome. *Acta Psychiatrica Scandinavica, 90*, 424–426.

Naranjo, C. A., Shear, N. H., & Lanctot, K. L. (1992). Advances in the diagnosis of adverse drug reactions. *Journal of Clinical Pharmacology, 32*, 897–904.

Nemeroff, C. B. (1994). Evolutionary trends in the pharmacotherapeutic management of depression. *Journal of Clinical Psychiatry, 55*(Suppl.), 3–15.

Nemeroff, C. B., DeVane, C. L., & Pollock, B. G. (1996). Newer antidepressants and the cytochrome P450 system. *American Journal of Psychiatry, 153,* 311–320.

Nestler, E. J. (1992). Molecular mechanisms of drug addiction. *Journal of Neuroscience, 12,* 2439–2450.

Neuvonen, P. J., Pohjola-Sintonen, S., Tacke, U., & Vuori, E. (1993). Five fatal cases of serotonin syndrome after moclobemide-citalopram or moclobemide-clomipramine overdoses [Letter]. *The Lancet, 342,* 1419.

Neuvonen, P. J., Varhe, A., & Olkkola, K. T. (1996). The effect of ingestion time interval on the interaction between itraconazole and triazolam. *Clinical Pharmacology & Therapeutics, 60,* 326–331.

New Wyeth gel filled temazepam capsules. (1990). *The Pharmaceutical Journal, 244,* 593.

Nilsson, A., Boman, I., Wallin, B., & Rotstein, A. (1994). The EMLA patch—a new type of local anaesthetic application for dermal analgesia in children. *Anaesthesia, 49,* 70–72.

Nimmo, W. S. (1990). The promise of transdermal drug delivery. *British Journal of Anaesthesia, 64,* 7–10.

Nordin, C., & Bertilsson, L. (1995). Active hydroxymetabolites of antidepressants. Emphasis on E-10-hydroxy-nortriptyline. *Clinical Pharmacokinetics, 28,* 26–40.

Obesity. (1996). *Prescriber's Letter, 3*(12), 68.

Ogbru, O. (1997). Drug interactions with grapefruit juice. *Drug Link, 1*(8), 59–61.

Olkkola, K. T., Backman, J. T., & Neuvonen, P. J. (1994). Midazolam should be avoided in patients receiving the systemic antimycotics ketoconazole or itraconazole. *Clinical Pharmacology and Therapeutics, 55,* 481–485.

O'Mara, N. B., & Nahata, M. C. (1995). Drugs excreted in human breast milk. In L. A. Pagliaro & A. M. Pagliaro (Eds.), *Problems in pediatric drug therapy* (3rd ed.) (pp. 245–335). Hamilton, IL: Drug Intelligence.

Oshika, T. (1995). Ocular adverse effects of neuropsychiatric agents. *Drug Safety, 12,* 256–263.

Owens, D. G. (1996). Adverse effects of antipsychotic agents. Do newer agents offer advantages. *Drugs, 51,* 895–930.

Pagliaro, A. M. (1985, October). Diet, vitamins, and nutrient interactions with drugs in the elderly. *Proceedings of the International Holistic Gerontology Symposium.* Ponoka, Alberta.

Pagliaro, A. M. (1995). Administering drugs to infants, children, and adolescents. In A. M. Pagliaro & L. A. Pagliaro (Eds.), *Problems In Pediatric Drug Therapy* (pp. 1–101). Hamilton, IL: Drug Intelligence.

Pagliaro, A. M., & Pagliaro, L. A. (Eds.). (1986). *Pharmacologic aspects of nursing.* St. Louis, MO: C. V. Mosby.

Pagliaro, A. M., & Pagliaro, L. A. (1996). *Substance use among children and adolescents: Its nature, extent, and effects from conception to adulthood.* New York, NY: John Wiley.

Pagliaro, A. M., & Pagliaro, L. A. (1997). Teratogenic effects of in utero exposure to alcohol and other abusable psychotropics. Chapter 2 in P. Budetti & M. Haack (Eds.), *Drug-dependent mothers and their children: Issues in public policy and public health* (pp. 31–63). New York, NY: Springer.

Pagliaro, L. A. (1985, October). Drug interactions in the elderly: Overview and basic principles. *Proceedings of the International Holistic Gerontology Symposium.* Ponoka, Alberta.

Pagliaro, L. A. (1986). Mechanisms of drug action. In A. M. Pagliaro & L. A. Pagliaro (Eds.), *Pharmacologic aspects of nursing* (pp. 71–77). St. Louis, MO: C. V. Mosby.

Pagliaro, L. A. (1994). Pharmacopsychology updates: Attention-Deficit/Hyperactivity Disorder. *Psymposium, 4*(3), 14–15.

Pagliaro, L. A. (1995). Pharmacopsychology updates: Drugs and sexual (dys)function. *Psymposium, 4*(6), 20–21.

Pagliaro, L. A. (1995). Pharmacopsychology updates: Psychotropic teratogens. *Psymposium, 5*(1), 18–19.

Pagliaro, L. A. (1995). The straight dope: A consideration of substance-induced disorders. *Psynopsis, 17*(Spring), 14.

Pagliaro, L. A. (1996). Pharmacopsychology updates: Drug prescription privileges for psychologists. *Psymposium, 5*(4), 11–12.

Pagliaro, L. A. (1996). Should Canadian psychologists follow the APA trend and seek prescription privileges?: Of course they should!—An invited critical commentary of Dozois and Dobson. *Canadian Psychology, 36*(4), 305–312.

Pagliaro, L. A. (1996). The effects of psychotropics on learning and memory: An overview. *Alberta Correctional Education Journal*, Special Issue: "Proceedings of the ACEA Conference '96", 8–15.

Pagliaro, L. A. (1997, Fall). Face to face: First nurses, now psychologists. *Innovation, 12.*

Pagliaro, L. A., & Benet, L. Z. (1975). Critical compilation of terminal half-lives, percent excreted unchanged, and changes of half-life in renal and hepatic dysfunction for studies in humans with references. *Journal of Pharmacokinetics and Biopharmaceutics, 3*, 333–383.

Pagliaro, L. A., Jaglalsingh, L. H., & Pagliaro, A. M. (1992). Cocaine use and depression [Letter]. *Canadian Medical Association Journal, 147*, 1636–1637.

Pagliaro, L. A., & Locock, R. A. (1992). Nutritional products. In *Self-medication: Reference for health professionals* (4th ed.). Ottawa, ON: Canadian Pharmaceutical Association.

Pagliaro, L. A., Maguire, T., & Pagliaro, A. M. (1997). Significant interaction between Librium® and Antabuse®. *The American Journal of Pharmacopsychology, 1*(2), 4–5.

Pagliaro, L. A., & Pagliaro, A. M. (Eds.) (1983). *Pharmacologic aspects of aging*. St. Louis, MO: C. V. Mosby.

Pagliaro, L. A., & Pagliaro, A. M. (1986). Adverse drug reaction index. In A. M. Pagliaro & L. A. Pagliaro (Eds.), *Pharmacologic aspects of nursing* (pp. 1727–1745). St. Louis, MO: C. V. Mosby.

Pagliaro, L. A., & Pagliaro A. M. (1986). Age-dependent drug selection and response. In A. M. Pagliaro & L. A. Pagliaro (Eds.), *Pharmacologic aspects of nursing* (pp. 130–139). St. Louis, MO: C. V. Mosby.

Pagliaro, L. A., & Pagliaro, A. M. (1986). Drugs used to treat psychotic disorders. In A. M. Pagliaro & L. A. Pagliaro (Eds.), *Pharmacologic aspects of nursing* (pp. 325–351). St. Louis, MO: C. V. Mosby.

Pagliaro, L. A., & Pagliaro, A. M. (1991). Drug induced automatism: Psychological aspects [Abstract]. *Canadian Psychology, 32*, 204.

Pagliaro, L. A., & Pagliaro, A. M. (1992). Alcohol metabolism in a native patient [Letter]. *Canadian Medical Association Journal, 146*, 2141.

Pagliaro, L. A., & Pagliaro, A. M. (1992). Drug induced aggression. *The Medical Psychotherapist, 8*(2–3), 9.

Pagliaro, L. A., & Pagliaro, A. M. (1992). Pharmacopsychology as distinct from psychopharmacology: The initial results of a historical and philosophical inquiry [Abstract]. *Canadian Psychology, 33*, 437.

Pagliaro, L. A., & Pagliaro, A. M. (1993). Carbamazepine-induced Stevens-Johnson syndrome. *Hospital and Community Psychiatry, 44*, 999–1000.

Pagliaro, L. A., & Pagliaro, A. M. (1995). Abuse potential of the antidepressants: Does it exist? *CNS Drugs, 4*(4), 1–6.

Pagliaro, L. A., & Pagliaro, A. M. (1995). Alcoholic cognitive impairment and reliability of eyewitness testimony: A forensic case report. *The Medical Psychotherapist, 11*(1), 9–10.

Pagliaro, L. A., & Pagliaro, A. M. (1995). Drug prescription privileges for Canadian psychologists: Attainable and necessary. *Canadian Clinical Psychologist, 5*(3), 2–5.

Pagliaro, L. A., & Pagliaro, A. M. (Eds.) (1995). *Problems in pediatric drug therapy* (3rd ed.). Hamilton, IL: Drug Intelligence.

Pagliaro, L. A., & Pagliaro, A. M. (1996). Alcohol and other substance use among the disabled. In K. Anchor (Ed.), *The disability analysis handbook* (pp. 107–137). Nashville, TN: American Board of Disability Analysts.

Pagliaro, L. A., & Pagliaro, A. M. (1997). Teaching clinical pharmacology to prescribing psychologists [Abstract]. *Clinical Pharmacology & Therapeutics, 61*(2), 219.

Pagliaro, L. A. & Pagliaro, A. M. (1998). *The pharmacologic basis of psychotherapeutics: An introduction for psychologists.* Washington, DC: Brunner/Mazel.

Pagliaro, L. A., & Pagliaro, A. M. (in press). *Psychologists neuropsychotropic drug reference.* Philadelphia, PA: Brunner/Mazel.

Pagliaro, L. A., & Pagliaro, A. M. (in preparation). *Clinical psychopharmacotherapeutics for psychologists.* Philadelphia, PA: Brunner/Mazel.

Pagliaro, L. A., Pagliaro, A. M., Henderson, D., Kirchen, M., & Uibel, B. (1997). The effects of drugs upon cognition, learning, and memory [Abstract]. *Canadian Psychology, 38*(2a), 4.

Perry, P. J. (1995). Clinical use of the newer antipsychotic drugs. *American Journal of Health-System Pharmacy, 52*(Suppl. 1), S9–S14.

Perry, P. J., Zeilmann, C., & Arndt, S. (1994). Tricyclic antidepressant concentrations in plasma: An estimate of their sensitivity and specificity as a predictor of response. *Journal of Clinical Psychopharmacology, 14*, 230–240.

Perucca, E., Gatti, G., & Spina, E. (1994). Clinical pharmacokinetics of fluvoxamine. *Clinical Pharmacokinetics, 27*, 175–190.

Petursson, H. (1994). The benzodiazepine withdrawal syndrome. *Addiction, 89*, 1455–1459.

Popli, A. P., Kando, J. C., Pillay, S. S., Tohen, M., & Cole, J. O. (1995). Occurrence of seizures related to psychotropic medication among psychiatric inpatients. *Psychiatric Services, 46*(5), 486.

Product withdrawals. *Drug Link, 1*(10), 1.

Prosser, T. R., & Kamysz, P. L. (1990). Multidisciplinary adverse drug reaction surveillance program. *American Journal of Hospital Pharmacy, 47*, 1334–1339.

Reiss, R. A., Haas, C. E., Karki, S. D., Gumbiner, B., Welle, S. L., & Carson, S. W. (1994). Lithium pharmacokinetics in the obese. *Clinical Pharmacological Therapeutics, 55*(4), 392–398.

Reynolds, G. P. (1994). Antipsychotic drug mechanisms and neurotransmitter systems in schizophrenia. *Acta Psychiatrica Scandinavica, 380*, 36–40.

Ritschel, W. A. (1983). Pharmacokinetics in the aged. In L. A. Pagliaro & A. M. Pagliaro (Eds.), *Pharmacologic aspects of aging.* St. Louis, MO: C. V. Mosby.

Robinson, D. S., Roberts, D. L., Smith, J. M., Stringfellow, J. C., Kaplita, S. B., Seminara, J. A., & Marcus, R. N. (1996). The safety profile of nefazodone. *Journal of Clinical Psychiatry, 57*(Suppl. 2), 31–38.

Robinson, T. E., & Berridge, K. C. (1993). The neural basis of drug craving: An incentive-sensitization theory of addiction. *Brain Research and Brain Research Reviews, 18*, 247–291.

Roose, S. P., & Glassman, A. H. (1994). Antidepressant choice in the patient with cardiac disease: Lessons from the Cardiac Arrhythmia Suppression Trial (CAST) studies. *Journal of Clinical Psychiatry, 55*(Suppl. A), 83–87.

Rose, J. E., Levin, E. D., Behm, F. M., Adivi, C., & Schur, C. (1990). Transdermal nicotine facilitates smoking cessation. *Clinical Pharmacology and Therapeutics, 47*, 323–330.

Ryder, M. A. (1993). Peripherally inserted central venous catheters. *Nursing Clinics of North America, 28*, 937–971.

Sachdev, P. (1995). The epidemiology of drug-induced akathisia: Part I. Acute akathisia. *Schizophrenia Bulletin, 21*, 431–449.

Sachdev, P. (1995). The epidemiology of drug-induced akathisia: Part II. Chronic, tardive, and withdrawal akathisias. *Schizophrenia Bulletin, 21*, 451–461.

Schmidt, C. J., Sorensen, S. M., Kehne, J. H., Carr, A. A., & Palfreyman, M. G. (1995). The role of 5-HT2A receptors in antipsychotic activity. *Life Sciences, 56*, 2209–2222.

Schneider, J. K., Mion, L. C., & Frengley, J. D. (1992). Adverse drug reactions in an elderly outpatient population. *American Journal of Hospital Pharmacy, 49*, 90–96.

Schneider, P. J., Gift, M. G., Lee, Y. P., Rothermich, E. A., & Sill, B. E. (1995). Cost of medication-related problems at a university hospital. *American Journal of Health-System Pharmacology, 52,* 2415–2418.

Schumock, G. T., & Thornton, J. P. (1992). Focusing on the preventability of adverse drug reactions. *Hospital Pharmacy, 27,* 538.

Segraves, R. T. (1995). Antidepressant-induced orgasm disorder. *Journal of Sex & Marital Therapy, 21,* 192–201.

Sharma, H., & Pompei, P. (1996). Antidepressant-induced hyponatraemia in the aged. Avoidance and management strategies. *Drugs & Aging, 8,* 430–435.

Sheiner, L. B., Benet, L. Z., & Pagliaro, L. A. (1981). A standard approach to compiling clinical pharmacokinetic data. *Journal of Pharmacokinetics and Biopharmaceutics, 9,* 59–127.

Slattery, J. R., Nelson, S. D., & Thummel, K. E. (1996). The complex interaction between ethanol and acetaminophen. *Clinical Pharmacology & Therapeutics, 60,* 241–246.

Small, J. G., Hirsh, S. R., Arvanitis, L. A., Miller, B. G., & Link, C. G. (1997). Quetiapine in patients with schizophrenia. *Archives of General Psychiatry, 54,* 549–557.

Smiley, R. M., & Finster, M. (1996). Do receptors get pregnant too? Adrenergic receptor alterations in human pregnancy. *Journal of Maternal-Fetal Medicine, 5*(3), 106–114.

Smith, M., & Buckwalter, K. C. (1992). Medication management, antidepressant drugs, and the elderly: An overview. *Journal of Psychosocial Nursing and Mental Health Services, 30*(10), 30–36.

Stahl, S. (1994). 5HT1A receptors and pharmacotherapy. Is serotonin receptor down-regulation linked to mechanism of action of antidepressant drugs? *Psychopharmacology Bulletin, 30,* 39–43.

Stahl, S. M. (1992). Serotonin neuroscience discoveries usher in a new era of novel drug therapies for psychiatry. *Psychopharmacology Bulletin, 28*(1), 3–9.

Stanton, J. M. (1995). Weight gain associated with neuroleptic medication: A review. *Schizophrenia Bulletin, 21,* 463–472.

Steward, D. J. (1993). Eutectic mixture of local anesthetics (EMLA): What is it? What does it do? *The Journal of Pediatrics, 22*(5, part 2), S21–S23.

Stock, M. J. (1997). Sibutramine: A review of the pharmacology of a novel anti-obesity agent. *International Journal of Obesity, 21*(Suppl. 1), S25–S29.

Stolley, P. D. (1990). How to interpret studies of adverse drug reactions. *Clinical Pharmacology & Therapeutics, 48,* 337–339.

Stowe, C. D., Ivey, M. M., Kuhn, R. J., & Piecoro, J. J. (1995). Administering intravenous drugs to infants and children. In L. A. Pagliaro & A. M. Pagliaro (Eds.), *Problems in pediatric drug therapy* (3rd ed.) (pp. 541–675). Hamilton, IL: Drug Intelligence.

Taddio, A., Nulman, I., & Reid, E. (1992). Effect of lidocaine-prilocaine cream (EMLA®) on pain of intramuscular Fluzone® injection. *The Canadian Journal of Hospital Pharmacy, 45,* 227–230.

Taddio, A., Robieux, I., & Koren, G. (1992). Effect of lidocaine-prilocaine cream on pain from subcutaneous injection. *Clinical Pharmacy, 11,* 347–349.

Tatro, D. S. (1991). Food-drug interactions—Part I. *Facts and Comparisons Drug Newsletter, 10*(6), 41–42.

Tatro, D. S. (1997). Clozapine/sertraline drug interaction: Increased plasma clozapine concentrations. *Drug Link, 1*(9), 68

Tatro, D. S. (1998). Increased plasma buspirone concentrations by erythromycin/itraconazole. *Drug Link, 2*(1), 5.

Tatro, D. S., Ow-Wing, S. D., & Huie, D. L. (1986). Drug toxicity. In A. M. Pagliaro & L. A. Pagliaro (Eds.), *Pharmacologic aspects of nursing* (pp. 180–187). St. Louis, MO: C. V. Mosby.

Taylor, D. P., Carter, R. B., Eison, A. S., Mullins, U. L., Smith, H. L., Torrente, J. R., Wright, R. N., & Yocca, F. D. (1995). Pharmacology and neurochemistry of nefazodone, a novel antidepressant. *Journal of Clinical Psychiatry, 56*(Suppl. 6), 3–11.

Taylor, D., & Lader, M. (1996). Cytochromes and psychotropic drug interactions. *British Journal of Psychiatry, 168,* 529–532.

Thomas, N. R. (1986). Review of the anatomy, physiology, and assessment of the central nervous system. In A. M. Pagliaro & L. A. Pagliaro (Eds.), *Pharmacologic aspects of nursing* (pp. 207–222). St. Louis, MO: C. V. Mosby.

Thomson, P. D., Rowland, M., & Melmon, K. L. (1971). The influence of heart failure, liver disease, and renal failure on the disposition of lidocaine in man. *American Heart Journal, 82,* 417–421.

Toth, P., & Frankenburg, F. R. (1994). Clozapine and seizures: A review. *Canadian Journal of Psychiatry, 39,* 236–238.

Ueda, C. T., & Hoie, E. B. (1995). Pediatric pharmacokinetics. In A. M. Pagliaro & L. A. Pagliaro (Eds.), *Problems in pediatric drug therapy* (3rd ed.) (pp. 713–735). Hamilton, IL: Drug Intelligence.

Varhe, A., Olkkola, K. T., & Neuvonen, P. J. (1994). Pharmacokinetics and drug disposition: Oral triazolam is potentially hazardous to patients receiving systemic antimycotics ketoconazole or itraconazole. *Clinical Pharmacology and Therapeutics, 56,* 601–607.

Volpicelli, J. R., Alterman, A. I., & Hayashida, M. (1992). Naltrexone in the treatment of alcohol dependence. *Archives of General Psychiatry, 49,* 876–880.

Watsky, E. J., & Salzman, C. (1991). Psychotropic drug interactions. *Hospital and Community Psychiatry, 42,* 247–256.

Weiner, M., & Weiner, G. J. (1996). The kinetics and dynamics of responses to placebo. *Clinical Pharmacology & Therapeutics, 60,* 247–254.

Williams, L., Davis, J. A., & Lowenthal, D. T. (1993). The influence of food on the absorption and metabolism of drugs. *Medical Clinics of North America, 77,* 815–829.

Wolfe, R. (1997). Antidepressant withdrawal reactions. *American Family Physician, 56,* 455–462.

World Health Organization (1992). *The ICD-10 classification of mental and behavioural disorders: Clinical descriptions and diagnostic guidelines* (10th ed.). Geneva, SZ: World Health Organization.

Yee, G. C., Stanley, D. L., Pessa, L. J., Dalla Costa T., & Beltz, S. E. (1995). Effect of grapefruit juice on blood cyclosporin concentration. *Lancet, 345*(8955), 955–956.

Yee, L. Y., & Lopez, J. R. (1992). Transdermal fentanyl. *The Annals of Pharmacotherapy, 26,* 1393–1399.

Zajecka, J., Tracy, K., & Mitchell, S. (1997). Discontinuation symptoms after treatment with serotonin reuptake inhibitors: A literature review. *Journal of Clinical Psychiatry, 58,* 291–297.

Zaleon, C. R., & Guthrie, S. K. (1994). Antipsychotic drug use in older adults. *American Journal of Hospital Pharmacy, 51,* 2917–2943.

Zimmer, R., Gieschke, R., Fischbach, R., & Gasic, S. (1990). Interaction studies with moclobemide. *Acta Psychiatrica Scandinavica, 360,* 84–86.

Appendix A: Pharmacologic Classification and Listing of the Psychotropics Included in This Text

ABUSABLE PSYCHOTROPICS

CNS DEPRESSANTS

Opiate Analgesics

anileridine ✣
buprenorphine *
butorphanol
codeine
dezocine *
fentanyl
heroin
hydrocodone
hydromorphone
levorphanol
meperidine
methadone
morphine
nalbuphine
opiate analgesics general monograph
oxycodone
oxymorphone
pentazocine
propoxyphene

Sedative-Hypnotics

Barbiturates

barbiturates general monograph
butabarbital
mephobarbital
pentobarbital

phenobarbital
secobarbital

Benzodiazepines

alprazolam
benzodiazepines general monograph
bromazepam *
chlordiazepoxide
clorazepate
diazepam
estazolam *
flurazepam
lorazepam
nitrazepam *
oxazepam
quazepam *
temazepam
triazolam

Miscellaneous Sedative-Hypnotics

buspirone
chloral hydrate
chlormezanone *
ethchlorvynol
meprobamate

CNS STIMULANTS

Amphetamines

amphetamines general monograph
amphetamines, mixed *
benzphetamine *
dextroamphetamine
methamphetamine

Amphetamine Derivatives and Related Central Nervous System Stimulants

dexfenfluramine * (voluntarily removed from U.S. market in September 1997)
diethylpropion
fenfluramine * (voluntarily removed from U.S. market in September 1997)
mazindol
methylphenidate
pemoline
phendimetrazine *
phentermine

Miscellaneous Central Nervous System Stimulants

nicotine

NONABUSABLE PSYCHOTROPICS

ANTIDEPRESSANTS

Monoamine Oxidase Inhibitors

moclobemide *
phenelzine
tranylcypromine

Selective Serotonin Re-Uptake Inhibitors

fluoxetine
fluvoxamine
paroxetine
selective serotonin reuptake inhibitors general monograph
sertraline
venlafaxine

Tricyclic Antidepressants

amitriptyline
amoxapine
clomipramine
desipramine
doxepin
imipramine
nortriptyline
proptriptyline
tricyclic antidepressants general monograph
trimipramine

Miscellaneous Antidepressants

bupropion *
maprotiline
mirtazapine *
nefazodone
trazodone

ANTIMANICS

carbamazepine
lithium
valproic acid

ANTIPSYCHOTICS

Atypical Antipsychotics

clozapine
olanzapine *
quetiapine
risperidone

Butyrophenones

haloperidol

Dibenzoxazepines

loxapine

Dihydroindolones

molindone *

Diphenylbutylpiperidines

fluspirilene ❦

Miscellaneous Antipsychotics

pimozide

Phenothiazines

chlorpromazine
fluphenazine
mesoridazine
methotrimeprazine
pericyazine ❦
perphenazine
phenothiazines general monograph

pipotiazine *
prochlorperazine
promazine
thioproperazine *
thioridazine
trifluoperazine

Thioxanthenes

flupenthixol *
thiothixene
zuclopenthixol *

ANTIDOTES AND MISCELLANEOUS DRUGS

disulfiram
flumazenil
naloxone
naltrexone

Pharmacologic classifications other than the one presented here can be used. However, the one selected for use in this text was developed by the authors and has been found, over the past two decades of publishing, researching, and teaching psychotropic pharmacology, to be both parsimonious and correct.

Some psychotropics, because of the nature of their action and/or chemical structure, may be classified into more than one category. These psychotropics have been assigned, in a somewhat arbitrary manner, to the category that we reasoned was most appropriate for this text. For example, clomipramine, which can be classified as either a selective serotonin re-uptake inhibitor or a tricyclic antidepressant, has been classified as a tricyclic antidepressant because of its chemical derivation, structure, and spectrum of pharmacologic action. For additional discussion regarding both the pharmacologic classifications used in this text and the individual pharmacologic classes of the psychotropics, see *The Pharmacologic Basis of Psychotherapeutics: An Introduction for Psychologists* (Pagliaro & Pagliaro, 1998).

Approximately half a dozen psychotropics, which were included in earlier drafts of this text, were deleted from the final version. Although these psychotropics continue to be available for prescription in North America, their use has decreased dramatically because of the availability of other safer and more efficacious drugs. The exclusion of these drugs allowed a significant number of pages to be used for more frequently prescribed and therapeutically important psychotropics. The deleted psychotropics and a brief rationale for their deletion follows.

Amobarbital (Amytal®), a barbiturate sedative-hypnotic, has been largely replaced by the benzodiazepines for the symptomatic management of sleep disorders. The benzodiazepines are as efficacious as amobarbital and generally are safer to prescribe because they possess a significantly higher therapeutic index and significantly lower abuse potential.

Amphetamine sulfate (available under its generic name) has been virtually totally replaced by other amphetamines (including the mixed amphetamines that contain amphetamine sulfate) for the adjunctive symptomatic management of A-D/HD and narcolepsy.

Glutethimide (formerly Doriden® and currently available under its generic name) has been almost totally replaced by safer and more efficacious sedative-hypnotics. Glutethimide's ADR and toxicity profile is very similar to that of the barbiturates. Thus, the benzodiazepines and some of the miscellaneous sedative-hypnotics that have much higher therapeutic indexes are preferentially recommended and prescribed.

Midazolam (Versed®), a benzodiazepine sedative-hypnotic, is primarily used prior to surgery to provide anxiolytic and sedative effects in conjunction with the use of a general anesthetic. Thus, it is unlikely that midazolam will be commonly prescribed by psychologists.

Paraldehyde (Paral®), a miscellaneous sedative-hypnotic, was used in the past primarily as adjunctive pharmacotherapy for the symptomatic management of alcohol withdrawal. However, its use was associated with an unpleasant odor and taste, as well as, gastritis. In addition, it possesses a significant ADR profile including metabolic acidosis, nephrosis, and toxic hepatitis associated with prolonged use. Although still available for use, paraldehyde should be considered obsolete. The benzodiazepines (e.g., chlordiazepoxide, diazepam) have totally replaced the use of paraldehyde for the treatment of alcohol withdrawal.

Appendix B: United States Drug Enforcement Agency Schedule Designations

USDEA SCHEDULE DESIGNATIONS[1]

Schedule I

No currently accepted medical use in the United States. Drugs in Schedule I are considered to have a high potential for abuse and cannot be legally prescribed. Examples of Schedule I drugs include heroin, LSD, and methaqualone.

Schedule II

Approved for medical use but are considered to have a high potential for abuse and a severe liability to produce physical and psychological dependence. Several states require that prescriptions for these abusable psychotropics be handwritten on special "triplicate" prescription pads. The prescriber writes the prescription, keeping a copy for his or her files, and the prescriber gives two copies (an original and a carbon copy) to the patient, who then must have the prescription filled within a certain specified number of days or it becomes invalid. The pharmacist retains the original copy of the prescription for the pharmacy files and forwards the carbon copy to the state regulatory agency, where it is put into a special database for purposes of monitoring and regulation. Prescriptions for drugs included in Schedule II cannot be renewed (i.e., refilled). A new prescription must be handwritten each time that it is needed. Examples of Schedule II drugs include methylphenidate (Ritalin®), morphine (M.O.S.®), and secobarbital (Seconal®).

Schedule III

Potential for abuse and physical or psychological dependence exists but is thought to be less severe than for Schedule I or II. Generally, this schedule contains abusable psychotropics from the same pharmacologic categories as found in Schedule II but often in combination products (e.g., codeine and aspirin; codeine and acetaminophen). Other examples from Schedule III include benzphetamine (Didrex®), butabarbital (Butisol®), and phendimetrazine (Prelu-2®).

---

[1] These categories are specified in the *Code of Federal Regulations*, Title 21, Volume 9, Part 1308 (revised as of April 1, 1996). They were first delineated in and remain a part of the "Comprehensive Drug Abuse Prevention and Control Act of 1970." Note that these categories are legal classifications and, as such, must be considered by all prescribers in the United States. However, they are *not* pharmacologic classifications. For detailed information and discussion of the pharmacologic classifications of the "controlled substances" (i.e., abusable psychotropics), readers are referred to the first text in this series, *The Pharmacologic Basis of Psychotherapeutics: An Introduction for Psychologists* (Pagliaro & Pagliaro, 1998) and the reference text, *Substance Use Among Children and Adolescents: Its Nature, Extent, and Effects from Conception to Adulthood* (Pagliaro & Pagliaro, 1996).

Schedule IV

Potential for abuse and dependence is considered to be low and is less than for drugs in Schedule III. The various benzodiazepines (e.g., chlordiazepoxide [Librium®], diazepam [Valium®]) are all included in Schedule IV. Other examples of abusable psychotropics from Schedule IV include chloral hydrate (Noctec®), meprobamate (Equanil®, Miltown®), phentermine (Fastin®), phenobarbital (Luminal®), and propoxyphene (Darvon®).

Schedule V

Potential for abuse and dependence is considered to be limited and is less than for drugs in Schedule IV. In some states, limited quantities of Schedule V drugs may be dispensed by a pharmacist *without* a prescription. In these cases, the purchaser must be at least 18 years of age and present valid identification. The pharmacist must limit the quantity of the drug dispensed and keep a permanent record of these transactions, including the name and address of the purchaser, date dispensed, and quantity of drug dispensed. Schedule V drugs consist primarily of mixed-formulation (i.e., multi-ingredient) anticough and antidiarrheal products containing relatively low doses of opiates.

Appendix C: Food and Drug Administration Pregnancy Categories

FDA PREGNANCY CATEGORIES

Category A

Controlled studies show no significant risk. Human studies have failed to demonstrate a risk in the first or later trimesters of pregnancy. The possibility of fetal harm is remote.

Category B

No available evidence of significant risk in humans. Animal studies have not demonstrated a fetal risk, and human studies are lacking. Alternatively, animal studies have demonstrated adverse effects, but these effects have not been confirmed by first trimester human studies, and there is no evidence of adverse effects in later trimesters.

Category C

Risk cannot be adequately ruled out. Animal and human studies have shown an adverse effect (i.e., teratogenic or embryo-lethal), but there are no adequate human studies.

Category D

Positive evidence of risk exists. There is evidence of a risk of harm to the human fetus, but benefits from use might outweigh the risk.

Category X

Contraindicated in pregnancy. Animal or human studies have demonstrated a significant risk of teratogenesis and that the risk is clearly greater than the benefits.

Appendix D: Abbreviations and Symbols

ADE	adverse drug event
A-D/HD	attention-deficit/hyperactivity disorder
ADRs	adverse drug reactions
AIDS	acquired immune deficiency syndrome
ANS	autonomic nervous system
ATP	adenosine triphosphate
AUC	area under the curve
CA^{++}	calcium ion(s)
cAMP	cyclic adenosine monophosphate
CDC	Centers for Disease Control
CL_R	renal clearance
CL_T	total clearance
cm	centimeter(s)
CNS	central nervous system
COPD	chronic obstructive pulmonary disease
C_p	plasma concentration
$C_{p\,ave}$	average plasma concentration
CPK	creatine phosphokinase
CR	controlled release; continuous release
CSCI	continuous subcutaneous infusion
CTZ	chemoreceptor trigger zone
CVS	cardiovascular system
D_2	dopamine-2 (receptor)
DEA	Drug Enforcement Agency
DNA	deoxyribonucleic acid
DNI	drug-nutrient interaction
DSM-IV	*Diagnostic and Statistical Manual of Mental Disorders* (4th ed.)
D_5W	dextrose 5% in water
EAC	Editorial Advisory Committee
ECG	electrocardiogram
ECT	electroconvulsive therapy
ED_{50}	average dose that is effective for 50% of the population
EICD	electronic infusion control device
EPRs	extrapyramidal reactions
F	fraction of the administered drug dose that is available to the systemic circulation
FDA	Food and Drug Administration
Fe^{++}	ferrous iron ion(s)
GABA	gamma-aminobutyric acid
GABA-T	gamma-aminobutyric acid transaminase
GI	gastrointestinal
HCl	hydrochloride; hydrochloric acid
HIV	human immunodeficiency virus

HPB	Health Protection Branch
hr	hour(s)
IAA	indole acetic acid
ICD	*International Classification of Diseases*
IHL	intermittent heparin lock
IIC	intermittent infusion control
IM	intramuscular
INR	international normalized ratio
IQ	intelligence quotient
IV	intravenous
Ka	rate constant of absorption
kg	kilogram(s)
L	liter(s)
LA	long acting
LD_{50}	average dose that is lethal for 50% of the population
MAOI	monoamine oxidase inhibitor
mEq	milliequivalent(s)
mg	milligram(s)
Mg^{++}	magnesium ion(s)
min	minute(s)
ml	milliliter(s)
mmol	millimole(s)
NAD	nicotinamide adenine dinucleotide
NAPQI	N-acetyl-para-benzoquinone
ng	nanogram(s)
nmole	nanomole(s)
NMS	neuroleptic malignant syndrome
N-REM	non-rapid eye movement
NS	normal saline
NSAIDs	nonsteroidal anti-inflammatory drugs
PABA	para-aminobenzoic acid
Pb^{++}	lead ion(s)
PCA	patient-controlled analgesia
PEL	polyethylene
pH	hydrogen ion potential
PICC	peripherally inserted central (venous) catheter
pKa	ion dissociation constant
PNS	peripheral nervous system
PO	by mouth; orally
PT	prothrombin time
PVC	polyvinylchloride
RBF	renal blood flow
REM	rapid eye movement
SAR	structure–activity relationship
SC	subcutaneous
SCOI	subcutaneous opiate infusion
SD	standard deviation
SDAs	serotonin–dopamine antagonists
SIDS	sudden infant death syndrome
SGOT	serum glutamic oxaloacetic transaminase; aspartate transaminase
SGPT	serum glutamic pyruvic transaminase; alanine transaminase

SR	slow release; sustained action
SSRI	selective serotonin re-uptake inhibitor
$T_{1/2}$	half-life of elimination
TBC	total body clearance
TCAs	tricyclic antidepressants
TD	tardive dyskinesia
TDDS	transdermal drug delivery system
TDM	therapeutic drug monitoring
TENS	transcutaneous electrical nerve stimulation
THC	delta-9-tetrahydrocannabinol
TI	therapeutic index
TR	time release
Vd	volume of distribution
V_{max}	maximum possible rate of drug metabolism
®	registered trademark symbol
°C	degree(s) Centigrade
°F	degree(s) Fahrenheit
>	greater than
<	less than
~	approximately
τ	tau (dosing interval)
μg	microgram(s)
μmol	micromole(s)
5-HIAA	5-hydroxyindoleacetic acid
5-HT	5-hydroxytryptamine; serotonin
5-HT2	serotonin-2 (receptor)
5-HTP	5-hydroxytryptophan

Index

A

C

E

P

U